MEDICAL TRANSCRIPTION
Fundamentals & Practice

Health Professions Institute

Linda Campbell, CMT
Ellen Drake, CMT
Sally Crenshaw Pitman, MA,CMT
Susan M. Turley, MA, CMT

Prentice Hall
Englewood Cliffs, NJ 07632

ART ACKNOWLEDGEMENTS:

Badasch, Shirley A., et al., *Introduction to Health Care Occupations, Third Edition.*Englewood Cliffs, NJ: Prentice Hall, 1993, p. 68, p. 153, p. 226.

Grant, Harvey D., et al., *Emergency Care, Fifth Edition.* Englewood Cliffs, NJ: Prentice Hall, 1993. p. 45, p.130. p. 177, p. 207.

Marshall, Judith, *Medicate Me, First Edition.* Modesto, CA: Health Professions Institute, 1987. p.4, p. 39, p. 59, p. 89, p. 97, p. 113, p. 172, p. 173.

The Prentice Hall Medical Assistant Kit, *Cardiology, Third Edition.* Englewood Cliffs, NJ: Prentice Hall, 1993. p. 165.

The Prentice Hall Medical Assistant Kit, *Dermatology, Third Edition.* Englewood Cliffs, NJ: Prentice Hall, 1993. p. 26.

The Prentice Hall Medical Assistant Kit, *Endocrinology, Third Edition.* Englewood Cliffs, NJ: Prentice Hall, 1993. p. 83, p. 194.

The Prentice Hall Medical Assistant Kit, *Gastroenterology, Third Edition.* Englewood Cliffs, NJ: Prentice Hall, 1993. p. 83, p. 194.

The Prentice Hall Medical Assistant Kit, *Neurology, Third Edition.* Englewood Cliffs, NJ: Prentice Hall, 1993. p. 265, p. 280, p. 293, p. 306.

The Prentice Hall Medical Assistant Kit, *Urology and Reproduction, Third Edition.* Englewood Cliffs, NJ: Prentice Hall, 1993. p. 238.

Production Editor: Lynne Breitfeller
Buyer: Ilene Sanford
Acquistions Editor: Mark Hartman
Editorial Assistant: Louise Fullam

© 1994 by Prentice-Hall, Inc.
A Simon & Schuster Company
Englewood Cliffs, New Jersey 07632

Printed in the United State of America
10 9 8 7 6 5

ISBN 0-13-016437-2

Prentice-Hall International (UK) Limited, *London*
Prentice-Hall of Australia Pty. Limited, *Sydney*
Prentice-Hall Canada Inc., *Toronto*
Prentice-Hall Hispanoamericana, S.A., *Mexico*
Prentice-Hall of India Private Limited, *New Delhi*
Prentice-Hall of Japan, Inc., *Tokyo*
Simon & Schuster Asia Pte. Ltd., *Singapore*
Editora Prentice-Hall do Brasil, Ltda., *Rio de Janeiro*

Contents

Acknowledgments

Medical Transcription Fundamentals and Practice was inspired by Mark Hartman, health professions editor at Prentice Hall Career & Technology. He asked our help in introducing medical assistants, medical record personnel, and other allied health students to the transcription of medical dictation by using authentic physician dictation.

The leaders in medical transcription education, we at Health Professions Institute are pleased with the opportunity to provide an up-to-date short course in medical transcription for a broad audience. This course complements the more extensive SUM Program for Medical Transcription Training which provides comprehensive training for medical transcriptionists in a thousand-hour program.

Medical Transcription Fundamentals and Practice is the work of the HPI staff and associates, namely, Linda C. Campbell, CMT, Director of Development, Modesto, Ca.; Ellen Drake, CMT, Director of Education, Modesto; and Susan M. Turley, MA, CMT, RN, Curriculum Director, Baltimore. The editorial assistance and computer graphics provided by Elaine Aamodt were invaluable. The professionalism evident in all their work is well demonstrated in this course.

Development of this course would not have been possible, however, without the expert assistance of John H. Dirckx, M.D., who has served as medical consultant to HPI since 1987, and our colleague Judith Marshall, MA, CMT, author of *Medicate Me* and many other fine essays originally printed in *Perspectives on the Medical Transcription Profession.*

What makes this transcription course unique is not only the inclusion of authentic physician dictation but also the pertinent medical readings by physicians, the interesting articles by medical transcriptionists about the profession, and the challenging exercises and learning tools.

We are most grateful to Mark Hartman for his vision, encouragement, and patience in working with us to produce this course, and for the generous support provided by Prentice Hall Career & Technology.

Sally C. Pitman, MA, CMT
Editor & Publisher
Health Professions Institute
Modesto, California

Lesson 1. Introduction

Medical

- Give three meanings for *diagnosis* in medicine.
- Discuss three ways in which the language of medical dictation differs from everyday language.
- List the various sections discussed in the History part of a History and Physical Examination Report.
- Discuss the features and advantages versus disadvantages of available drug reference books.
- Give five reasons why physicians order lab tests.
- Describe the purpose and content of each of the types of medical reports.

Fundamentals

- Describe the role of the medical transcriptionist as a member of the healthcare team.
- List two characteristics of medical transcriptionists that make them ''special people.''
- Explain the statement, ''Medical transcriptionists are the mind behind the machine.''
- Cite two reasons why laughter is important in medical transcription.
- Describe the advances made in the technology that medical transcriptionists use today.
- Discuss the features and advantages versus disadvantages of commonly available drug reference books.
- Describe common wordsearching techniques.

Practice

- Describe the skills coordination process necessary in transcribing medical dictation.
- Become familiar with six categories of transcription errors and how to avoid or minimize them.

A Closer Look

The Medical Transcription Profession

The professional healthcare team includes physicians, nurses, therapists, technicians, dieticians, and other healthcare support staff. A vital member of this team is the medical transcriptionist. While not as visible to the general public as those members of the team providing hands-on care, the medical transcriptionist plays an important role in documenting the quality of patient care.

Medical transcriptionists provide an important service to both physician and patient by transcribing dictated medical reports that document a patient's medical care and condition. These may include office chart notes, history and physical examinations, consultations, letters, memos, admission notes, emergency department notes, operative reports, discharge summaries, and many specialized laboratory tests and diagnostic studies. Medical transcriptionists transcribe reports from a variety of medical specialties, and each day's work presents a unique challenge and opportunity for learning.

Medical transcriptionists contribute to quality patient care through their commitment to excellence. Because each dictated report represents a part of a patient's life, the medical transcriptionist transcribes it with care, demonstrating an extensive knowledge of medical terminology, anatomy, pharmacology, human diseases, surgical procedures, diagnostic studies, and laboratory tests in order to produce an accurate and complete permanent medical record.

A mastery of English grammar, structure, and style, a knowledge of transcription practices, skill in typing, spelling, and proofreading, and the highest professional standards contribute to the medical transcriptionist's ability to interpret, translate, and edit medical dictation for content and clarity.

Medical transcriptionists work in a variety of settings, including medical centers, general and specialty hospitals, clinics and group practices, radiology and pathology offices, government facilities, insurance companies, home offices, and other environments. Some medical transcriptionists combine their transcription skills with clinical skills to work as medical assistants. Others become supervisors, managers, and college teachers.

Medical transcriptionists' earnings vary according to geographic area, skill level, place of employment, and method of compensation. Transcriptionists working in large metropolitan areas generally earn more than those in smaller cities. Transcriptionists who are paid on production often earn more than those who are compensated on an hourly basis. Some facilities have incentive pay plans where transcriptionists are paid a bonus over and above the minimum production level and base pay for that facility. Generally speaking, entry-level transcriptionists can expect to earn at least twice the hourly minimum wage in larger cities, perhaps less in other areas. Experienced transcriptionists and those paid on production usually earn significantly more.

There is a critical nationwide shortage of qualified medical transcriptionists; consequently, there are many more job openings than qualified transcriptionists to fill them. Job opportunities exist all over the United States and Canada and in American hospitals in foreign countries. In addition to choice of work setting, transcriptionists can often find part-time or full-time employment with flexible scheduling.

What Is a Medical Transcriptionist?

by Judith Marshall, MA, CMT

Medical transcriptionists are very special people. We are workers who sign our initials on each finished product; we are craftspersons in a modern age. We are the experts in the complicated machinery of today—word processing units, computers, cathode ray tubes, mag cards, memory banks.

But more importantly, we are the practitioners of communication. We are the magicians of medical terminology, the masters of grammar and punctuation, and our expertise flows through related areas of pharmacology and the sophisticated new instruments from the operating room. We are the trained ears who create sense out of many diverse accents, and sometimes, just plain **non**sense.

And one of the hallmarks of a medical transcriptionist is the willingness to share. Like the great cooks of the world who share their recipes, we try to help the newcomer, the student fledgling, and each other with the tricks of the trade—how to flip through the *PDR* or the *ADI,* how to check under "ph" when the word sounds like it begins with "f," how to find something under "disease" or "syndrome" when all we hear is a proper name.

I think we all evidence, to a great degree, a commonality of compassion. Marching across our view each day are life and death, struggle with disease, social problems, and sometimes (thank goodness) the human comedy.

We have our ethics and we have our morals. Medical transcriptionists know more about a patient than anyone else except the physician. We practice discretion. We wade through gallons of urinalyses and rivers of blood samples, and we know the chemical state of the patient as well as the most intimate details of the social history.

Although we may be half-crazed after a morning of thirty T&A's or cataract extractions, or thirty chest x-rays (all of which were normal), we just *appear* to have a glazed, bored look.

But when we transcribe a birth record, often the medical transcriptionist breathes a silent "welcome on board, kid" to the new arrival. When a discharge summary becomes a death summary, often we are saddened, no matter how old the patient.

When transcribing surgery, major or minor, when we hear "The patienttoleratedtheprocedurewellandleft theoperatingroomingoodcondition," we often think, "Good," not just because the report is over but because it was a successful surgery.

And in the medical offices, how fortunate the patient is to have a friendly personal relationship with the guardian of the medical record, the medical transcriptionist. Like the personnel in the drug company, the insurance company, and the laboratory, the dedicated professional in transcription serves the health-care consumer—the patient.

So, if you know that *café au lait* is not a Spanish cheer, that *peau d'orange* is not orange sauce for a duck, that *bilirubin* is not the name of a little boy, that a *CABG* patch has nothing to do with Br'er Rabbit, that *Takahashi* is not a new Japanese car, and if you know the great tunnels of Boston and New York, the Callahan Tunnel, the Sumner Tunnel, and the *carpal tunnel*—you speak the language of medical transcription professionals.

The Mind Behind the Machine

by Vera Pyle, CMT

Let me introduce you to medical transcription and medical transcriptionists. You will notice that I use the term "transcriptionist," not transcriber. A transcriber is the machine that plays a dictated report through our headsets so that we may transcribe it. It is NOT the person who transcribes. A medical transcriptionist is "the mind behind the machine."

If there is one thing that transcriptionists are known for, it is our love for words. This is the common thread in our profession. It is what gives us a kinship, and it is one of the things that makes us professionals.

If I were cast away on a desert island, the book I would probably want to take with me is an unabridged English dictionary, and I could be happy for years. Transcriptionists can get lost in a dictionary. We look up a word and we see something else that looks interesting, and then we look up another word, and so on. Words are truly exciting. I would much rather have a dozen new medical words all researched and defined than a five-pound box of candy. I hope that you too will come to share this feeling.

Some years ago I was transcribing the manuscript of a textbook by a physician for whom I had worked in the past. He is a well-educated, extremely literate person. He is a published poet, a musician, a composer, a teacher—a real Renaissance man. So it was with some trepidation that I presumed to suggest changes. I transcribed the page the way he dictated it, and then I gave him my version as well. He read it and beamed. "This is a tremendous improvement," he said. "You know, Vera, together we could rule the world."

It was a charming proposition. However, it is not my ambition to rule the world. All I want is recognition for what I know and how accurately and intelligently I can convey that information—my contribution to the delivery of the best possible healthcare for a patient.

Some 25 years ago, our hospital got the prototype of one of the first word processing machines. Our medical record director brought in a group of interns and residents to see this marvel. Pointing to the machine proudly, she said, "And this is the machine that transcribes your reports." Not so, I thought then, and now. The machines we use are simply tools. Without the knowledge contained in the mind of the transcriptionist, the machines are impotent. The transcriptionist is the mind behind the machine.

Humor in Medicine: Bloopers

by Sally C. Pitman, MA, CMT

Most medical transcriptionists have a lively sense of humor, and we hear much to laugh about in a typical day's dictation. A sense of humor is essential for longevity in the field of medical transcription. While we are not insensitive to the gravity of the medical reports that we are transcribing, nevertheless we enjoy the comic relief afforded by the humor in medicine. Laughter helps us maintain a sense of balance and perspective.

Practically every transcription office has a central Funny File where the medical transcriptionists routinely record some of the misstatements, malapropisms, slips of the tongue, dangling modifiers, and other bits of humor in medical dictation. When an experienced medical transcriptionist occasionally has a lapse in consciousness—or takes a shortcut between the ears and the keyboard without the dictation going through the mind—an embarrassing gaffe can occur. Instead of typing "senile cataract," the transcriptionist may type "penile cataract"—a blooper.

Doctors and medical transcriptionists alike can be guilty of Freudian slips, and the results provide a good laugh when shared with one's colleagues. In fact, sharing a laugh with someone who understands the joke intensifies the fun of the error in dictation or transcription. When I am transcribing alone and have no one around to share the laughter with, my enjoyment is diminished. When a doctor dictated, "This is the second hospital admission for this 66-year-old white male who was found under the bed in his hotel room and was admitted to the hospital for evaluation of this problem," that struck me as hilarious. It would not have been nearly so funny if I had not been able to share it with someone.

Many years ago I was transcribing x-ray reports for hours on end, and doing it very mechanically by the end of the day. Suddenly, a sentence I had just transcribed registered in my brain. The radiologist had said, "The glenoid fossa is well-seated in the acetabulum," and I had typed exactly what he said. I burst into laughter at the image this evoked and called the radiologist to tell him what he had dictated. Undaunted, he roared, "Yeah, you should've SEEN that guy!"

The incident shows what can happen when even an experienced medical transcriptionist unthinkingly or mechanically types what doctors **say** rather than what they **mean.**

Surely every doctor has at one time or another said something like, "The patient smokes two beers a day and drinks two packs." Most physicians know they are not infallible and appreciate the transcriptionist's medical knowledge and editing ability. Though they may dictate half asleep in the middle of the night or after ten hours of surgery, they are counting on us to be alert and, when necessary, to correct their mistakes.

Lest you think we are putting anyone down, let me say that we are not deriding doctors who make mistakes in dictation, or students or trainees who guess wrong in transcription, or experienced medical transcriptionists who occasionally err. We don't mean to offend anyone. But one reason these dictation and transcription bloopers are funny is that they are "inside jokes." We have to know the correct medical terms and have a vivid imagination for the quotes to be funny. The medical transcriptionist has to know that the glenoid fossa is in the shoulder joint and cannot be well-seated in the hip—without grotesque results!

Doctors don't always just accidentally say funny things in the dictation, however. Frequently they crack jokes in an aside to the medical transcriptionists. We fondly remember the bicentennial tape dictated by our favorite radiologist in 1976. Also, the physician who dictated a clinic note on the Great Pumpkin one Halloween Day was clearly out to entertain us.

And the transcriptionist can *hear* the laughter in the voice of the physician who dictated, "The only complaint of this 74-year-old woman is that the wind keeps blowing her off her motorcycle and she suffers aches and pains because of this."

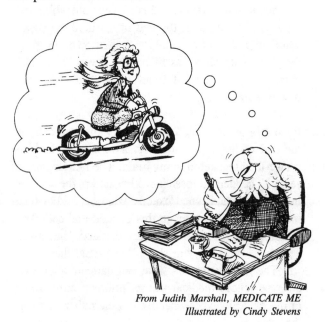

From Judith Marshall, MEDICATE ME
Illustrated by Cindy Stevens

Why are **bloopers** funny? Why is it funny when someone types "x-rays of the vertebral column show **bunny fur** formation" (instead of "bony spur")? I think lapses from correct medical terminology are funny when they evoke **concrete sensory images** that in context are humorous. The image of bunny fur on the spinal column is so incongruous that, when pictured on the x-ray, it evokes laughter.

Does humor have a place in medicine? Medical transcriptionists believe it does. Laughter can be the best medicine for whatever ails us. We can be tired, frustrated, overworked, depressed, and even ill, and something funny in the dictation—whether intentional or not—can make us laugh and bring us out of the doldrums. Laughter can renew our spirits and help us to work with renewed energy. It's the best medicine.

Medical Transcription Equipment

by Bruce Tennant, CMT

As physicians depend on their stethoscopes, scalpels, and tongue depressors, medical transcriptionists are also indebted to the tools of their trade—the typewriter or word processor and the transcribing machine. Let's take a look at the evolution of this equipment and see how far we have come in just a decade or two.

Although the first typewriters came out in the middle 1850s, it wasn't until the early part of this century that such machines were reliable enough to firmly establish them in all clerical fields. Indeed the QWERTY keyboard (named for the six keys just above the left hand's home row) was designed so that it would be more difficult to type fast. To type too fast back then meant jammed keys and wasted time. Even so, to be proficient in typing was a tremendous asset to your clerical resumé. An interesting quirk in this new career was that the people who used these machines were called typewriters. A job description in a 1910 newspaper listed more than 50 jobs for "typewriters who must be able to type 50 words per minute."

Although we now call the machines typewriters and the operators typists, this syndrome has continued to this day. Ads in local papers still refer to a need for medical *transcribers* rather than medical *transcriptionists* (MTs). A real change towards denoting MTs as a separate entity from the machines they use began to catch on in the 1970s.

The real next step in technology was the IBM Selectric typewriter, introduced in the early 1960s. It replaced individual internal mechanical keys with an "element" which was a spherical ball with all the necessary letters of the alphabet on it. The ball moved back and forth across the page, eliminating the need for a carriage. The typing speeds of good typists skyrocketed. In 1972 the first of the self-correcting Selectric typewriters contained lift-off tape so that errors could be more quickly lifted off the page. This increased production time even more. Most MTs now over 40 started their careers on this type of machine, even though it meant the continued use of carbon paper if copies were needed.

In the late 1970s the electronic typewriter was introduced. This was a crude forerunner to the word processing machines of today. Essentially it could "remember" a few lines of what had been typed. It also added stylistic touches such as bold typeface for emphasis. In addition, you could make a correction while looking at the line display (such as in a calculator), and correct any mistakes before they were typed or printed.

Real word processors and computers began to be available in the late 1970s. An MT could input an entire page, check for errors, and then print that page, producing perfect pages (and perfect carbons). Currently the real emphasis is on personal computers (PCs) equipped with a variety of word processing software.

The machines used to record dictation can be traced right back to Thomas Edison's invention of the phonograph. President Warren Harding's inaugural address was recorded, and through a crude relay system it was dutifully transcribed by a typist and sent to the major newspapers.

Up until the 1930s and 1940s, physicians either wrote all the records directly in the chart or dictated in person to secretaries. The ability to understand and write in shorthand was much more valued during this time for medical secretaries doing medical transcription. However, here and there transcribing machines began to be manufactured directly for clerical use. Although they were poor in sound quality and difficult to use, physicians could then dictate their letters, hospital records, and any other data at any time anywhere.

The great explosion in transcriber efficiency came with the mylar tape machines. The advantage to transcriptionists was a great leap forward in sound quality. The transcription you will be doing in this course is performed with the help of the standard cassette introduced in 1970, measuring 4 by 2½ inches. Its main advantages were size and the fact that the tape was fully contained in a plastic box. No more would MTs have to work directly with feeding tape from one spool to another. Standard cassette tapes were easily produced, took much less room, and created the smallest dictating machines to date.

I have spoken of the *standard* cassette tape, but others have also been introduced in the last few years. The *minicassette* was introduced more than 25 years ago. It essentially was the same as the standard-sized cassette in construction, but it measured a scant 2¼ by 1¼ inches. This required a very small spool of tape and became popular for portable dictating machines. Although these tapes are still used by many, the industry standard for small-sized cassettes is the *microcassette*. The microcassette measures exactly 2 inches in length, but is otherwise unchanged from the original "mini" design.

Now there is a system that eliminates even mylar recording tape: digital dictation. Many of you either own or know of someone who has a compact disc player for music. The compact disc reproduces sound using digital technology that is extremely complicated; however, the end result is a disc that is without any background noise, hiss, or other extraneous sounds found on regular mylar tape.

What's in store for medical transcription in the next century? Considering how far we've come in the last two decades, it's safe to say that medical transcriptionists have a great deal to look forward to, as the equipment they operate becomes more and more helpful to their medical tasks.

Medical Readings

The History and Physical Examination

by John H. Dirckx, M.D.

The term *diagnosis* (from Greek *diagignosko,* to judge, discriminate) has several closely related meanings in medicine, which few of us take the trouble to distinguish in practice. Diagnosis means, first, the intellectual process of analyzing, identifying, or explaining a disease. In this sense, diagnosis forms the subject matter of the branch of medicine called Physical Diagnosis. Secondly, in a more concrete sense, diagnosis means the explanation proposed for a given patient's problems. Thus we speak of "arriving at a diagnosis'' or of ''making a tentative diagnosis of pancreatitis.'' Thirdly, *diagnosis* is often used synonymously with *disease* or the name of a particular disease: ''Her diagnosis is multiple sclerosis.'' ''Patients with this diagnosis often progress to renal failure.''

The techniques used by the physician to gather data for a diagnosis are embodied in the two procedures known as history and physical examination. The history or anamnesis is the patient's own account of his experiences and observations of his illness—his *symptoms*—elicited by careful, methodical questioning. Physical examination is the process whereby the physician seeks and observes objective changes and abnormalities—the *signs* of illness. It is not generally understood by lay persons that in a typical case, a skillfully obtained history supplies both a larger number of diagnostic clues and more useful and specific ones than the physical examination.

By convention, the term *physical examination* includes only those procedures performed directly by the physician relying on his own senses, with the aid of a few simple, hand-held instruments. Although x-ray and laboratory studies, electrocardiography and electromyography, various kinds of scans, or other elaborate techniques may be absolutely essential to a precise and accurate diagnosis, they are not considered part of the physical examination.

The scope and nature of the history and physical depend on several variables. The patient's complaints give direction and focus to both history-taking and examination. The physician's field of specialization often determines the type and extent of diagnostic maneuvers he employs. The setting of the examination—doctor's office or clinic, hospital emergency department, intensive care unit, or the patient's home—will have a bearing on what is done and not done. The patient's condition—whether alert, confused, belligerent, or unconscious—will influence the type of history that can be obtained and the degree of cooperation that can be enlisted during examination. Much may depend on formally established, quasi-legal requirements—forms to be filled out for a prospective employer or insurer, or hospital staff bylaws to be complied with.

Usually there is some overlapping of content between the history and the physical examination. The physician does not wait to start observing the patient until he has finished taking the history, nor does he stop asking questions once he has begun the examination.

The report of a thorough history and physical contains more negative than positive statements: ''He has had a mild chronic cough for many years but denies hemoptysis, purulent sputum, chest pain, dyspnea on exertion, orthopnea, asthma, bronchitis, or emphysema.'' This is because the physician is not concerned merely with compiling a list of abnormalities. In order to establish a complete picture of the patient's condition he must also say what common or relevant symptoms and signs are not present.

The language in which a physician writes or dictates a history and physical contains many recurring terms, phrases, and formulas. Some of these pertain to formal medical terminology, while others are highly informal, perhaps regional, institutional, or even individual, and do not appear in conventional medical reference works. An important characteristic of this language is its rigid economy, its tendency to abbreviate and condense wherever possible. It must be remembered that even a physician who dictates many pages of medical records a day probably produces at least as many pages of longhand in hospital charts and office or clinic records. Hence written abbreviations crop up constantly in dictated material, as when the physician dictates, ''a mass in the subQ'' for ''a mass in the subcutaneous tissue,'' or ''nocturia times three'' (which he would write ''nocturia x 3''), meaning that the patient gets up three times a night to urinate.

Compression of ideas and omission of connectives and even of whole phrases yield a terse and seemingly incoherent style of prose. ''The heart is regular at 82 without murmurs, clicks, or rubs.'' ''The face is symmetrical and the tongue protrudes in the midline.'' The physician who passes abruptly from a description of a painful, red, light-sensitive eye to the remark that the patient gives no history of pain or swelling in joints has not slipped a mental cog. He has merely omitted a connecting phrase rendered unnecessary by the fact that any other physician reading his remarks will know that iritis (the tentative diagnosis) occurs in several syndromes along with arthritis.

Adding to the abstruseness of the workaday language of physicians is its heavy use of long, arcane, abstract words. This is not the place to explore the reasons why physicians feel compelled to say ''experienced epistaxis'' instead of ''had a nosebleed,'' but the fact must be recognized that, in clinical records, technical words and phrases often replace simpler and plainer forms of expression.

As in nonmedical settings, the grammar of dictated material tends to be exceedingly loose, with many incomplete sentences and syntactic breaks. The extent to which a transcriptionist amends and refurbishes what is dictated will depend on local conventions and institutional guidelines.

History. As a rule, the physician compiles the medical history by questioning the patient. At times, however, much or all of the information must be obtained from someone else; considerable historical material may be drawn from written records. With experience, a physician learns to word questions so that they can be understood by a person of average intelligence, do not give offense or provoke hostility, elicit a maximum amount of relevant information with a minimum expenditure of time and effort, and do not suggest or invite specific answers. (A question like ''You haven't had any sexual problems, have you?'' virtually demands a negative reply.) Often the patient's response to one question determines what will be asked next, or how it will be asked. Little by little, a tolerably complete understanding of the patient's medical status, *as he perceives it,* emerges.

It must be emphasized that, although a standard format is almost always followed in recording the patient's history, the information may have been obtained in much different order, perhaps even on more than one occasion or from a variety of sources. The answer to a dozen questions may be compressed into a single telling phrase. The physician often translates the patient's statements into medical jargon. Thus, ''I threw up at least five times'' becomes, ''He experienced emesis times five.'' On the other hand, the physician may make a point of quoting the patient's words exactly: ''It feels like my intestines are all tangled around my heart.'' Or he may fall into a colloquial style of dictation, unconsciously echoing the language actually used in interviewing the patient: ''Since then he has had no more bellyache and is eating fine.''

Introduction to Pharmacology References

Drug reference books are an important resource for medical transcriptionists. Experienced transcriptionists often purchase their own drug reference books every year or every other year to keep up to date on new drugs.

Drugs are used to treat many medical and surgical conditions. Some people, particularly those who are elderly, take multiple (sometimes as many as ten or more) medications each day. Therefore, it is critical that medical transcriptionists be familiar with drugs, their indications and dosages, and how to research new or unusual drug names in drug reference books.

Pharmaceutical companies use three different names to describe a drug: the chemical name (which is a complicated formula describing the drug's molecular structure), the generic name (a shorter name assigned to the drug chemical), and the trade or brand name (the copyrighted name selected by the pharmaceutical company). The trade or brand name is easy to pronounce, may indicate what the drug is used for or how often it is taken, and is selected for its appeal to prescribing physicians. A generic drug may have several trade names copyrighted by different manufacturers.

Generic drugs are always written in lowercase letters, while trade name drugs have an initial capital letter. Some trade name drugs also have internal capitalization (such as pHisoHex).

There are several drug references available for medical transcriptionists. Most physicians' offices have current copies of the *Physicians' Desk Reference* (published annually by Medical Economics Company), well-known as the *PDR*. This is a standard drug reference that contains various sections of drugs. Those of most interest to medical transcriptionists include the yellow pages which list generic names of drugs, the pink pages which list brand names of drugs, the blue pages which list drugs by their therapeutic category, and the white pages which give a complete description of the listed drugs including indications and dosages. Not all drugs are listed in the *PDR*; only those that the manufacturer pays to have listed are included. Therefore, it can be difficult to find certain types of drugs. It is also important to note that the *PDR* contains only prescription drugs; a separate publication for nonprescription drugs is available.

Another standard drug reference is the *American Drug Index (ADI)*, by Norman and Shirley Billups, published annually by Facts and Comparisons, J. B. Lippincott Company. This comprehensive reference lists both generic and trade name drugs and prescription and nonprescription drugs in alphabetical order throughout. Unfortunately, it lists every drug name in all capital letters rather than in initial capitals and lowercase letters. Generic drugs are preceded by a small black dot, and trade name drugs list the name of the manufacturer, thus alerting the transcriptionist that the drug is to be capitalized.

A new drug reference book to be updated annually was first published in 1992: *Saunders Pharmaceutical Word Book*, by Ellen and Randy Drake (published by W. B. Saunders). It is not just a listing of drugs, as the title implies, but an A to Z listing of medications with generic drugs in lowercase letters and trade names capitalized, as the transcriptionist must type them. Also, each entry states briefly what the drug is for and the usual methods of administration. Brand names are cross-referenced to generics. Of special help to transcriptionists is the appendix list of Sound Alikes, 879 pairs of drugs that sound enough alike to be confusing.

Understanding Pharmacology, by Susan Turley, published by Regents/Prentice Hall, is an easy-to-read, enjoyable textbook used in many pharmacology classes. It is especially useful to medical transcriptionists seeking a greater understanding of drugs and their uses. Drugs are discussed by medical specialty or body system, and the book contains a glossary of over 1200 commonly used drugs. Excerpts from *Understanding Pharmacology* are included in the Pharmacology section of each lesson in this course.

It is important to remember that there are drug names that sound very much alike but their uses are completely different. Example: Xanax (used to treat anxiety) and Zantac (used to treat stomach ulcers). Drug reference books are valuable not only because they provide the correct spelling of a drug name, but because they help transcriptionists to select the correct drug name based on its indications for use.

Words such as tablet, capsule, solution, elixir, and cream are not part of the trade name of a drug and should not be capitalized when transcribed.

Introduction to Laboratory Tests

In the past decade there has been a dramatic increase in both the number of new diagnostic laboratory tests as well as in the complexity of the tests offered. This explosive growth in the field of laboratory medicine has been due to the demand by physicians for new and improved diagnostic procedures, combined with the ever-expanding capacity of modern technology to meet the demand with increasingly sophisticated laboratory methods and equipment.

On a daily basis medical transcriptionists come in contact with dictation which details the results of laboratory tests performed on patients. In order to accurately transcribe this material, it is important to be familiar with the names and abbreviations of many laboratory tests, the reasons they are offered, and the meaning of the results.

Laboratory tests can be performed in many different settings: clinics, physicians' offices, health fairs, and sometimes even at home by patients themselves, though the greatest number of laboratory tests are performed within the hospital setting. Hospital laboratories are equipped with the most technologically advanced and automated equipment to handle hundreds of tests each day. The largest hospitals perform all standard laboratory tests, as well as many uncommon ones, which may be requested by smaller hospitals or clinics whose facilities are not equipped to handle unusual tests.

The laboratory of a hospital is divided into many smaller departments which perform specialized laboratory tests. This division of labor is also reflected to a great extent on the average laboratory slip which is used to report the results of laboratory tests. Various sections on the lab slip include hematology, blood bank, chemistry, coagulation, urinalysis, stool examination, microbiology, and cytology.

Hematology is concerned with the study of the formed components or cells of the blood. These cells include mature red blood cells, white blood cells, and platelets, as well as their immature forms. The function of the red blood cell is to carry oxygen from the lungs to the body tissues. The function of the white blood cell is to fight any foreign substances that enter the body, such as bacteria. Platelets function along with the coagulation factors in the blood to form a blood clot at the site of tissue injury. White blood cells are further differentiated into groups which have diagnostic value. These include lymphocytes, monocytes, neutrophils, eosinophils, basophils, and bands or immature neutrophils.

There are many brief forms, slang, and special terms associated with the blood. Brief forms are acceptable in medical reports, but transcriptionists should always spell out in full any slang words which are dictated. For example, *monos* is an acceptable brief form for monocytes, but *lytes* is a slang term that must be translated *electrolytes* in medical reports.

A complete blood count (CBC) includes tests which measure red blood cell and white blood cell levels. A CBC with differential also measures the levels of all of the different types of white blood cells. Other common tests are the hemoglobin and hematocrit (often dictated as H&H and must be written out in full), which are indicative of the oxygen-carrying capacity of the blood as well as the percentage of red blood cells per blood sample. Normally the hematocrit is about three times greater than the hemoglobin level for the same patient, so that if the patient's hemoglobin level was reported as 15, you could expect that the hematocrit would be approximately 45.

The chemistry section of the laboratory performs tests on many different electrolytes, fats, and other substances found in the serum, or clear fluid which separates from a clotted blood sample. Blood chemistries include tests for electrolytes: sodium, potassium, calcium, and chloride. Fats include cholesterol, triglycerides, and LDL (low-density lipoproteins). Other substances tested include bilirubin, SGOT, SGPT, and LDH which are used to evaluate liver function. BUN and creatinine are useful indicators of kidney function. Uric acid levels are tested to diagnose the medical condition of gout. Often the physician orders a combination of tests under one name. For example, by checking a box next to the entry "serum lipid profile" on the laboratory slip, the physician can order the tests for cholesterol, triglycerides, total lipids, and lipoproteins. An elevated serum acid phosphatase is useful in detecting prostatic cancer.

The microbiology department of the laboratory identifies infectious organisms through the use of microscopes and culture and sensitivity testing. Specimens for testing are obtained from urine, stool, blood, sputum, wound drainage, or other body fluids. A sample of the specimen is smeared onto a culture medium and incubated at 37°C for sufficient time to allow bacterial growth to occur. Antibiotic discs placed on the media of the culture plates permit evaluation of the sensitivity of the bacteria cultured to specific antibiotics. Antibiotic discs to which the bacteria are sensitive are surrounded by a ring or zone of inhibition of bacterial growth. Bacteria that are resistant to an antibiotic will show no inhibition of growth around the disc.

A rapid method to tentatively identify a pathogenic bacterium is to smear a sample on a slide and then stain the slide with the Gram stain. This stain differentiates between organisms that are gram-positive and gram-negative. The shape of the bacterium can provide further clues to the identity of the organism. The acid-fast stain is used to identify mycobacteria specifically.

Physicians order laboratory tests to be performed on patients for a variety of reasons:
1. To diagnose disease in a patient who is ill.
2. To screen for hidden diseases. Well-known examples include use of the Pap smear to identify cervical cancer, and the self-administered test for occult or hidden blood in the stool as an indicator of colon cancer.
3. To assess the extent of damage from disease processes.
4. To monitor the effectiveness of treatment prescribed by the physician.
5. To monitor blood levels of certain medications. Periodic blood samples can insure that drug levels in the blood remain within the therapeutic range.
6. To monitor the course of a disease.

Laboratory test results are measured and reported most often using the metric system. Common units of measure include centimeters, millimeters, cubic centimeters, milliliters, grams, milligrams, micrograms, milliequivalents, and percentages.

Laboratory test values are reported as numerical values. If the value falls within the range observed in normal individuals, it is considered normal. If it falls outside of this range, it is considered abnormal. The age and sex of a patient cause variation in the normal range of laboratory values.

The accepted normal range for a particular laboratory test varies from one laboratory to another, due to differences in equipment and methodology used in testing. Therefore, lab slips usually give the accepted normal range for that particular facility. The normal value is printed next to the blank space for the reported value for the individual patient. When transcribing, it is not unusual for the medical transcriptionist to hear the physician say, "Normal for our laboratory is . . . ," after dictating a patient's test result.

The transcription of laboratory test terminology presents certain challenges for the medical transcriptionist. Correctly transcribing the name of a laboratory test or its abbreviation is just the first step. Numerical results must be transcribed with absolute accuracy. Care must be taken to place decimal points accurately and to transcribe units of measure correctly.

It is also necessary to understand why a test was ordered and what the results indicate. Some dictations contain considerable detail concerning the test process, the use of special stains or dyes, as well as the significance of the results.

As a student, you will want to study this critical area of medical transcription diligently. As a practicing medical transcriptionist, you will always be increasing your knowledge of laboratory tests and procedures, as the technology of medicine increases daily.

Anatomy/Medical Terminology

Wordsearching in Medical References

Medical transcriptionists are known for their love of words and their use of medical references. Today, unlike ten years ago, there are many excellent reference books available for the medical transcriptionist—medical dictionaries, medical specialty word and phrase references, medical abbreviation references, and medical style manuals.

Each type of reference fills a particular need. A medical dictionary provides definitions to help the medical transcriptionist differentiate between similar-sounding words; however, it does not contain many specialty words, abbreviations, and surgical instruments. Medical specialty word and phrase references contain terms from one medical specialty and include slang, surgical instruments, drugs, new and unusual terms, abbreviations, and laboratory tests for that specialty. Medical abbreviation references contain common and unusual abbreviations and their definitions from all medical specialties. Medical style manuals give suggestions on how to handle questions of format, punctuation, grammar, and spelling in medical reports.

Not all unfamiliar dictated words are medical, however. It is important to remember that many physicians have an extensive vocabulary and may dictate English words that are new to the transcriptionist.

The following medical references form the basis of a library for medical transcription students and practitioners.

Dorland's Illustrated Medical Dictionary, 27th ed., 1988. Published by W. B. Saunders Co., Philadelphia.

Stedman's Illustrated Medical Dictionary, 25th ed., 1990. Published by Williams & Wilkins, Baltimore.

Current Medical Terminology, 4th ed., by Vera Pyle, 1992. Published by Health Professions Institute, Modesto, CA.

The Medical Word Book, 3rd ed., by Sheila Sloane, 1991. Published by W. B. Saunders Co., Philadelphia.

Medical Phrase Index, 2nd ed., by Jean Lorenzini, 1989. Published by PMIC, Los Angeles.

Word and phrase reference books published by Health Professions Institute in the specialties of Cardiology, Gastroenterology, Orthopedics/Neurology, Pathology, Psychiatry, and Radiology.

A standard English dictionary, such as *Webster's Ninth New Collegiate Dictionary,* by Merriam-Webster.

A valuable source of information for transcriptionists are drug reference books, including:

American Drug Index, by Billups and Billups. Published annually by J. B. Lippincott Co., St. Louis.

Physicians' Desk Reference. Published annually by Medical Economics Co., Des Moines.

Saunders Pharmaceutical Word Book, by Ellen and Randy Drake. Published annually (beginning in 1992) by W. B. Saunders, Philadelphia.

If a reference book cannot provide the answer to a drug question, the medical transcriptionist may even seek help from a pharmacist.

No medical transcription practitioner or student should be without up-to-date reference sources. Take time to examine the medical reference books available to you as you begin this course. Wordsearching, or locating the medical word that is correct in both spelling and meaning, is a skill that takes time and practice to develop.

Following are some suggestions to help you improve your wordsearching skills.

1. If you are unable to locate a word in your reference books, it could be that the word in question has an initial letter other than the sound you heard. For instance, the phonetic pronunciation of *v* sounds very much like that of *f*, the letter *m* may sound like *n*, and so on. The *z* sound you hear may actually be an *x* (*x*iphoid) and the *k* might be *ch* (is*ch*emic). Medical terms that contain silent letters (*euthyroid, herniorrhaphy, pneumonia*) or are frequently mispronounced (*menstruation*) also present a challenge.

As you gain experience using available resources, you will become familiar with the techniques of determining sound-alikes and efficient in locating terms with silent letters.

2. If you are unable to locate a phrase under a particular entry, try looking under a related entry.

Many structures have a Latin as well as an English name. If you are looking for the name of a muscle, look under both *musculus* and *muscle.* Other Latin-English entries include *ligamentum* and *ligament, tendo* and *tendon, fissura* and *fissure, arteria* and *artery.*

Look under a related term to find additional subentries. If you can't find the correct term under the entry *operation,* look under *procedure.* If you can't find the correct term under *disease,* look under *syndrome.* If you can't find the correct term under *sign,* look under *test.*

3. When you hear a phrase that you cannot understand, look first under the noun, not the adjective. The noun usually follows the adjective. For example, to find *bullous emphysema,* you would look under *emphysema* (the noun), not *bullous.* To find *Parkinson's disease,* you would look under *disease.*

One exception is that in Latin phrases the noun is followed by the adjective: fascia lata, ligamentum flavum. Look under the first word. Another exception is bacterial names; the genus is given first, followed by the species: *Neisseria gonorrhoeae.*

If you are unable to locate a term after consulting all available medical references, you have several options. You may ask your instructor to assist you or you may flag the term and attach a note to the report. On the job, a medical transcriptionist would (1) seek another transcriptionist's opinion, (2) refer to the patient's chart (if available), (3) contact the dictating physician for clarification, or (4) leave a blank in the report and attach a note so that the dictator may insert the correct word.

A flag is a note that is paperclipped or attached in some way to the report. It lists all blanks left in the report, giving the page and line number for ease of identification, and may also give a phonetic spelling of what the word sounded like to the transcriptionist. This will assist the dictator or supervisor in filling in the blank.

When wordsearching, it is important to remember: *Never guess* at a word just to fill in a blank. A blank does not reflect poorly on the medical transcriptionist who has thoroughly researched the question. Leaving a blank is the correct thing to do when all reference books and other sources have been exhausted. Remember, the integrity and accuracy of the medical record is far more important than never leaving a blank. The latter is not a realistic goal, even for experienced medical transcriptionists.

Prefixes and Suffixes

The following matching exercise reviews common prefixes and suffixes and their meanings as encountered in dictation from all medical specialties.

Medical transcriptionists are confronted daily with the need to select the correct prefix or suffix based on the medical meaning of the report, even when what is dictated is unclear.

Correctly identifying and spelling medical prefixes and suffixes is extremely important. In particular, note those prefixes and suffixes which can sound essentially the same when dictated: *intra-* and *inter-, -tomy* and *-stomy, -scopy* and *-scope.* Failing to differentiate between *hypo*kalemia (low blood potassium) and *hyper*kalemia (elevated blood potassium) in transcribing is a serious medical error. Likewise, failing to differentiate between gastro*scopy,* gastro*tomy,* and gastro*stomy* will convey an entirely wrong medical meaning.

Inexperienced medical transcriptionists often incorrectly transcribe **inter**venous instead of **intra**venous or **inter**operative instead of **intra**operative. Note that *intra-* means "within" and *inter-* means "between." Thus, an intravenous line is within a vein, not between veins; the term *intraoperative* indicates the time within or during surgery, not between surgeries.

A strong foundation in basic terminology will greatly assist you in completing this course. Subsequent chapters will review additional prefixes and suffixes specific to particular medical specialties. Test your basic knowledge of this material by completing the following exercise.

Instructions: Match the prefix or suffix in Column A with its definition in Column B.

Column A   *Column B*

A. -itis   __D__ the study of
B. auto-   _____ a tumor
C. post-   _____ toward
D. -logy   _____ development or form
E. -tomy   _____ inflammation of
F. -pathy   _____ pain
G. intra-   _____ without
H. -algia   _____ discharge
I. -scopy   _____ enlargement of
J. supra-   _____ across
K. -graph   _____ self
L. a-   _____ a disease condition
M. -megaly   _____ within
N. -plasty   _____ new opening created surgically
O. trans-   _____ beside or near
P. -oma   _____ cutting out
Q. ad-   _____ increased in amount
R. -osis   _____ an abnormal condition
S. dys-   _____ an instrument used to record
T. -stomy   _____ painful or difficult
U. pseudo   _____ a surgical repair
V. -plasia   _____ process of examining visually
W. hyper-   _____ located above
X. -ectomy   _____ making an incision into
Y. para-   _____ coming after
Z. -rrhea   _____ false

Transcription Guidelines

Style. The transcription of medical reports (medical or technical writing) differs in technique from the production of essays and manuscripts (formal writing for publication). The latter requires strict adherence to prescribed forms, style, and syntax, and often the writer generates several draft copies before arriving at a finished, polished document for publication.

Medical reports, in contrast, contain many abbreviations, brief forms, shortcuts, and word coinages that are an integral part of the language of medicine. A first-time final copy of a medical report is expected, and it is simply not feasible or necessary for the production-oriented medical transcriptionist working in a fast-paced environment to attempt to convert a medical document into a piece of formal writing or a polished essay.

Medical transcriptionists are expected to produce clean, neat, and accurate documents for every medical report dictated and to follow certain suggested stylistic guidelines studied in this course.

Many stylistic factors determine proper editing, punctuation, and grammar. Even respected reference materials vary and may contradict one another and themselves. Additionally, the transcriptionist's employer may mandate specific rules of grammar, style, and format to be followed, and in that case the transcriptionist will follow the employer's requirements.

Editing. Every dictator has at one time or another misspoken and said something like, "The patient smokes two beers a day and drinks two packs," or refers to the surgery on the *left* leg in one paragraph and the *right* in the next. Dictating physicians are counting on the medical transcriptionist to be alert and, when necessary, to correct their mistakes.

The experienced medical transcriptionist, with a firm grasp of medical language and terminology, and familiarity with the dictating physician's preferences, may edit in various ways throughout a report; however, the student should transcribe the reports verbatim, **as dictated,** making changes only to correct obvious errors, to comply with standard grammar and punctuation guidelines, or to add headings and paragraphing where appropriate.

Where warranted, the transcriptionist may add conjunctions (and, but, for, or, nor), prepositions (of, to, with), articles (a, an, the), pronouns and nouns as the subject of a sentence, and verbs to complete a sentence.

| Dictated: | No tenderness present over chest. |
| Transcribed: | No tenderness is present over the chest. |

| Dictated: | Came in with chest pain. |
| Transcribed: | The patient came in with chest pain. |

| Dictated: | No tenderness on palpation. |
| Transcribed: | No tenderness was elicited on palpation. |

It is acceptable, however, to type all of the above as dictated, to preserve the style of the dictator.

As a general rule, the history portion of medical reports is dictated in the past tense. Some physicians, however, dictate in the present tense even when discussing past events. While some expect the transcriptionist to change the report to past tense, other dictators want the report to be transcribed as dictated. When the dictator's preference is not known, the transcriptionist may either edit for consistency or transcribe as dictated.

Some dictators switch tenses within a report. In this case, the transcriptionist may elect to transcribe as dictated or edit the report to one tense for consistency, if the dictator's preference is not known.

Editing also includes watching for medical inconsistencies within a report, such as a hysterectomy reportedly done on a man, or different ages given for the same patient within one report, or a surgery that begins on the left leg and ends on the right leg.

All editing should be done with a light hand, and the distinctive style of the individual dictator should be preserved in the report. As Vera Pyle noted in "The Editing Function of the Medical Transcriptionist," *Journal of AAMT* (Summer 1982), p. 42:

In editing dictation, we do not go charging in, doctoring up reports in an aggressive way, in an intrusional way. It has to be done so subtly, so delicately, so carefully, that we get a favorable response from the dictator. . . .

We must be so involved with what we are transcribing that we know what is going on and can detect something that is dictated that does not make sense, that does not flow, that does not add up. We must listen with an educated ear, with an intelligent ear, so that we can produce an accurate, intelligent, clear document, always remembering the fine line between editing and tampering.

Transcription Tips

Homonyms. Homonyms are words that are pronounced in the same way but are spelled differently and have different meanings.

Well-known English homonyms include:

flower	flour
sight	site
bare	bear
stationary	stationery
principal	principle
their	there

Medical homonyms are presented in the Transcription Tips sections for each body system or medical specialty in this course. Common medical homonyms include:

humeral	humoral
ileum	ilium
viscus	viscous
elicit	illicit
perineal	peroneal

Sound-alike words. Sound-alike words are similar to homonyms but may have a slightly different pronunciation. Sound-alike words are, however, quite difficult to distinguish when dictated on tape. Therefore, distinguishing sound-alike words and selecting the one with the correct meaning is a critical skill for medical transcriptionists listening to a dictated report.

Common sound-alikes include prefixes such as *intra-* and *inter-*, *hypo-* and *hyper-*, as well as suffixes such as *-tomy, -ostomy, -ectomy,* and *-scope, -scopy.* Making the wrong choice of prefix or suffix can drastically change the medical meaning of a word.

Common sound-alike words include:

advice	advise
affect	effect
coarse	course
than	then
in	on
prostate	prostrate
oral	aural
abduction	adduction
bile	bowel
ascitic	acidic
facial	fascial
perineal	peritoneal
ureteral	urethral

Sound-alikes Exercise

Instructions: In the following sentences circle the correct sound-alike from the words in parentheses.

1. The patient was (counseled, councilled) to get psychiatric help.

2. The patient expressed strong (decent, descent, dissent) to the recommended bypass operation.

3. Venous (access, assess, excess, axis) was needed for I.V. administration of antibiotics, so a heparin lock was placed.

4. (Accept, except) for a slight weakness in the left arm, the patient had no residual symptoms of stroke.

5. The patient's wife made an (allusion, elusion, illusion) to possible alcoholism by stating that the patient drank a six-pack a day, but the patient denied a drinking problem.

6. Because penicillin was not (affective, effective), the patient was put on another antibiotic.

7. My (advice, advise) to the patient was to drink plenty of liquids, get lots of sleep, and take aspirin for pain.

8. The patient complained of (a symptomatic, asymptomatic) cough for the last month, but it was nonproductive.

9. I would (assess, access, excess, axis) his chances of surviving the operation at 50/50.

10. The surgical (cite, sight, site) was dressed with a sterile bandage.

11. The patient was not (conscious, conscience) after the head injury.

12. Moderate exercise would certainly (complement, compliment) the patient's post-CABG therapy.

Sample Reports

Medical Reports

There are a variety of medical reports generated every day in physician offices, clinics, and hospitals. Medical transcriptionists should be familiar with those dictated in each work setting.

Physicians in private practice frequently dictate office chart notes, letters, initial office evaluations, and history and physical examinations.

Medical reports dictated in hospitals and medical centers are numerous in category; however, they invariably include dictations from the "basic four" reports: History and Physical Examination, Consultation Report, Operative Report, and Discharge Summary. Emergency Department Reports, hospital progress notes, and diagnostic studies are often dictated as well.

Chart Note. The chart note (also called progress note or follow-up note) is dictated by a physician after talking with, meeting with, or examining a patient, usually in an outpatient setting, although progress notes are occasionally dictated on hospital inpatients. The chart note contains a concise description of the patient's presenting problem, physical findings, and the physician's plan of treatment, and may also include the results of laboratory tests.

Chart notes can vary in length from one sentence to one or more pages, with the average note being two to four paragraphs long. Chart notes are sometimes dictated in an informal, staccato style using clipped sentences, abbreviations, and brief forms.

There are numerous formats for dictated chart notes. SOAP notes are those dictated in the SOAP format (an acronym for Subjective, Objective, Assessment, and Plan—headings within the note).

Letter. Physicians frequently dictate letters to communicate patient information to other physicians, insurance companies, and government offices. Medical transcriptionists need to be familiar with the various standard business letter formats. An employer may express a preference for a specific letter format, although the full-block format (with the parts of the letter lined up on the left margin) is the one most commonly used.

Referral letters and consultation letters are not mere business letters; they are medical documents in letter form and as such should be transcribed with the same high degree of skill and accuracy as other medical reports.

Initial Office Evaluation. Performed in the physician's office or clinic setting, the initial office evaluation is dictated after the physician sees a patient for the first time. It contains essentially the same information as the history and physical examination, although the physical examination in an initial office evaluation may be limited to specific areas of disease.

History and Physical Examination (H&P). Shortly before or after a patient is admitted to the hospital, the physician obtains the patient's subjective history and conducts an objective physical examination. These findings are then dictated by category and usually include the patient's Chief Complaint (presenting problem), History of Present Illness (events leading to the patient's hospitalization), Past Medical History (medical and surgical problems from childhood to the present, medications, and allergies), Family History (the medical condition of parents and other family members), Social History (the patient's occupation, lifestyle, and habits), Review of Systems (the medical condition of the patient's major organs), and the Physical Examination.

The Physical Examination details the physician's objective findings on examination of the patient. The following subheadings are usually dictated: General Appearance, Vital Signs, Skin, HEENT (Head, Eyes, Ears, Nose, and Throat), Neck, Chest, Breasts, Heart, Lungs, Abdomen, Back, Extremities, Genitalia or Pelvis, Rectum, Neurologic Exam, and occasionally Mental Status Exam. In addition, this report includes an Admitting Diagnosis, and sometimes a proposed Treatment Plan. The History and Physical report is also known as the Admission History and Physical.

Emergency Department Report. An Emergency Department Report is much like an Initial Office Evaluation, except that the patient is seen and treated in an Emergency Department of a hospital or acute-care clinic. The Presenting Complaint, Present Illness, Physical Examination, and Course of Treatment are usually dictated. Sometimes the patient's condition is serious enough to warrant admission to the hospital, but more often the patient is seen, evaluated, treated, and then released to home with a recommended treatment plan.

Consultation. Consultations result when one physician requests the services of another (usually a specialist) in the care and treatment of a patient. The Consultation Report usually contains the subheadings Brief History of the Present Illness, Findings, Pertinent Laboratory Work, Working Diagnosis or Impression, and a Recommended Course of Treatment. The Consultation Report may be dictated in letter format and is to be transcribed on the stationery of the physician's office or the medical facility or on preprinted consultation forms.

Operative Report. After a surgical procedure is performed, a detailed description of the operation is dictated. Surgical procedures are carried out in hospitals, outpatient surgery centers, and occasionally in a physician's office. The Operative Report usually contains information at the beginning that is obtained from written records, including the date of operation, the duration of anesthesia and operation times, and names of the operating surgeon and assistants. The dictation includes Preoperative Diagnosis, Postoperative Diagnosis, Title of Operation, Findings, and Procedure. The dictation of the Procedure includes a detailed description of the operation itself, including anatomic landmarks, surgical instruments, suture materials used to close the incision, estimated blood loss, complications encountered, condition of the patient at the end of the procedure, sponge and needle count at the end of the procedure, and, if applicable, tourniquet time, blood and fluids administered, drains placed, and medications given. Some surgeons also dictate a Postoperative Plan.

Discharge Summary. By the time a patient is ready for discharge from the hospital, a variety of treatment modalities have been carried out. The Discharge Summary is the medical document that summarizes the patient's course in the hospital and may be short if the patient's stay in the hospital was brief and uncomplicated. Most reports include a summary of the admission and discharge diagnoses, procedures or operations performed (if any), brief review of the patient's history, the physician's findings on physical examination, a report of laboratory work performed and pertinent findings, the patient's hospital course, discharge medications, and the discharge plan or disposition.

The Healthcare Record

by Pamela K. Wear, MBA, RRA

The healthcare record is chronological, documented evidence of a patient's initial database, initial evaluation, identified problems and needs, objectives of care, prescribed treatment, and end results.

The healthcare record is the property of the hospital or the medical facility or office in which it originated, and it cannot be removed from the premises without a subpoena or court order. It is maintained in a Health Information Department usually headed by an RRA (registered record administrator) or an ART (accredited record technician).

"Medical record," the terminology that was used for over fifty years, is now evolving to "healthcare record" to denote both illness and wellness. The Medical Record Department is likewise changing to the Health Information Department with the advance of technology, and the Director of Medical Records is changing to Director of Health Information. RRAs and ARTs are called Health Information Managers and are certified by the American Health Information Management Association (AHIMA), formerly called the American Medical Record Association (AMRA).

Purpose of the healthcare record. The healthcare record is a measurement of care rendered in a medical facility. It is utilized to plan, communicate, and evaluate the quality of care given to each patient. It is "proof of work done," containing documentation to meet federal, state, and JCAHO (Joint Commission on Accreditation of Healthcare Organizations) standards and regulations as well as those for reimbursement and third-party payer requirements.

The healthcare record is maintained for medical-legal protection for the patient, facility, staff, and physician. It is used for research, compiling statistics, and evaluation of healthcare delivery.

Origin of the healthcare record. In hospitals, the healthcare record begins in the Admissions Department, Outpatient Registration, or the Emergency Department. Patients having surgery as outpatients check in at Outpatient Registration, which registers elective surgery outpatients and clinic patients. These patients, after observation, may also be admitted. Patients may also enter the hospital after evaluation in the Emergency Department.

The major role of these departments is to collect patient identification and demographic information. The correct spelling of the patient's legal name and birthdate are critical elements to determine positive patient identification. This information is used to assign a healthcare record number that is maintained for the lifetime of the patient and should be recorded on all transcribed reports.

Additional identification entries on patients are address, next of kin, birthplace, social security number, occupation, sex, marital status, ethnic origin, religious preference, and admitting diagnosis. Financial entries include the patient's employer, job title, address of company, insurance company, person responsible for emergency notification and payments, type of coverage, insurance identification number, and type of payment plan.

All this information is recorded on an admission sheet or patient demographic face sheet. The hospital is required by federal law to collect a minimum amount of information, and this sheet is usually available in some format to the transcriptionist to assist in patient identification.

Consents. These departments also have responsibility for obtaining a Conditions for Admission form which includes the patient's consent for treatment, outline of patient's responsibilities, including billing, and the assurance that confidentiality will be protected. Throughout a patient's care, additional informed consents for surgery, procedures, invasive diagnostic tests, transfer, etc., will be obtained as appropriate.

Medical Entries

1. *Physician orders*: A patient is admitted and treated only on the order of an attending physician. The admission includes orders for diagnostic tests, medications, and treatments. These forms are usually multipart with a copy for the pharmacy. Depending on the physical layout of the transcription department, the physician's orders can be used as a reference for identification of the patient's medications and other data.

2. *Diagnostic tests*: From the physician's orders, the nurses generate a requisition for diagnostic tests. These are sent to the appropriate department, whose personnel perform the tests and document the results. Typical diagnostic results include the following. Laboratory: Lab slips include the results of urinalyses, complete blood counts, electrolytes, chemistries, specimens, and blood transfusions. Pathology and autopsy results are also the responsibility of this department. Radiology: Dictated reports include the clinical history, findings, and conclusion for any x-rays performed. Cardiology: Electrocardiograms, Holter monitor, and exercise stress test results are dictated, or reports are machine generated. Neurophysiology: Electroencephalograms, electromyograms, and sleep disorder results are dictated or machine generated.

3. *Nursing entries*: Nurses assess patients on admission by completing an admission history and physical, establish a patient care plan, and set up forms for documentation of graphic information such as vital signs (temperature, pulse, respiration, blood pressure, and weight). Intake and output of fluids, diet and hygiene records, medication records, as well as specialized forms for monitoring diabetes, operating room check lists/operating room record/recovery room record, and nurses' notes/observations become a part of every patient's healthcare record.

4. *Physician entries*: The physician dictates the patient's History and Physical, which includes the Chief Complaint, History of Present Illness, Past Medical History, Family History, Social History, Review of Systems, Physical Examination, and Plan.

The physician may call in consultants as appropriate to assist in the patient's care. The consultant writes or dictates a consultation which includes a comprehensive review of the healthcare record and/or complete physical examination and recommendations.

The physician writes or dictates progress notes which include all pertinent plans and observations during the patient's care.

If the patient has a diagnostic procedure or a surgical procedure performed, the physician dictates preoperative and postoperative diagnoses, the name of the procedure, assistant, findings, technique, and outcome. The anesthesiologist completes a pre-anesthesia and post-anesthesia evaluation.

At the conclusion of the patient's hospitalization the physician writes or dictates a comprehensive discharge summary which includes a brief history, course of the hospitalization, conclusions, follow-up instructions and discharge medications, diagnoses, complications, and any surgical procedures.

5. *Therapists' entries*: Physical, occupational, speech, vocational, and recreational therapists, and social workers who might be requested to assist in the patient's care write or dictate an initial evaluation and plans, ongoing progress notes, and a final summary with follow-up instructions.

6. *Ancillary personnel entries*: Dietary personnel, discharge planners, utilization review managers, and others participating in the patient's care record progress notes on each of their visits.

Emergency record. Patients evaluated and treated only in the Emergency Department receive a condensed version of the inpatient healthcare record, which includes demographic information, nursing assessment, physician's evaluation, treatment, and conclusions. A comprehensive visit might include a dictated note with diagnostic test results, consents, and instructions.

Physician's office healthcare records. The healthcare records maintained in a physician's office include many, but not all, of the records and forms contained in the hospital healthcare record. The patient's records include an initial history and physical exam, office visits, progress notes, diagnostic test results, copies of acute hospitalization reports, letters to insurance companies, consultation letters, etc. These records have a higher percentage of handwritten notes, although many physicians dictate on all their patients' visits.

Conclusion. A patient's healthcare record is made up of important, accurate, and timely data entries that communicate illness and wellness information that a healthcare provider must have in order to treat the patient. Thus, the health information department and medical transcription are vitally linked in the delivery of healthcare.

Transcription Practice

As you transcribe, remember that you are beginning a new physical skill that requires the coordination of your eyes, ears, fingers, and foot (if you use a foot pedal). You may already be an accomplished typist and that will give you an advantage. We recommend that students have a copy typing speed of at least 45 words per minute before attempting to transcribe. However, the skills needed to copy type and transcribe are somewhat different, and you should expect your transcription to be slow and halting in the beginning.

Try this exercise: Cross your arms across your chest in a way that is comfortable. You may have your right arm uppermost or your left arm, depending on what is customary for you. Now try to cross your arms so that the other arm is uppermost. This can be quite awkward for some people. You may find yourself repeatedly trying to ''arrange'' your arms to get them right.

Just as it feels unfamiliar to cross your arms in a different way than you are accustomed to, it may also feel awkward to transcribe what you hear rather than copy type what you see. Although the keyboard is the same, the way in which you interact with it is significantly different, requiring coordination of timing of the eyes, ears, fingers, and use of a foot pedal or hand control connected to the transcriber.

As you begin to transcribe, do not try to type fast at first, but strive first for accuracy of medical words, grammar, punctuation, and format. All of these constitute another group of new variables that you must constantly consider, evaluate, and take time to master. Understanding the scope and details of all of these variables in the transcription process can seem overwhelming at first, but your diligence will be rewarded later as you add speed to your new skill of accuracy.

Transcribe each dictation carefully, stopping as often as necessary to look up new and unfamiliar words for spelling and meaning. Wordsearching time is time well spent and is NEVER wasted, as it strengthens and builds one of the most important skills you bring to transcription.

Start slowly and proceed carefully and thoughtfully, taking advantage of every opportunity to learn, memorize, and understand new medical material. Most importantly, be encouraged by your progress. Speed will come naturally as you gain knowledge and experience, and soon you will see the fruits of your efforts as you transcribe new reports confidently, accurately, and quickly.

Error Analysis

The most common errors committed by students include omitting important dictated words, selecting the wrong words (both medical and English), misspellings, typographical errors, and grammatical and punctuation mistakes. The solutions listed below will help you assess the kinds of errors you are making and show you how to minimize them.

Omitted dictated word. Listen carefully to the dictation and slow your pace. Do not attempt to increase your transcription speed until these errors are minimized.

Wrong word. Take care in checking word definitions. The definition must match the context of the report.

Misspelled word. Mentally spell the corrected word several times. Highlight it in your dictionary or write the word in your personal notebook so that you will be aware of it each time you look it up.

Typographical error. Your proofreading is at fault. Allow time to elapse between the time you transcribe the report and the time you proofread it.

Grammatical error. If a physician makes a grammatical error, you are expected to correct it. If your transcription contains a significant number of these types of errors, a review of basic English is in order— for you, not the physician, unfortunately.

Punctuation error. The most serious punctuation errors are those that alter medical meaning. If you make a significant number of these kinds of errors, a review of basic punctuation would be useful. There may be several acceptable but different ways to punctuate some sentences without changing the medical meaning.

Learning Objectives

Medical

- List some of the dermatologic symptoms and diseases in the Review of Systems of an H&P.
- List common physical findings of dermatologic disease found in a physical examination.
- Give the names of six different forms in which drugs are manufactured.
- Discuss the purpose and technique involved in performing common dermatologic laboratory tests and surgical procedures.
- Given a cross-section illustration of the structure of the skin, memorize the anatomic structures.
- Demonstrate knowledge of anatomical, medical, pharmacological, adjectival, and sound-alike terms by accurately completing the exercises in this lesson.

Fundamentals

- Describe three ways in which silent letters in the spelling of English words complicate the process of medical transcription.
- List the four steps involved in proofreading.
- Describe six common transcription errors.
- Given a medical report with errors, identify and correct the errors.
- Describe how the transcriptionist can edit report headings.

Practice

- Accurately transcribe authentic physician dictation from the specialty of dermatology.

A Closer Look

Is Medical Transcription What I DO or What I AM?

by Judith Marshall, MA, CMT

Every summer I sit on the sand and ponder the cosmic questions of life, as the water laps my aging toes. Who am I, what am I, what does it all mean, and who cares?

There are drinks in the cooler. When I bought the ice for the beach, I recognized the clerk. "So, Geraldine, you work for the Lil Peach now?"

"No," she snapped, her voice like those little pops in phone static. "This is what I do; it's not what I AM."

Geraldine was hot and tired but I got her drift. I'm a medical transcriptionist—is it what I do or is it what I am? Just an old-fashioned transcriptionist. The kind who knows how to spell all the OLD diseases: poliomyelitis, syphilis, gonorrhea. The kind that people buttonhole with questions of health. Daily living is, after all, wellness and sickness, and in-between, okay-I-guess, fine-I-guess. Saying "Hi" in America means hello, how are you. Once in a while someone really tells you how they are.

A friend or relative steps on my shoelaces and says, "Say, Judith, you know that medical stuff. What is this medicine I am taking?" . . . "I have a rash. What does it mean?" . . . "The doctor says I have hyper, hyper something. Now what could that be?"

If I had a dollar for every time someone asked if I am a nurse, I could wallpaper the spare room. And have you noticed how disappointed people are when you tell them you're not a nurse?

After I moved to Massachusetts from Ohio, I went to the voter registration office and filled out a computer form. Occupation: Medical Transcriptionist. The gum-chewing clerk gave me a petulant look. "It doesn't fit in the boxes. What else are you besides this very long word? How about Secretary? How about Typist?''

"No, I'm not a typist in the *pure* sense.''

By this time she was out of patience and I was out of control.

"Pure or impure, what shall it be? Do you want to vote in this country or not?''

Yes, I surely did want to vote, so for the government, for the Commonwealth of Massachusetts, for God and the flag, I became a *MED SEC.* Now I fit in the boxes.

Ten years later the census office in my home town sent us a computer form. Our household is listed as "One retired male, one spayed dog, one neutered dog, one MED TRANS.'' It took ten long years to move from MED SEC to MED TRANS and the dogs get better billing.

Is a TRANS better than a SEC? The next time I voted, one of the inquisitive election workers asked me what sort of medicine I transport and isn't it nice that women can be anything they want to be, even truck drivers.

Dizzy Gillespie, My Brother, and Me

Kathy Rambo, CMT

When I was a high school freshman and my sister was a senior, my mother bought us a typewriter. Sis was already taking her second year of typing, and I was planning on at least two years myself, so Mom thought we should have our own machine. Well, sophomore and then junior years rolled around, and somehow, with the French and Latin and chemistry courses, I had no time for typing class.

Then came senior year. I had room for an extra class in my schedule and was looking forward to finally learning how to type. On the first day of the school year, I walked into the office of the 86-year-old nun who was to be senior counselor and handed her my tentative class schedule. She looked it over quickly, then handed it back, pointing to one item on the list and saying, "You're too smart for this.''

"Too smart for what?'' I asked.

"Typing,'' she replied. "You're too smart to waste your time and intelligence in a typing class. You should take something more challenging.''

"Like what?''

"Like calculus. Or more chemistry. Or a third year of Latin.''

English I excelled at. History wasn't too bad. But a second year of chemistry? I had come too close to blowing up my lab partner last year to want that challenge again. Or calculus? I had learned only one good thing from algebra and geometry—how to cheat without getting caught. No way was I going to take more math.

That left only a third year of Latin. The *Iliad*. The *Odyssey*. The pits. However, it was 1963, and one didn't challenge one's superiors, especially if the superior was a nun. And so I found myself at graduation ready to go out and *amo*, *amas*, *amat* the world, but not ready to type. Assured, however, that nuns really do know what's best, even if they are 86 years old and have lived most of their lives in a convent, I departed for Marygrove College. The typewriter came along with me, just in case—which was fortunate, since the list of requirements I received at orientation included a mandate that all class papers turned in must be typed.

Every night after dinner, while my roommate and friends were down in the lounge listening to Peter, Paul and Mary, the Limeliters, and a new British group called the Beatles, I was at the typewriter, banging away as fast as I could, trying to type my homework. By the end of the year, I had become pretty fast and was missing only the first 45 minutes or so of lounge time.

The following year I transferred to a state college closer to home and also found a job on the Action Line column at the local newspaper office. They liked my writing; they never asked about my typing. And the first time I visited the editorial offices, I realized I'd come home—every single reporter in that room was sitting at a typewriter, one finger of each hand racing all over the keys. Not one of them was typing the correct way. When I had the nerve to mention this a few weeks later to a co-worker, he said, "Hey, Dizzy Gillespie doesn't play his horn right either, blowing his cheeks out like that. But it doesn't stop him from being one of the best trumpet players of all time.''

Four years later, my sister in California called. Would I like to come out and stay with her? I was young, it was 1969, and visions of love-ins beckoned. How could I refuse? Once there, though, I found newspaper jobs hard to come by. Then Sis, a hospital nurse, came home one day with the news that the radiology department was looking for an orderly/receptionist. Since the stories of Ben Casey and Dr. Kildare were still fresh in my mind, I thought doctors and hospitals were exciting places, so I applied. Six months later, the woman who typed the x-ray reports retired, and my boss asked me if I wanted to try it. Eager for something other than wheeling patients and answering the phone, I agreed—and then remembered I couldn't type the correct way. But the x-ray typist had a room all to herself and no one ever came there except to drop off the doctors' tapes, so I decided to take the job and not say anything about my handicap. Besides, after four years in a newspaper office, I had learned to hunt and peck quickly and accurately. And I was one up on the reporters—I could use *two* fingers on one hand.

Back in Ohio on vacation later that year, I confessed my shortcoming to my brother, and he just laughed. Pat had spent most of his life playing drums, from the Navy band to Juilliard School of Music and on to Broadway musicals. He was well known and well respected for his talent. And he reminded me that, because of an injury to his hand and arm when he was a kid, he didn't play drums the way drummers were supposed to—he couldn't hold the sticks in the "correct" position. But there he was on Broadway anyway, making lots of money and having lots of fun. And no one cared about his "handicap."

The rest is history, as they say. I went from job to job, always a better position, always more pay. Nobody gave me a typing test, so nobody knew how I typed. They only knew I could get the work done, well and quickly. I finally received my B.A. in English. My specialty became doctors who were foreign born, with thick accents and poor grammar skills. And then computers arrived.

"That'll put an end to the hunt-and-peckers," a co-worker smugly told me one day (I sat behind her, so she wasn't aware of my unique typing method). That scared me. A screen in front of me? How could I look at a screen instead of focusing on the center of the keyboard? Was my secret finally going to come out? Deciding to face my fear, I got a job in a hospital that had just converted to computers. Once again, I was safe. The screen proved no more formidable than the piece of paper that used to stare at me from the typewriter. I just didn't stare back. As a bonus, I discovered computers have something else typewriters don't—spellchecking software, which speeded up my proofreading chores. No one noticed how I typed. They only saw the caliber of my work and they were pleased.

The other day, when one of those unexplainable blue spells descended and I didn't care if Dizzy Gillespie was the best horn player or my brother made lots of money on Broadway; a day when I just knew that if the people in my business networking group ever found out I couldn't type the "correct" way, they'd laugh me out of the organization and I wouldn't be able to get another account no matter how experienced I was

in every other way, my husband saw my mood and brought me a cup of tea.

"By the way, Hon," he said, "did you know Def Leppard's drummer has only one arm?"

Dictation and Transcription: Adventures in Thought Transference

Part 1

by John H. Dirckx, M.D.

The pronunciation is the actual living form or forms of a word, that is, the word itself, *of which the current spelling is only a current symbolization. . . .*

General Explanations
The Oxford English Dictionary

Every time I read this passage, I am struck anew by the realization that the sequences of letters we put down on paper are not words, but only visible representations of those evanescent sequences of vocal sounds that are the only true words. When we speak of "the written word," we are indulging in metaphor: words are heard but not seen. Indeed, most of the world's three thousand languages are exclusively spoken languages having no writing systems.

I offer these reflections to introduce an inquiry into the nature of the dictation-transcription process, a form of communication unique among human activities. The dictator expresses thoughts in speech (which is electronically recorded) and the transcriptionist puts those thoughts on paper by converting sounds heard to conventional symbols.

The product of the transcriptionist's effort is not, however, a mere phonetic record of what is heard on the tape but rather a rendering of the dictator's thoughts in finished English prose. That is, instead of making a perfectly faithful record of speech sounds heard, the transcriptionist performs various analytic and interpretive functions and modifies the record by a complex series of deletions, additions, alterations, and emendations. Moreover, this editorial activity is performed simultaneously at several levels: phonetic (recognition and interpretation of speech sounds and their correct representation in writing), conceptual (monitoring of word choice, grammar, and style), and formal (punctuation, consistency of form, appropriate units of measure). Even at what I have called the phonetic level, the transcriptionist constantly discriminates and amends on the basis of context, so that even here there is nothing mechanical or automatic about the transcription process.

Studying exactly how the sounds of language are metamorphosed into a written transcript affords valuable insights into the physiology of speech and the psychology of communication, and should add an element of interest and even excitement to the most humdrum dictation.

Sound judgments. On the purely phonetic level, the transcriptionist is called upon to insert letters and symbols not corresponding to anything audible on the tape, to delete certain sounds that are heard, to discriminate between various possible representations of a sound or group of sounds, and to alter or amend erroneous or inappropriate sounds.

Some of these changes are made necessary by the nature of our English alphabet and spelling system, some by the structure and limitations of the human speech apparatus, and some by various lapses and errors made by dictators. Let's look at each of these factors in turn.

The ideograms of the Chinese language, the heart shape used to represent the word *love* on bumper stickers, and the so-called Arabic numerals (1, 2, 3 . . .) are nonphonetic writing symbols. That is, they refer to ideas rather than to sounds. Speakers of mutually unintelligible dialects of Chinese can readily correspond in writing even though they pronounce the symbols differently. (More accurately, they use different spoken words to express the ideas represented by the symbols.) If Italians or Swedes were to incorporate the heart sign into a message on a bumper sticker, they would pronounce it ''amo'' or ''elskar'' rather than ''love.'' The number signs are understood around the world, but whereas we pronounce 5 ''five,'' others say ''cinque,'' ''fem,'' and so on.

In contrast, the Latin alphabet, which is used with various modifications by most modern Western languages, is a phonetic writing system in the sense that each of its symbols represents one or more speech sounds rather than the ideas behind the words. All the same, in English at least, the system is fraught with redundancy and ambiguity. For example, each of the vowels can stand for three or more different sounds, and so can some consonants (lose, see, sugar) and groups of letters (ache, arch, charade). Conversely, the same sound may be spelled in a variety of ways: agent, joint, soldier; acid, base; rose, raze; sugar, fissure, share; colon, keel, physique; self, sylph, slough.

Silent letters may not be the most difficult feature of English spelling, but they are surely the most paradoxic. For a phonetic writing system to include symbols that are essential to the spelling of certain words and that nevertheless represent no sounds heard in those words is a palpable absurdity. Yet there is hardly a letter in our alphabet that does not figure in the spelling of some word without being represented in its pronunciation.

Most modern Western languages have adopted spelling rules that rigorously exclude silent letters. (The silent initial *h* of Spanish, Italian, and Portuguese is a notable exception.) Why do we have them? Silent letters in English spelling may be divided into two main groups: those that were formerly sounded but have dropped from the pronunciation of words while being retained in their spelling, and a few that were introduced into the spelling of certain words by misguided scholars or other bunglers even though they were never a feature of the pronunciation of those words.

To the first group belong most of our silent initial letters (gnome, hour, knife, mnemonic, pneumonia, wrench), silent *gh* (bough, caught), and silent final *b, e,* and *n* (climb, come, column). All of these letters stand for sounds that were heard in these words at some period in their history but have now been dropped, largely because they are awkward.

A smaller group of silent letters were inserted between the fifteenth and the eighteenth centuries into the spelling of some words even though at no time had they been sounded in those words. Scholars who saw in the English spelling of certain Romance words a debasement of the Latin originals changed *dette* (ultimately from the Latin *debitum)* into *debt* and *suttle* into *subtle* (from *subtilis)*. Other changes along the same lines resulted from errors as to the origin of words. Thus, *iland,* from Old English, was mistakenly associated with *isle,* from Latin *insula,* and encumbered with a useless *s: island. Rime* became *rhyme* solely through the example of the etymologically unrelated but semantically kindred *rhythm.*

A third type of silent letter is silent only in the pronunciation of certain speakers or classes of speakers. In some regional dialects, the final *r* is typically dropped (''beta blockah''). Many persons say ''in'' or ''een'' for the sound represented by final *-ing,* while others vowelize final *l,* saying something like ''naso'' and ''normo'' for *nasal* and *normal.* Most of us drop unstressed short vowels from the middle of some words: ''fact'ry,'' ''priv'lege,'' ''tet'nus.''

Many other oddities of English spelling might be mentioned. Suffice it to say that the relation between speech sounds and the symbols that convention requires us to use to represent them is erratic, almost haphazard. That is why the transcriptionist cannot simply match a symbol to a sound heard, as in making a stenographic (shorthand) record, where, for example, *f, ph,* and *gh* (in *enough)* are all represented by the same symbol, while the *b's* of *doubt* and *subtle* are not represented at all.

(Part 2 of this article appears in Lesson 3.)

Medical Readings

The History and Physical Examination

by John H. Dirckx, M.D.

Review of Systems: Skin. The dermatologic history is usually omitted unless the patient has cutaneous complaints or a condition in which such complaints might be expected. The skin is subject to numerous injuries and local diseases and often reflects systemic disease as well.

The patient is questioned about prior diagnosis of severe or chronic cutaneous disease and any treatments used for them in the past or at present. Since patients often erroneously diagnose themselves as having psoriasis, fungal infection, or hives, the interviewer must be cautious in accepting such diagnoses. Lay persons are also prone to treat their own skin problems with a limitless variety of remedies, many of which can create further symptoms. Hence the physician inquires carefully about all such treatments.

The commoner skin complaints are local or general eruptions or rashes, itching, dryness or scaling, pigment changes, and solid tumors of various kinds. Disorders of the hair (abnormal appearance of the hair, excessive hair, hair loss) and nails (deformity, discoloration) are also part of the dermatologic history. Lay persons are notoriously inept at describing their own skin lesions and rashes. If the problem is still present, the physician will usually not waste time in getting a garbled, secondhand description of something that he can see for himself.

On the other hand, the physician will carefully question the patient about the duration of the problem; whether it comes and goes, remains unchanged, or is gradually getting better or worse; whether it is spreading from one area to others; whether the patient can suggest any reason for the problem (he usually can, rightly or wrongly); and whether anything seems to make the problem better or worse.

Physical Examination: Skin. Dermatologists like to say that the skin is the largest and most conspicuous organ of the body.

In assessing the skin, the physician ensures adequate exposure of the surface by removing clothing, dressings, bandages, and ointments. He uses bright natural or artificial light and, as needed, a magnifying lens.

Examination of the skin is not carried out by inspection alone. The examiner palpates any area of skin that appears abnormal and observes its temperature, texture, tenseness or laxness, moistness or dryness. He also looks for tenderness and crepitation. When a zone of normally lax skin, such as on the abdomen, is gently picked up between thumb and finger and then released, it should flatten out again immediately. Failure to do so (tenting) indicates poor skin turgor, a sign of significant dehydration.

In evaluating skin color, the examiner considers the intensity and distribution of normal pigment (melanin) and any abnormal coloration (cyanosis, erythema, jaundice, bronzing). When local or diffuse redness is present, a diascope can be used to distinguish capillary dilatation from other causes. A diascope is a small flat piece of clear glass or plastic, which is pressed firmly against the reddened skin. Blanching indicates that dilated capillaries have been compressed. Redness due to hemorrhage or abnormal pigmentation will not fade on pressure.

Very small hemorrhagic lesions of the skin (less than 2 mm) are called petechiae. Areas consisting of larger lesions (2-5 mm) are called purpura, and still larger lesions are called ecchymoses. Localized or generalized loss of pigment is also noted, as well as any tattoos and surgical or traumatic scars.

Although disorders of the skin can produce an almost infinite variety of abnormal patterns, the basic structural changes can be reduced to a manageably small range of possibilities. Macules, papules, vesicles, bullae, pustules, wheals, and nodules are called primary lesions because they can all appear without previous evidence of cutaneous abnormality.

Scales, crusts, excoriations, fissures, ulcers, scars, and lichenification are known as secondary lesions because they result from evolution of primary lesions. Any or all of these can be present in a given case of dermatitis, depending on its cause and course. Any of them can also result from noninflammatory conditions of the skin.

Cutaneous diagnosis depends on a consideration of many factors: the type, number, grouping, and location of lesions; combinations of features occurring together; signs of evolutionary change, secondary infection, or the effects of treatment; and the presence of associated symptoms such as fever, headache, or pain in the joints or abdomen.

While many skin problems (acne, warts, poison ivy, ringworm) arise in the skin and stay there, many others (hives, the eruptions of measles, chickenpox, and lupus erythematosus) are signs of systemic disease.

Malignant tumors of the skin are not uncommon in older persons, particularly on sun-exposed parts of the body such as the face and neck. In addition, a very small percentage of pigmented lesions in younger persons prove to be highly malignant melanomas. For these reasons all skin tumors and pigmented lesions are subjected to critical scrutiny.

In most cases of trauma, the skin is affected in some way. Open injuries are described as abrasions (due to scraping away of the skin surface), incised wounds (due to sharp, blade-like objects), punctures, and lacerations (bursting of skin due to blunt trauma). Closed injuries are generally contusions, sometimes with hematoma formation.

Burns may be described as partial- or full-thickness burns, or graded: first degree, erythema; second degree, blistering; third degree, charring.

Infections of the skin and immediately subjacent soft tissues are common, resulting usually from penetrating injury but occasionally from invasion of diseased tissue by opportunistic bacteria. The examiner notes the pattern of lesions, the degree of inflammation, and any pus or exudate present.

Pharmacology: Drug Forms

1. **Tablet.** This drug form contains dried powdered active drug as well as binders and fillers to provide bulk and ensure proper tablet size. A **scored** tablet has an indented line running across the top. It can be easily broken into two pieces with a knife to produce two doses. **Enteric** tablets are covered with a special coating which resists stomach acid but dissolves in the alkaline environment of the small intestine to avoid irritating the stomach (example: Ecotrin). **Slow-release** tablets are manufactured to provide a continuous, sustained release of certain drugs. Often this is abbreviated as SR (slow release) or LA (long acting) in the trade name of the drug (examples: Procan SR and Entex LA). **Caplets** are easy-to-swallow coated tablets in the form of capsules. Tablets can also be designed to be dissolved in water before being taken orally (example: Klorvess effervescent tablets). Some over-the-counter drugs come in the form of **lozenges.** These tablets are formed of a hardened base of sugar and water containing the drug and other flavorings. They are never swallowed, but are allowed to dissolve slowly in the mouth and release the drug topically to the tissues of the mouth and throat (example: Cepacol lozenges). In prescriptions, *tablet* is sometimes abbreviated as *tab* or *tabs*.

2. **Capsule.** This drug form comes in two varieties. The first is a soft gelatin shell manufactured in one piece in which the drug is in a liquid form inside the shell (examples: Atromid-S and fat-soluble vitamins such as A and E). The second form of capsule is a hard shell manufactured in two pieces which fit together and hold the drug which is in a powdered or granular form. Many nonprescription cold remedies and pain medications were manufactured in this form until some Tylenol capsules were reported to be contaminated with cyanide in the early 1980s. Subsequently, many companies now manufacture their nonprescription pain medications in a tablet or caplet form. Many prescription drugs, however, are still manufactured as capsules. In prescriptions, *capsule* is sometimes abbreviated as *cap* or *caps*.

3. **Cream.** A cream is a semisolid emulsion of oil (such as lanolin or petroleum) and water, the main ingredient being water. Emulsifying agents are added to keep the oil and water well mixed. Many topical drugs are manufactured in a cream base (example: hydrocortisone cream).

4. **Ointment.** An ointment is a semisolid emulsion of an oil (such as lanolin or petroleum) and water, the main ingredient being oil. Many topical drugs are manufactured in an ointment base (example: Kenalog ointment). Specially formulated ophthalmic ointments are made to be applied topically to the eye without causing irritation. Most creams and ointments are applied to the skin without precise measurement; however, nitroglycerin ointment (used to prevent angina) is precisely measured in inches on a specially marked applicator paper which is taped to the patient's skin.

5. **Lotion.** A lotion is a suspension of an active drug in a water base for external use (examples: Keri lotion, calamine lotion).

6. **Powder.** A powder is a finely ground form of an active drug. Powdered drugs can be contained in

capsules but can also be found in glass vials where they must be reconstituted with water before being injected (example: intravenous ampicillin). Powders can also be reconstituted for oral use (example: Metamucil).

7. **Liquid.** Liquids come in the form of either solutions or suspensions. Solutions contain the drug fully dissolved in a base. Solutions never need to be mixed as the drug-to-water concentration is always the same in every part of the solution, even after prolonged standing. **Solutions** come in many forms: elixirs, syrups, tinctures, liquid sprays, and foams.

Elixirs contain an alcohol and water base with added sugar and flavoring (example: Tylenol elixir). Elixirs are commonly used for pediatric or elderly patients who cannot swallow the tablet or capsule form of a drug. **Syrups** contain no alcohol, being a concentrated solution of sugar, water, and flavorings. Syrups are sweeter and more viscous (thicker) than elixirs. Most over-the-counter cough medications have a syrup base which not only carries the drug but acts to soothe inflamed mucous membranes in the throat. **Tinctures** have an alcohol and water base (example: Merthiolate tincture).

Liquid sprays contain a solution of the drug combined with water or alcohol to be sprayed by a pump or aerosol propellant. Spray liquid drugs are commonly used for topical application (examples: Afrin nasal spray, Primatene Mist spray, Benadryl spray.) Nitroglycerin is available in a spray form for application under the tongue during anginal attacks. Certain over-the-counter contraceptives are available as **foams**.

Suspensions contain fine, undissolved particles of a drug suspended in a liquid base. After prolonged standing, these fine particles will gradually settle to the bottom of the container. Therefore it is always important to shake suspensions well before using, a fact that is noted on the label of these drugs (example: Maalox and other antacids). An **emulsion** is a suspension in which fat particles are mixed with water (example: Intralipid intravenous fat solution).

Two general terms used to describe a liquid are **aqueous** (from the Latin word *aqua,* water), meaning of watery consistency, and **viscous**, which designates a nonwatery or thick liquid.

8. **Suppositories.** Suppositories contain a solid base of glycerin or cocoa butter containing the drug. They are manufactured in appropriate sizes for rectal or vaginal insertion and also come in adult and pediatric sizes. Vaginal suppositories are most often used to treat vaginal infections but can also be used orally to treat yeast infections in the mouth. Rectal suppositories can be used to administer drugs to patients who are vomiting (example: Tylenol suppositories).

9. **Transdermal.** The transdermal form of drugs is relatively new. It consists of a multi-layered disk containing a drug reservoir, a porous membrane, and an adhesive layer to hold it to the skin. The porous membrane regulates the amount of drug released to the skin (example: Transderm-Nitro for prevention of angina). These drugs are often known as transdermal patches.

Dermatology Drugs

Because of the superficial nature and location of most dermatologic diseases, they respond well to topical drug therapy. Mild cases of skin diseases such as acne, psoriasis, poison ivy, contact dermatitis, superficial infections, herpes simplex infections, lice, and diaper rash can be successfully treated with topical agents. However, drugs which act systemically may be necessary when dermatologic diseases become widespread or particularly severe.

Acne drugs. Various creams, lotions, and gels are used topically to cleanse away oil and dead skin (keratolytic action), to close the pores (astringent action), to inhibit the growth of skin bacteria (antiseptic action), and to kill skin bacteria (antibiotic action).

Prescription antibiotics may be used topically to treat more serious cases of acne vulgaris. These include:
    clindamycin (Cleocin T)
    meclocycline (Meclan)
    tetracycline (Topicycline)
Tetracycline may also be prescribed orally for systemic treatment of acne vulgaris.

Severe cystic acne which may be unresponsive to antibiotic treatment may be treated with topical tretinoin (Retin-A), a form of vitamin A. It causes skin cells to multiply more rapidly. This rapid turnover prevents pores from becoming clogged and infected. A structurally related drug, isotretinoin (Accutane), is prescribed orally for the same purpose.

Acne rosacea, an adult form of acne not caused by excessive oil but exacerbated by heat, stress, and skin irritation, is treated with metronidazole (Metro-Gel).

Psoriasis drugs. Various topical agents are used to treat psoriasis. Among them are **coal tar** lotions, gels, and shampoos that cleanse away dead skin (keratolytic action) and decrease itching (antipruritic action). These trade name products include Balnetar, Denorex, Estar, Tegrin, and Zetar.

Topical corticosteroids. Topical corticosteroids, both over-the-counter and prescription, are indicated for the relief of contact dermatitis, poison ivy, insect bites, and to treat psoriasis, seborrhea, and eczema. Oral corticosteroids may be given to act systemically in cases of severe inflammation or itching.

Topical corticosteroids come in several strengths as indicated by a percentage following the trade name. Some common over-the-counter and prescription generic and trade name topical corticosteroid agents are:

    amcinonide (Cyclocort)
    betamethasone (Diprosone, Uticort, Valisone)
    clocortolone (Cloderm)
    desonide (Tridesilon)
    desoximetasone (Topicort)
    dexamethasone (Decaderm, Decadron)
    fluocinolone (Lidex, Synalar)
    flurandrenolide (Cordran)
    halcinonide (Halog)
    hydrocortisone (CaldeCort, Cortaid, Cortef, Cortril, Hycort, Hytone)
    triamcinolone (Aristocort, Kenalog)

Note: The endings *-sone, -olone,* and *-onide* are common to some generic corticosteroids.

Laboratory Tests and Surgical Procedures

The following laboratory tests and surgical procedures may be found in dermatology dictation. Review these terms and their definitions.

biopsy, excisional Complete excision or removal of a skin lesion. In addition, some adjacent, normal-appearing tissue is also removed for comparison.

biopsy, incisional Partial removal of a lesion by making an incision into the lesion and removing a section of it as well as some adjacent, normal-appearing tissue for comparison.

biopsy, punch Removal of one section of a lesion using a sharp surgical instrument known as a punch.

biopsy, skin Removal of all or part of a skin lesion. The tissue is sent to the pathology laboratory to determine whether it is malignant or benign.

Bx Abbreviation for *biopsy.*

cryosurgery The application of liquid nitrogen (at a temperature of -196°C) to destroy superficial skin lesions.

fulguration The application of an electrical current to destroy superficial skin lesions.

electrodesiccation See *fulguration.*

intradermal test The injection into the intradermal layer of the skin of a chemical or other type of substance known to produce an allergic reaction in sensitive individuals. This creates a wheal which is outlined in pen and/or measured. The area is examined again in 30 minutes. A reddened, enlarged area at the site of the injection indicates a positive allergic reaction to that chemical or allergen.

KOH test KOH (potassium hydroxide) and methylene blue dye are applied to scrapings from the skin to detect, under the microscope, the presence of a fungal infection.

patch test The application to the skin of a piece of filter paper containing a chemical or other type of substance known to produce an allergic reaction in sensitive individuals. Many patches are taped to the skin and labeled. After 24-48 hours, the skin underneath is examined. Reddened, raised areas of skin indicate a positive allergic reaction to that chemical or allergen.

potassium hydroxide test See *KOH.*

scratch test The application, to a superficial scratch made in the skin, of a chemical or other type of substance known to produce an allergic reaction in sensitive individuals. Many scratches are made in the skin, and the area is examined again in 30 minutes. Reddened, raised areas of skin indicate a positive allergic reaction to that chemical or allergen.

skin scrapings Removal of a thin layer of skin cells by lightly scraping the skin with a scalpel and placing the cells on a slide for examination under the microscope after they have been stained.

skin testing See *patch test, scratch test,* and *intradermal test.*

Anatomy/Medical Terminology

Anatomy: Structure of the Skin

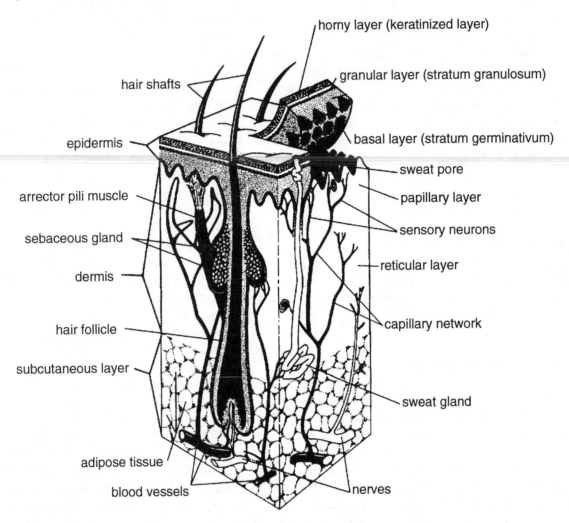

horny layer (keratinized layer)

granular layer (stratum granulosum)

hair shafts

basal layer (stratum germinativum)

epidermis

sweat pore

arrector pili muscle

papillary layer

sensory neurons

sebaceous gland

reticular layer

dermis

hair follicle

capillary network

subcutaneous layer

sweat gland

adipose tissue

blood vessels

nerves

Adjective Exercise

Adjectives are formed from nouns by adding adjectival suffixes such as *-ac, -al, -ar, -ary, -eal, -iac, -ic, -ical, -oid, -ous, -tic,* and *-tous.* In addition, some adjectives have a different form entirely from the noun, which may be either Latin or Greek in origin.

Test your knowledge of adjectives by writing the adjectival form of the following dermatology words. Consult a medical dictionary to select the correct adjectival ending as necessary.

 1. epidermis   _epidermal, epidermoid_
 2. epithelium   _____
 3. integument   _____
 4. erythema   _____
 5. seborrhea   _____
 6. xanthoma   _____
 7. macule   _____
 8. cyst   _____
 9. papule   _____
10. vesicle   _____
11. eczema   _____
12. psoriasis   _____
13. callus   _____

Medical Terminology Matching Exercise

The skin (and all its structures), hair, and nails comprise the integumentary system. This matching exercise will test your knowledge of the root words, anatomic structures, symptoms, and disease processes encountered in dermatology.

Instructions: Match the term in Column A with its definition in Column B.

Column A

A. wart
B. pruritus
C. tinea
D. psoriasis
E. sebum
F. adipose tissue
G. wheal
H. alopecia
I. keloid
J. melanocyte
K. pustule
L. scabies
M. lipoma
N. epidermis
O. onycho-
   mycosis
P. vesicle
Q. comedo
R. Kaposi's
   sarcoma
S. macule
T. petechiae

Column B

__A__ skin growth caused by a
    virus
____ itching
____ fungal infection of skin
____ noninfectious disease of
    scaly patches
____ infectious disease caused by
    mites
____ pigment-containing tissue
    cells that determine skin
    color
____ most superficial layer of skin
____ fat
____ oil secreted by skin glands
____ benign tumor of
    subcutaneous fat
____ fungal infection of the nails
____ malignant skin growths seen
    in AIDS
____ produced by an allergic
    reaction
____ skin lesion filled with clear
    fluid
____ abscess containing pus
____ red, flat skin lesion
____ hair loss
____ tiny skin hemorrhages
____ blackhead
____ enlarged scar tissue

Lay and Medical Terms

Lay Term	*Medical Term*
athlete's foot	tinea pedis
baldness	alopecia
black-and-blue mark	ecchymosis
blackhead	comedo
blister	vesicle
boil	furuncle
hives	wheal or urticaria

Sound-alikes Exercise

Instructions: Circle the correct term from the sound-alikes in parentheses in the following sentences.

1. Stomatitis and (abscess, aphthous) ulcers made it almost impossible for the patient to eat.

2. After observing the silvery gray, scaling patches on the patient's skin, the dermatologist diagnosed (cirrhosis, psoriasis).

3. The patient had an allergic rash of unknown origin which was diagnosed as (atopic, trophic, ectopic) dermatitis.

4. The bedridden patient had a chronic, weeping, (atopic, trophic, ectopic) ulcer on his ischial (eminence, imminence).

5. The patient had an obvious bee sting which was surrounded by an inflamed halo of (edema, erythema, arrhythmia).

6. From ankles to knees, the patient had a weeping, brawny (edema, erythema, arrhythmia).

7. Both great toenails were deformed by (fundal, fungal) growths.

8. Because the patient had a solitary boil or (carbuncle, caruncle, furuncle) on her left buttock, she could not sit.

9. Without treatment, the physician feared that the solitary boil would expand, creating a cluster of boils or (carbuncle, caruncle, furuncle).

10. The patient had violaceous papules with a fine, shiny, scaly appearance that resembled (lichen, liken) planus.

11. The flat, molelike lesion had a (melenic, melanotic) appearance.

12. The dermatologist removed the numerous, small (palpations, palpitations, papillations) from around the patient's neck because they were constantly irritated by her necklaces.

13. The patient complained of an intense (parietes, pruritus) associated with the poison ivy rash.

14. The (varicose, verrucous) warts were benign and no treatment was needed.

15. The child's feet and ankles were covered with numerous, small (vesicals, vesicles) from the red ant bites.

Drug Word Search

Locate and circle the dermatology terms hidden in the puzzle horizontally, vertically, and diagonally, forward and backward. A numeral following a term in the word list indicates the number of times it can be found in the puzzle.

```
M  B  Q  R  D  I  P  R  O  S  O  N  E
E  E  T  W  P  S  O  R  A  L  E  N  A
T  T  R  O  C  I  P  O  T  N  O  M  C
R  A  O  O  T  R  O  C  O  L  C  Y  C
O  D  C  O  G  F  K  S  O  O  H  N  U
G  I  I  N  L  A  I  N  A  K  I  I  T
E  N  P  E  Z  L  I  L  E  R  B  T  A
L  E  O  E  A  C  T  N  O  P  I  A  N
Y  L  T  V  M  A  A  P  E  G  C  C  E
B  A  I  A  R  L  S  K  I  N  L  I  Z
R  V  I  D  O  O  N  A  L  C  E  M  J
C  R  Q  G  E  N  I  T  C  A  N  I  T
T  M  I  N  O  X  I  D  I  L  S  V  W
```

Accutane
Aveeno
Betadine
coal tar
Cyclocort
Diprosone
Hibiclens
Kenalog
Lidex
Meclan
MetroGel

Micatin
minoxidil
Neosporin
psoralens
Rogaine
skin
Tinactin
Topicort (2)
triamcinolone
Valisone
Zetar

How to Proofread

Professional medical transcriptionists function with minimum supervision while producing maximum results in both quantity and quality. While the majority of working transcriptionists have an immediate supervisor responsible for quality control, the attitude of transcriptionists should be one of independence and responsibility for their work. Professionals take pride in the accuracy and completeness of their own work and gain satisfaction from a job well done, both in quality and quantity.

Proofreading is a critical skill for medical transcriptionists. Proofreading involves looking for mistakes of all types in the transcribed document and correcting them. The usual types of errors that occur include omitting important dictated words, selecting the wrong English or medical word, misspelling words, and making typographical, grammatical, or punctuation errors.

As with all other skills, proofreading skills can be improved with practice. As your instructor points out errors in your transcripts, you may begin to see trends in the errors you make. If you find that you miss few medical words but misspell many English words, you will know to pay particular attention to English words as you proofread your next transcript.

Most students proofread too superficially when they begin transcribing. Here is a four-step method to help you achieve the best results from your proofreading.

1. The conscientious use of reference books is the first step toward good proofreading. Look words up as you encounter them. Do not save all your word searching until the end of the report when you will have forgotten how some of the words sounded at the beginning of the dictation.

2. Lightly proofread what you are transcribing as it appears on the screen of your word processor or the paper you are typing on. Your eyes will begin to do this automatically as you perfect your proofreading skills. This method helps you catch missed words and typographical errors as they occur. Print out your transcript on paper if you are using a word processor. It is much easier to proofread the transcript on paper than it is on the screen.

3. If you cannot find a word, leave a blank of appropriate length depending on how long or short the

word sounds. Attach a flag (a sheet of paper clipped to the transcript or a sticky note placed on the transcript) which identifies all blanks, which lines of the transcript they are located on, and what the dictated word sounded like to you. On the job, these flags may be returned to you with the correct word written in by the physician or supervisor. It is a good habit to begin making legible and complete flags now as you transcribe each report. (See Lesson 3 for more information on the practice of flagging.)

4. As a final step in proofreading, use a medical or English spellchecker if your word processor has one and your instructor allows you to do so. Be aware, however, that the spellchecker will not catch errors such as transcribing *no* instead of *not* or transcribing *ilium* instead of *ileum.*

Proofreading is a skill that requires continual practice to perfect. There are several components to proofreading, all of which must be mastered by the medical transcriptionist. Careful proofreading is the key to eliminating the following errors.

Omitting important dictated words. Beginning medical transcriptionists often try to improve their transcription speed too soon—before they are able to listen and remember blocks of dictation. As they try to keep up with the dictating voice, they inadvertently omit some of the dictated words. By adjusting the speed control on the transcriber unit, the transcriptionist can begin slowly, assure that no dictated words are overlooked, and then slowly increase the speed of the tape which will, in turn, increase transcription speed.

Selecting the wrong English or medical word. Because the quality of a tape recording does not perfectly reproduce the human voice, it is easy for words and phrases to be garbled or to sound like something quite different from what they are. Therefore, transcriptionists never just transcribe what they think they hear; they transcribe only what makes sense in the context of the report. By careful wordsearching and verifying word definitions, medical transcriptionists avoid selecting the wrong English or medical word.

A wrong medical word can convey a wrong diagnosis for a patient, and that error is carried in the patient's permanent medical record. The professional medical transcriptionist NEVER transcribes anything that does not make sense and/or cannot be verified in a reference book.

Misspelling words. The misspelling of a medical word can be as serious an error as selecting the wrong medical word. Misspellings of both medical and English words can be avoided by careful proofreading and by using the spellchecker function on the word processor. Experienced medical transcriptionists know that electronic spellcheckers cannot be relied upon to locate all of the errors in a document.

Typographical errors. Typographical errors are often the result of carelessness or attempting to type fast rather than focusing on accuracy. You will catch most of these errors through careful proofreading, especially if some time elapses between the time of the transcription and the time of proofreading. Word processing spellcheckers will also help to catch transposed letters and other kinds of typos.

Grammatical errors. Subject-verb agreement errors and other grammatical errors are commonly made by dictating physicians, and it is the job of the transcriptionist to correct them. Sometimes grammatical errors are hard to catch when transcribing, and thus must be identified through careful proofreading.

Punctuation errors. Punctuation is an important part of a correctly transcribed sentence. Incorrectly placed commas can, at times, actually change the medical meaning of a sentence. Each lesson in this course has Transcription Guidelines to review the grammar, punctuation, style, and format rules that contribute to the correct transcription of a medical report.

Proofreading cannot be done quickly or haphazardly. It is often more productive to proofread your transcript several hours or even a day after you type it so that errors will become more obvious. This is a trick that beginning medical transcriptionists can use to strengthen their ability to find errors; however, on the job, transcriptionists are expected to proofread their work as they are transcribing it and do a final proofreading check as soon as they finish the entire document.

Proofreading Exercise

Instructions: In the paragraphs below, circle or identify misspelled and missing medical and English words and write the correct words in the numbered spaces opposite the text. Consult medical and English dictionaries as necessary.

1	The labratory testing of blood, urine, and	1 _____laboratory_____
2	other body fliuds and waste products plays a	2 _____
3	miner roll in modern diagnostic medicine. The	3 _____
4	number availabel tests increases almost daily,	4 _____
5	and the range of diseases and conditions	5 _____
6	amenable to labratory study continually	6 _____
7	broadens. Some mention of labratory test	7 _____
8	results appears frequently in history and	8 _____
9	physical examintion reports and nearly always	9 _____
10	in hospital discharge summarys. Accordingly,	10 _____
11	the medical transcirptionist must be familiar	11 _____
12	with the general conceps of labratory medicine	12 _____
13	as well as with specific tests. Diagnostic	13 _____
14	labratory procedures may be called tests,	14 _____
15	studies, or simply work ("lab studies," "lab	15 _____
16	word"). Phisicians may report that they	16 _____
17	ordered, got, ran, did, or (in the case of	17 _____
18	blood work) drew a test.	18 _____
19	Crohn's disease is a chronic disease which	19 _____
20	consists of inflamation of the GI track—most	20 _____
21	commonly inflamation of the terminal ilium.	21 _____
22	The exact cause is unknown, but possible	22 _____
23	causes are allerges, imune disorders, and in-	23 _____
24	fections. Labratory tests have not detected any	24 _____
25	bacteria or virus responsable for causing	25 _____
26	Crohn's disease. The patient experiences	26 _____
27	cramping, abdominal pain, nausea, diarhea,	27 _____
28	abdominal tenderness, and weekness. Patience	28 _____
29	may be given intervenous fluids to provide	29 _____
30	nutrition while resting the bowl. Some patients	30 _____
31	even require surgery if the bowel perferates,	31 _____
32	obstructs, or if there is massive hemorrage.	32 _____

BLOOPERS

Incorrect	Correct
Keratosis was removed by defecation.	Keratosis was removed by desiccation.
A 28-year-old white male, a beast, complaining of an itchy rash in the groin.	A 28-year-old white male, obese, complaining of an itchy rash in the groin.
Cultures showed Mexican flora.	Cultures showed mixed skin flora.

Transcription Tips

1. A patient consulted a dermatologist for a skin problem. ''What do I have, Doctor?'' the patient asked anxiously. The dermatologist examined the man carefully and after a few moments said, ''It looks like a maculopapular erythematous eruption.'' ''Oh, my!'' the patient exclaimed. ''What is that?'' ''A rash,'' the doctor replied.

   There is a difference between describing a condition and determining a diagnosis. As you study medical terminology you will encounter terms which describe symptoms, body parts, positions, anatomic structures, diseases, and surgical procedures. Make sure you understand the difference between words that describe symptoms and those that describe a disease or surgical procedure.

2. Both the Romans and the Greeks studied the body and disease processes extensively. Similar medical terms in English are derived from different Latin and Greek root words. Both root words *cutaneo-* (cutaneous, subcutaneous) and *dermato-* (dermatitis, dermatologist) mean *skin*. The Latin word for skin is *cutis*, the Greek *derma*. Both root words *onycho-* (onychomycosis) and *unguo-* (subungual) mean *nail*. *Onycho-* is from Greek, *unguo-* from Latin.

3. *Callus* is a noun which describes a localized growth of a hard, horny epithelium, as ''There is a callus on the palm of the hand, near the ring he is wearing.'' *Callous* is an adjective meaning hard, as ''There is a callous area on the heel of the left foot.''

4. There is no official single brief form for the term *subcutaneous.* If the physician dictates the brief form, the transcriptionist may transcribe *subcu* or subQ.

5. The term *pruritus* (from Latin *prurire,* to itch) is frequently misspelled *-itis* because of the mistaken impression that it ends in the suffix *-itis* (inflammation of).

6. *Psoriasis* and *psoriatic* are difficult to spell and even more difficult to find in a medical dictionary because of the initial silent *p.*

7. Memorize these hard-to-spell dermatology terms:

callus	psoriasis
eczema	verrucous
onychomycosis	xanthoma
pruritus	

8. Note these hard-to-spell dermatology drugs:

   gentamicin (the generic name ends in *-micin*)
   Garamycin (the trade name ends in *-mycin*)
   interferon alfa-2b (note the unusual spelling of *alfa,* unlike the spelling of the Greek word *alpha*)
   pHisoHex (unusual for its lowercase initial letter and internal capitalization—patterned after *pH,* which indicates acid/alkaline parameters)

9. Directions can be expressed as adverbs by adding the suffix *ly.*

Direction	*Adverb*
anterior	anteriorly
posterior	posteriorly
inferior	inferiorly
superior	superiorly
distal	distally
proximal	proximally
lateral	laterally
medial	medially

10. Two directions used together to designate a direction can be either hyphenated or combined into a single word. Notice the spelling changes in the combined form. Note: This is the physician's option, not the transcriptionist's. The transcriptionist should transcribe what is dictated.

anterior-posterior	*or*	anteroposterior
anterior-lateral	*or*	anterolateral
posterior-anterior	*or*	posteroanterior
posterior-lateral	*or*	posterolateral
superior-lateral	*or*	superolateral

11. The direction *transverse* is an adjective. Do not confuse it with the verb *traverse* meaning ''to go across.''

    A transverse incision was utilized.
    The scar traversed the entire abdomen.

Terminology Challenge

Instructions: The following terms appear in the dictation on Tape 1A, Dermatology. Before beginning the medical transcription practice for Lesson 2, become familiar with the terminology below by looking up each word in a medical or English dictionary. Write out a short definition of each term.

advancement flap
afebrile
amphotericin B
anterior
antibiotic
aspirated
asymptomatic
athlete's foot
Augmentin
b.i.d.
benign
Benzagel
Betadine
blackhead
Burow soaks
Candida albicans
Cefobid
cellulitis
Clark's level 3
cocci
coloration
comedo
confluent
contact sensitivity
cosmetic removal
culture
cyst
demineralization
dermatitis
digit
disfigurement
dorsum
eczema
ENT
ERYC
erythematous
Ethilon suture
extremity
foreign body
frozen control

fungal
gelatinous
Gram stain
gram-negative
gram-positive
griseofulvin
group D strep
Hibiclens soaks
inflammatory reaction
interdigital web space
Keflex
Kenalog
ketoconazole
Komed
laceration
Lactobacillus
LCD
left lower quadrant
lesion
local anesthesia
Lotrimin cream
lymphadenopathy
malignant
medial aspect
melanoma
mid-pretibial area
mixed flora
motor status
Neosporin
nonpruritic
obese
osteomyelitis
p.r.n.
Pernox
plaque
potassium
  permanganate
pruritic
Pseudomonas
psoriasis

pustular
q.i.d.
q.o.d.
resonant
scapulae
secondarily infected
sensory
staph
streptococcus
synovial cyst
systolic murmur
tobramycin

toe web
topically
triamcinolone cream
ulceration
unresectable
Valisone cream
vascular
wartlike lesion
white count
whitehead
wide margin resection
Xylocaine

Sample Reports

Format

Various medical report formats and styles exist nationwide. For example, the examination portion of a routine History and Physical report might be transcribed in block paragraph form or with indentations, hanging paragraphs, with subheadings in all capitals, and with subheadings in upper and lowercase letters. The physician's dictating style may determine the appropriate format, or a particular medical facility may mandate certain standard formats. Thus, individual report formats may vary from dictator to dictator, report to report, and setting to setting.

The transcriptionist may add headings and subheadings to a dictated report as appropriate. The transcriptionist should be alert for important headings that are not dictated but are a vital part of the report, such as Diagnosis or Final Diagnosis or Impression in a History and Physical Examination report or Discharge Summary, and Preoperative Diagnosis and Postoperative Diagnosis in an Operative Report. If any of these headings are not dictated, the transcriptionist should supply them and flag the report to the attention of the dictator so that the diagnosis can be stated.

Doctors may take shortcuts by dictating abbreviations, even for report headings, such as *CC* (Chief Complaint) and *HPI* (History of Present Illness). These headings should always be spelled out in full. Note: Do not confuse a *CC* dictated for Chief Complaint with the other definitions of the abbreviation *cc*: cubic centimeter and carbon copy.

If a physician dictates a narrative portion that belongs under a particular heading but fails to dictate the heading, the transcriptionist should insert the proper heading. For example, it is not uncommon for physicians to finish dictating the Physical Examination section of a Discharge Summary and begin to dictate laboratory test results or x-ray results without giving a heading for a new section. The transcriptionist should paragraph after the Physical Examination and insert an appropriate paragraph heading such as Laboratory Data or Laboratory and X-ray Data before transcribing the information.

Dictated:

> PHYSICAL EXAMINATION: The fracture site was tender to palpation. He had good sensation and circulation in the leg. Multiple views of the tibia revealed there was a stairstep-type fracture at the distal portion of the tibia. The CBC and differential were normal.

Transcribed:

> PHYSICAL EXAMINATION: The fracture site was tender to palpation. He had good sensation and circulation in the leg.

> LABORATORY AND X-RAY DATA: Multiple views of the tibia revealed there was a stair-step-type fracture at the distal portion of the tibia. The CBC and differential were normal.

If a physician dictates the singular form Diagnosis and then lists several diagnoses, the transcriptionist may use either Diagnosis or Diagnoses to head the list.

Physicians frequently number the diagnoses and want them listed vertically for ease in reading. The transcriptionist may elect to enumerate a long list of diagnoses, whether or not numbers are dictated. Occasionally a dictator will begin to number the diagnoses and then give only one diagnosis; in that case, omit the number (no need for a 1 without a 2). Be aware that in listing several diagnoses, dictators often lose track of the next number. They may inadvertently give the wrong number (which should be corrected by the transcriptionist) or delegate the numbering to the transcriptionist by saying "number next" to indicate the next diagnosis.

There are many acceptable formats for the set-up of medical reports and even alternative acceptable formats for the same sentence.

Dictated:	Extremities are unremarkable.
Transcribed:	The extremities are unremarkable.
	EXTREMITIES: Unremarkable.
	EXTREMITIES are unremarkable.

Transcribe paragraphs as dictated unless paragraphing would alter the medical meaning or continuity of the report. In addition, paragraphing may be added to break up long reports appropriately, to set up a new heading and its accompanying paragraph, and to separate the Findings from the Operative Procedure. Be aware that when some physicians dictate "new line," they mean to begin a new paragraph.

With the advent of computers, many hospitals and clinics have instituted standard format outlines for each type of report dictated. These are stored in the computer's memory as templates which can be "pulled up" by the transcriptionist. This practice has introduced greater conformity in format style within an institution and has made adjusting and remembering formats painless.

At the end of each lesson there are samples of reports in the medical specialty studied in that lesson, illustrating a variety of formats. Students should refer to these samples often and use them as guidelines to transcribe the dictations on the tapes in this course.

Sample dermatology reports appear on the following pages.

Transcription Practice

After completing all the readings and exercises in Lesson 2, transcribe Tape 1A, Dermatology. Use both medical and English dictionaries and your Quick-Reference Word List at the back of this book as resource materials for finding words. Proofread your transcribed documents carefully, listening to the dictation while you read your transcripts.

Transcribe (*NOT* retype) the same reports again without referring to your previous transcription attempt. Initially, you may need to transcribe some reports more than twice before you can produce an error-free document. Your ultimate goal is to produce an error-free document the first time.

[SAMPLE LETTER, BLOCK FORMAT]

June 28, 1993

Blue Cross Insurance
2334 Wilshire Blvd.
Los Angeles, CA 95634

Re: Billy Rubin

Gentlemen:

The patient returned to our office and had 17 intracutaneous tests to reaffirm that he was allergic or not allergic to some additional allergens. We also performed a set of allergy tests by the epicutaneous method. We discussed giving allergy injections for those allergens which were unavoidable. I then gave him his first allergy shot, divided up into his left and right arm.

I felt that I had communicated why he was going to be getting allergy injections and why we were going to try to improve his chronic sinusitis problem. The next day the patient stopped payment for his $76 charge.

I think that, as a practicing allergist who is board-certified, I personally provided an adequate examination as well as adequate allergy testing, both epicutaneous and intracutaneous, as well as consultation services. He was also given his first allergy injection and he was made fully aware of all the problems related to injections.

I hope that this establishes some additional information concerning this problem.

Sincerely yours,

N. E. Day, M.D.

NED:hpi

CHART NOTE

Billy Rubin   June 28, 1993

The patient was seen for three visits because of recurrent episodes of urticaria. He was started on treatment with ephedrine, Periactin, and Sinequan, and his hives are almost but not completely gone.

It is my feeling that acute urticaria (in our definition an urticaria that has been present for less than 3 months) should not be evaluated for cause unless that cause is apparent, but rather should be treated only with drug therapy, since at least 70% of patients with acute urticaria will have the urticaria clear spontaneously and because the possibility of finding the cause is so small. His urticaria has not been present for longer than 3 months, and therefore I have elected to treat him only with drug therapy. His hives seem to have almost cleared, and I think that we should continue his drug therapy for a period of time before pursuing any further evaluation. He is on the same three medicines noted above and is to call me in a week for follow-up.

NED:hpi

CHART NOTE

Susan Sommer   Age 43   April 13, 1994

This is a follow-up. It was my impression that she had the skin reaction on her buttocks due to a drug hypersensitivity, the most likely drug being Pronestyl and the secondary drug being either Aldactone or hydrochlorothiazide or both. She was treated both with penicillin and with prednisone, and I have now followed her for a period of 2 months. Her symptoms have completely cleared and there has been no recurrence, and this is an alteration of the previous pattern in which she had episodes every 2 to 3 weeks.

It is impossible to skin test for any of these drugs, and the reaction indeed may not be an IgE-mediated reaction, in which case skin testing would be negative at any rate. We therefore need to draw some conclusions which perhaps may be incorrect but which are at least reasonable. I would recommend that she be given no more Pronestyl or Aldactazide and would be very hesitant at giving her any of the sulfonamide-based diuretics or at using sulfa-type drugs in the future. If she does not have a recurrence, I am not planning to see her again.

_____

N. E. DAY, M.D.

NED:hpi

Shirley U. Jezt   #123456789   Admitted 1/24/94   R. Skinner, M.D.

HISTORY AND PHYSICAL EXAMINATION

HISTORY: This 17-year-old was admitted via the emergency department. She gives a history of shooting crank. Since that time the left antecubital space has been infected.

PAST HISTORY: The patient has been shooting for at least a year. She denies use of drugs other than crank. The patient has a 2-year-old child and a 3-week-old child and has been in the hospital only for that. Denies accidents, injuries, or other infections.

SOCIAL HISTORY: The patient is a 17-year-old I.V. drug user.

PHYSICAL EXAMINATION: Temperature 102.2°. Pulse 112. Respirations 20. Blood pressure 104/60.
GENERAL: Well-developed, well-nourished, English-speaking Caucasian 17-year-old.
EENT: No gross abnormalities. Pupils constricted. Fair dental repair.
NECK supple, no palpable nodes.
CHEST: Lungs are clear. Heart regular, not enlarged, no murmurs. Breasts normal.
ABDOMEN soft, no palpable masses.
PELVIC AND RECTAL: Not done.
ORTHOPEDIC: Examination of the left antecubital space reveals there is a generalized area of tender cellulitis with a moderate amount of swelling on the left as compared with the right.

X-RAYS: No x-rays are available for review.

DIAGNOSIS:
1. Chronic intravenous drug user.
2. Cellulitis, left arm.

PLAN: The patient should be admitted to the hospital for I.V. antibiotics and possible opening of the wound.

_____

ROSALIND SKINNER, M.D.

RS:hpi
d:1/24/94
t:1/24/94

Ida Wannagh   #987654321

Admitted: 6/1/93

Discharged: 6/10/93   **DISCHARGE SUMMARY**

ADMISSION DIAGNOSES:
1. Left lower leg cellulitis.
2. Left lower leg ulceration.
3. Diabetes mellitus.
4. Possible psoriasis.

DISCHARGE DIAGNOSES:
1. Left lower leg cellulitis.
2. Left lower leg ulceration.
3. Diabetes mellitus.
4. Lichen simplex chronicus.

BRIEF HISTORY: This is a 48-year-old white female with obesity and diabetes who has had a smoldering left lower extremity cellulitis for the past 2 to 3 months. It is possibly related to her pruritus and psoriasis. She has been treated in the past with Coumadin and IV antibiotics. On the day of admission she presented to my office with worsening of the cellulitis and a new 2 cm ulceration, and was admitted for IV antibiotics and further evaluation.

EXTREMITIES revealed bilateral edema 1 to 2+ to the knees, with erythema and diffuse excoriations with erythema from the ankle to the midshin area on the left lower extremity. She had a 2 x 2 cm superficial ulcer on the lateral aspect of the ankle.

LABORATORY on admission revealed sodium was 138. Electrolytes were normal. BUN and creatinine were normal. The creatinine was 1.4, which is probably acceptable for this obese woman. PT was slightly elevated at 15.6, PTT was normal. A subsequent chem panel was essentially normal. CBC revealed a white blood cell count of 6,000, hemoglobin 12, hematocrit 35 with 345,000 platelets, and a normal smear.

HOSPITAL COURSE: The patient was seen in consultation by the dermatologist who confirmed my diagnosis of cellulitis. She was placed on IV Kefzol for 48 hours with marked improvement in her cellulitis. Her skin condition was consistent with lichen simplex chronicus, and she was begun on Topicort cream b.i.d. Her Coumadin was not continued, as she had no venogram or Doppler evidence of deep venous thrombosis in the past. As well, she seems to feel that the Coumadin made her rash worse.

DISCHARGE MEDICATIONS: Glyburide 2.5 mg q.d., Keflex 500 mg p.o. q.i.d., Lasix 20 mg q.d., Mellaril 50 mg q.h.s., Topicort cream to affected areas b.i.d., and normal saline and dressing changes for wound care.

N. E. DAY, M.D.

NED:hpi
d:6/10/93
t: 6/11/93

Lesson 3. Urology

Learning Objectives

Medical

- Describe the contents of these sections of the H&P: Chief Complaint, History of Present Illness, Family History, Social History, and Habits.
- List common urologic symptoms and diseases in the Review of Systems section of an H&P.
- Trace the formation of urine from the renal artery to the urinary meatus.
- List common findings of genitourinary disease found in a physical examination.
- Describe the action of these classes of drugs: thiazide diuretics, loop diuretics, potassium-sparing diuretics, and potassium supplements.
- Given a cross-section illustration of the urinary tract and kidney, memorize the anatomic structures.
- Demonstrate knowledge of anatomical, medical, pharmacological, adjectival, and sound-alike terms by accurately completing the exercises in this lesson.

Fundamentals

- Discuss the correct use of flagging to obtain information in order to fill in blanks in transcribed reports.
- Describe the ways in which homonyms and variations in pronunciation of medical words complicate the process of medical transcription.
- Given a medical report with errors, identify and correct the errors.

Practice

- Accurately transcribe authentic physician dictation from the specialty of urology.

A Closer Look

Flagging

Flagging a report is what medical transcriptionists do when they have to leave a blank or have some other question about a report, such as a lab value, age, date, or medical discrepancy, or questionable comments by the dictator.

As a hospital or clinic transcriptionist, you can learn much from the physicians who readily respond to flags. You will learn the most if you work directly for the physicians whose dictation you transcribe. A physician employer often gives lengthy explanations, illustrating or demonstrating a procedure with models.

Most supervisors insist that their transcriptionists leave blanks rather than be creative and make up dictation to avoid leaving a blank. You should always learn your department's or employer's policy for handling questionable dictation.

Hospitals and clinics will probably have a policy similar to the following. When presented with a questionable word or phrase:

1. Seek the supervisor's opinion or that of another MT.
2. Refer to the patient's chart if available.
3. Contact the dictating physician to ask about the word in question. (This must be done with great tact and is often handled by the supervisor or lead transcriptionist.)
4. Leave a blank in the report and attach a flag to the dictator's attention.

Some physicians go out of their way to let the transcriptionist know what the word in question is; physicians have been known to copy whole articles out of texts or journals to answer an MT's questions.

Other physicians simply write the word directly into the typed document without giving the transcriptionist any feedback. One hospital solved the latter problem by asking the chart analysts and coders to report to the transcription supervisor any physician-made corrections they spotted.

Attaching notes, however, can present problems. Post-It notes or notes paperclipped to the report can fall off. Communication in writing is much more difficult than speaking, and notes must be worded in an extremely tactful manner. The person to whom the note is directed can take offense when none is intended.

If possible, the note should include a phonetic rendering of the missing word or phrase to help the physician remember or identify the missing part. Generally speaking, the shorter the note or more impersonal it is, the better for avoiding offense. You may have better luck, however, getting written responses from the physician when including some type of compliment or requesting specific information.

Another problem in this computer age is that many MTs never see the printed copy of their reports. The printer is in another location, and a clerk handles the sorting and charting. The solution has been for hospitals to create a standard memo to accompany the report just like another page of the report. It contains the patient's name and other pertinent information in case the two get separated. It usually has boxes or blanks to check for the problem encountered and a place to fill in a "sounds like."

Whether your employer uses individual notes or a standard memo form, it is important to recognize that leaving a blank is the behavior of a professional who desires to produce the most accurate, highest quality report possible and who is always, above all, wanting to learn.

Card Sharks

by Judith Marshall, MA, CMT

We regret to inform you, Dr. Bungler, that twelve charts must be redictated. That wasn't a microphone you were using; you dictated into our new electric pencil sharpener.

Love and kisses,
jm in Transcription

This is an example of the medical transcriptionist (MT) writing a note to communicate with a physician. It is variously called carding, flagging, tagging, or marking.

Carding is a delicate issue and there are problems. Transcription is a "from their mouth to our ears" situation and many people think MTs, like children, should be seen and not heard. Some supervisors systematically

rip the messages from the transcript with the justification of "Let's not bother our physicians." Supervisors in some private transcription services read each card going out to a client and either rewrite it or throw it away.

Carding is a chance for the transcriptionists to say something, ask something, or prevent something.

Prevention could mean corralling every new batch of interns and residents, locking them in a room, and teaching them how to dictate. In practice, even in hospitals where an orientation program is devised, the new physicians arrive by bus, plane, or car at 4 a.m. and begin their new year half dead. (Don't ever go to an Emergency Department on July 1.) Physicians on rotation are given up as lost causes before they can even sneeze into their first microphone. We would like to warn them, we want to lecture them in risk management, we want to nip their little buds. But we can't. We are lucky to catch a glimpse of them.

Working off premises, we once transcribed the dictation of a particular resident. His summaries included not only all the laboratory data, day by hospital day, but all of the normal laboratory ranges, repeated for each day. We called the director of medical records who said that this doctor was on a six-week rotation and that it was not our place to make any suggestions; if the senior supervising physician read the summaries and disapproved of their length and content, it was up to him to take action. Talk about hazardous waste!

Obviously we have more latitude in the private business sector of transcription. But I don't think there

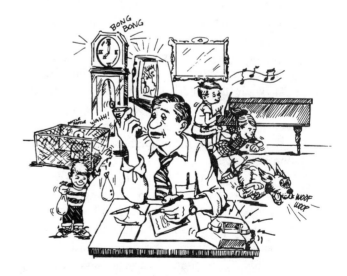

I want to write, "Look, Dr. Yahoo, if you expect me to extract your voice from that mob around the telephone, your pilot light is on low."

Judith Marshall, MEDICATE ME
Illustrated by Cindy Stevens

is any point in asking the doctor not to dictate in a car or plane. I do card if the car radio is on or if the plane noises of pilot's voice and ding-ding-dings are easier to transcribe than the dictation. I will card if the dictation was done at the beach with the children or in the garden with the bluejays.

I will card if the dictation was done at home simultaneously with family conversation. Give me a break from the dinner menu and problems with the children, the piano practice, and the family dog. I want to write, "Look, Dr. Yahoo, if you expect me to extract your voice from that mob around the telephone, your pilot light is on low."

When some word is really new and we can't find it in our good reference library, we spell it phonetically and ask what it is. We hope for an answer and usually we get one. Once, however, I wrote, "It sounds like _____" and typed the word. The answer was, "It sounds like you don't know what you are doing!" You can't win them all.

Some things should never be said, let alone written down. There are unique situations requiring tact and discretion. One such case was the Bedtime Story Caper in a metropolitan hospital. All of us were transcribing frantically to meet a deadline and the dictation tanks kept filling up. We were exhausted and irritable. And there it was. One of our residents had taken a little boy who could not sleep into the dictation room on the ward to show him the telephone "toy." It was 3:30 a.m. For more than thirty minutes the kind physician soothed and entertained the child. He told him stories and sang him lullabies, all into the "toy." The youngster was then taken to bed by a nurse and the physician continued regular dictation.

Were we to forget about our wasted time and to praise the caring doctor, or communicate to him somehow that while this interlude was heartwarming, it should not be repeated. What good would a note have done and why involve a supervisor? A brief chat with the new resident ended the midnight serenades on the dictation equipment.

It is hard to resist the urge to straighten out a physician, especially an arrogant or patronizing one. Dr. Malaprop fancies herself a multilingual marvel. She dictated that the patient took "a menage of drugs." We transcribed "melange" and did not card it. Dr. Fossil is a forty-year veteran in practice and the chief of a service. He is adroit and skillful in surgery but botches and mangles words. If we hear "allergic to plantation," we change it to "plantain." "There are no advantageous breath sounds" we silently change to

"adventitious." When it comes to the English language, he is a great but sloppy dictator. It is our responsibility to produce the most perfect record through careful medical editing. It is not our responsibility to rub his nose in his mistakes or ask him to change.

I have equally strong feelings against cuteness. Some cards I read are too clever, too droll, and even downright flirtatious. Some of the messages list four or five books checked and places called, all supposed to somehow impress the doctor that we work so hard. Doctors don't have time for that sort of thing and they don't really care.

If some piece of dictation is particularly superior, why not card it and say so? Send a cigar, a silver dollar, a single carnation, or a fancy chocolate bar, rather than "Why, Dr. Whippersnapper, you clever devil, how DO you manage to know so many new words, you rascal, you!"

People do have strange names and we can usually verify them. Nicknames should be spelled by the physician and when they are not, we card them. We asked how to spell Brammie, Ivy, Lolly, Pudge, Nanook, Kip, and Pip. One day we heard a no-nonsense doctor recounting the clinic visit of little Hitler so-and-so. What? We had no chart or patient list. Could parents really name a child this name? They could and did, the response came back. (The family was visiting America from a foreign land.) Never assume a doctor is kidding with a name.

My *imaginary* cards include, "Dr. Chutzpah, you ignorant jerk. Shape up or all your tapes will go through the magnetic bulk eraser." Or "Dr. Goodwrench, make up your mind which knee you operated on. Either dictate or get off the phone." One sharp-as-a-marble doctor actually received a rebuke for his constant sarcastic references to every obese female as "that porker."

And do let us stamp out sweetness. Some MTs are so gosh-awful nice and darling in their cards. The doctors have given them a bad report, a bad hour, a bad day, and a bad headache. It's enough to give me diabetes when I read the card:

Dr. Wunderkind: You have no patient names or numbers or dates, you mumbled and ate lunch all through this. But you are such a great healer and you are up for canonization, I hear. It is my fault there are blanks and I am sorry and will never do it again and please walk on me, I am a doormat.

Your humble and obedient servant
Mary Jane

See what I mean? Mary Jane's niceness will get her no earthly reward but a well-trodden appearance. There is nothing wrong with an occasional card with a little bite to it.

Dictation and Transcription: Adventures in Thought Transference

Part 2

by John H. Dirckx, M.D.

The same, only different. A frequent source of difficulty in transcription is the existence of homonyms or, more precisely, of homophones. Homonyms are two or more words that are spelled and pronounced the same but differ in meaning—for example, *mole* 'small mammal,' *mole* 'pigmented nevus,' *mole* 'uterine neoplasm,' *mole* 'breakwater,' *mole* 'unit of measure based on molecular weight.' Strictly speaking, a set like this should cause no trouble, because even if the transcriptionist should mistake the meaning, the spelling would be the same.

Similarly, homographs (words spelled the same but pronounced differently) should create no ambiguity in dictation. A special kind of homograph results from variation in placement of syllable stress: tínnitus-tinnítus, ángina-angína, fácet-facét. The American transcriptionist may sometimes be startled by a British dictator's placement of stress in such words as cervícal, éphedrine, labóratory, and skelétal.

But it is homophones that demand alertness and judgment—words that sound the same but are spelled differently. Sometimes the difference is plain from the context ("I guessed he was a guest when he discussed his disgust") and sometimes it is not ("Dr. Templeton is losing his patience/patients"). Many homophone pairs are created by our custom of reducing unaccented vowels to a neutral "uh" sound. We hear this sound, for example, in the second syllables of both *callus* and *callous, mucus* and *mucous, villus* and *villous.* Only the context tells the transcriptionist whether to type the noun form in *-us* or the adjective form in *-ous.* In the same way, *instillation* may be indistinguishable from *installation, perineal* from *peroneal, have* from *of.*

Styles of pronunciation that are characteristic of certain regional or ethnic dialects may create homophones in the dictation of some speakers. One person may fail to distinguish between *finally* and *finely,* another between *then* and *than,* a third between *his* and

he's, a fourth between *long* and *lung.* The practice of dropping final *l* or *r* or both can erase the differences between such pairs as *sulfa/sulfur* and *femoral-popliteal/ femoropopliteal,* and place the transcriptionist in peril of creating such monstrosities as *musculodystrophy* and *normal tensive.*

In my part of the country, a sizable segment of the populace practices itacism. This term, originally denoting an analogous dialectal variation in Greek, refers to a raising of the short e sound in a tonic (stressed) syllable so that it sounds like short *i.* Thus, for example, *attend, get, men,* and *shelter* are pronounced as if they were spelled *attind, git, min,* and *shilter.* Although this causes little or no inconvenience in the examples I have used, the wholesale disappearance of tonic short *e* does create some ambiguities that must be averted by further modifications of the language. For instance, persons who pronounce *pen* exactly like *pin* customarily distinguish the former word by saying *inkpen* (pronounced "inkpin"). (Less than a week after making notes for the above paragraph, I saw in a local antique shop a box of old fountain pens labeled "Inkpins $1.00.")

Homophony is not confined to pairs of words. A phrase may sound almost exactly like another phrase of entirely different, even opposite meaning. Two notorious examples—*had no carcinoma* for *adenocarcinoma* and *prepped and raped* for *prepped and draped*—have passed into legend. Whole books of such blunders, many of them no doubt spurious, have been published. A frequent source of difficulty is the unaccented *a* at the beginning of words: *atonic bladder* vs. *a tonic bladder, a symmetric swelling* vs. *asymmetric swelling.*

Besides discriminating between homophones, the transcriptionist performs a variety of what might be called normalizing operations, that is, recognizing variant pronunciations and reducing them to their conventional or normal forms before putting them on paper. The range of such deviations is enormous. Some result from congenital or acquired speech impediments such as tongue-tie or obstruction of the nasal passages by hypertrophic adenoids or chronic allergic rhinitis. Some are due to dialectal variations (a few of which I have already mentioned) or to speech habits learned in childhood, such as substituting a glottal catch (momentary closure of the vocal cords) for *t* at the end of a syllable.

A large number of deviant pronunciations arise from the structure of the human vocal apparatus and the difficulty or awkwardness of producing certain sound sequences. The omission of the first *d* sound in *Wednesday* and the rearrangement of sounds in *comfortable* (="comftorble") are examples of such changes. In rapid speech, *cysts* and *tests* often come out "cyss" and "tess." We also tend to insert extraneous sounds into our speech to smooth certain transitions. Some of these inserted sounds are virtually standard (*compfort, intsulin*), some are dialectal (*hematoma-r of the rectus sheath, mower* [=more]), and some are decidedly substandard (*athaletic, drownding*).

Frank mispronunciations include both the mishandling of English phonetics by non-native speakers and isolated errors (most of them acquired by imitation) such as *phalynx, larnyx, ishium,* and *meninjocele.* Here may also be mentioned certain recurring deviations from correct pronunciation that have been adopted as an affectation by certain speakers. Among these are the bizarre plurals *abscesses, processes,* and other words pronounced to rhyme with *neuroses,* and the compulsive gallicization of words having no connection with French (*centimeter, centrifuge, difficile,* and *mitrale*).

To recapitulate, in turning a phonetic (speech) record into a written one, the transcriptionist inserts "silent" letters, suppresses extraneous sounds (including "uh"), selects the correct one of several alternative spellings, and recognizes deviant pronunciations—all in the light of a sustained monitoring of the context and a thorough understanding of medicine, medical terminology, dictating conventions, and human frailty.

(Part 3 of this article appears in Lesson 4.)

Medical Readings

The History and Physical Examination

by John H. Dirckx, M.D.

Chief Complaint and History of Present Illness. The statement of the patient's chief (or presenting) complaint (or complaints) and a narration of the course of the illness up to the moment when the history is taken far outweigh the rest of the history in importance. In fact, the other parts of the history may be dealt with perfunctorily or even omitted altogether in the case of a simple, clear-cut illness or injury.

Some physicians prefer to state the Chief Complaint exactly in the patient's words ("I can't sleep," "My left arm is numb"), while others strive for maximum conciseness and precision ("Insomnia," "Hypesthesia of the dorsum of the left forearm"). Often the statement of the chief complaint includes an indication of its duration or other features: "Intermittent pain and pressure in the epigastrium for one week." Sometimes several apparently related complaints are mentioned together: "Fever, vomiting, diarrhea, and severe headache." Even when the patient himself cannot give any history, the heading "Chief Complaint" is still used: "Sudden loss of consciousness at home and deepening coma."

The History of the Present Illness is the heart of the medical history, for it contains all historical details leading up to and in any way pertaining to the patient's current status. If, for example, a patient is hospitalized for pneumonia, the history of present illness might include mention of his smoking habits, current medicines, previous treatments or hospitalizations for respiratory disease, and all negative and positive answers to questions about the respiratory tract, even though this material would probably appear in other parts of the history if the patient had appendicitis instead of pneumonia. In an acute illness, the history of present illness may consist of just a sentence or two, but if the patient's current problem is the culmination of months or years of chronic, evolving illness, this part of the history may occupy a whole page or more.

The narrative of the course of an illness follows a certain pattern, basically chronological. By convention, the physician starts with a brief description of the patient, including age and sex and often race and social status. He then records the date (or time) and nature of onset of the first symptoms and traces the progress of the illness—the appearance of additional symptoms, their effect on the patient's lifestyle and well-being, and the results of treatment, physician-prescribed or otherwise—finally reporting the events that prompted the present consultation or hospitalization. This part of the history may contain an almost limitless variety of information, including diagnoses and the names of drugs and operations.

Nonspecific symptoms such as fever, chills, loss of appetite, headaches, muscle aches, lethargy, drowsiness, decline in exercise tolerance, and inability to concentrate can herald the onset of a broad variety of diseases.

No matter what the initial or presenting symptom,

the physician will try to learn when it started; whether it came on gradually or abruptly; whether it has continued unchanged, waxed and waned, or intermittently disappeared; and whether the patient can suggest any reason for it. The duration of a symptom is of the utmost importance in analyzing its meaning. A 12-hour history of constant, agonizing, unilateral headache with blurred vision and vomiting might indicate cerebral hemorrhage, encephalitis, meningitis, or brain abscess, among other possibilities. A 20-year history of such headaches recurring at intervals could not possibly be due to any of these. Similarly, the suddenness with which a symptom appears and the pattern of its subsequent behavior may supply essential clues to its significance.

The physician usually carries the history of present illness down to the present by describing the circumstances that led to his involvement in the case. At this point, all historical data considered relevant to the patient's present condition have been recorded. By convention, however, the examiner goes on to review a number of other historical points, both for the sake of completeness and because unsuspected clues and relationships are frequently uncovered in the process.

Family History. The importance of the family history lies in the fact that many developmental abnormalities, diseases, and tendencies to disease are not only hereditary (genetically transmitted from parent to child) but familial (occurring in some or all members of a family). In addition, a thorough family history can provide clues to unwholesome environmental influences or exposure to communicable disease.

The complete Family History includes the age and state of health (or age at death and cause of death) of each member of the patient's immediate family (parents, siblings, and children), selected data about other blood relatives, and a general statement regarding family history of certain conditions. In practice the Family History is often passed over as noncontributory.

Social History. This part of the history includes any personal information about the patient's past or present life which, though nonmedical, may have a bearing on his health. The ideal Social History would include data on the patient's birth, upbringing, academic career, marital history and present status, spouse's health history, military service, occupations past and present, avocations and hobbies, social and cultural pursuits, political and religious activities, foreign travel or residence, financial status, police record, and current family structure, living arrangements, and personal responsibilities.

Seldom does the physician have time or motivation to extract such a voluminous mass of nonmedical and doubtfully relevant information from a patient, except in the course of psychotherapy. Hence the Social History is often omitted.

A history of travel in the tropics can lead to the explanation of an unusual case of fever or diarrhea.

A complete occupational history includes dates of all jobs held by the patient, with attention to exposure to hazardous chemicals, noise, psychological stress, and other adverse conditions; industrial illnesses or injuries, workers' compensation claims filed, and disability allowances; medical or other restrictions on work assignments.

Habits. Under this heading comes information about the patient's lifestyle, specifically his regular or customary practices with respect to eating, sleeping, exercise, recreation, and the use of prescription and nonprescription medicines, caffeine, nicotine, alcohol, and other substances of abuse.

Dietary habits need to be investigated if the patient has a weight problem or digestive tract symptoms.

The sleep history includes hours of sleep each night, ease of falling asleep, tendency to awaken during the night, restfulness of sleep, use of sleeping medicines, daytime napping, nightmares, and sleepwalking.

A person's habits regarding exercise, recreations, and vacations from work may supply clues to risk-taking, compulsive, or excessively sedentary lifestyles.

A useful unit for recording lifetime cigarette smoking history is the pack-year, which is the equivalent of smoking one package of cigarettes a day for one year. Hence a person who smoked 1½ packages of cigarettes a day for 24 years would be called a 36-pack-year smoker.

Persons who abuse alcohol or drugs are notoriously unreliable historians. The more searching the interrogation, the more likely they are to conceal or distort the truth about their drinking or drug use and other elements of their health history that may be in any way related.

Review of Systems: Genitourinary. The kidneys and urinary tract (ureters, bladder, and urethra) and the reproductive system are considered together because of their close anatomic association and the frequency with which one disease affects both organ systems.

A thorough review of genitourinary history includes past diagnoses of congenital anomalies of the urinary or genital tract; urinary tract infections; stone in a kidney, ureter, or bladder; sexually transmitted (venereal) diseases; genitourinary surgery; and menstrual and reproductive history.

Symptoms suggesting renal or urinary tract disease are pain in one or both flanks, increase in frequency of urination (as opposed to increase in urine volume), nocturia (being awakened at night by the urge to void), burning or pain on voiding, difficulty voiding, diminution in the urinary stream, incontinence of urine, bedwetting in an older child or adult, blood in the urine, and any other marked change in the appearance of the urine.

Men are questioned about urethral discharge or burning; itching, rash, ulcers, or other lesions of the genitals; pain or swelling in the testicles; scrotal masses; and infertility.

Examination of the Groins, Rectum, and Anus. The abdominal examination concludes with palpation of femoral pulses and an assessment of the groins for dermatitis, enlarged lymph nodes, and hernias. A hernia is the protrusion of some normally contained structure through a weakness or defect in a body wall. Most hernias occur in the groin and contain loops of small intestine. A true inguinal hernia lies above the inguinal ligament, a femoral hernia just below it at the top of the thigh. In the male an indirect inguinal hernia can descend into the scrotum. With recumbency a hernia often reduces; hence the subject is examined for hernias while standing, if possible. The physician places his fingers over each groin in turn and asks the subject to cough vigorously. In examining a male patient he approximates his finger to the external inguinal ring by invaginating a portion of the scrotal skin.

At this point in the examination of a male patient the physician proceeds to the external genitalia. With the patient still standing he inspects the penis and scrotum for dermatitis, ulcers, scars, and other cutaneous lesions. The penis is assessed for developmental anomalies and the foreskin, if present, is retracted for inspection of the glans. The urethra may be milked to express any discharge. The scrotal contents are palpated and any masses, testicular enlargement or deformity, or tenderness is noted. If one or both testicles are not felt in the scrotum, an attempt is made to locate them in the inguinal canals (undescended testis). Scrotal masses are assessed by transillumination. A bright focal light is placed behind and in contact with the scrotum, and the room lights extinguished. A cyst or hydrocele will transmit light; a solid tumor or hernia will not.

The examination of this region in the male concludes with a rectal examination. The physician performs a digital rectal examination not only to gather data about the rectum and anus but also to evaluate the pelvic walls and pelvic organs, particularly the prostate in the male, for evidence of tenderness or masses.

The patient may stand and bend forward with his arms resting on the examining table, or lie on his left side or on his back with his knees drawn up. The examiner first inspects the anus and perineum for swellings, masses, hemorrhoids, fissures, cutaneous lesions, fistulous tracts, or signs of inflammation. He then gently inserts a gloved and lubricated finger into the rectum, noting sphincter tone and any tenderness, scarring, or masses in the anal canal, and palpating the interior of the rectum as far as he can reach. He observes any masses, thickening, or fixation of the rectal walls and also the amount and consistency of any stool present. He palpates the pelvic walls and all structures within his reach, including the prostate and the seminal vesicles. After withdrawing his finger he notes any stool, blood, pus, or mucus adhering to the surface of the glove and may perform a simple chemical test for occult blood before discarding the glove.

Pharmacology: Urinary Tract Drugs

Urinary tract drugs include diuretics (used to treat hypertension), urinary tract antibiotics and other anti-infection agents, urinary tract analgesics, urinary antispasmodics, and potassium supplements taken concurrently with many diuretics to counteract their potassium-wasting effect.

Diuretics. Diuretics increase the natural excretion of sodium (and therefore also water). By causing extra sodium and water to be excreted from the circulating blood volume, diuretics are useful in the treatment of hypertension.

Diuretics are divided into several groups on the basis of their action within the nephron of the kidney: thiazide diuretics, loop diuretics, and potassium-sparing diuretics.

Thiazide diuretics act at the site of the distal renal tubule within the nephron. They increase the excretion of sodium (and therefore water) in the urine. The thiazide diuretics include:

chlorothiazide (Diuril)

hydrochlorothiazide (HCTZ) (Esidrix, HydroDIURIL, Oretic)

methylclothiazide (Enduron)

Note: The ending -iazide is common to generic thiazide diuretics.

Other diuretics closely related in structure and action to the thiazide diuretics are:

chlorthalidone (Hygroton)

metolazone (Zaroxolyn)

Loop diuretics act at the site of the proximal and distal tubules as well as the loop of Henle (hence their name). They block the reabsorption of sodium into the bloodstream so that it is excreted along with water into the urine. The loop diuretics include furosemide (Lasix)

Both thiazide and loop diuretics cause sodium and water to be excreted. Sodium is a positive ion (Na^+). The action of these diuretics also causes potassium, another positive ion (K^+), to be excreted. The excessive loss of potassium can cause serious side effects, including cardiac arrhythmias. Patients who need to take a thiazide or loop diuretic may also be given potassium supplements, or they may take a potassium-sparing diuretic alone or in combination with the other diuretics to offset the potassium-wasting effect.

Potassium-sparing diuretics include:

spironolactone (Aldactone)

triamterene (Dyrenium)

Some products combine a thiazide diuretic with a potassium-sparing diuretic in one tablet. These combination products include:

Aldactazide (hydrochlorothiazide and spironolactone)

Dyazide (hydrochlorothiazide and triamterene)

Maxzide (hydrochlorothiazide and triamterene)

Moduretic (hydrochlorothiazide and amiloride)

Potassium supplements. Potassium supplements are frequently prescribed for patients taking thiazide and loop diuretics to avoid potassium depletion. Although some foods, such as bananas, are rich in potassium, dietary sources alone are usually not sufficient to replenish potassium loss from diuretics. Potassium supplements are manufactured as liquids (patients often object to the taste), powders and effervescent tablets (to be mixed with water), capsules, and tablets. Dosages are measured in milliequivalents (mEq). Trade name potassium supplements include:

Kay Ciel	K-Dur
K-Lor	Klorvess
Klotrix	K-Lyte
K-Tab	Micro-K
Potage	Slow-K

Note: The *K* in trade names for potassium supplements refers to the chemical symbol for potassium (K^+).

Anatomy/Medical Terminology

Anatomy: The Urinary System; A Kidney

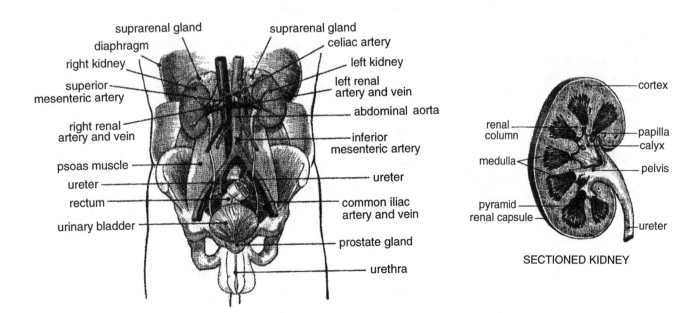

SECTIONED KIDNEY

Urology Fill-in Exercise

Instructions: The following paragraphs describe the process by which urine is formed. The numbered blanks correspond to the numbers in the narrative paragraphs. Fill in the blanks with the correct term from the word list below.

During the process of metabolism, proteins taken into the body are broken down into (1). This nitrogenous waste must be removed continuously by the kidneys. Other nitrogenous waste products removed by the kidney include creatinine and uric acid. In addition, the kidneys regulate blood electrolytes by excreting or retaining sodium and potassium. Circulating blood (carrying urea, creatinine, uric acid, sodium, and potassium) flows through the (2), which enters the kidney through a small depression on the medial aspect of the kidney called the (3). The renal artery divides into arterioles and then into capillaries within the cortex of the kidney.

Special capillary tufts called (4) are where the process of urine production actually begins. These capillary tufts are surrounded by a cuplike structure called (5) that collects filtrate taken from the capillary blood. This filtrate contains water, waste products, and electrolytes. The combination of the capillary tuft and the cuplike collecting tube is known as a (6), which is considered the functional unit of the kidney.

As the filtrate passes through the proximal convoluted tubule, the (7), and the distal convoluted tubule, water and electrolytes needed to maintain body functions are absorbed back into the blood. At this point, the filtrate is urine. The many renal tubules containing urine empty into cuplike collecting areas in the renal pelvis known as the (8). The collected urine then flows through the hollow tubes known as (9) into the urinary bladder.

The bladder has three orifices within it: one opening from each of the two ureters and one opening leading to the urethra. The triangular area within these three openings is called the (10). The urethra ends at the (11) where the urine is expelled from the body.

The process of urination is also known as (12) and (13). In the male, the urethra passes through a gland at the base of the bladder, called the (14) gland. This gland often enlarges in elderly men and can block the flow of urine.

1. urea _____
2. _____
3. _____
4. _____
5. _____
6. _____
7. _____
8. _____
9. _____
10. _____
11. _____
12. _____
13. _____
14. _____

Bowman's capsule
calices or calyces
glomeruli
hilum
loop of Henle
micturition
nephron
prostate
renal artery
trigone
urea
ureters
urinary meatus
voiding

Medical Terminology Matching Exercise

The kidneys, ureters, bladder, and urethra comprise the genitourinary system. Complete the following matching exercise to test your knowledge of the word roots, anatomic structures, symptoms, and disease processes encountered in the medical specialty of urology.

Instructions: Match the term in Column A with its definition in Column B.

Column A

A. retroperitoneal
B. trigone
C. micturition
D. hilum
E. pole
F. glomerulus
G. Bowman's capsule
H. nephrolithiasis
I. meatus
J. glomerulonephritis
K. calix (or calyx)
L. pyelo-
M. nocturia
N. oliguria
O. anuria
P. pyuria
Q. incontinence
R. dysuria
S. hematuria

Column B

____ blood in the urine
____ cuplike structure that surrounds the glomerulus
____ urge to urinate during the night
____ inflammation of the glomerulus
____ kidney stones
____ decreased production of urine
____ painful urination
____ no urine production
____ collection of capillaries shaped like a ball in the kidney
____ upper or lower end of kidney
____ area where blood vessels and nerves enter the kidney
____ triangle in the bladder formed by end of ureters and entrance to urethra
____ opening of urethra to outside of body
____ region where urine collects within the renal pelvis
____ position of kidneys in body
____ pus in the urine
____ voiding
____ inability to hold urine in the bladder
____ root word meaning renal pelvis

Lay and Medical Terms

Lay Term	*Medical Term*
pass water, pee	urinate, micturate, void
kidney stone	renal calculus, nephrolithiasis

Adjective Exercise

Adjectives are formed from nouns by adding adjectival suffixes such as *-ac, -al, -ar, -ary, -eal, -ed, -ent, -iac, -ial, -ic, -ical, -lar, -oid, -ous, -tic,* and *-tous.* In addition, some adjectives have a different form entirely from the noun, which may be either Latin or Greek in origin.

Test your knowledge of adjectives by writing the adjectival form of the following urology words. Consult a medical dictionary to select the correct adjectival ending as necessary.

1. urine   _____
2. kidney   _____
3. bladder   _____
4. ureter   _____
5. urethra   _____
6. hilum   _____
7. calyx   _____
8. glomerulus _____
9. incontinence _____
10. uremia   _____

Root Word and Suffix Matching Exercise

Instructions: Combine the following root words with suffixes to form words that match the definitions below. Fill in the blanks with the medical words that you construct.

Root Word	Suffix
oligo-	-oscopy
cyst-	-itis
noct-	-iasis
nephro-	-uria
litho-	-ectomy
glycos-	-ology
pyo-	
uro-	

A. the study of the urine

_____

B. inflammation of the bladder

_____

C. the urge to void at night

_____

D. scanty production of urine

_____

E. using a scope to visualize the bladder

_____

F. surgical removal of a kidney

_____

G. pus (white blood cells) in the urine

_____

H. sugar in the urine

_____

I. condition of kidney stones
   (Tip: Use 2 root words and 1 suffix.)

_____

Drug Word Search

Instructions: Locate and circle the urology drugs and terms hidden in the puzzle horizontally, vertically, or diagonally, forward or backward. A numeral following a drug or term indicates the number of times it can be found in the puzzle.

```
Q  E  T  Y  L  K  S  L  O  W  K  Z  K
Y  H  R  A  A  E  K  A  Y  C  I  E  L
R  E  N  E  S  E  D  D  P  C  D  K  O
E  P  I  L  I  J  O  I  U  I  N  O  R
N  Y  L  O  X  O  R  A  Z  R  E  R  V
I  R  L  M  A  N  E  A  A  X  Y  C  E
S  I  N  A  B  S  T  B  P  I  A  I  S
I  D  O  Z  N  C  I  W  S  Q  U  M  S
R  I  R  D  A  E  C  X  O  U  K  K  V
T  U  U  D  I  U  R  E  T  I  C  D  F
N  M  L  E  D  I  M  E  S  O  R  U  F
A  A  A  E  D  I  Z  A  Y  D  B  R  K
G  E  S  I  D  R  I  X  C  D  R  U  G
```

Aldactazide	K-Lyte
Cystospaz	Lasix (2)
diuretic	Maxzide
drug	Micro-K
Dyazide	Oretic
Esidrix	Pyridium
furosemide	renal
Gantrisin	Renese
Kay Ciel	Saluron
K-Dur (2)	Slow-K
kidney	Zaroxolyn
Klorvess	

Proofreading Skills

Proofreading Exercise

Instructions: In the report below, circle the errors. Identify misspelled and missing medical and English words and write the correct words in the numbered spaces opposite the text. Review proofreading guidelines on pages 28-29.

#	Text	#	Answer
1	HISTRY AND PHSYICAL EXAMINATION	1.	HISTORY PHYSICAL
2		2.	
3	HISTORY: This 38-year-old mail was	3.	
4	admitted threw the emergency department with	4.	
5	a hsitory of less than one day of a cute	5.	
6	urethral colic on the left side. The patient had	6.	
7	an IBT in the emergency department earlier	7.	
8	today which shows partial to complete	8.	
9	destruction of the left ureter at the urethro-	9.	
10	vesical junction with a large stone approxi-	10.	
11	mately 8 x 5 mm lodged at the UB junction.	11.	
12	The patient has no other clacifications visible.	12.	
13	The patinet denies any previous history of	13.	
14	urinary track stones or other GU problems	14.	
15	except for prostratitis a cuople of years ago.	15.	
16	The patient has no other significant medical	16.	
17	problems.	17.	
18		18.	
19	FAMILY HISTORY: No familial history of	19.	
20	kidney stones or other significant hereditary	20.	
21	diseese.	21.	
22		22.	
23	PHYSICAL EXAM reveals a well-nourished,	23.	
24	well-developed male in no acute distress.	24.	
25	Pupils equal, round, react to light. Ears, nose,	25.	
26	and throat clear. Neck supple, no JB	26.	
27	distention or bree. Lungs clear to T&A.	27.	
28	Heart: Regular rythm, no murmur. Abdomen	28.	
29	soft, slight left CBA tenderness, slight left	29.	
30	lower quadrant tenderness, no rebound.	30.	
31	Genitalia is within normal limits. Penis:	31.	
32	Normal male. Extremities: No cyanosis,	32.	
33	clubing, or edema. Neurologic: Oriented x 3	33.	
34	with no gross deficits.	34.	
35		35.	
36	IMPRESSION: Left lower urethral stone with	36.	
37	obstruction.	37.	

Transcription Tips

1. Both the Romans and the Greeks studied the body and disease processes extensively. Often different medical terms describe the same anatomic structure because the root words were derived from either the Latin or Greek language.

   Both root words *ren-* (renal) and *nephr-* (nephrolithiasis) refer to the *kidney*. *Ren-* is Latin and *nephr-* is Greek.

   Both root words *vesic-* (vesical neck) and *cyst-* (cystoscopy) refer to the *urinary bladder*. *Vesic-* is Latin and *cyst-* is Greek.

   Both root words *test-* (testosterone) and *orchi-* (orchiectomy) refer to the *testicle*. *Test-* is Latin and *orchi-* is Greek.

2. Do not confuse the term *prostate* (a gland of the male reproductive system through which the urethra passes) and the term *prostrate* (an adjective describing a posture of submission, exhaustion, or extreme grief).

3. The abbreviation *UA* (urinalysis) is acceptable and commonly known. The combined form *urinalysis* is used rather than *urine analysis*.

4. Distinguish between *ureter/ureteral* and *urethra/urethral*, which refer to two totally different anatomical structures.

5. Some words have more than one acceptable spelling. The preferred spelling always appears as the main entry followed by the definition in the dictionary. For example, *calix/calices* is preferred, *calyx/calyces* an acceptable alternative. Preferred spellings may vary among English and medical references.

6. *Cath* is a slang term for *catheterization*, *cysto* for *cystoscopy*. Slang terms should be translated in medical reports.

7. The accent falls on different syllables in *CYS'to scope* and *cys TOS'copy*.

8. Spelling tips for urinary tract drugs:

   Dyazide (spelled *Dy*, not *Di*)
   NegGram (unusual for internal capitalization)
   HydroDIURIL (unusual use of all capital letters for the second part of the drug)
   Kay Ciel (trade name for *KCl*, an abbreviation of the chemical name *potassium chloride*)
   Urispas, Anaspaz, Cystospaz (similar-sounding trade names ending in different letters)

9. Urine specific gravity is always written as the number 1 followed by a decimal point and three other numbers. Normal values range between 1.001 to 1.030. A dictated value which sounds like "ten ten" is correctly transcribed as 1.010.

10. **Spelling.** A mnemonic (pronounced "ne-mon-ic," rhymes with "demonic") device is a memory aid that helps link the unfamiliar to the familiar. Our brains use a number of mnemonic devices consciously and unconsciously. Using mnemonic devices and learning how to construct our own will help us remember the spellings of many of the new words we have to learn in medical transcription.

    First-letter cues. To learn to spell long or difficult words, construct sentences that are easily remembered, with the initial letters spelling out the word in question. For example, the spelling of "rhythm" is difficult to remember; thus, constructing the sentence, "**R**uby **h**ad **y**ams, **T**ommy **h**ad **m**uffins," serves as a unique and effective spelling aid. Medical students remember the Hallpike caloric stimulation response with "Caloric testing produced COWS"; COWS stands for **c**old to the **o**pposite, **w**arm to the **s**ame.

    Imagery link. Linking words that evoke mental images make them easier to remember. "Dysphagia" and "dysphasia" are frequently confused but are more easily remembered by linking "dysphagia" with "gag" and "dysphasia" with "speech." The words "discrete" and "discreet" present a spelling challenge at times. In the sentence "There were large, discrete nodules noted in the neck," an easy way to remember the correct spelling of "discrete," which means separate, is that the "t" **separates** the two *e*'s.

Keyword link. This involves linking two unrelated words in a similar way. For example, the words "principle" and "principal" are often confused. An effective solution is to link "principle" with "rule" (one's principles are one's rules), and *all other uses* are spelled "principal" (meaning the chief or foremost, a school administrator, and principal and interest). Another example is "stationery" as in "letter."

Pronunciation tricks. Mentally changing the pronunciation of a word will assist spelling. For example, "hors d'oeuvre," which is correctly pronounced "or-derve," is easier to spell when pronounced as spelled: "hors-doe-uv-re."

Association of spelling with "logical order." A difficult spelling to remember is that of "mittelschmerz," the medical term for intermenstrual pain. Is it "mittle" or "mittel"? By associating the word with **alphabetical order** ("e" comes before "l" in the alphabet and "e" comes before "l" in "mittelschmerz"), the appropriate spelling is easier to remember.

Another example of logical order is **order of appearance.** For example, to remember the spellings of "perineal" and "peroneal," one can associate them with their order of appearance in the body: from head to toe, the perineum (torso) comes before peroneal (leg).

Terminology Challenge

Instructions: The following terms appear in the dictation on Tape 1B, Urology. Before beginning the medical transcription practice for Lesson 3, become familiar with the terminology below by looking up each word in a medical or English dictionary. Write out a short definition of each term.

Achilles reflex
acute
adnexa
ampicillin
amylase
antihypertensive
appendectomy

asymptomatic
atrophic
autologous
b.i.d.
band neutrophils
benign
bilaterally

bladder floor
bladder outlet
bladder suspension
blind vaginal pouch
blood panel
BPH (benign prostatic hypertrophy)
bruit
BUN (blood urea nitrogen)
calcium
calculus
cervix
chloride
cholecystectomy
cholesterol
chronic
clubbing
complexity
constipation
creatinine
crevice
CT scan
CVA (costovertebral angle)
cyanosis
cyst
cystocele
cystogram
cystoscopy
deficit
dialysis
diarrhea
diffuse
dilatation
disposition
distal
distention
diverticulum
dysuria
edema
elective
end-stage
endoscopic
enlargement
Ex-Lax
extremities
fatigue
flank (noun)
focal tenderness
fungal

glucose
gm
gross examination
guaiac
heart gallop
heart rub
HEENT
hematocrit
hematuria
heme
hemoglobin
hydrochlorothiazide
hydronephrosis
hydroureter
hypertrophy
hypoglycemia
hysterectomy
incontinence
IVP (intravenous pyelogram)
JV (jugular venous)
kidney
KUB (kidneys, ureters, bladder)
LDH
malaise
Marshall test
McBurney's point
mg
Minipress
murmur
nausea
needle suspension
nephrolithiasis
nephrologist
neurological
nocturia
nontender
obesity
obstructive
organomegaly
oriented x 3
P&A (percussion and auscultation)
pallor
palpable
periodic
phosphorus
postvoid residual
potassium
prophylactic coverage

prostate, prostatic
proximal
q.a.m.
q.i.d.
quadrant
radiate
radiopaque
reactive
rectocele
recurrent
renal failure
rhythm
segmented neutrophils
Septra DS
SGOT
SMA-20
sodium
sputum
stool
stress incontinence
sulfa
supple
symptom
TFTs (thyroid function
   tests)

triglycerides
trilobar
TURP (transurethral
   resection of prostate)
ultrasonography
unremarkable
uremia
ureter
urethral
urge incontinence
uric acid
urinalysis
urinary force
urinary hesitancy
urinary stream
urinary terminal dribbling
urinary urgency
urologic
UTI (urinary tract
   infection)
varices
vesical neck
vital signs
yeast infection

Sample Reports

Sample urology reports appear on the following pages, illustrating a variety of different formats.

Transcription Practice

After completing all the readings and exercises in Lesson 3, transcribe Tape 1B, Urology. Use both medical and English dictionaries and your Quick-Reference Word List at the back of this book as resource materials for finding words.

Proofread your transcribed documents carefully, listening to the dictation while you read your transcripts.

Transcribe (*NOT* retype) the same reports again without referring to your previous transcription attempt. Initially, you may need to transcribe some reports more than twice before you can produce an error-free document. Your ultimate goal is to produce an error-free document the first time.

BLOOPERS	
Incorrect	**Correct**
An undefended testicle.	An undescended testicle.
Some suggestion of impudency.	Some suggestion of impotency.
Exophthalmos of prostate, normal.	Examination of prostate, normal.

CHART NOTE

Patty Pashunt   June 1, 1993

SUBJECTIVE: This is a 24-year-old white married female who complains of urinary burning and frequency beginning approximately five days ago. She denies any prior urinary problems. She has had no chills, fever, flank pain, or hematuria. She has noted nocturia x 3 since the onset of her symptoms. She has had no nausea or abdominal pain. She denies vaginal discharge or itching. Last menstrual period began 17 days ago. She is on Demulen 1/35-28 for birth control but has taken no other medicines. She is sexually active in a stable and apparently exclusive marital relationship. Her general health is good, and she denies recent URI. She has never been pregnant.

OBJECTIVE: Temperature 98.6, pulse 72 and regular, blood pressure 116/80. The patient is alert and in no distress. Her skin is pale, warm, and dry. There is no costovertebral angle tenderness, and palpation of the abdomen indicates no masses or organomegaly. The bladder is not palpable or tender. On pelvic exam, there is no evidence of vulvar edema or erythema and no discharge. The cervix is clean and only scant mucoid material is seen in the vault. She had a negative (class 1) Pap smear about 8 months ago. Bimanual exam reveals a normal size uterus which is slightly retroflexed. The adnexal areas are normal. There are no masses or abnormal tenderness, and the rectal examination is negative.

A clean-voided urine shows 15 to 20 white blood cells per high-power field, 8 to 10 red cells, 4+ occult blood, 1+ protein, negative for sugar, pH 5.5.

ASSESSMENT: Acute cystitis.

PLAN:
1. Septra DS 1 b.i.d. x 7 days.
2. Pyridium 200 mg q.4-6h. p.r.n. burning.
3. Increase oral fluids.
4. I discussed the probable origin of her condition with the patient and advised her to make a practice of voiding immediately after intercourse in the future.
5. The patient is to report back in one week for repeat urinalysis and to see me and is to call in the day after tomorrow if she has any persisting symptoms.

ABG:hpi

Mitchell Twitchell   #987123456   Admitted 6/1/93   P. Harder, M.D.

HISTORY AND PHYSICAL EXAMINATION

HISTORY: This 43-year-old male was admitted through the emergency department with a history of less than one day of acute ureteral colic on the left side. The patient had an IVP in the emergency department earlier today which shows partial to complete obstruction of the left ureter at the ureterovesical junction with a large stone approximately 8 x 5 mm lodged at the UV junction. The patient has no other calcifications visible. The patient denies any previous history of urinary tract stones or other GU problems except for prostatitis a couple of years ago. The patient has no other significant medical problems.

PAST MEDICAL HISTORY: Otherwise negative.

ALLERGIES: None.

MEDICATIONS: None. Follows usual diet.

FAMILY HISTORY: No familial history of kidney stones or other significant hereditary disease.

PHYSICAL EXAM reveals a well-nourished, well-developed male in no acute distress.
HEAD & NECK: Eyes: Pupils equal, round, react to light. Ears, nose, and throat clear. Neck supple, no JV distention or bruit.
CHEST: Lungs clear to P&A.
HEART: Regular rhythm, no murmur.
ABDOMEN: Soft. Slight left CVA tenderness, slight left lower quadrant tenderness, no rebound.
GENITALIA: Within normal limits. Penis: Normal male.
EXTREMITIES: No cyanosis, clubbing, or edema.
NEUROLOGIC: Oriented x 3 with no gross deficits.

IMPRESSION: Left lower ureteral stone with obstruction.

RECOMMENDATION: Hydration, analgesia, observation, and if the stone does not pass within 72 hours or less, will probably recommend patient for ureteroscopy and stone basketing, and if needed, ultrasonic lithotripsy. If the stone cannot be mobilized downward, push-back and ESWL might be considered.

_____

PAUL HARDER, M.D.

PH:hpi
D: 6/1/93
T: 6/2/93

Mitchell Twitchell

#987123456

June 1, 1993

Medical 701B

CONSULTATION

HISTORY: Apparently this patient presented to the emergency department last night about midnight with excruciating left flank pain radiating down into the left groin and testicle, chills, nausea, vomiting, and slight urinary burning, all of about two hours' duration, and a stat urine showed 60 to 80 red cells. Apparently he was given Stadol 2 mg IM for analgesia and some IV fluids, and he had an emergency IVP run which showed a radiopaque stone measuring about 0.5 cm partially blocking the left ureter at a point about 3 cm below the UP junction. There was moderate hydronephrosis without appreciable dilatation of the caliceal system, and some dye was getting down into the distal ureter. I have reviewed these films, and they show normal urinary tract anatomy on the right and on the left, except as noted.

When I examined him about 10 a.m., he was still in considerable distress, although noticeably obtunded by a dose of Demerol given about one-half hour prior to my visit. He was sufficiently alert, however, to give a good clear history. Apparently this man has had two previous episodes of left-sided ureteral colic followed by spontaneous passage of stones, once while on military service in Turkey and once since then, but on neither occasion were the stones preserved for analysis.

His general health is good and he takes no medicine. He has never had a urinary tract infection. There is no known family history of renal lithiasis, gout, or bone or joint disease; however, he is adopted. He is 41 years of age, married, with two daughters, and is employed as a manager of a bowling alley.

EXAMINATION: Temperature is 99.2, pulse 100, blood pressure 150/80. Physical exam is quite benign except that he is pale, sweating, restless, and in considerable distress and tender at the left CVA and in the left upper quadrant over the kidney and ureter. External genital exam is unremarkable. I did not attempt to do a rectal exam. He has an IV running, even though he is now taking oral fluids and he is not nauseated. He is voiding painlessly, and his urine is being strained. I did not see his urine, but according to the patient and the attendant, it is not grossly bloody.

DIAGNOSIS: Left ureterolithiasis with partial ureteral obstruction and hydronephrosis.

RECOMMENDATIONS:
1. Continue analgesia and hydration.
2. Continue straining urine and preserve any solid material passed for chemical analysis.
3. Clean-voided midstream urine for culture and sensitivity.
4. After this has been obtained, start Cipro 500 mg q.12h. orally.

(Continued on page 2)

Mitchell Twitchell

#987123456

June 1, 1993

Page 2

CONSULTATION

RECOMMENDATIONS (continued)

5. He is now about 12 hours post onset of symptoms, but there is still a good statistical chance that he will pass his stone spontaneously. We are going to get another IVP at 4 p.m., and if he is still obstructed, I think we had better attempt to bring this stone down with a snare before he gets enough local edema to obstruct completely or gets into trouble with a red-hot ascending pyelonephritis.
6. In any event, he needs a biochemical diagnosis of his problem, and depending on that, he may need dietary or drug prophylaxis against future calculus disease.

Thank you for the privilege of collaborating in the care of this patient.

_____

MILTON ROCKHARD, M.D.

MR:hpi
d:6/1/93
t: 6/2/93

DATE OF SURGERY:	June 4, 1993
PREOPERATIVE DIAGNOSIS:	Recurrent bladder neck obstruction.
POSTOPERATIVE DIAGNOSIS:	Same.
TITLE OF OPERATION:	Cystoscopy and transurethral resection of the prostate.

TECHNIQUE: Upon administration of satisfactory spinal anesthesia, the patient was placed on the cystoscopy table in the lithotomy position. The external genitalia were prepped and draped in the usual manner for endoscopy. The #24 Wappler instrument was passed under direct vision, revealing a normal distal urethra. There is no evidence of stricture or other localized lesion. As one enters into the prostatic urethra, he has a normal-appearing verumontanum. There is a small apical growth on the patient's left side, but this is not impressive. He has a very large, obstructing-appearing lobe coming in from the right side, mainly superiorly, with only a relatively small amount near the floor. As one enters the prostatic urethra, there is a slightly scarred bladder neck contracture apparent; however, it is of wide caliber and would not be considered significant. The instrument was then entered into the bladder and again about 1000 cc of fluid was removed. The bladder was then irrigated, and cystoscopy was done with both right-angle and Foroblique lens systems. The main thing one sees here is a heavily trabeculated bladder, multiple bands and ridges, no true diverticulum. No stones are identified. There is no evidence of inflammation or tumor.

At this point, the McCarthy Storz Foroblique resectoscope sheath was introduced, size 28 in character, after accepting comfortably 28 and 30 van Buren sounds. A standard transurethral resection of the prostate was done. The ureteral orifices sat nicely back from the bladder neck, and I instilled indigo carmine just for security. Once the bladder neck was cut down on the bladder side, I then started at 11 and subsequently 1 o'clock cutting lateral lobe tissue out bilaterally and then cut the tissue as it fell in. Because of his decompensating bladder, I did a fairly radical and deep transurethral resection of the capsule throughout. I did stay within the verumontanum, but took out apical lobes as safely as I could. At the end of the resection, there was some venous bleeding but no evidence of arterial bleeding. The prostatic urethra was wide open. All chips were then irrigated from the bladder, and a 26 three-way Foley inserted. It was inflated to 55 cc. We observed him for venous bleeding; this stopped almost immediately and remained clear. At that point, he was transferred to the recovery room with vital signs stable, in good general condition.

_____

H. R. PILES, M.D.

HRP:hpi
d: 6/4/93
t: 6/5/93

DESERT MEDICAL CENTER
Joshua Tree, California 90000

OPERATIVE REPORT

Samuel Senn

#082741

Surgery 400-C

Lesson 4. Urology

Learning Objectives

Medical

- Describe eight routes of administration of drugs.
- Discuss the purpose and technique involved in performing common urologic laboratory tests and surgical procedures.
- Describe the procedures done in a urinalysis.
- Given a cross-section illustration of the male reproductive tract, memorize the anatomic structures.
- Define common urologic abbreviations.
- Differentiate between various urologic homonyms and sound-alike terms.
- Differentiate between the preferred and alternative spellings of medical words.
- Demonstrate the correct plural formation of Latin nouns.

Fundamentals

- Discuss two important points in accepting and dispensing criticism.
- List two reasons why medical transcriptionists will not be replaced by technology.
- Describe the ways in which the medical transcriptionist must edit mispronunciations, slips of tongue, malapropisms, and other dictating errors.

Practice

- Accurately transcribe authentic physician dictation from the specialty of urology and urologic surgery.

A Closer Look

Criticism

by Marcy Diehl, BVE, CMT, CMA-A

Criticism first became a subject for conversation in my life about 25 years ago when I went to work for a prominent thoracic and cardiovascular surgeon. During the course of the interview, he asked me if I were able to take criticism gracefully. Well, I was stumped. No one had ever asked before; they had just handed it out, and I really didn't know how gracefully I had accepted what I had had so far. It depended on who was dishing it out, I guess.

I thought about my response, worrying that my prospective job somehow hinged on what I had to say one way or the other. I felt he would have liked for me to say something like ''Oh, I love criticism,'' or even ''I never need it!'' Evidently I gave the right answer, however (he did hire me), when I replied, ''Well, I guess we'll have to find out, won't we?'' This answer implied to him that he would hire me and that we would both see how his criticism and my acceptance of it went along.

But I was now on the alert. I was forewarned that criticism was, in fact, a big possibility, and I worked very hard against the day when ''we'' would find out how gracefully I could accept it. I really didn't know where it would come from. There were a lot of possibilities; the day seemed fraught with them.

That was just the first day.

By the second day, I found out. That was the day my first transcripts were returned. Large permanent blue-black ink circles covered the many carefully prepared documents. It was hard to be graceful when I looked at the ruination of a half-day's labors (actually, half a night, too, as I had spent long hours at home researching unfamiliar words).

We had weeks of that, and I was getting discouraged; still graceful, I presume, but discouraged. The errors were becoming fewer and fewer, but that didn't seem to help much, since I wanted them to disappear. It was harder and harder to face up to them somehow, now that I was feeling more secure in the job. Grace was wearing thin. He never said anything. I never said anything. I just retyped. A lot.

Now two things happened. The surgeon's wife came into the office on Saturday morning when he proofread and busily marked up my work. She watched, appalled. Monday morning shortly after I arrived for work, she called "to see how you're taking it." "Fine," I said. She was relieved, and reported that she had talked to him about it, feeling that he had been too harsh. "Well, she won't learn if I don't teach her, and she's worth teaching."

I learned about grace that day. He took his precious time to teach and to help me. He had a B.S. in journalism and knew his Greek and Latin roots to a fine degree as well. I was pretty much humbled by his constant criticism, his love of perfection, and his belief in my potential for growth.

All of our lives we are both subjected to and the dispensers of criticism. If we can remember to accept it with the spirit in which it is given, realizing it took some time to critique our performance and that it was done because of our ultimate potential, we then must accept it not only with grace but with thanks.

Secondly, we must try to remember to give our criticism only with graciousness, knowing that we can help someone in whom we see the potential for personal or professional betterment, and not criticize to showcase our own skills. If we cannot criticize fairly, with love and in private, then we need to withhold it.

This is a lifelong relationship—us and criticism. We never should feel we have outgrown the need. If we protect ourselves by not doing anything new anymore, sticking to only what we do perfectly, then we will no longer grow in grace and wisdom.

Tape Dancing

by Judith Marshall, MA, CMT

Whenever medical transcriptionists get together and talk about our work, we often chat about "that rhythm," those perfect blends of great physicians, mellifluous tones, equipment without snaps and crackles in the headset and without sticky keys and broken

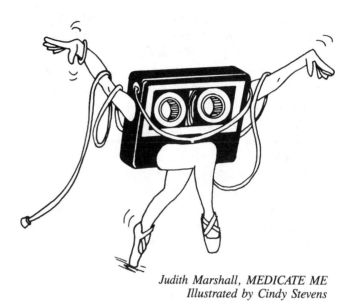

Judith Marshall, MEDICATE ME
Illustrated by Cindy Stevens

pedals—that rhythm. When every word you hear, you know, when every spelling is there in your head or at your fingertips in the proper reference source—whizzing along, getting that upbeat feeling, *that* rhythm. Each of us has felt it. Fortissimo, pianissimo, largo or molto vivace, on it goes.

Perhaps a romantic point of view, but why not? There is such a paucity of knowledge about what we do and how we do it that most of the emphasis has been on that four-letter word, TYPE.

Read any Sunday's *Boston Globe* in the Want Ad section and there it is, "Medical Transcriptionist Wanted. Must be able to type 60 wpm and have some knowledge of medical terminology." Where's the romance in that?

In movies, books, or television, have you ever seen the profession represented? In ten years of watching General Hospital, the closest I ever got was Dr. Steve asking Jessie for the chart. In the popular series starring Jack Klugman, we see Quincy poised over the deceased and dictating into an overhead microphone, but that is it. Has Johnny Carson ever interviewed a medical transcriptionist?

So where's the music? It's all in our perspective. It's how *we* view it first. A mining expedition? A treasure hunt each day in an ocean of words? A challenge? Do your days pass in a blur of disco-like beat or hum along in ballad form? It doesn't matter. What matters are the voices, whether they are staccato or monumentally dull-pitched. The voices form the very fabric of what we do.

We have to be alert and oriented x 3 even when the dictating physician isn't. And typing speed, while nice to possess, isn't the answer. All the technology in the world isn't going to make that medicolegal document correct—only you can do that with your expertise.

Ah, technology, the boon and bane of all of our lives. Personally I have a great respect and probably an equal amount of fear related to technology. We have all heard of the Bell Laboratory proclamations from time to time on the new equipment which will transcribe automatically from the spoken word.

In the world of advertising exists a machine of which Vance Packard wrote in *The New and Still Hidden Persuaders:* "There are also machines that offer voice-pitch analysis. First, our normal voices are taped and then our voices while commenting on an ad or product. A computer reports whether we are offering lip service, a polite lie or a firm opinion."

In twenty years, they say, the medical transcriptionist will go the way of the elevator operator and the buggy whip salesman. Nonsense. Hogwash. T'aint so.

We don't just know medical terminology. We understand it. We can sling around "medicalese" or "medicant" any old time, and in our own way we regulate and stimulate that language, for it is indeed a language. We are in the key positions. We break the sound barrier every day. We have a surgical precision all our own, a knife-like wit at times, and our own scalpel-sharp intelligence. We have sensitivity, humor, a sense of responsibility and ethics, and most importantly, we have excellence.

We strive for excellence daily in a society which does not fire the bad worker and does not fail the bad student. Yes, we strive for excellence in communication. We are the significant others. We are those small initials.

When their participles are dangling, we are there to prop them up. We clip and tidy and prune in a forest of gerunds and adjectives and adverbs and abbreviations and we toil mightily in the gardens of nomenclature.

We are the people who listen intently—not just hear, but listen. If the eyes are the mirror of the soul, so are the voices, and we carry those voiceprints in our minds, attuned to the pauses, the idiosyncratic nuances.

So, at times, when we all suffer from the methylene blues, on those days when life is just one rewind, during those weeks when we do not pass GO and we definitely do not collect $200, we can take renewed encouragement in our profession.

Richard Blue, of Sunshine Unlimited, spoke in January of 1981 in Framingham, Massachusetts. He said, "Successful people do what other people don't

want to do." What could we personally do besides attend professional meetings for continuing medical education? A myriad of possibilities. But we do. Because we are professional and because we want to learn. We have already paid our dues.

Like Rumpelstilskin who spun gold out of straw, we make beautiful music from the spoken word. Oh, we do indeed **tape dance,** and the sweetest sounds we sometimes hear are "end of dictation, thank you."

Dictation and Transcription: Adventures in Thought Transference

Part 3

by John H. Dirckx, M.D.

In other words. Although nearly everyone takes it for granted that the kinds of editing I have been discussing thus far are part of the transcription process, many question the propriety of the transcriptionist's judging and altering the factual content of a dictation, correcting the dictator's grammar and syntax, and touching up the style to improve clarity and coherence. Yet such adjustments are manifestly necessary, not only in dictation by non-native speakers of English but in the vast majority of all dictations.

By choosing to dictate a document rather than write it out, the dictator not only sidesteps many of the mechanical tasks associated with composition but implicitly delegates these tasks to the transcriptionist. No dictators have such perfect powers of concentration that they never accidentally repeat themselves, never inadvertently substitute one word for another, never leave a sentence unfinished. Sooner or later the most alert and cautious dictator makes each of these mistakes, and others besides.

Clearly these normal human lapses ought not to be reproduced in the transcript, and just as clearly the duty of identifying and correcting them devolves on the transcriptionist. The following survey of errors in dictation and remedies applied by the transcriptionist includes a number of authentic examples taken from The SUM Program for Training Medical Transcriptionists, published by Health Professions Institute.

Just as mispronounced words and names must be spelled correctly by the transcriptionist, erroneous spellings supplied by the dictator must be ignored. (It is my impression, based on a review of all the tapes in The SUM Program, that about 25% of the spellings supplied by dictators for technical terms and eponyms are wrong.)

From time to time everyone says one word when another is intended. These so-called slips of the tongue are actually, of course, slips of the mind. Often a "wrong" word is conceptually related to the word it replaces: "Examination of the carotid [coronary] arteries confirmed the presence of complete occlusion of the right coronary artery." A relevant word may slip in by anticipation and displace another word: "The staples [skin] of the chest was also closed with staples."

When the intrusive word sounds something like the right one, it is called a malapropism (after Mrs. Malaprop, a character in an eighteenth-century comedy by Sheridan). Some malapropisms evidently result from momentary lapses: *pericardial infusion* (for *effusion*). Others are permanent features of the dictator's vocabulary, as was the case with Mrs. Malaprop: *melanotic* (for *melenic*) *stools*; *with regards* (for *regard*) *to*.

Numerous other kinds of verbal errors can creep into a dictation, including the use of illegitimate words ("transversing [traversing] the toe at the level of the interphalangeal joint"; "a Kelly forcep" [forceps]), incorrect medical Latin ("genu varus [varum]"; "tensor fascia lata [fasciae latae]"), irrational jargon ("normal axis deviation [normal axis]"), and inadvertent redundancies ("postoperatively he had an uneventful postop course"; "the right shoulder shows a well-healed four-inch scar over the anterior aspect of the right shoulder").

One of the medical transcriptionist's greatest challenges is dealing correctly with slang terms used by dictators. These terms vary in propriety; some may be left in the record while others must be replaced with more formal terminology. The transcriptionist must therefore not only distinguish the acceptable from the inappropriate but also understand the latter and be able to supply suitable alternatives.

The great majority of slang terms requiring "translation" are just shortened forms of technical words, and the transcriptionist's role is simply to expand them to their normal form: *lytes* to *electrolytes, H and H* to *hemoglobin and hematocrit, V tach* to *ventricular tachycardia, nitro* to *nitroglycerin, regurge* to *regurgitation*. Similarly, in the interests of clarity the transcriptionist must often elaborate on a dictated laconism such as the following: "The patient had stable gases on 50% face mask" (on 50% oxygen by face mask).

Among the few vestiges of grammatical inflection in modern English are changes in the form of nouns and verbs to signify whether they are singular or plural:

one stitch, two stiches; he stitches, they stitch. Not surprisingly, most of the purely grammatical errors committed by dictators are faults of subject-verb agreement. Such errors are common in everyday speech and even writing. As the mind constructs a sentence phrase by phrase, grammatical forms are apt to be selected on the basis of ideas rather than of words. Often a singular noun is used when the speaker is actually "thinking plural" and goes on to use a plural verb: "The right and left lung (lungs) are congested." "No definite site of his occult GI bleeding were (was) identified."

In a long or inverted clause or sentence, the true subject may be lost sight of and the verb may be made to agree with the wrong noun or pronoun, or with some idea not expressed: "Examination of sections of both right and left lungs shows severe vascular congestion but are (is) otherwise unremarkable." "There is (are) demonstrated fractures of the second, third, and fourth ribs."

As we move out of the realm of pure grammar and into that of style, the standards of correctness become less clear-cut and the remedies applied by the transcriptionist less automatic. Yet even here it should be obvious that hopeless syntactic jumbles must somehow be resolved, and grossly inelegant phrasing amended.

A permanent medical document dictated by one professional and transcribed by another is expected to conform to certain norms of precision, clarity, coherence, and taste. Where the dictator's competence or diligence falls short, the transcriptionist must supply the deficiency. Again the task requires a broad base of knowledge about the subject of the dictation and considerable skill in composition and editing. Most transcriptionists perform this operation so deftly and unobtrusively that the majority of dictators never even suspect that their dictation has undergone revision (or that it needed it).

A matter of form. The third level at which the transcriptionist exercises a discriminating and editorial function is that of format or layout, including punctuation and consistency in the use of abbreviations, numerals, and units of measure. In general the transcriptionist's decisions on these points are unrelated to anything heard in the dictation. It is true that dictators often supply directions for formatting and punctuation, but many of these (such as calling each new line a "paragraph" or separating complete sentences with a "comma") must simply be ignored by the transcriptionist. Other directions, while not actually incorrect, may violate the canons of English composition or introduce inconsistencies.

Armed with basic typewriting skills and a knowledge of the rules of punctuation, the transcriptionist creates the format of a report and supplies commas and periods as needed in the very act of transcribing the dictation. Numerals and units of measure are typed according to established conventions and in consistent fashion regardless of how they occur in the dictation. Thus "six tenths" becomes *0.6* and "four and a half milliliters" becomes *4.5 ml (mL)*.

No one can master the lore of a craft so perfectly as never to be at a loss for a word, a meaning, a rule, a spelling. A crucial requirement for the practice of most professions is knowing where to look up what one doesn't remember or can't understand. The medical transcriptionist depends heavily on dictionaries, drug references, word books, and personal files or notebooks to supply authoritative answers to questions raised by the dictation.

But not every ambiguity and perplexity can be resolved by recourse to reference books or by consultation with associates. Repeated hearings may not suffice to enlighten the transcriptionist as to whether an enigmatic sound is a word or a hiccup. Even with due consideration of the context, some homophones will remain equally probable. "Kay see ell" may be either the chemical formula KCl or the drug name Kay Ciel, which is meant to sound exactly like it, and does. In cases such as this the transcriptionist does not make a stab in the dark but leaves a blank for the dictator to complete with the appropriate material.

My purpose in discussing various linguistic and psychological dimensions of the dictation-transcription process has not been to swamp the reader in complexities but to give some notion of the extent to which transcription differs from mere phonetic rendering of what is said by the dictator. Just as it is possible to go through life using language constantly without ever gaining much insight into phonetics or semantics, it is possible to learn and practice so exacting a profession as medical transcription without ever appreciating fully the complexity of the field.

While it is all too easy for transcriptionists and dictators alike to take it for granted that transcription is "writing down what somebody said," it should be evident from my remarks that it is only by penetrating and sharing the dictator's thoughts that the transcriptionist can produce an accurate and otherwise fully satisfactory transcript.

Fuller awareness of the breadth, intricacy, and difficulty of medical transcription should heighten the respect of dictators and others outside the profession for those who practice it. Transcriptionists themselves can be proud of their hard-won and socially valuable competence in a field demanding both technical and intellectual virtuosity.

Medical Readings

Pharmacology: Routes of Administration

There are various routes of drug administration. Some drugs are approved for use via more than one route and are manufactured in different forms appropriate for those different routes. Each route of administration has distinct advantages and disadvantages as discussed below. A drug given by one route will be therapeutic; given by another route, it may be ineffective, harmful, or even fatal.

1. **Oral.** The oral route is the most convenient route of administration and the most commonly used. Tablets, capsules, and liquids are all given orally. Even patients who have difficulty swallowing a tablet or capsule can usually take the liquid form of a drug without problems. Infants are given drugs in a liquid form mixed with a small amount of formula in a nipple. Even unconscious patients can be given liquid medication through a nasogastric (NG) tube. The oral route is routinely abbreviated as *PO* or *p.o.* (Latin for *per os,* meaning *through the mouth).*

There are some disadvantages of the oral route, however. Some drugs, most particularly certain penicillins, are inactivated by stomach acid and cannot be given orally. After oral administration, some drugs are so quickly metabolized by the liver as they pass through the portal circulation that a therapeutic blood level cannot be achieved in the systemic circulation. Therefore, these drugs are given intravenously (example: lidocaine [Xylocaine] for cardiac arrhythmias). Some drugs cannot be taken with certain foods and drinks as they either combine chemically to form an insoluble complex or interact to produce adverse side effects (example: tetracycline cannot be taken with dairy products).

2. **Sublingual.** Sublingual administration involves placing the drug (usually in a tablet form) under the tongue and allowing it to slowly dissolve. The tablet is not swallowed (this would then become oral administration). The drug is absorbed quickly through oral mucous membranes and into the large blood vessels under the tongue. The sublingual route provides a faster

therapeutic effect than the oral route (example: nitroglycerin tablets or spray for treating angina attacks).

3. **Rectal.** Absorption of a drug via the rectal route of administration is slow and often unpredictable. This route is reserved for certain clinical situations, such as when the patient is vomiting and unable to take medications which cannot be given by injection (example: Tylenol suppositories). The exception to this is when drugs are administered rectally to relieve constipation or treat hemorrhoids.

4. **Vaginal.** The vaginal route is used to treat vaginal infections and vaginitis by using creams and suppositories (examples: Monistat suppositories, Premarin vaginal cream). Over-the-counter contraceptive foams are inserted vaginally as well.

5. **Topical.** When a drug is applied directly to the skin or to the mucous membranes of the eye, ear, nose, or mouth, it is administered via the topical route. The effects of the drug are generally local, not systemic (throughout the body) (examples: bacitracin antibiotic ointment, Sudafed nasal decongestant spray, Timoptic eye drops for glaucoma).

Sites of topical administration are abbreviated as follows:

Abbrev.	Latin Meaning	Medical Meaning
A.D.	*auris dextra*	right ear
A.S.	*auris sinistra*	left ear
A.U.	*auris utraque*	each ear
O.D.	*oculus dexter*	right eye
O.S.	*oculus sinister*	left eye
O.U.	*oculus uterque*	each eye

6. **Transdermal.** This relatively new route of administration differs from the topical route in that the drug is applied to the skin via physical delivery through a porous membrane, with the therapeutic effects felt systemically, not just at the site of administration. Drugs delivered by the transdermal route are usually manufactured in the form of a patch. Worn on the skin, the patch releases the drug slowly over a 24-hour period, providing sustained therapeutic blood levels (example: Transderm-Nitro for prevention of angina).

7. **Inhalation.** This route of administration involves the inhaling of a drug in a gas or liquid form. The drug is absorbed through the alveoli of the lungs (examples: nitrous oxide, a general anesthetic; albuterol [Proventil], a bronchodilator).

8. **Parenteral.** Parenteral is a general term, taken from the Greek words *para* and *enteron,* which literally mean *apart from the intestine.* Technically, *parenteral* means all routes of administration other than by mouth; but in clinical usage, parenteral commonly includes just the following routes of administration: intradermal, subcutaneous, intramuscular, intravenous, and the other less frequently used routes of intra-arterial and intrathecal.

Intradermal administration involves the injection of a liquid into the dermis, the layer of skin just below the epidermis. The epidermis itself is less than 1/20 of an inch thick; therefore, when an intradermal injection is correctly positioned, the tip of the needle is still plainly visible through the skin (example: Mantoux test for tuberculosis).

Subcutaneous administration involves the injection of liquid into the subcutaneous tissues, the fatty layer of tissue just under the dermis of the skin but above the muscle layer (example: insulin, heparin, allergy shots). There are few blood vessels in this layer, so drugs are absorbed more slowly than when given by intramuscular injection. Diabetics who inject insulin utilize approximately 10-12 different areas on the upper arm, thigh, and abdomen to rotate the site of daily subcutaneous insulin injections. The term *subcutaneous* is abbreviated in various ways as *subQ, SQ,* and *subcu*; there is no one official abbreviation.

Intramuscular (abbreviated *I.M.* or *IM*) administration involves the injection of a liquid into the **belly** (area of greatest mass) of a large muscle. The large muscles of the body are well supplied with blood vessels, and drugs are absorbed more quickly than following subcutaneous injection. There are only five intramuscular injection sites which can be used; other sites invite damage to adjacent nerves and blood vessels.

- Deltoid, located on the upper arm, lateral aspect.
- Vastus lateralis, located on the midthigh, lateral aspect.
- Rectus femoris, located on the midthigh, anterior aspect.
- Ventrogluteal, located on the side of the hip over the gluteus muscle, between the anterior superior and posterior superior spines of the iliac crest.
- Dorsogluteal, located over the gluteus minimus and edge of the gluteus maximus muscles in the upper outer quadrant of each buttock.

Some drugs cannot be given by intramuscular injection because they are not water soluble (example: Valium, Librium).

Examples of drugs given intramuscularly: Demerol for pain; vitamin B_{12} for pernicious anemia; Garamycin for bacterial infections.

Intravenous (abbreviated *I.V.* or *IV*) administration of a drug involves the injection of a liquid directly into a vein and may be done in one of three ways. The injection of a single dose of a drug (**bolus**) may be given through a **port** (rubber stopper) into an existing intravenous (I.V.) line. This is often referred to as **I.V. push** because the drug is manually pushed into the I.V. line in a very short period of time. A drug may also be mixed with the fluid in an I.V. bag or bottle and administered continuously over several hours. This is known as **I.V. drip.** A drug may also be mixed in a very small I.V. bag or bottle and administered over an hour or less by I.V. drip. This small secondary I.V. bag or bottle is connected through tubing to a port in the existing primary I.V. line. This method is known as **I.V. piggyback** administration.

Laboratory Examination of Urine

by John H. Dirckx, M.D.

The history of clinical pathology began with the observation that the urine and stools of sick persons are often abnormal. Pathologic changes in the urine and stool are mentioned frequently in the works of Hippocrates and Galen. Medieval physicians often limited their diagnostic investigations to feeling the patient's pulse and holding a flask of urine up to the light.

In the modern clinical laboratory, microscopic examination and chemical analysis of urine and stool specimens can yield information not only about the excretory and digestive systems but also about other body systems, water and acid-base balance, nutrition, and the presence of toxic substances. A major advantage of urine and stool examinations is that, under ordinary circumstances, both of these materials are readily available, and obtaining specimens calls for no invasive procedures or elaborate equipment.

For most of the tests done in the **urinology** laboratory, the preferred specimen is 60 to 90 mL of freshly voided urine. Although a random specimen is usually suitable, a **first-voided specimen** (the first urine passed after arising in the morning) may be more satisfactory in testing for trace substances because it is usually more concentrated.

A **clean-voided specimen** (clean catch) is one obtained after cleansing of the area around the urethral meatus (usually with liquid soap and cotton balls) to prevent contamination of the specimen with material from outside the urinary tract.

A **midstream specimen** is one that contains neither the first nor the last portion of urine passed. It is obtained by introducing a specimen container into the urine stream after voiding has begun and removing it before voiding ceases. The purpose of this procedure is to obtain as pure as possible a sample of bladder urine, with minimal admixture of cells or other material from the urethra.

A **catheterized specimen** is obtained by urethral catheter (less often by suprapubic needle puncture of the bladder), either because the patient cannot void or to prevent contamination of the specimen. A **24-hour urine specimen** consists of all the urine passed by the patient during a 24-hour period.

A urine specimen is usually collected in a clean, dry bottle or cup of glass, plastic, or waxed or plasticized paper. The container need not be sterile except for bacteriologic work. Examination of urine is carried out as soon as possible after the specimen is obtained because blood cells in urine rupture early and bacterial growth in a standing specimen may alter its chemical composition. When a delay is expected, the specimen is refrigerated. A one- or two-gallon jug is used to collect a 24-hour urine specimen. The jug may be kept on ice during the collection period, and one of several preservatives may be placed in the jug before collection begins.

The principal diagnostic procedure in urinology is the **urinalysis,** a set of routine physical and chemical examinations. In most laboratories, the urinalysis includes direct observation of the specimen for color, turbidity, and other obvious characteristics; determination of specific gravity; microscopic examination of sediment for cells, crystals, and other formed elements; determination of pH; and chemical testing for glucose, protein, occult blood, and perhaps bilirubin and acetone.

Variations in color and clarity of urine usually reflect variations in concentration of solutes, including pigment. Because the daily solute load is fairly constant, changes in concentration are nearly always due to changes in volume of water excreted. Turbidity (cloudiness) may be due to the presence of phosphates, which are insoluble in alkaline urine. A smoky brown color ("Coca-Cola urine") often indicates the presence of hemolyzed blood. Color changes may be due to abnormal waste products (bilirubin, porphyrins), drugs (methylene blue, phenazopyridine), or pigments from foods (beets, blackberries). Mucus shreds, fragments of tissue, or calcareous material may be grossly evident in the specimen.

Microscopic examination of the urine is usually preceded by centrifugation of the specimen to concentrate any cells or other formed elements present. A polychrome stain such as the Sternheimer-Malbin stain (crystal violet and safranin in ethanol) may be added to the sediment to enhance the distinctive features of various cells, but is not essential. Microscopic examination is carried out on a small volume of fluid urine placed on a slide and covered with a cover slip. Dried smears of urine are not ordinarily suitable for examination.

Formed elements frequently found in urine are red blood cells, white blood cells, casts, crystals, bacteria, epithelial cells, and amorphous sediment. Cell counts are recorded as cells per high-power field, obtained as an average after examination and counting of several fields. A small number of red and white blood cells are present in normal urine.

A finding of more than 1 or 2 **red blood cells** per high-power field (RBC/hpf), called microscopic hematuria, indicates either bleeding in some part of the excretory system or contamination of the specimen with blood, possibly menstrual. Hematuria occurs in acute glomerulonephritis, urolithiasis, hemorrhagic diseases, infarction of the kidney, tuberculosis of the kidney, benign or malignant tumors of any part of the urinary tract, and many cases of simple cystitis. The presence of more than 1 or 2 **white blood cells** per high-power field (WBC/hpf), known as pyuria, usually indicates infection in some part of the urinary tract.

Casts are microscopic cylindrical bodies that have been formed by concretion of cells or insoluble material within renal tubules and subsequently excreted in the urine. Casts are always abnormal. They are reported as the number counted per low-power field. Hyaline and waxy casts are homogeneous casts varying in refractility. They consist of coagulated protein and are found in conditions associated with leakage of protein through glomeruli: nephritis, nephrotic syndrome (including lupus nephrosis and Kimmelstiel-Wilson disease), toxemia, and congestive heart failure. Granular casts are formed by aggregation of red or white blood cells or both in renal tubules and occur in many of the same conditions as hyaline and waxy casts.

A variety of **crystals** may be found on microscopic examination of the urine. Their chemical composition can usually be deduced from their shape. Crystals of uric acid, cystine, calcium oxalate, and triple phosphate may appear in the urine of persons who excrete abnormal quantities of these materials and are subject to stone formation. **Bacteria** in significant numbers in a freshly voided specimen (bacteriuria, bacilluria) suggest urinary tract infection. Some squamous **epithelial cells** (squames) are often found in urine and have little

significance. **Amorphous sediment** is a general term for ill-defined solid material seen on microscopic examination of urine. It consists of chemical and cellular debris and is of no diagnostic importance.

Routine chemical testing of urine is usually performed with a "dipstick," a commercially produced strip of plastic or paper bearing a series of dots or squares of reagent, each designed to assess a specific chemical property of urine. The dipstick is immersed briefly in the urine and the test squares are observed for color changes. These tests are semiquantitative and are read by comparing the degree of color change in each square with an appropriate color chart. Results of dipstick tests other than pH are reported as either positive on a scale of 1 to 4 (1+, 2+, 3+, 4+) or negative.

The **pH** of urine (traditionally called the "reaction") is normally about 5.5. The urine may be alkaline (pH 8) in vegetarians and in persons with urinary tract infection due to urease-producing organisms such as *Proteus*, which split urinary urea to ammonia in the bladder.

The presence of **protein** in the urine (proteinuria) is usually due to leakage of albumin from the glomeruli. Hence it is often termed albuminuria, even though routine tests for protein in urine do not distinguish which proteins are present. Protein loss from the kidney occurs in glomerulonephritis, nephrotic syndrome, renal infarction, fever, and toxemia. In addition, most chemical tests for protein are positive in the presence of hematuria or pyuria.

Normally all of the plasma glucose that appears in glomerular filtrate is reabsorbed in the renal tubules. The detection of **glucose** in the urine (glycosuria) generally indicates an abnormal elevation of plasma glucose. The renal threshold for glucose is about 180 mg/dL. That means that at plasma levels above 180 mg/dL, more glucose appears in glomerular filtrate than can be reabsorbed by the tubules. Glycosuria is a cardinal finding in diabetes mellitus. It also occurs after rapid absorption of dietary glucose (alimentary glycosuria) and in some persons with abnormally low renal thresholds for glucose (renal glycosuria).

Occult blood refers to blood present in insufficient quantity to alter the color of the urine. A positive test for occult blood has generally the same significance as the finding of red blood cells in urine. **Acetone** and other ketones appear in the urine in diabetes mellitus with acidosis, in starvation, thyrotoxicosis, and high fever. Only bilirubin that has been conjugated with glucuronic acid is soluble in water. Hence the appearance of **bilirubin** in the urine (bilirubinuria, choluria) is noted in obstructive jaundice, in which conjugated bilirubin enters the blood stream from bile, but not in jaundice due to hemolysis or liver disease, in which only unconjugated bilirubin is elevated in the plasma.

Laboratory: Urinary Tests and Procedures

17-ketosteroids   Urinary breakdown products of adrenal cortical hormones, increased in certain disorders of the adrenal gland.

24-hour creatinine clearance   See *creatinine clearance, 24-hour.*

24-hour urine collection   See *urine, 24-hour.*

5-HIAA (5-hydroxyindoleacetic acid), urinary   The major urinary breakdown product of serotonin, increased in carcinoid syndrome.

acetone, urinary   Acetone is the principal serum ketone. Acetone in urine can be detected in a urinalysis or with a urinary dipstick. Small amounts are found in starvation and other abnormal metabolic states, larger amounts in uncontrolled diabetes mellitus. See also *ketones, urinary.*

acid phosphatase   An enzyme whose level in the serum is often increased in prostatic carcinoma.

amorphous sediment   Unformed and generally insignificant debris seen in a urine specimen under microscopic examination.

BUN (blood urea nitrogen)   The serum level of urea nitrogen, a waste product of protein metabolism. Normal BUN is 10 to 20 mg/dL. Elevation indicates impairment of kidney function. The abbreviation *BUN* does not need to be translated in medical reports.

casts   Cylindrical masses found on microscopic examination of the urine. They are formed by the aggregation of cells or coagulation of abnormal materials in renal tubules, from which they take their shape. Casts are always abnormal. Types of casts: hyaline, granular, waxy.

catheterization   Passage of a flexible tube or catheter up the urethra into the bladder to remove urine. Common catheters include a red rubber Robinson catheter (which is withdrawn after the bladder is drained) and a Foley catheter (which has an inflatable balloon at the tip, keeping the catheter in the bladder and allowing it to continuously drain urine).

Chemstrip GK   A dipstick used to measure glucose and acetone.

Chemstrip 5   A dipstick used to test urine for blood, glucose, acetone, and protein, and to determine pH.

creatinine clearance, 24-hour   A measure of kidney function, calculated from the serum creatinine level and the amount of creatinine excreted in the urine in 24 hours. Do not confuse *creatinine* with *creatine.*

cystoscopy   Procedure for examining the urethra and internal structures of the bladder using a hollow, lighted scope (cystoscope).

dialysis   The process of removing waste products from the blood when the kidneys are unable to do so. Hemodialysis removes the waste by passing the patient's blood directly through an artificial kidney machine. Peritoneal dialysis introduces fluid into the abdomen through a catheter. This fluid uses osmosis to draw waste from capillaries in the peritoneal cavity. The fluid or dialysate containing the waste products is then removed via the catheter.

dipstick   A commercially produced strip of plastic or paper bearing one or a series of pads of reagent, each of which is designed to test for a specific substance in urine or blood. After exposure to the specimen, any color changes in reagents are interpreted by comparison with a standard chart. Results are usually reported as either negative or positive on a roughly quantitative scale from 1 to 4 (1+, 2+, and so on).

E. coli (*Escherichia coli*)   A gram-negative bacterium normally found in the intestine, responsible for most urinary tract infections. Some strains may cause diarrheal disease. *E. coli* is usually the form dictated and does not need to be translated in medical reports.

electrolytes, urinary   Sodium, potassium, and chloride ions in the urine. Determination of their concentration may help to explain abnormalities of serum electrolytes due to renal or metabolic disease.

enterococcus   A streptococcus normally found in the intestine and sometimes responsible for urinary tract infections.

glucose, urinary   See *glycosuria.*

glycosuria   The presence of glucose (blood sugar) in the urine. This occurs only when serum levels of glucose are very high and the excess is excreted or "spilled over" into the urine. Glucose in the urine is strongly suggestive of diabetes mellitus. Glycosuria can be detected in a urinalysis or with a urinary dipstick.

intravenous pyelogram (IVP)   An x-ray involving the intravenous injection of contrast medium which, as it is excreted by the kidney, outlines structures of the urinary tract.

ketones, urinary Ketones or ketone bodies are wastes formed when fat is metabolized rather than glucose to provide energy. Urinary ketones are found in patients with diabetes mellitus and those on starvation diets. Ketonuria can be detected with a dipstick or in a urinalysis.

KUB An x-ray of the kidneys, ureters, and bladder taken without contrast dye. A common abbreviation that does not usually need translation.

nitrazine paper Reagent paper used to determine the pH of urine and other body fluids by color change.

nitrites, urinary Breakdown products of urinary nitrites due to the action of bacteria on urine in the bladder. When detected in urine they are presumptive evidence of bacterial infection of the urinary tract.

N-Multistix A dipstick for determining the presence of bilirubin, blood, glucose, ketones, nitrites, protein, and urobilinogen in urine as well as determining pH.

protein, urinary Any amount of protein in the urine is considered abnormal and usually indicates renal disease. Proteinuria can be detected in a urinalysis or by urinary dipstick.

Pseudomonas aeruginosa A gram-negative bacterium that causes infections of the urinary tract and soft tissues.

pyuria The presence of a large number of white blood cells (pus) in the urine, pyuria is indicative of a bacterial infection.

specific gravity The weight of a substance per unit of volume, compared to pure water which is assigned a value of 1.000. The specific gravity of urine is a rough measure of the amount of material dissolved in it. The urine specific gravity is reported as the number 1 followed by a decimal point and three other digits. A dictated specific gravity of "ten ten" would be correctly transcribed 1.010.

Tes-Tape A strip of paper impregnated with reagent, used to detect glucose in the urine.

TNTC (too numerous to count) An indication of a very large number of red or white blood cells in a urine specimen.

TURBT (transurethral resection, bladder tumor) A surgical procedure to remove a bladder tumor, it involves inserting a cystoscope through the urethra and into the bladder.

TURP See *transurethral resection of the prostate.*

transurethral resection of the prostate (TURP) A surgical procedure to alleviate difficulties urinating, it involves inserting a cystoscope through the urethra to remove hypertrophied prostatic tissue obstructing the urethra.

UA See *urinalysis.*

urinalysis (UA) A group of tests performed on a urine specimen, including naked-eye observation for color and turbidity, specific gravity, pH, chemical testing for glucose, protein, occult blood, and sometimes acetone and bilirubin, and microscopic examination for cells, crystals, and casts. The combined form *urinalysis* is used rather than *urine analysis.*

urine, 24-hour A collection of all urine passed by a patient during a 24-hour period.

urine, catheterized A specimen of urine obtained by passing a sterile catheter into the bladder.

urine, clean catch or clean-voided A urine specimen obtained after cleansing the area around the urethral opening to prevent contamination of the specimen with material from outside the urinary tract.

urine, first-voided The first urine passed on arising in the morning.

urine, midstream A urine specimen that includes neither the first nor the last part of the urine passed during voiding.

urine, suprapubic A specimen of urine obtained by inserting a sterile needle through the abdominal wall into the bladder.

Uristix A dipstick used to detect glucose and protein in the urine.

white blood cells, urinary The finding of more than one or two white blood cells per high-power field in a specimen of urine usually indicates urinary tract infection. This condition is also known as pyuria.

Anatomy/Medical Terminology

Anatomy: The Male Reproductive System

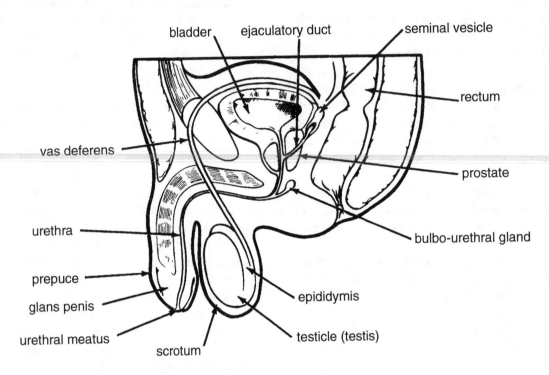

Abbreviations Exercise

Common abbreviations may be transcribed as dictated in the body of a report. Uncommon abbreviations should be spelled out, with the abbreviation appearing in parentheses after the translation. All abbreviations (except laboratory test names like VDRL and SGOT) must be spelled out in the Diagnosis or Impression section of a medical report.

Instructions: Define the following common urologic abbreviations. Then memorize both abbreviations and definitions to increase your speed and accuracy in transcribing dictation from urology.

BPH   _____
BUN   _____
ESWL   _____
GU   _____
IVP   _____
KUB   _____
TNTC   _____
TURBT _____
TURP   _____
UA   _____
UTI   _____
VCUG   _____

Sound-alikes Exercise

Instructions: Circle the correct term from the sound-alikes in parentheses in the following sentences.

1. Genitalia: The patient has hypospadias and (chordae, chordee).
2. The mother brings her 10-year-old son in today because of frequent, nighttime (anuresis, enuresis).
3. Intravenous pyelogram revealed bilateral, poorly functioning (atopic, atrophic, ectopic) kidneys.
4. Clear (efflux, reflex, reflux) of urine was seen coming from both ureteral orifices.
5. It was felt the (anuresis, enuresis) was caused by severe prostatic hypertrophy, completely obstructing the prostatic urethra.

(Continued on following page)

Sound-alikes Exercise *(cont.)*

6. Due to benign hyperplasia of the (prostate, prostrate), a decision was made to do a prostatectomy.
7. A (ureteral, urethral) discharge was present, and gonococcus ws diagnosed.
8. Both (urethras, ureters) were patent on intravenous pyelogram.
9. The (vesical, vesicle) neck of the bladder was obstructed by prostatic hypertrophy.
10. Vesicoureteral (efflux, reflex, reflux) was felt to be the cause of the patient's recurrent urinary (track, tract) infections.

Transcription Tips

Spelling

1. Some words have more than one acceptable spelling, and the preferred spelling may vary from reference to reference. In a dictionary the preferred spelling is followed by the definition and possibly by subentries; the alternative spelling directs the reader to the preferred spelling. Examples:

annulus	anulus
bur	burr
calix	calyx
curet	currette
disk	disc
distention	distension
long-standing	longstanding
transected	transsected

2. Some medical words have a different spelling when their form is changed.

Achilles tendon	tendo Achillis
fascia lata	tensor fasciae latae
inflamed	inflammation
tendon	tendinitis

Spelling Exercise

1. Look up each of the following words in a medical dictionary and circle the preferred spelling.

aneurism	aneurysm
calices	calyces
caesarean	cesarean
dysfunction	disfunction
fetal	foetal
fontanel	fontanelle
hydroma	hygroma
leucocyte	leukocyte
liter	litre
orthopaedic	orthopedic
tocolysis	tokolysis
trepanation	trephination
venipuncture	venopuncture

Do you see that stopping at the first word that appears alphabetically without looking at the definition is not always wise? The same is true of many sound-alike words.

2. Find the noun form (singular and plural) of the following adjectives.

luminal	_____
foraminal	_____
phalangeal	_____
salpingeal	_____

Combined Forms

1. Physicians frequently dictate combined forms. It is acceptable to use either the combined form or the standard (often hyphenated) form when it is uncertain which is dictated. Examples:

femoral-popliteal	femoropopliteal
inferior-lateral	inferolateral
tracheal-bronchial	tracheobronchial
metatarsal-phalangeal	metatarsophalangeal
anterior-lateral	anterolateral
ureteral-pelvic	ureteropelvic
medical-legal	medicolegal
abdominal-perineal	abdominoperineal

Combined Forms Exercise

Instructions: Make combined words out of the following compounds.

costal-vertebral _____

genital-urinary _____

posterior-lateral _____

rectal-vaginal _____

superior-lateral _____

ureteral-pelvic _____

ureteral-vesical _____

urethral-vesical _____

ventricular-peritoneal _____

vesical-ureteral _____

Plural Forms

1. Most Latin nouns ending in -us form their plurals by changing -us to -i. Most nouns ending in -a form their plurals by changing -a to -ae. Nouns ending in -um form their plurals by changing -um to -a.

Singular	Plural
bronchus	bronchi
vertebra	vertebrae
diverticulum	diverticula

2. The terms *diverticulum* (singular) and *diverticula* (plural) cause a great deal of confusion in gastro-intestinal dictation. Physicians may pronounce the plural form "di-ver-tik-u-la," "di-ver-tik-u-lee," or even "di-ver-tik-u-lay." No matter how the physician pronounces the word, however, there is only ONE correct spelling of the plural—*diverticula*.

3. Generally medical words derived from Latin or Greek are pluralized according to guidelines in the recommended references. However, some physicians prefer to pluralize Latin terms as they are in English. Transcribe them as dictated unless they are incorrect.

Latin	English
fistulae	fistulas
lumina	lumens
cannulae	cannulas
axillae	axillas
medullae	medullas

Plurals Exercise

Instructions: Give the plural form of the following words. If the plural can be formed in more than one way, give both.

acetabulum _____

atrium _____

cornea _____

focus _____

fossa _____

labium _____

malleolus _____

nucleus _____

ostium _____

pleura _____

plexus _____

septum _____

sequela _____

vertebra _____

Terminology Challenge

Instructions: The following terms appear in the dictation on Tape 2A, Urology. Before beginning the medical transcription practice for Lesson 4, become familiar with the terminology below by looking up each word in a medical or English dictionary. Write out a short definition of each term.

ADH (antidiuretic
  hormone)
anesthetic
  general
  spinal
anterior
antibiotic
Bartter's syndrome
biopsy
borderline
calix
catheter
  5 French
  8 French
  18 French
  acorn-tipped
  angle-tipped

catheter *(cont.)*
  Foley
  ureteral
cellulated
circumcision
concentrating defect
constrict
debris
deficiency
diabetes insipidus
diagnostic
diverticular
double-J stent
double-voided urine
dressing
  2 x 2
  collodion

dressing *(cont.)*
  Steri-strips
dysuria
edema
electrolytes
  chloride
  CO_2
  potassium
  sodium
endocrinologist
endotracheal
enuresis
excretion
external oblique fascia
extracorporeal shock-
  wave lithotripsy
  (ESWL)
extubate
fellow
fibers
filling defect
fluoroscopy
foreskin
fragmentation
fulguration
gantry
glans penis
granuloma
gravity drainage
hematoma
hemostasis
hernia
herniorrhaphy
hydrocele
hydrocelectomy
hypokalemia
hyposthenuria
incision
internal inguinal ring

inverted
juvenile
KV reading
lithotriptor
loading dose
localized
lower pole calix
manipulated
mEq/L
metastatic
mg/dl
negligible
nephrology
nephronophthisis
objectives
obstruction
orchiectomy
orifice
osmolality
p.r.n.
palliative
patent
pathology
pediatric
phimosis
polydipsia
polyuria
position
  dorsal lithotomy
  lithotomy
posterior
postoperative
preoperative
processus vaginalis
proctitis
prostatic bed
prostatic chips
proximal, proximally
radiation cystitis

radiation therapy
recanalization
redundant
renal pelvis
residual
retraction, retracting
retrograde pyelogram
sac
scope
  11.5 French
  22 French
  28 Storz
  cystoscope
  resectoscope
  ureteroscope
scrotum
Segura stone basket
specific gravity
spermatocytic
spun hematocrit

stage D3 adenocarcinoma
stone basketing
subcutaneous tissue
submucosal tunnel
suture
  4-0
  5-0
  subcutaneous
  subcuticular
  Vicryl
testicle and cord
trabeculated
transected
transitional cell carcinoma
uptake
urine dipstick
vasectomy
verumontanum
vessel loop
void (verb)

Transcription Practice

After completing all the readings and exercises in Lesson 4, transcribe Tape 2A, Urology. Use both medical and English dictionaries and your Quick-Reference Word List as resource materials for finding words. Proofread your transcribed documents carefully, listening to the dictation while you read your transcripts.

Transcribe (*NOT* retype) the same reports again without referring to your previous transcription attempt. Initially, you may need to transcribe some reports more than twice before you can produce an error-free document. Your ultimate goal is to produce an error-free document the first time.

Lesson 5. Gastroenterology

Learning Objectives

Medical

- List common gastrointestinal disease conditions mentioned in the Review of Systems section of a History and Physical Examination Report.
- List common physical findings of gastrointestinal disease found during a physical examination.
- Describe the action of these classes of GI drugs: H_2 blockers, antidiarrheals, laxatives, and antiemetics.
- Given a common generic GI drug, match it to its correct trade name.
- Given a category of GI drugs, indicate which drugs belong to that category.
- Given a cross-section illustration of the gastrointestinal tract (the digestive system), memorize the anatomic structures labeled.
- Describe the path of digestion from the mouth to anus.

Fundamentals

- Explain why *not* transcribing verbatim is "the wonder and headache of medical transcription."
- Discuss the most common errors of grammar made by ESL physicians and how the medical transcriptionist corrects them for accuracy and completeness.
- Discuss the guidelines for transcribing eponyms in medical dictation, including capitalization, accent marks, particles, short forms, and the possessive *'s* form.

Practice

- Accurately transcribe authentic physician dictation from the specialty of gastroenterology.

A Closer Look

If You Don't Know the Words, Just Hum

by Judith Marshall, MA, CMT

Dot and I were enjoying a summer luncheon of poached salmon and egg sauce, first having slipped into a dry martini. "It was one of those weeks," she sighed. "Either the dictating physicians didn't know what they were saying or the transcriptionists made up words and tried to flim-flam the proofreader."

"Not OUR transcriptionists," I retorted.

"No, of course not," she said, "but that sort of thing gets my gander up."

"Your what? Don't you mean 'dander'?"

"Oh, whatever. Same word, isn't it?"

I thought of that old joke, "Why does a hummingbird hum?" Answer: "Because it doesn't know the words."

Maddening medico-babble can begin with one little word. A doctor was pontificating about leg pains. "They were of unclear etiology and not clearly ischemic though not clearly not ischemic either." My "gander" rose a bit but I transcribed that verbatim because, frankly, I didn't know what else to do. Lest one think a young resident said that, nay, nay. It was a "Hah-vahd" man with a distinguished reputation in one of those fashionable troika practices, Lawton, Crest, and Lipton, or as we call them, Larry, Curley, and Mo. The young women call them Larry, Darryl, and the other Darryl.

Some people say they transcribe everything verbatim because "I give it like I get it." This implies we are dispatchers who relay messages and call taxis without any actual thought process. Humbug! *Not* transcribing verbatim is the wonder and the headache of medical transcription.

A brilliant doctor dictated explosively like a skier going out of a chute. In neurosurgery he was a vocabulary master, but let him stray into another specialty and he wobbled. We covered for him until the case of the Courvoisier uterus; that's what he called the incision. Checking *Dorland's* yielded the *Couvelaire uterus,* named for a Paris obstetrician. It made sense to us, so we changed it. Dr. Brain returned the report and said we were mistaken; the word was *Courvoisier.* We sent him a photocopy of the dictionary page. He rolled it into a ball and sent it back with his secretary. Somewhere in New England is a discharge summary with a brandied uterus. I know he will go to his grave saying JOHN Hopkins University and Julia CHILDS.

Another physician recited that the patient had a positive *Legitimes* sign. I thought, how odd; Sophocles, Aristotle, Euripides I know, but who is this ancient Greek? The lovely doctor was very brave in admitting she didn't know how to pronounce it and said, "Operator, just spell *Legitimes* any way you like." Since the patient suffered electric-like shocks down the back, she must have meant *Lhermitte's* sign. From the record, the patient could have had either cord compression or multiple sclerosis. We typed Lhermitte's sign, adding a note about pronunciation. We never heard from the doctor so we hope she approved, but perhaps she thought the matter too humdrum to respond.

But by golly, being right doesn't always endear us to the dictator or make us respected. A lengthy report from a malpractice insurer dealt with an anaerobe manometer. The work was tedious and boring, all about engineering and instrumentation. Something kept nagging at me, page after page. Finally, I recognized that *anaerobe* was incorrect. I looked for *manometer* in *Dorland's* and there was *aneroid manometer,* a device that measures pressure in a system as compared to that of a vacuum. The entire summary was revised to reflect the change from *anaerobe* to *aneroid.* The clerical supervisor of the client telephoned to register protest. We were NEVER to do that again, that if we ever even THOUGHT we PERCEIVED an ALLEGED error, to INDICATE such on a note, but NEVER tamper with the dictation. So there, Ms. Smarty-Pants Marshall.

Sometimes we are embarrassed for our dictators who wander off the mark: the novice who always wants Medical Records to *ascertain* copies of reports, who told us that the patient was complaining of pain as a *rouge* to get narcotic medication; a social worker who consistently worries that the patient will suffer the *stigmata* of admission to the detox unit.

I rather like some of the more colorful dictation. "The patient was stiff as hell." Now that's succinct and descriptive. "The thyroid was out of whack."

"The patient was not feeling up to snuff." Condition on discharge: "The patient was hanging in there."

Like a candle, dictation has two ends. Here are some humdingers by transcriptionists: downgoing *panther* (plantar) responses; non-*genetic* medication; pain in the upper *asparagus* (esophagus); diminished sensation in *Apache* (a patchy) distribution; *decor* (the cor) is distant; *insolent*-dependent diabetes; and *tupelo (two-pillow)* orthopnea. And one charming Transylvanian looking for lesions of the *oral fangs* (oropharynx).

When the patient was an eminent professor of poetry and held the Siegal Chair (yes, the doctor spelled it), our protégée, no doubt dreaming of the Cape, typed *seagull chair.*

It took a four-letter word to prick my sanctimonious defenses. A prospective client called and asked if I knew how to transcribe the SOAP system. "Yes," I lied. I can transcribe anything. Lemme at it. I know my stuff. All night long I lay awake wondering what this system was and why didn't I know the word SOAP. At 8 a.m. in the doctor's office they showed me what they meant: Subjective, Objective, Assessment, and Plan. It was a humbling experience.

Shortly afterward I visited my therapist to help cope with my obsessive-compulsive fascination with words and my passion, yes, passion, for precision in medical language.

My doctor leaned forward conspiratorially and said, "I understand completely and I agree with you. Where would we be without clarity? So, Judith, get your ducks in a row, clear your decks, and do what is appropriate and don't do what is inappropriate. Are you comfortable with that?"

The sound of humming filled the room and I felt a pain beginning in my upper asparagus.

The ESL Physician and the Art of Medical Transcription

Mary Ann D'Onofrio, AMLS, CMT, ART

Great emphasis today is placed upon the need for the medical transcriptionist to have a proficient understanding of anatomy and physiology, and a thorough knowledge of medical, pharmacologic, and laboratory terminology. It is essential to master the "science" of medical transcription to be successful in this career. However, seldom is the "art" of medical transcription more apparent, and more important, than when transcribing for the ESL physician, i.e., the physician who speaks English as a second language.

Physicians are intelligent, well educated, and expert in their particular medical specialties; the ESL physician is no exception. Likewise, the medical transcriptionist who is a *true professional* is intelligent, well educated, and an expert in the fields of English grammar, medical terminology, anatomy and physiology, and language in general. Formal or informal study of Latin and Greek as the roots of the language of medicine fosters an understanding of how plurals are formed, and makes sense out of the seemingly contradictory medical phrases with adjectival components. Expertise in these areas enables the MT to transcribe the physician's dictation into an accurate medical report that is grammatically correct. Likewise, a knowledge of the vocabulary and grammar of a modern foreign language enhances the MT's ability to understand better and to transcribe more accurately the ESL physician's dictation.

In focusing on the unique editing problems encountered in transcribing the physician who speaks English as a second language, I wish to emphasize that not all ESL physicians present editing problems for the medical transcriptionist. Many such physicians actually have a knowledge and skill in using proper English equal to or exceeding that possessed by the average American college graduate.

This article focuses on those ESL physicians whose ability to dictate a formal medical report according to the rules of English composition is not on a par with their conversational speech. In addition to grammatical and nongrammatical editing problems encountered in transcribing the ESL physician, I shall briefly discuss many of the variances in pronunciation of the English language among ESL physicians. At all times, however, transcriptionists should realize that the doctors know what they mean to say, and that the doctors most likely are speaking according to the correct grammatical and phonetic rules of their native language.

The most common errors of grammar made by the ESL physician are (1) failure to use the definite or indefinite article before a noun, (2) misplacement of prepositional phrases, (3) redundancy, and (4) non-agreement of parts of speech. These problems will be more readily apparent through examples.

Let me illustrate the first problem with an example from my experience transcribing for a physician from Asia. Many such physicians are unaccustomed to the use of the indefinite and definite articles, *a*, *an*, and *the*. A sentence similar to the following is often encountered:

Patient is 47 years old man.

The thought is perfectly clear; however, the grammar needs editing. It can easily be changed to:

The patient is a 47-year-old man.

A few years ago I came upon a number of grammatical problems all in the same piece of dictation. This is what the ESL physician dictated:

Patient is 52 years old obese white male for past 25 years. He denies ever drug or alcohol abuse. He is cooperative and having no difficulty of verbal communication.

Has the patient been male for just the past 25 years? Hardly. This is how I transcribed the paragraph:

The patient is a 52-year-old white male, obese for the past 25 years. He denies drug or alcohol abuse. He is cooperative and is having no difficulty with verbal communication.

It would also be correct to transcribe that last sentence:

He is cooperative and has no difficulty with verbal communication.

The following psychiatric admission note is another example of an ESL physician's redundancy and confusion concerning proper English grammar:

This is a 14-year-old white Caucasian female who is admitted by her mother voluntarily complaining of situational problems resulting in acting-out behavior by her.

Eliminating the redundancy and repositioning the descriptive clause, I transcribed:

This is a 14-year-old Caucasian female, admitted voluntarily by her mother, who complains of situational problems resulting in her acting-out behavior.

However the medical transcriptionist chooses to resolve

grammatical problems in dictation, it is of the utmost importance to keep as much to the *letter* as to the *spirit* of the thought communicated via dictation.

The medical transcriptionist who transcribes for the ESL physician will usually find that the nongrammatical editing problem is one of the following: (1) diction, (2) mistaken identities (homonyms, synonyms, antonyms, eponyms), or (3) slip-of-the-tongue errors. It is essential that the medical transcriptionist be constantly on the alert for these problems.

Let us first consider **diction**. This is a common problem when transcribing the ESL physician who has a decided accent. For now, let us deal with the hesitancy factor often present. I refer specifically to the use of *uh* and *er* as they are interjected before a precise word is selected by the ESL physician in dictation. This is a problem for the medical transcriptionist because *uh* can be mistaken for the indefinite article *a* or for the first syllable of a word that begins with *a*. The sound *er* is often mistaken for the conjunction *or.* Let me illustrate with some examples from my own transcription experience:

> The lesion was located . . . uh . . . proximally to the extensor hallucis longus muscle.

In this example, it is necessary to differentiate between *uh . . . proximally* and *approximately*—two different ideas. This is especially difficult when transcribing ESL physicians because they may inadvertently substitute the *-mately* ending when *-mally* is intended.

The other side of this coin is seen when the ESL physician hesitates slightly in the pronunciation of the word *atypical* and similar words which begin with *a* as the first syllable. Here is an example:

> Clinical findings reveal the patient to have a— typical angina pectoris.

Did the physician actually say "uh . . . typical angina pectoris"? Be sure before you type.

Let us now consider the interjection of *er* before a dictated word, and the conjunction *or.* For example, the physician dictates:

> Physical examination at this time fails to reveal any right . . . er . . . left inguinal hernia.

In this instance, the physician has had a change of thought! He dictated *right*, hesitated by saying *er*, then continued (without indicating verbally to the transcriptionist what he was doing) by substituting the word *left* before *inguinal hernia*. Since the distinct possibility exists that the physician wishes to say that the physical exam fails to reveal any *right or left inguinal hernia*, it is imperative that the transcriptionist listen carefully. If any doubt exists regarding precisely what the physician intends, the transcriptionist should relisten to the dictation; check the patient's chart for additional verification of what the patient's condition or treatment has been; or, if necessary, write the physician a note requesting clarification of the problem passage.

Research of this type takes time. Even if one's payment for transcribing is based solely on line production, a professional medical transcriptionist will take the time to verify the accuracy of the dictation, and not risk creating an error in a patient's medical record. In any event, don't be "clever" and guess. You may be wrong.

Like us all, the ESL physician is not exempt from **mistaken identities**; that is, pronouncing one word but meaning to use another term, be it homonym, synonym, antonym—even eponym. Doctors and medical transcriptionists alike must be alert to the nuances of such similar-sounding words as *tortuous* and *torturous*, *turbid* and *turgid*, *pars* and *parts*, *evulsion* and *avulsion*, *Reynolds* and *Raynaud's*.

Few English words pose more difficulty for the ESL physician than the words *look* and *see*. *Webster's New Collegiate Dictionary*, Ninth Edition, includes these definitions:

> **look**—to exercise the power of vision; to ascertain by the use of one's eyes.

The above definition describes physical activity. But compare:

> **see**—to perceive by the eye; to form a mental picture of; to perceive the meaning or importance of; to be aware of.

That definition indicates mental activity, reaching a conclusion. I recall an ESL physician with limited familiarity with the English language dictating the following:

> He seemed to look himself as a victim of other people.

I knew what the doctor meant to say; I also knew he

would expect his precise meaning to be conveyed in proper English. Therefore, I transcribed:

> He seemed to see himself as a victim of other people.

That same ESL physician might be further confused with these complex idiomatic uses of the verb *look*: *look after* (meaning to minister to), *look forward to* (to anticipate); *look in on* (to visit); *look on* (to observe); or *look over* (to examine).

Another type of nongrammatical problem which I have found while transcribing for the ESL physician is the **slip-of-the-tongue error**, common to all of us. Still, it must be recognized and reckoned with. One such error is obvious and presents no real problem if a patient list or the medical record is readily available: the inversion of a patient's name. Medical records usually have the patient's surname recorded first, followed by the given name. It is not uncommon for the dictator to misread this order of names, especially when hurried or tired. With the availability of a computerized central database for patient information, this can be a moot problem for both dictator and transcriptionist.

Other such errors are more difficult to ascertain since they require that the transcriptionist be aware of a discrepancy in the dictation. A simple example of this is the physician's substitution of *right* for *left*, or vice versa, in describing an x-ray finding of a patient's arm fracture. There usually is additional information the transcriptionist can readily research to determine if an error in dictation has been made.

A more serious problem for the transcriptionist presents itself, however, when a physician inadvertently substitutes one suffix for another. I encountered the following dictation, describing a patient with Valley Fever, a respiratory disease caused by the fungus *Coccidioides immitis:*

> The patient was admitted to the hospital for treatment of coccidioidomyoma.

My computer spellchecker verified that no such word was in its database. My other references confirmed that the term for Valley Fever was *coccidioidomycosis*. I typed this term in the report I was transcribing but attached a note to the physician indicating the word he had dictated and requesting verification of the word I had typed. This, for me, was the proper risk management procedure to follow. In this case the term *coc-*

cidioidomyoma was an obvious mispronunciation on the part of the physician.

In today's environment, with coding so critical to the reimbursement process, a correct typing of what actually is a real but inappropriately dictated medical term on the part of the ESL physician just might lead to an error in coding, and even to inaccurate hospital reimbursement. Just consider these two bona fide medical terms: leiomyo**fibr**oma (a benign tumor of the smooth muscle and fibrous connective tissue) and leiomyo**sarc**oma (a malignant neoplasm of the smooth muscle tissue.) Of course, there would need to be some suspicion by the medical transcriptionist that an error exists before questioning the use of one of these terms over the other; however, responsibility for risk management by MTs is even more critical when transcribing for the ESL physician.

As I mentioned previously, physicians who speak English as a second language may display an inability to pronounce certain English sounds, or to pronounce them with difficulty. As often happens, the ESL physician's use of a particular word or combination of words is not ill chosen; it's just that the pronunciation of a particular word sounds much like some other English word to the medical transcriptionist. For example, the ESL physician from a middle European country may pronounce the English *th* sound like *ze* wherein the resultant dictation *the aerophagia* meaning "the swallowing of air" becomes to the transcriptionist's ear *xerophagia* with the entirely different meaning of "eating of dry food only."

An ESL physician with a Spanish or Latin American heritage may interchange the *v* and *b* sounds with the resultant *bolar* for *volar* or *Boyd* for *void*, and the like. They may also substitute *es* for the English *s* or *x* sounds in some words. This would present a particular problem for differentiating between certain words such as *essential* and *sensual*, *esotropia* and *exotropia*. The final syllable *us* may be pronounced by the ESL physician as *oose*; thus, the English word *sinus* may become *sin'yoose* to the transcriptionist's ear and be transcribed in the medical report as *sinews,* a vastly different meaning from the one intended. Each medical transcriptionist has encountered many additional examples of such problem words while transcribing for the ESL physician. It is always advisable to keep a record of these sound-alikes as they are encountered.

Transcribing for the physician who speaks English as a second language is one of the most challenging and rewarding areas of medical transcription. It requires very careful listening. It often entails researching the medical record and consulting medical references; and when one must consult the physician, it requires tact. Knowing that the physician has confidence in your ability to transcribe his or her dictation into a grammatically perfect report makes this "art" of medical transcription genuinely satisfying.

Transcribing Gastroenterology Dictation

by Bron Taylor

Transcription of gastrointestinal system dictation is relatively straightforward, which isn't to say it can be mastered overnight. We can work for years in this area and still be challenged by hearing strange and wonderful new things from the doctors.

Patients with GI complaints are in considerable distress, not only from the painful and sometimes life-threatening conditions themselves, but also from the embarrassment many of them can cause. Physicians working with these problems have learned to put the patients at ease and acquire, if they didn't start out with it, a good sense of humor.

The relief that many patients obtain from correct diagnosis and treatment of GI problems is considerable, too, and all of this, plus the many organ systems involved in these problems and the interfaces with other specialties, make this a very dynamic and ever-changing field, with new drugs and new treatments being constantly introduced.

GI transcription problems. The problems we face in transcribing GI dictation are those all transcriptionists face, and the same solutions apply. Acquiring good reference material; establishing links with other transcriptionists, with physicians, with nurses in the Endoscopy Room and staff who work in Central Supply; keeping an accurate personal notebook; reading medical journals—all help one to master and stay on top of this material.

There are several specific GI questions that baffle most beginners, such as the *perineal/peritoneal/peroneal* sound-alikes. Careful listening will often distinguish *peritoneal* from *perineal*, and in an operation such as an abdominoperineal resection (in which both terms appear), one has to be alert to this. The word *peroneal*, referring to the area of the outer side of the leg, is much less likely to appear in GI dictation.

Another problem is *ileum/ilium*, and I'm indebted to Vera Pyle for a mnemonic device for distinguishing these. The "e" in ileum is a letter made with a loop, like the loops of bowel of the ileum.

Another frequent source of confusion is the word *ascitic,* from ascites. It sounds like *acidic,* and the only way to resolve this one is by context. An *ascitic wave* is the fluid wave seen on palpation of the abdomen in patients with ascites. I have seen students transcribe "acidic wave" and insist "that's what the doctor said." Similarly, in the early stages of doing this work, one can confuse *cirrhosis* with *serositis,* and again, context saves the day.

Here, as with all transcription, the more one learns about the anatomy and what's going on, the more interesting and enjoyable the work is and the less likely one is to make such errors.

As with transcription of any type, dictators can sometimes lead us astray. One of the typical dictation errors is the plural of diverticulum, which is *diverticula,* not *diverticulae, diverticuli, diverticulee,* or *diverticulas.*

Another source of confusion from the physicians is when they "helpfully" (and sometimes it is) dictate punctuation, without any warning that they've deviated from the body of their reports to talk to us directly. One dictator where I work baffled many of us for months in talking about the retroflexion maneuver used in endoscopy, also called the *J-turn maneuver.* He'd say, very fast, "with the J, that's-J-as-in-the-letter-J turn maneuver." (When we finally deciphered this, we immediately wrote the term on our bulletin board, which is a good practice to follow so that others won't have to reinvent the wheel.) Also, the dictated punctuation mark *colon* can cause a problem in gastrointestinal dictation, much of which concerns the colon itself.

General transcription problems. All of us face the same problems when working with this material, but we have many tools to cut through the confusion. Reference books are our best friends. My list of the absolute minimum references includes the latest *Dorland's,* the latest *American Drug Index,* and *Current Medical Terminology.*

Beyond these basics, I like to use the most recent *Merck Manual* I can find, especially for laboratory values. Look up what your patient has in the index in the back, then look under the laboratory findings section of that disease. Under each disease entity is a short essay covering etiology, symptoms and signs, laboratory findings, diagnosis, and treatment. It also has a table of normal values, and many other sections which can tell one a lot about what's going on in the dictation.

I prefer the *American Drug Index* (*ADI*) to the *Physicians' Drug Reference* (*PDR*) for drugs because it's more comprehensive in scope and faster to use with its A to Z format.

Some transcriptionists are unclear on how to use the *ADI*. There is a belief in the transcription community that drugs with the little dot or bullet in front of their names are generic, which is true, but, as the "special note to medical transcriptionists" in the Preface points out, the most accurate and fastest way to tell if a drug is generic is to look for a manufacturer's name in parentheses immediately after the name of the drug; if it's not there, the drug is generic. This trick always works and is very fast and accurate.

As for medical journals, beginners may be intimidated by them, but as one progresses and learns the language of medicine, there comes a point when one can read journal articles of interest just as if they were in plain English. This is one of the rewards of learning transcription, as it opens up the world of the scholarly physician, some of whom write beautifully, and all of whom are interesting. Dr. Largen's article (in Lesson 6) is an example of the kind of article one can find in journals. Sometimes the letters to the journal editor are the best part, sometimes the essays. Many doctors are interested in the history of medicine and have an amazing number of odd and wonderful stories, and they share them in the journals.

Editing. Editing should be done in transcription to enhance clarity. Until a transcriptionist acquires a sense of what the dictator *means,* which comes with practice and experience, and until one is *sure* about this, editing should be confined to changing only the very obvious mistakes dictators make when they're tired.

Slang should be edited out. A dictator who's tired or in a bad frame of mind may talk about "mets," for metastases, but really doesn't want to see that brief form later on rereading the record. Similarly, obvious errors resulting from fatigue can be edited. One should try to have the transcription be a perfect record of what the dictator *intended* to say, which is not always what he or she actually said. Determining this is a difficult matter, and until one has heard the procedure in question dictated over and over and one is absolutely certain what was intended, it's better not to edit too much.

The basic rule when editing is NEVER GUESS. There is nothing dishonorable about leaving a blank in a report. Nobody can be expected to understand everything every dictator says, or immediately know every new drug, tool, and procedure. Guesses are especially hazardous now that many transcriptionists are using word processors and turning out beautifully printed reports; a guess which turns out to be wrong still looks elegant and credible. This is particularly hazardous when guessing about drug names, as medications with very similar names can have wildly different effects. Guessing the wrong word is the kind of thing that can wake you up in the middle of the night. It's much safer to leave a blank, when you have an unintelligible mumble and you've exhausted all your sources in the time you have.

The dictators themselves are a good source of answers to our questions, although their spelling should always be taken as a starting point, not the last word. One has to use common sense, courtesy, and sensitivity about asking questions of busy physicians. Not every physician is willing at any point in his or her day to be interrupted with our questions, but good times do occur and those opportunities should be seized. Some of my most memorable learning experiences have occurred spontaneously when a willing physician (who loved to teach) was caught at an opportune moment and took the time to explain a procedure or help me to research a difficult spelling.

If confronting physicians isn't to one's taste, or if the transcription is done in an area where one just doesn't run into doctors, sending a note with a question regarding the dictation with some kind of easily returned envelope has worked for me very well, either in hospital mail or stamped and addressed regular mail. I do all the work for them so that they only have to check a box and drop the envelope in the mail, and almost always I get a response. Sometimes they write at some length, if the question catches their interest and they have the time.

Once we have an unusual word confirmed by a physician, something not in reference material, it's a good practice to share it with other transcriptionists on a bulletin board or through a memo. Finally, it should go into your personal notebook, with a note that it's an unconfirmed doctor's spelling (if that's the case), but it should be written down so the source doesn't have to be asked the same question over and over.

Most of the terms in GI dictation are in the printed references, but the very newest techniques are not, for a time, and surgeons have a habit of referring to anatomical landmarks and surgical techniques by eponyms, which are sometimes specific to the medical center where they trained.

A note about speed. Beginners can be intimidated by listening to experts transcribe at high speed, and can be overwhelmed by real-world expectations of productivity. It can all seem hopeless, when first listening to the tapes, many of which seem to be dictated in a foreign language. How can one be expected to do meticulous, accurate work—as *fast* as it has to be done?

It's one thing to say NEVER GUESS, look up everything if you have any doubt, and ask everyone questions—and another to produce work *fast*. And if that's not confusing enough, medical transcriptionists are expected to edit errors in the dictation, as they become capable and experienced.

Editing requires great delicacy, sensitivity, and knowledge. The official policy in some medical record departments is that the transcriptionists must never edit what the doctors say; they must type exactly what the dictators say. When confronted directly about editing, many doctors will tell you NOT to edit their dictation, yet when they meet you in the hall, they'll thank you for making their work read so beautifully. And when a beginner asks an experienced transcriptionist or supervisor how to handle an obvious error in dictation or inappropriate language, they will often tell the beginner to type what the dictator *means* rather than *says* in that particular instance. It can all be incredibly confusing.

Gaining speed in spite of all these pressures and areas of potential conflict is not hopeless. It's *knowledge of medicine* that increases speed and accuracy, not learning to move one's fingers faster on the keyboard. By understanding what's going on in the dictated procedures, by knowing the anatomy well, by being familiar with the most frequently used medications, you eventually arrive at the point where you almost know what's going to be dictated before the doctor says it, and that's the point where speed comes almost before you know it. Suffering through the learning process, not being tempted to take shortcuts—this is the real road to speed. You'll get to the point where you don't have to look up words so often because you understand how the dictator is thinking.

The foreign accent problem, which is formidable for beginners, solves itself by the same method. You will get to the point where you KNOW what the dictator wants to say, no matter how odd the words sound, and people will tell you you have a wonderful ear. This really will happen, although it has to be taken on faith at the beginning.

One of the satisfactions of this work is the degree to which you can teach yourself about medicine. You don't have to formally enroll in an anatomy course or become a pharmacy student, if you keep your ears and eyes open and soak up all the medical information you can, all the time. The amount of anatomy to be learned is finite—there are a certain number of muscles and bones and nerves to learn, and no more, and anatomy can be learned so well that using it becomes automatic. New drugs and procedures are being constantly introduced, but once one knows the bulk of them, most of the work is done.

We don't want to give the impression that there is so much new information to be learned with every report that the transcriptionist must spend every day in a time-consuming search for new information. There are patterns that underlie what the dictators are saying, and it all makes good sense, and it's a great satisfaction to learn these—by any means. The reports themselves will teach you a great deal.

It's especially important in the beginning stages to resist pressure to *guess* and thus avoid leaving blanks in reports. Unfortunately there *are* supervisors who encourage guessing and who will not allow blanks in reports, who think that pages without gaps are "good enough." You have to resist this pressure because it is just not safe to guess when you're working on a patient's permanent medical record.

Too many words sound alike. One of the best tools you can develop is a little bell of doubt that rings for you when you're really not sure what you're transcribing. When this bell goes off, trust it—if you have a hunch it might be wrong, it probably IS wrong. Look it up, ask someone, and, if you have to leave a blank, do that—and attach a note to the dictator.

With study and experience, one acquires a picture of what's happening behind the dictation, and everything starts to make sense. Mumbles become clear, your questions to the doctors become more astute and generate more interesting answers, you catch more mistakes, and you begin to see the bigger picture and realize how it all fits together. Some days you'll have the satisfaction of having a new procedure or drug already in mind before it's dictated, which is a nice "a-ha" feeling and brightens your day.

Starting out as a beginning transcriptionist, it may all seem complex and without pattern or reason, but once you have a good grasp of the anatomy and the disease processes and the rationale behind the doctor's approaches to these problems, it all sorts itself out.

Not every day will be fascinating, for much of the dictation will be repetitive, but there are many rewards hidden in the tapes.

Medical Readings

The History and Physical Examination

by John H. Dirckx, M.D.

Past Medical History. The Past Medical History provides a survey of all medical information not covered in the History of Present Illness, containing useful information about the patient's past illnesses, injuries, surgeries, chronic diseases and disabilities, allergies, and immunizations.

Because most patients have difficulty recalling all of their prior illnesses, the physician customarily asks if the patient has ever had any of the following serious diseases: diabetes, tuberculosis, asthma, pneumonia, high blood pressure, heart attack or heart disease, stroke, epilepsy, ulcer, cancer, anemia, arthritis, kidney disease, nervous or mental disease. An affirmative answer prompts the physician to inquire further as to the date of the illness, severity, treatment, and complications.

Usual childhood diseases are included in this section, although only chickenpox remains usual; all others, including measles, mumps, rubella, whooping cough, polio, and diphtheria have been virtually eliminated by routine immunization of children.

Past injuries include fractures, dislocations, severe sprains or strains, open wounds or burns, loss of a body part, and significant trauma to internal organs. Injuries from falls and automobile accidents are common. In addition, industrial accidents and injuries sustained while in the military may be mentioned. However, patients often conceal or lie about injuries sustained in a fight or while engaged in criminal activities.

Even the most minor surgical procedures can result in changes of structure or function that may later be mistaken for signs of disease. Therefore, a thorough surgical history is important. However, patients are seldom conversant with the technical details of their operations and tend to forget childhood operative procedures such as tonsillectomies.

Chronic diseases that are not directly related to the present illness are also reviewed with the patient. Chronic conditions such as diabetes, hypertension, rheumatoid arthritis, coronary artery disease, or mental illness would be mentioned. In addition, significant functional impairments, such as blindness and paralysis,

belong in the Past Medical History section of the History and Physical Examination.

Any prior history of allergy or sensitivity, especially to medicines, should be part of the patient's written records. Usually such information is prominently displayed on the front of a hospital chart or medical office record to prevent inadvertent administration of that medicine.

Routine childhood immunizations must usually be taken for granted unless written records are available to provide verification.

Review of Systems: Gastrointestinal. The digestive system, like the respiratory system, begins at the lips. However, symptoms affecting the mouth, teeth, tongue, salivary glands, and throat are usually considered in other parts of the history. The gastrointestinal history is concerned mainly with two types of symptoms: abdominal pain of any type or degree (though abdominal pain often results from nondigestive causes) and any disturbances of digestive function, including anorexia, nausea, vomiting, and diarrhea. Symptoms due to disorders of the liver or biliary tract, the pancreas, or the rectum or anus are also included here.

In reviewing the past digestive tract history, the examiner inquires about previous diagnoses of hiatal hernia, ulcer, gallstones or gallbladder disease, pancreatitis, colitis; any tumors of the alimentary canal or associated structures; results of gastrointestinal x-rays or other diagnostic studies; operations on the digestive organs, including appendectomy and hemorrhoid surgery; and use of antacids, laxatives, enemas, or prescription medicines for digestive symptoms.

Abdominal pain may be described as burning, crampy, or dull. It may be constant, intermittent, or of varying intensity. It may remain in one place or radiate or migrate to another, perhaps in the back or chest. It may be brought on, aggravated, or relieved by eating, not eating, drinking, defecation, or assuming certain positions. It may be provoked by eating certain foods; a record of any food intolerances is an important part of the digestive history.

Symptoms besides abdominal pain that draw attention to the digestive system are anorexia, nausea, pain or difficulty in swallowing that seems to originate below the pharynx, vomiting, flatulence, constipation, diarrhea, abnormal appearance of the stools, weight loss, jaundice, and anorectal pain, swelling, or bleeding. A history of vomiting prompts inquiries about its frequency and the volume and character of emesis. Blood that is mixed with gastric contents often has a characteristic coffee-grounds appearance. Jaundice, a yellow color of the skin, mucous membranes, and ocular sclerae, indicates an excessive quantity of bile pigment in blood and tissues. It can result from intrinsic liver disease (hepatitis, hepatic failure) or from obstruction of the biliary tract by a gallstone or a tumor.

Because constipation and diarrhea mean different things to different people, the interviewer must carefully determine the frequency and consistency of the patient's stools. Even with normal bowel habits, an abnormal stool color can indicate disease. Clay-colored stools occur in obstruction of the biliary tract because bile does not reach the intestine. Blood that has passed through much of the intestine before appearing in the stool may look tarry black (melena) because of digestive changes in blood pigment.

Inguinal hernia may also be considered with the gastrointestinal history because most hernias contain loops of bowel and eventually affect digestive or eliminative function. The patient is asked about swelling or bulging in the groin or scrotum that is accentuated by coughing or straining and diminishes or disappears in the recumbent position.

Physical Examination of the Abdomen and Rectum. Palpation of the abdomen is performed to assess muscle tone, to determine the size, shape, and position of the abdominal and pelvic organs, and to detect any masses or tenderness. The physician starts with light palpation, which provides information about the abdominal wall and any zones of tenderness, and then progresses to deep palpation to study the internal organs and search for masses. An area of pain or tenderness known to the physician is examined last.

Throughout the examination, the physician closely observes the patient's face for signs of distress. Rebound tenderness, a transient stab of pain when the abdomen is pressed and then suddenly released, denotes local or generalized peritoneal irritation. The physician may look for tenderness in the liver or gallbladder by gentle fist percussion over the right lower ribs or by hooking a finger under the right costal margin and asking the patient to inhale deeply. Costovertebral angle tenderness occurs in inflammation or infection of the kidney or ureter.

Most normal intra-abdominal structures cannot be distinctly felt through the abdominal wall. By vigorous palpation of a very thin patient, one can feel parts of the normal liver, spleen, and kidneys, but ordinarily these organs must be enlarged before they can be palpated. No part of the digestive tract can normally be felt, nor can the pancreas, gallbladder, or ureters. In an obese patient, even gross abnormalities can escape detection by palpation.

Percussion can be used to measure the liver span (the width of liver dullness between lung and bowel resonances) and to distinguish between a solid organ or tumor, which yields a dull or flat note, and bowel distended by gas, which yields a hollow or resonant note. It can also confirm the presence of ascitic fluid by detecting a change in the percussion note as the patient rolls from his back to his side (shifting dullness).

The physician uses auscultation to evaluate the bowel sounds and to listen for bruits. Normal intestinal activity produces characteristic gurgling sounds at intervals of a few seconds. Bowel sounds are reduced or absent in ileus and peritonitis, hyperactive in diarrhea and intestinal obstruction. Bruits (abnormal sounds or murmurs) can be heard over narrowed segments of large arteries, including the aorta. The presence of both fluid and gas in the abdominal cavity can be demonstrated by hearing a succussion splash with or without a stethoscope when the patient is shaken.

Pharmacology: GI Drugs

Gastrointestinal drugs are prescribed to treat disease conditions of the stomach and intestines such as ulcers, diarrhea, constipation, ulcerative colitis, irritable bowel syndrome, or gallstones.

Ulcer drugs. Antacids were the original, and for many years the only, treatment for peptic ulcers. They are weak bases which exert a therapeutic effect by neutralizing acid. By raising the pH, they also inhibit the action of pepsin. They contain aluminum, magnesium, calcium, sodium, or a combination of these as the active ingredients.

Antacids are available over-the-counter without a prescription and include Alka-Seltzer, Bromo Seltzer, Di-Gel, Gelusil, Maalox, Mylanta, Riopan, Rolaids, and Tums.

The release of gastric acid is triggered by histamine which acts on special histamine receptors (known as H_2 receptors) in the gastric parietal cells lining the stomach. Drugs which block these receptors and prevent the release of acid are known as H_2 blockers and are used to treat ulcers. H_2 blockers currently prescribed to treat ulcers include:

> cimetidine (Tagamet)
> famotidine (Pepcid)
> nizatidine (Axid)
> ranitidine (Zantac)

A unique anti-ulcer drug unrelated to either antacids or H$_2$ blockers is sucralfate (Carafate). This drug acts topically on the ulcer surface. It is attracted to injured areas of the mucous membrane which are draining fluid high in protein. The drug binds directly to these areas, forming a protective layer or bandage over the ulcer, allowing it to heal.

Antidiarrheal drugs. Antidiarrheal drugs produce a therapeutic effect by slowing peristalsis in the intestinal tract or by absorbing the extra water in diarrhea stools and forming a gel. Some antidiarrheal drugs exert their effect because they contain opium or related substances. Although opium and related compounds have pain-relieving properties, a common side effect of that group of drugs is constipation. This side   effect becomes a therapeutic effect in treating diarrhea.

Drugs for diarrhea which contain opium or related substances are classified as narcotics and may be controlled substances depending on the actual addictive qualities of that particular drug. Examples: difenoxin (Motofen), diphenoxylate (Lomotil), loperamide (Imodium), tincture of opium (paregoric). Other antidiarrheal drugs contain non-opiate substances such as kaolin and pectin which absorb water. Examples: Donnagel, Kaolin, Kaopectate.

Laxatives. Prescription laxatives are used for short-term treatment of constipation, with attention also given to adequate water intake, dietary fiber/bulk, and other measures to promote regularity. Over-the-counter laxatives are frequently overused and even abused. Classifications of laxatives include magnesium laxatives, irritants, bulk-producing laxatives, stool softeners, and mechanical laxatives.

Magnesium laxatives include the active ingredient of magnesium which attracts water from the bloodstream into the intestines to soften the stool. These drugs include Epsom salt, M.O.M. (milk of magnesia), and Phillips' Milk of Magnesia.

Irritant laxatives act directly on the intestinal mucosa to stimulate peristalsis. Examples: Dulcolax and Ex-Lax.

Bulk-producing laxatives hold water that is normally absorbed into the bloodstream from the intestines. Their laxative action is the most natural and safest of all of the laxatives. Examples: Fiberall, Metamucil, Perdiem.

Laxatives which act as stool softeners are emulsifiers which allow water and fat in the stool to mix. Examples include Correctol, docusate (Colace, Surfak).

Mechanical laxatives include suppositories (such as glycerin suppositories) which directly stimulate the urge to defecate by their presence in the lower colon.

Bowel preps or enemas may be prescribed to evacuate the colon prior to surgical or endoscopic procedures. These include Fleet enema and polyethylene glycol/electrolyte solution (CoLyte, Evac-Q-Kit, GoLytely, X-Prep).

Antiemetics. Antiemetic drugs are used to control nausea and vomiting which can arise from bacterial or viral illnesses of the GI tract; as a side effect of drugs, surgery, radiation, or chemotherapy; or from vertigo and motion sickness. Vomiting patients are often given antiemetics in rectal suppository form because they cannot keep the oral medications down.

For severe nausea and vomiting, chlorpromazine (Thorazine) and prochlorperazine (Compazine) are prescribed. For moderate nausea and vomiting, promethazine (Phenergan), thiethylperazine (Torecan), and trimethobenzamide (Tigan) are prescribed.

Vertigo is caused by irritation to the inner ear (from labyrinthitis or vestibular neuritis) which upsets balance and stimulates the vomiting center. Motion sickness arises from repeated motions, such as in a car, which also overstimulate the inner ear.

Drugs used to treat vertigo and motion sickness include dimenhydrinate (Dramamine), meclizine (Antivert, Bonine), and scopolamine (Transderm-Scop). All of these drugs are given orally with the exception of scopolamine (Transderm-Scop) which is manufactured as a small transdermal patch worn behind the ear.

Anatomy/Medical Terminology

Drug Matching Exercise

Instructions: Match the generic name drug in Column A with its trade name in Column B. Note: Generic names may be used more than once.

Column A	Column B
A. cimetidine	____ Surfak
B. famotidine	____ Compazine
C. sucralfate	____ Carafate
D. docusate	____ Thorazine
E. dimenhydrinate	____ Antivert
F. prochlorperazine	____ Tagamet
G. meclizine	____ Zantac
H. chlorpromazine	____ Pepcid
I. ranitidine	____ Colace
	____ Dramamine

Anatomy: The Gastrointestinal Tract

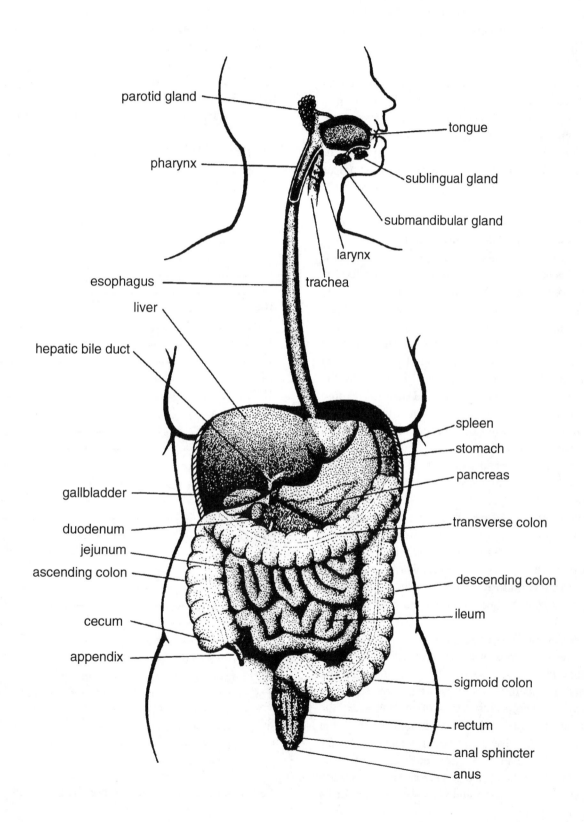

Fill-in Exercise: Digestion

Instructions: The numbered blanks correspond to the numbers in the narrative paragraphs. Fill in the blanks with the correct entry from the word list on the following page.

Digestion begins in the (1), where food is chewed thoroughly, a process known as (2). There it is mixed with saliva. Saliva contains the digestive enzyme (3), which begins the digestion of starch. The food then passes through the (4), or throat, where it is swallowed, a process known as (5). From the throat, food passes through a long tube known as the (6), through the (7) sphincter, and finally into the stomach.

The body of the stomach is called the (8). Folds in the stomach wall are known as (9). Within the stomach, gastric glands secrete (10) acid and pepsin, which digest proteins. The partially digested food is then moved by wavelike contractions known as (11) through the pyloric sphincter into the small intestine.

The first part of the small intestine is the (12). The digestion of fats takes place there as bile, which is produced in the (13) and stored in the (14), and is mixed with food. The pancreatic enzyme (15) completes the digestive process for fats. The food then moves into the second and third parts of the small intestine, the (16) and (17). The walls of the small intestine contain microscopic projections of mucous membrane called (18) that allow digested food to pass through the intestinal wall and into capillaries for distribution throughout the body.

Waste products from food digestion continue to pass through the digestive tract, passing from the ileum through the (19) valve and into the first part of the large intestine, the (20). A long, wormlike structure known as the vermiform (21) is found here; its purpose is unknown, but if it becomes inflamed, it must be surgically removed.

Food waste then moves progressively through the large intestine as more water is absorbed and the waste becomes firmer. The section of large intestine that follows the cecum is the (22). It has three segments that are named according to their orientation within the abdomen. The (23) colon ascends upward from the cecum toward the liver. Under the liver it bends, forming the (24) flexure. It then continues across the abdomen; this section is the (25) colon. When it reaches the spleen, the (26) colon turns downward and forms the splenic flexure.

The next segment of the large intestine is the (27) colon, named for the S-shape resembling the Greek letter *sigma*. The last segment of the large intestine is the (28). Waste passes through a final sphincter at the base of the rectum called the (29), or (30) sphincter. The final solid waste product excreted from the body is known as (31) or (32). The process of excretion is called (33). The entire digestive tract is also known as the (34) canal or (35) tract, and the small and large intestines are known by the general term (36).

1. oral cavity _____
2. _____
3. _____
4. _____
5. _____
6. _____
7. _____
8. _____
9. _____
10. _____
11. _____
12. _____
13. _____
14. _____
15. _____
16. _____
17. _____
18. _____
19. _____
20. _____
21. _____
22. _____
23. _____
24. _____
25. _____
26. _____
27. _____
28. _____
29. _____
30. _____
31. _____
32. _____
33. _____
34. _____
35. _____
36. _____

Select words from the word list on the following page.

Fill-in Exercise: Digestion *(continued)*

alimentary	hepatic
amylase	hydrochloric
anal	ileocecal
anus	ileum
appendix	jejunum
ascending	lipase
bowel	liver
cardiac	mastication
cecum	oral cavity
colon	peristalsis
defecation	pharynx
deglutition	pyloric
descending	rectum
duodenum	rugae
esophagus	sigmoid
feces	stool
fundus	transverse
gallbladder	villi
gastrointestinal	

Adjective Exercise

Adjectives are formed from nouns by adding adjectival suffixes such as *-ac, -al, -ar, -ary, -eal, -ed, -ent, -iac, -ial, -ic, -ical, -lar, -oid, -ous, -tic,* and *-tous.* In addition, some adjectives have a different form entirely from the noun, which may be either Latin or Greek in origin.

Test your knowledge of adjectives by writing the adjectival form of the following gastroenterology words. Consult a medical dictionary to select the correct adjectival ending as necessary.

1. liver _____
2. esophagus _____
3. stomach _____
4. intestine _____
5. pylorus _____
6. ileum _____
7. colon _____
8. appendix _____
9. feces _____
10. nausea _____
11. jaundice _____
12. constipation _____
13. anorexia _____

Lay and Medical Terms

Lay Term	*Medical Term*
vomiting	emesis
belching	eructation
heartburn	GE reflux (gastroesophageal)
piles	hemorrhoids
gallstones	cholelithiasis
chewing	mastication
gas in stomach	flatulence
fart	flatus

Transcription Guidelines

Eponyms

1. An eponym is a place or thing which takes its name from a person (living or dead, real or imaginary). In the language of medicine, eponyms abound. Surgical instruments, medical devices, operative procedures, and anatomic structures are frequently named after the person who made the discovery or invention. An eponym that is used as an adjective is usually capitalized; the noun which follows is not.

Alzheimer's disease	Down syndrome
Tinel's sign	Kirschner rod
Buck's fascia	Achilles heel

2. A word derived from an eponym is generally not capitalized.

   cesarean section (from Julius Caesar)
   parkinsonism (from Parkinson's disease)
   kocherized (from Kocher clamp)

3. Avoid using an apostrophe and *s* with eponyms of surgical instruments and medical devices.

   Fogarty catheter (*not* Fogarty's catheter)
   DeBakey clamp (*not* DeBakey's clamp)

4. The use of the apostrophe and *s* with other eponyms is determined by common usage, as demonstrated in the examples above. The transcriptionist should consult a medical dictionary to determine current

usage, if the dictating physician's preference is not known.

Kasai operation	McBurney's incision
Apgar score	McMurray's maneuver

Exception: Hyphenated eponyms do not show possession.

Abbe's operation	Abbe-Estlander operation
Chiari's disease	Budd-Chiari syndrome

5. Various medical dictionaries and style references often disagree with each other about whether a particular eponym should have an apostrophe and s to show possession; thus, in many instances there may be more than one acceptable style.

Lasègue sign	Lasègue's sign
Cushing syndrome	Cushing's syndrome
Babinski reflex	Babinski's reflex
Graves disease	Graves' disease

6. If *a, an,* or *the* precedes an eponym, it is not necessary to use the possessive apostrophe and *s*.

She was placed in the Trendelenburg position.
A McBurney incision was made in the right
   lower quadrant.
The Bassini hernia repair was accomplished
   without difficulty.

Eponym Exercise

Instructions: Circle the correct eponym in the following sentences.

1. The patient experienced a (Jacksonian, jacksonian) seizure last week.

2. X-ray examination revealed (Osgood-Schlatter, Osgood-Schlatter's) disease.

3. We then inserted a (Rush's, Rush) rod into the tibia.

4. The abdomen was opened through a (Pfannenstiel, Pfannenstiel's) incision.

5. A (Jackson-Pratt, Jackson-Pratt's) drain was inserted for drainage.

How to Transcribe Eponyms

by John H. Dirckx, M.D.

The independent transcriptionist or transcription supervisor should adopt and follow certain basic styling guidelines, including some pertaining to eponyms. The following are suggested as being in accord with standard practice and as likely to be found acceptable by the vast majority of dictators.

1. **Capitalization.** Capitalize the first letter of a name that retains its character as a proper name (Fowler's position, tetralogy of Fallot).

Do not use a capital letter for a proper name that has been converted to a common noun (atlas) or a unit of measure (ampere).

Do not use a capital letter for a derived noun (coxsackievirus), adjective (gram-positive), or verb (kocherize).

2. **Accent marks.** Know and use accent marks appropriately if your typewriter or word processor has them. If not, do not write them in with a pen.

If you have no umlaut (ä, ö, ü), it is acceptable practice to insert an *e* after the umlauted vowel of a German or Scandinavian word or name (Friedlaender for Friedländer, Schoenberg for Schönberg, Schueller for Schüller). This cannot, however, be used instead of the dieresis of French, as in Laënnec.

3. **Particles.** Transcribe what you hear: Recklinghausen's disease or von Recklinghausen's disease, Quervain's disease or de Quervain's disease. Follow a standard reference work for capitalization of particles.

4. **Short forms.** Distinguish standard abridgments of names (Pap smear, K wire) and short forms of eponyms ("the Romberg is negative") from nonstandard slang forms (Mets for Metzenbaum scissors, Mik pad for Mikulicz pad). Type the former as dictated and expand the latter.

5. **Possessive 's form.** Transcribe what you hear: Alzheimer disease or Alzheimer's disease, Bartholin gland or Bartholin's gland (but not, of course, Lyme's disease).

After a name ending with an *s* or *z* sound, when a separate *s* is not normally heard in speech, it is acceptable to show the possessive with an apostrophe alone, omitting the *s* (Graves', Homans', Vleminckx'). Note, however, that a name ending in a silent *s* or *z* does not come under this rule (Duroziez's disease, François's syndrome—*Dorland's* to the contrary notwithstanding) and that some speakers do add a second *s* sound, particularly after names of one syllable (Betz's area, Fox's disease).

The last topic deserves some elaboration. Difficulties, inconveniences, and uncertainties regarding the *'s* possessive form in eponyms have prompted some medical editors and lexicographers to try to legislate it out of existence. According to one argument, this form is irrational because the persons named do not own the cells, structures, or tissues, or did not suffer from the diseases, syndromes, or signs, named after them. But look wherever you will in our language, you will find examples of the *'s* possessive (and the *of* possessive) in numerous cases where the possession is neither physical nor legal, but rather arises from discovery, invention, authorship, or publication.

Some editors, while acknowledging that the *'s* form is a natural and idiomatic feature of technical language, have sought to justify its abolition on the grounds of expediency, as part of that typographic simplification characteristic of newspaper styling, other features of which are the omission of periods and spaces from abbreviations (eg, MD) and of accent marks from foreign words and phrases.

A third argument for the wholesale exclusion of the *'s* form is that this form is inconsistently used. Much of the inconsistency is only apparent, however. The *'s* form is seldom used with compound names or with terms denoting instruments or other objects customarily preceded by the definite article (the Apgar score) or the indefinite article (an Erlenmayer flask, a Bassini repair—but a Cooper's ligament repair). It is also less common with terms denoting a plurality of objects (Kupffer cells, Kussmaul respirations). In many instances the *'s* has vanished because the proper name ends in an *s* or *z* sound (Coats disease, Graves—or Graves'—disease), or the following word begins with an *s* or *z* sound (Goodpasture syndrome, Wernicke zone).

Granted that there are exceptions to all of these rules, inconsistent use of the *'s* possessive form in eponyms is just one of a thousand irregularities and eccentricities in everyday language, including technical and formal language. An editor's function is to know and conserve the forms used by careful and cultivated speakers and writers, not to invent precepts out of thin air, in the pursuit of some elusive notion of linguistic homogeneity, that render idiomatic English illicit.

Certainly there is no justification for a rule that requires transcriptionists to omit the *'s* even when it is heard in dictation. The editorial function of the transcriptionist should be limited to the correction of errors and the application of well-founded and generally accepted rules of form and style. It should not be extended to include the imposition of arbitrary rules of usage on every dictator's choice of words. Moreover, the rule cannot always be put into effect by simply omitting the *'s*. "Dissection was carried down to Treitz's ligament." A change to "down to Treitz ligament" is not English, and "down to the Treitz ligament" is no better. The only acceptable variation is "down to the ligament of Treitz," and then what has become of all the arguments in favor of excluding *'s*? We still have a possessive expression; the *of* form (as contrasted with the null form seen in *Gram stain*) is just another inconsistency; and in typing *the* and *of* we have used more strokes than would have been needed to transcribe the term as dictated.

Transcription Tips

1. There are several sound-alike terms encountered in gastroenterology. Some common examples:

   peritoneal (refers to an area inside the abdominal cavity)
   perineal (pertains to the area between the genitalia and rectum)
   peroneal (pertains to the fibular bone in the leg)

2. Translate the following slang terms when dictated:

Slang	Translation
bili	bilirubin
procto	proctoscopy
tic	diverticulum

3. The following abbreviations should be translated for clarity when encountered in dictation.

Abbreviation	Translation
BE	barium enema
LFTs	liver function tests
RUQ	right upper quadrant
RLQ	right lower quadrant
LUQ	left upper quadrant
LLQ	left lower quadrant

4. Spelling tip: Spleen has two *e*'s, but *splenectomy* (removal of the spleen) has just one *e*.

5. Physicians commonly say *melanotic* when what they really mean is *melenic* (the passage of dark bloody stools). *Melanotic* refers to the presence of melanin (pigment), usually in the skin, and is not related to the stool or bowel.

6. Memorize the spelling of these difficult gastro-intestinal terms:

   cirrhosis
   borborygmus (the sound of gas moving through the
      intestine)
   intussusception

7. The following word has more than one acceptable spelling:

Preferred spelling	*Acceptable alternative*
distention	distension

8. Note the spellings of these challenging gastro-intestinal drugs:

   Dulcolax (the first *l* is often not pronounced by the
      dictator)
   Maalox (double *a*)
   Mylanta (*y*, not *i*)
   Mylicon (*y*, not *i*)
   Zantac (not to be confused with *Xanax*, an anti-
      anxiety drug)

Terminology Challenge

Instructions: The following terms appear in the dictation on Tape 2B, Gastroenterology. Before beginning the medical transcription practice for Lesson 5, become familiar with the terminology below by looking up each word in a medical or English dictionary. Write out a short definition of each term.

1+ bacteria	Hemoccult
acute	hemorrhage
antacid	high-power field
antibiotic	hyaline casts
appendectomy	jugular venous distention
Bactrim DS	lymphs (lymphocytes)
bands (banded	Maalox
neutrophils)	midepigastric
bile	monos (monocytes)
bilirubin	Naprosyn
bowel sounds	nausea
cholecystitis	niacin
cholelithiasis	nocturnal
codeine	organic disease
dehydration	p.r.n.
Di-Gel	palpitations
diet	Pepcid
BRAT	Percodan
clear liquid	peripheral edema
diffusely	Phenergan
Donnatal	phlegm
dyspeptic	pleural effusion
dysphagia	pleurisy
Ecotrin	prednisone
elixir	profuse
endoscopy	reflux
enteric-coated aspirin	regurgitation
eos (eosinophils)	segs (segmented
Epstein-Barr (EB)	neutrophils)
Excedrin	stool culture
Flexeril	substernal
gastroduodenal	Tagamet
gastroenteritis	temporally
gastrointestinal	Tigan
Gram stain	Torecan
guaiac	Tylenol No. 3
hematemesis	tympanitic
hematocrit	upper GI x-ray

Sample Reports

Sample gastroenterology reports appear on the following pages, illustrating different formats.

Transcription Practice

After completing all the readings and exercises in Lesson 5, transcribe Tape 2B, Gastroenterology. Use both medical and English dictionaries and your Quick-Reference Word List as resource materials for finding words.

Proofread your transcribed documents carefully, listening to the dictation while you read your transcripts.

Transcribe (*NOT* retype) the same reports again without referring to your previous transcription attempt. Initially, you may need to transcribe some reports more than twice before you can produce an error-free document. Your ultimate goal is to produce an error-free document the first time.

Humor: Doctors Learn and Grow

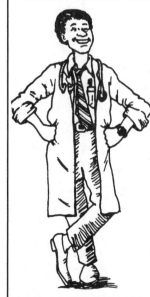

A favorite topic of medical transcriptionists is how physicians dictate reports. The difference between the dictating pattern of an eager young resident and that of an experienced practitioner is captured humorously in *MEDICATE ME* by Judith Marshall and illustrated by Cindy Stevens in the following excerpt.

How sweet doctors were in their youth. They sounded like this:

This is Dr. Cackleberry. Good evening. I am about to do my first physical, testing, testing, hope you can hear me. I want to do this right. I will spell all the medical words for you. This is a 36-year-old white female with BP 120/70 make a capital B and a capital P and the number 120 and a diagonal line, that is, uh, slash, I think, over the 70. That is 7–0.

Doctor learned and grew and became a successful physician in private practice, dictating to the same old transcriptionist—me:

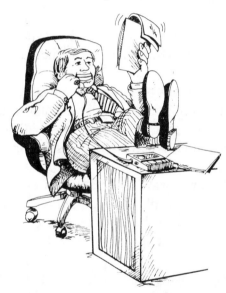

This is the big C here with a letter to, what date is this, the 7th of October, no, the 8th, 6th, whatever, you check that. Letter to looks like S. Voinovich, somewhere in Newton, look it up, re that Blount woman, I forget her name. Dear so and so, thank you for referring this pleasant 74-year-old female to me who was complaining of cardiac symptoms with no other problems. Then fill in the usual blah blah and so forth, normal exam, add the meds from the front of the chart, that's a good girl, signature, so and so and a copy to Frankel in Chicopee, he is some sort of osteopath. And I told you I'm in to my broker and not in to my wife, not the other way around. Now a letter to—

July 3, 1993

A. Sterling Workman, M.D.
3567 Union Avenue
Laborville, CA 93025

Re: Kent Feinditte

Dear Dr. Workman:

I was embarrassed to find out that through a clerical slip-up, this consultation note was not dictated promptly as it should have been. Please accept my apology.

I personally reviewed the air contrast barium enema. The radiologist's impression was that there was a soft tissue mass in the terminal ileum. My impression was that this could possibly be a Meckel's, although this would be very unusual. This is probably lymphoid hyperplasia and is unimpressive.

My impression is irritable bowel syndrome and possibly a Meckel's diverticulum. Therapeutically, I suggested he go on a high-fiber diet, and our nursing staff talked to him extensively about the use of bran. He was given three Hemoccult test cards and these were returned, and all three were negative.

Unless symptoms recur, I do not believe a further invasive workup is necessary at this time.

Thank you very much for referring me this patient, and again I apologize for the delay in sending you this note.

Sincerely,

Damon Fieckelith, M.D.

DF:hpi

Joe Bleaux   #82741   July 4, 1992   Medical 502B

GASTROENTEROLOGY CONSULTATION

The patient received multiple transfusions for his multiple vascular surgeries. There was no history of any jaundice following any of these transfusions, although he relates some jaundice many, many years ago with the etiology at that time being unclear. He has manifested no symptoms referable to liver disease and generally remains asymptomatic in this regard. There is no history of significant alcohol intake, recent travel, and the only drug one could implicate in his hepatitis is Aldomet, which he has been on for only one year.

His physical examination revealed that his liver extended 3 to 4 fingerbreadths below his right costal margin and was firm; however, no other signs of liver disease, namely, spider angiomata or palmar erythema, were present. We have found that his SGOT was elevated at least as far back as February. Several repeat blood tests have shown varying degrees of elevation of the bilirubin and transaminases. Additionally, his globulins have been elevated and his pro time has been mildly prolonged to approximately 50% of control.

It seems likely that Mr. Bleaux has chronic liver disease from his transfusions in the 1970s, the etiology being non-A non-B. It is unlikely that Aldomet is contributing to his elevated transaminases, as the elevations have been documented prior to the Aldomet usage. The possible chronic liver diseases include chronic persistent hepatitis, chronic active hepatitis, and the possible development of cirrhosis. I am concerned about the development of cirrhosis in view of the prolonged pro time and the elevated globulin level, although one cannot be sure regarding this diagnosis without a liver biopsy. In view of his mild enzyme elevations and his asymptomatic state in regard to his liver disease despite a liver biopsy showing chronic active hepatitis, I could not imagine treating him with immunosuppressive therapy in view of his age and general medical condition. Additionally, it is still unknown at this time what the natural history of this disease is as well as whether there is any significant response to steroid therapy in terms of prognosis. As well, with his mildly prolonged pro time, this would pose a slightly increased risk for the liver biopsy that at this time I do not feel is warranted in view of the unlikelihood of any treatment based on the liver biopsy findings.

We will simply watch him and have repeat liver tests in approximately 3 months. Should the disease progress in any way or he become symptomatic or new data become available on the use of steroids in the treatment of non-A, non-B chronic liver disease, then we may reassess the need for the liver biopsy at that time.

DAMON FIECKELITH, M.D.

DF:hpi
d: 7/4/92
t: 7/5/92

CHART NOTE

Ida Wannagh   February 25, 1992

The patient has primary biliary cirrhosis. I refilled the patient's colchicine. Articles were sent to the patient on primary biliary cirrhosis. The patient should have LFTs and a serum cholesterol drawn q. 8 months. I ordered a chem-25, CBC, iron, and TIBC. The results of these tests were within normal limits with the following important exceptions: serum iron was 45, which is low; TIBC was 433, which is high; and percent iron saturation was 10, which is low. Her ferritin was 10, which is also low. These results taken together indicate that the patient was iron deficient, and so I started her on Feosol one p.o. b.i.d. Her GGT was 105, which is elevated, and alkaline phosphatase was 209, which is also elevated. A CT scan of the abdomen had been done and was negative.

She continued to have abdominal pain. I gave her a trial of Reglan 10 mg p.o. q.i.d. and also scheduled an upper GI with small-bowel follow-through. The upper GI showed hesitancy in opening of the duodenal bulb, but the bulb was intrinsically normal and the duodenum was normal as well. The remainder of the upper GI series and small bowel series was normal. I don't believe the hesitancy in the opening of the duodenal bulb to be significant.

I saw the patient again with continued complaints of abdominal pain. At that time her friend had just died of colon cancer. She complained of fatigue and malaise as well as new symptoms of reflux and heartburn.

My impression is that she has irritable bowel syndrome as well as esophageal reflux. I gave her a prescription of Sinequan 25 mg q.d. and a sample supply of Tagamet 400 mg b.i.d. The Tagamet improved her symptoms, as she called in for a refill.

DF:hpi
d: 2/25/92
t: 2/26/92

Colin Bloom   #90438   Admitted: 6/1/92   Medical 302C

HISTORY AND PHYSICAL EXAMINATION

ADMISSION DIAGNOSIS: Metastatic colon cancer.

HISTORY OF PRESENT ILLNESS: A 61-year-old white male who is status post sigmoid resection and segmentectomy of the liver for colon cancer, who presents because of liver metastasis on CT scan despite one year of 5-FU therapy. He is without complaint of loss of appetite, weight loss, nausea, vomiting, jaundice, melena, or hematochezia. He denies change in bowel habits since the operation but does chronically have bulky stools.

PAST MEDICAL HISTORY: Resection of the sigmoid with segmentectomy of the left lobe of the liver, secondary to metastases, and a primary colocolostomy. Metastases were also noted to the regional and retroperitoneal lymph nodes which were also resected. 5-FU therapy was given as above.

MEDICATIONS ON ADMISSION: None.

ALLERGIES: None.

FAMILY HISTORY: There is no family history of cancer.

SOCIAL HISTORY: The patient does not smoke or drink.

PHYSICAL EXAMINATION:
VITAL SIGNS: Blood pressure 110/70, pulse of 60, respiratory rate 18, temperature 36.
GENERAL: This is a well-developed, well-nourished white male in no acute distress.
HEAD & NECK: HEENT unremarkable. Neck is supple without JVD, adenopathy, or bruit.
CHEST: Lungs are clear. Heart, regular rate and rhythm.
ABDOMEN is soft, nondistended, and nontender. Liver is approximately 8 to 10 cm in span and does not descend below the right costal margin. There is no splenomegaly or masses.
LYMPH NODES: There is no palpable adenopathy throughout.
RECTAL: Normal anal sphincter tone. No masses. Heme negative.
NEUROLOGICAL: Neurologically the patient is intact.

ADMISSION LABORATORY: Hemoglobin 14.4. White blood cells 6.9 with 66 segs, 19 lymphs, 5 monos, 9 eos, and 1 baso. Platelets 295,000. ASTRA was within normal limits. The profile showed an alkaline phosphatase of 141, AST of 29, total bilirubin of 0.5, total protein 7.5, albumin 3.9. PT is 11.5 and PTT is 28.1. Chest x-ray showed a small, approximately 1 cm nodule in the right lower lung and was otherwise normal.

PRINCIPAL DIAGNOSIS: Metastatic colon cancer.

_____
DAMON FIECKELITH, M.D.

DF:hpi
d: 6/1/92
t: 6/1/92

DATE OF SURGERY: July 5, 1993

PREOPERATIVE DIAGNOSIS: Symptomatic chronic cholecystitis and cholelithiasis.

POSTOPERATIVE DIAGNOSIS: Symptomatic chronic cholecystitis and cholelithiasis.
     Possible cyst or adenomyoma of the gallbladder.

OPERATION: Cholecystectomy with operative cholangiograms.

OPERATIVE PROCEDURE: Under satisfactory general anesthesia the abdomen was prepped with Betadine and draped, and a right subcostal incision was made. Bleeding was controlled by electro-coagulation. On exploration the liver margins were sharp. The gallbladder was not thick-walled. It was somewhat tense and stones could not definitely be palpated within it. The cystic duct was fairly long and quite small in diameter, and the common duct was of normal size. The stomach, spleen, kidneys, and pancreas were essentially normal to palpation although the right kidney seemed quite small. It was difficult to palpate in the lower abdomen. From prior surgery there were adhesions, and I did not feel anything in the lower half of the abdomen.

After packing the gut out of the way, the cholecystoduodenal ligament was opened. The cystic duct was fairly long and was milked up with a right-angle clamp and a Weck clip placed on it at its junction with the gallbladder. The cystic artery was easily identified, and it was cleaned and three Weck clips placed on it, and it was divided, leaving two clips on the proximal end of the artery. The gallbladder was dissected out from above downward and bleeders in the bed electrocoagulated as they were encountered.

A small opening was made in the cystic duct, and with some difficulty a cystic duct Cholangiocath was placed down into the common duct and a special clamp used to hold it in place. There was free flow of saline, and then dye was injected and two films were taken. On the first film there was a suggestion of a round mass just below the tip of the catheter. On the subsequent film I was not able to identify that. Subsequently a third film was taken, and most of the dye had gone into the duodenum and there was no shadow there that would suggest a stone. It was therefore felt that this most likely represented an air bubble.

The Cholangiocath was removed. The cystic duct was clipped with two Weck clips. The subhepatic area was irrigated with saline and aspirated and inspected, and there was no significant bleeding.

CLOSURE: Peritoneum and posterior rectus sheath with running 0 Vicryl. Anterior rectus sheath with running 0 Vicryl. The wound was irrigated, and the subcutaneous tissue was approximated with interrupted 3-0 Vicryl, and the skin was closed with clips.

Condition of patient at the end of operation was satisfactory. Estimated blood loss was approxi-mately 50 cc. The prognosis should be excellent.

DAMON FIECKELITH, M.D.

DF:hpi d&t: 7/6/93

MOUNTAIN MEDICAL CENTER Live Oak, California 90010 **OPERATIVE REPORT**	Thomas Ratley #802741 Surgery 400-C

DATE OF SURGERY: October 1, 1990

ANESTHESIA TIME: 7:30 a.m.-8:30 a.m.
OPERATION TIME: 7:35 a.m.-8:30 a.m

PREOPERATIVE DIAGNOSIS: Recurrent right inguinal hernia.

POSTOPERATIVE DIAGNOSIS: Recurrent right inguinal hernia.

TITLE OF OPERATION: Right inguinal hernia repair.

PROCEDURE: After the patient was placed supine on the operating table and proper level of anesthesia was attained, the abdomen was prepped and draped in the usual sterile fashion.

A right groin incision was made and carried through the subcutaneous tissue, through Scarpa's fascia, and to the external oblique fascia. The external oblique fascia was opened from the internal inguinal ring to the external inguinal ring. The ilioinguinal nerve was identified and preserved. The cord was mobilized and a defect was found medially. This was a direct inguinal hernia recurrence. The floor was entirely opened up, and a hernia repair was carried out by reapproximating the conjoined tendon down to Cooper's ligament with a running 0 Prolene stitch. This was carried out until a transition suture was placed, and then the conjoined tendon was reapproximated to the shelving edge until the internal inguinal ring was snug. The external oblique was closed over the cord with a running 3-0 Vicryl suture, the subcutaneous tissue with 3-0 plain, and the skin with a running 4-0 subcuticular Dexon stitch. The patient's wound was dressed, and he was sent to the recovery room in satisfactory condition.

_____

H. R. PILES, M.D.

HRP:hpi
d: 10/2/90
t: 10/3/90

MOUNTAIN MEDICAL CENTER
Lone Tree, California 90000

OPERATIVE REPORT

Samuel Senn

#802741

Surgery 400-C

Lesson 6. Gastroenterology

Learning Objectives

Medical

- Describe the causes of and treatments for common GI diseases.
- Discuss the purpose and technique involved in performing common GI laboratory tests and surgical procedures.
- Given a GI root word, symptom, or disease, match it to its correct medical definition.
- Define common GI abbreviations.
- Given a category of GI drugs, indicate which drugs belong to that category.

Fundamentals

- Discuss how the dictating practices of some physicians impact the transcription process.
- List some of the reasons why surgical procedures are performed.
- List identifying or background information included in the heading of an operative report.
- Discuss the correct use of capitals in editing medical sentences.
- Given a medical report with errors, identify and correct the errors.

Practice

- Accurately transcribe authentic physician dictation from the specialty of gastroenterology.

A Closer Look

Birds of a Feather

by Judith Marshall, MA, CMT

People and birds, I think, have a lot in common in the way they look and sound. For example, my uncle Felix looks like a parakeet and sounds like a hawk. (He also jaywalks.) However, in medical transcription I seldom see the dictating physicians, but that does not deter me from thinking of their voices as birdsong. No field glasses needed, just a place to perch and true grit to translate the hoots and wails, whistles, trills, and rolling twitters into intelligible medical documents.

I have pigeonholed some dictating birds (apologies to Audubon), some for whom I would leave a trail of breadcrumbs to my typewriter and some for whom I would buy a very large cat.

Consider the **Golden-Throated Boomer.** Its call is a loud repetition of its name. This is no timid chirp but a jovial "Hello, this is Dr. John J. Hunter, H-U-N-T-E-R." The Boomer's harmonics are liquid and flowing and its tempo perky. How good it is to hear that sort of forthright pronunciation. The Boomer never assumes the transcriptionist has been there for forty years and knows all physicians on the staff. Would that there were more Boomers in the Aviary!

Boomers stick to the point, unlike the **Wandering Tattler.** Tattlers have rapid tinkling notes and can be spotted in elevators, in the hall, and in the cafeteria where they discuss cases and use patient names. Tattlers dictate and talk to everyone around them at the same time. They can be useful in providing stock tips as they speak with a colleague or make other illuminating personal comments. Amazingly they never seem to know that we are out there listening, and listen we must, for at any moment they will again begin dictating.

Pink-Plumed Chucklers are at a premium in my work. No one can resist their wit. Humor is too rare in life and the Chuckler's humor never hurts anyone, especially the patient. The Chuckler is fun and jolly, but the cheer never detracts from the integrity of the medical record and certainly adds life to a tedious six-page report.

The **Red-Faced Hotdogger** does not mean to be funny but he is. This dictator just doesn't know he doesn't know and is not always a first-year resident. The senior staff member who is an expert in one major field and whose patient suffers from an ailment outside this area of expertise snatches at the word and misses. That's all right, Hotdogger. We know what you mean and we will get it right.

Silver-Tongued Wagtails are distinct and courteous. They have realistic expectations, empathy with the transcriptionist, and they know what they want to say. If you have any of these around, take them to lunch, give them an award, say thank you, write a complimentary note, and cherish them. They are on the endangered species list right now.

Wagtails have a foreign variety too. English may be their second or third language, but Wagtails are precise. They can spell anything correctly, including their names, and they sense when I **want** them to spell. Regional accents can be a problem but not with Wagtails. From Tennessee Warbler to Boston Brahminbird, it is possible to make beautiful music. The accent just adds grace notes to the dictation.

The **Black-Bellied Ring-Necked Loon** has a romantic call but is usually silent in the winter. There is a good reason. They hatch all their dictation in the spring. In the same group of quiet dictators is the **Hooded Roseate Spoonbill** who is nearly always silent—even with the microphone in hand. The long, lamentable pauses between sentences are irritating. But they are the only group that allows me a chance to stand up, headset on, and stretch my legs. The Spoonbill never seems to understand that in a voice-activated dictation system, silence will cut him off. At least **Ruffled Skimmers** make a little noise. They flip charts, rustle paper, and manage a snack while dictating. I know they are out there. I hear them breathing.

A little rascal who inhabits medical facilities is the **White-Rumped Clicker.** His call is a rapid clicking while in flight. Clickers never learned to use any equipment correctly. They are so busy going backwards they almost never go forward. They are ubiquitous and they have developed some little antibodies which make them impervious to advice from anyone.

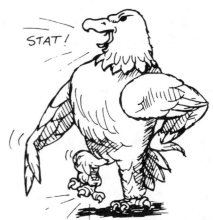

Judith Marshall, *MEDICATE ME*
Illustrated by Cindy Stevens

The **Snowy-Tufted Backdater** comes on the line on October 23 but wants all the dictation dated September 21. The Horned variety, when dictating letters, usually blames the office staff for losing and misfiling charts or blames the transcription service for losing dictation. Almost as frustrating is the **Ruby-Throated Statfoot,** named after its infamous call "Stat! Stat! Stat!" If they rule the roost, they do get what they cry for. The Statfoots differ from the Wagtails and Boomers in that most of their emergencies are self-made. Statfoots procrastinate or they forget to do their dictation. Backdaters and Statfoots do intermarry.

The **Snake-Eyed Abbreviator** lurks everywhere. The SEA uses every legal and authorized abbreviation in medical history and then improvises on the wing. HEENT and PERRLA and ASHD and CHF are trifles to this bird. "TPWWAC," says he, and the best minds in transcription are stunned. We look at the chart, confer among ourselves, and puzzle over it. We leave it blank and flag it. At the end of the summary there it is again and not a clue in sight. "TPWWAC," says he. We ask the SEA, who can't remember. Three months later the patient is readmitted and the history and physical is dictated by someone else who says, "The patient walked with the aid of a cane." Of course. How could we miss it? The SEA is called a turkey in plain English because its English never is.

Have you ever been tempted to punch someone in the beak? The most likely candidate would be the **Yellow-Crowned Changer.** "Correction, correction." I pause, I wait, thinking to trap him, listening ahead to anticipate the change. The Changer outwits me every time, sometimes clipping through four pages with scarcely an intake of breath. Once I am off guard and speeding along, the Changer stops me cold. "Take out that last paragraph." (Picture him roasted with carbon paper stuffing—oh, savory revenge.)

Orange-Tufted Nitpickers ignore medical transcriptionists for months on end. We transcribe marvelously, capture every nuance, and our copy is superb. We never hear a peep from the Nitpicker. Then without warning Nitpickers swoop down and nip. "You left out the capital C in New York City." "You didn't sign me off with my middle initial on this one report."

Nitpickers are distinct from **Red Pencilbirds** in that Nitpickers are correct in what they find, minuscule as it may be. Pencilbirds revel in editing. They have changed their minds and have practically rewritten the note and say, "Now take a look at this. This is what I said in the first place." "Not-suetable" is their call.

We can't fling our less than favorites from the nest but we can enjoy their diversity and we can learn from all of them. We could fly the coop ourselves, but most of us are here to stay. We have progressed. For the most part we do not copy from hen scratchings. Try dictating for an hour. It is humbling. Then make the best of it, feed the birds (popcorn and apples are always welcome), make friends with them, cajole them, advise them, but, above all, serve them. Their songs are not ordinary.

Surgery and Surgical Dictation

Part 1

John H. Dirckx, M.D.

Transcribing operative reports with maximum accuracy and facility calls for a knowledge of surgical terminology, a grasp of basic surgical principles, and some insight into the purpose and nature of surgical dictation. To a great extent, skill in this field can only be acquired through experience. My purpose here is to lay the groundwork for the development and refinement of such skill by imparting some fundamental information about how and why surgeons do what they do, and what factors determine the nature and content of surgical dictation.

Surgery—some basic concepts and principles. Surgery, if I may attempt a somewhat unconventional definition, is the science and art of correcting or ameliorating health problems with tools. Although the word *surgery* goes back to a Greek term meaning "working with one's hands," the implication has always been that those hands held tools, except in a few cases such as the reduction of fractures and dislocations where tools are not needed.

Modern surgeons use hundreds of highly specialized instruments, including some that are for purely diagnostic purposes. Although many surgical procedures can be performed through natural body orifices such as the mouth or the vagina, most of them involve making an artificial opening, usually an incision (cut) through the skin. This is so integral to the modern concept of surgery that a diagnostic or therapeutic procedure involving no cutting and no blood loss is generally not considered truly surgical.

Surgical procedures form a significant part of the practice of many medical specialties. The scope of general surgery varies from one area or institution to another, but generally includes operations on abdominal organs and the breast, the repair of hernias of the abdominal wall, and the surgical treatment of infections and neoplasms of the soft tissues. Orthopedic surgery is concerned with diseases and injuries of bones, joints, and muscles. Plastic and reconstructive surgery includes the repair of injuries, particularly those involving the skin of the face, and the prevention or correction of disfigurement or functional impairment due to congenital malformations, trauma, infection, malignancy, or previous surgery. The respective provinces of thoracic and cardiovascular surgery, neurosurgery, ophthalmology, otolaryngology, gynecology, and proctology are evident. Some surgeons specialize in the treatment of children, others in the treatment of patients with malignant diseases, still others in a single procedure such as cataract extraction with implantation of an artificial lens.

There is no sharp distinction between major and minor surgery. Generally speaking, a procedure that takes less than an hour, involves no vital organs or serious threat to life, and can be carried out by a single operator would be considered minor surgery. The term would also be applied to most procedures performed under local anesthesia or on an outpatient basis. Outpatient surgery is becoming increasingly popular, partly because of the high cost of hospital care. Although this type of surgery is usually performed in a hospital, with immediate access to the full range of diagnostic and therapeutic equipment and services available there, the patient is not admitted for an overnight stay. The limiting factor with outpatient surgery is often the time needed for the patient to recover from the effects of anesthesia.

It may be helpful to list some of the reasons for which surgical procedures are commonly performed, with examples of procedures performed for each type of reason.

Correction of congenital defects
   Repair of tracheoesophageal fistula
   Repair of cleft palate
   Strabismus repair
   Closure of spina bifida
   Derotation osteotomy for tibial torsion
Repair of injury or degenerative change
   Surgical closure of skin laceration
   Inguinal herniorrhaphy
   Laminectomy with excision of herniated
     nucleus pulposus
   Extraction of foreign body
   Debridement of burns
Removal of neoplasms and other abnormal growths
   Mastectomy for carcinoma of breast
   Resection of colon for carcinoma
   Excision of sebaceous cyst of back
   Extraction of ureteral stone
   Amputation of limb for osteogenic sarcoma
   Debulking of invasive and otherwise
     inoperable abdominal neoplasm
Procedures for treatment of localized infection
   Incision and drainage of furuncle
   Incision and drainage of subphrenic abscess
   Marsupialization of Bartholin abscess
Removal of an organ or tissue damaged or destroyed
by acute or chronic inflammation
   Appendectomy for acute appendicitis
   Cholecystectomy for chronic cholecystitis
     with cholelithiasis
   Oophorectomy for salpingitis
Removal, repair, or replacement of damaged or worn
structures
   Repair of cardiac valve
   Replacement of femoral head
   Cataract extraction
   Aortofemoral bypass graft
Revision or reconstruction of anatomy for improved
function
   Portacaval shunt for esophageal varices
   Hydrocephalus shunt
   Coronary artery bypass graft
   Billroth II anastomosis
Diagnostic procedures
   Arthroscopy
   Laparoscopy
   Exploratory laparotomy
   Open biopsy
Destructive procedures
   Castration in prostatic cancer
   Tubal ligation for prevention of conception

   Stellate ganglionectomy for posttraumatic
     ischemia of forearm
   Vagotomy for intractable peptic ulcer disease
Cosmetic surgery
   Breast augmentation
   Breast reduction
   Liposuction
   Remodeling of nose or chin

It should be evident that there are close parallels between many of the procedures listed above and the maintenance, repair, or reconditioning of a piece of machinery, such as an automobile. To carry the parallel a step further, when you have mechanical repairs done on your car's engine or transmission, much of the labor time you pay for is involved in disassembly and re-assembly. Similarly, although it takes but a single stroke of the knife to sever a diseased appendix or gallbladder, the surgeon must spend many minutes in gaining access to the site of the trouble and many more in putting everything back together after the essential work of the operation is done.

Surgical dictation—the what and the why. Most of the reasons for including a detailed operative report in the hospital, office, or clinic records of a surgical patient will occur to any intelligent person with some knowledge of medical matters. First, this information is essential to the completeness of a surgical patient's record and is often the most important thing in that record. Secondly, like any other medical record, the operative report may acquire importance as a legal document. It may, for example, be required to justify the fee charged by the surgeon for the procedure, particularly when, as is nearly always the case, the fee is to be paid by an insurance company or government agency. In case of litigation, the record will supply evidence in court on such matters as the indications for surgery and for the choice of procedure performed, the names of persons who participated in or witnessed the operation, and the exact nature and sequence of techniques employed.

Third, the information included in the operative report may be of crucial importance in the future medical and surgical care of the patient. Simply recording that the patient had a right inguinal herniorrhaphy or a right hip arthroplasty leaves unanswered many questions of technique. Exactly what condition was found by the surgeon at the time of operation? Which of various possible techniques were used, and why? What was removed? How were things put back together? Were grafts, implants, or other foreign materials left in the patient, and if so what was their nature, origin, and exact placement? Were any unusual problems encountered in the course of the surgery, and if so, how were they dealt with? The surgeon himself cannot be expected to remember details like these from every operation he performs. Other physicians and surgeons can only guess what exactly took place on the day of surgery if, later on, they are called upon to diagnose and treat delayed complications, problems arising with grafts or implants, or perhaps a recurrence of the condition for which surgery was performed. Finally, the prompt dictation of a detailed and accurate narrative of each operation performed is part of the intellectual discipline and lifelong learning process of the surgeon, whether he is a first-year resident or a seasoned veteran.

The format used by the surgeon in dictating an operative report will depend to some extent on the specialty and training, on the nature of the procedure, and on local conventions and institutional guidelines. The following discussion is based on an idealized format, some parts of which would be appropriate only for certain types of surgery. In addition, some pieces of information presented here under separate headings are regularly included by some dictators as part of the account of the operative procedure.

Identifying data and basic background information. Often a printed form is used for operative reports containing a heading with spaces for entering the following information.

Identifying data. The operative report must contain, as an absolute minimum, the name of the patient and any case or admission number assigned by the hospital for record-keeping purposes; the name of the surgeon; and the date on which the procedure was performed.

Name of procedure. Generally, standard procedural terminology must by used, and in addition to the name of the operation, a code number, for insurance and statistical purposes, may be required to be entered by the surgeon or by a clerk.

Preoperative diagnosis. The surgeon's provisional assessment of the patient's condition before beginning the operation, including the disease or condition that is the principal reason for the surgery. Again, standard terminology is required, followed by appropriate coding.

Postoperative diagnosis. A more definitive and precise diagnosis established at or after operation, but often the same as the preoperative diagnosis.

Names of surgeon(s) and anesthesiologist(s). The surgeon, any surgical assistants, and the anesthesiologist(s) are ordinarily identified somewhere in the operative record. The name of the person dictating the operative report (who may not be the principal surgeon) will also appear at the end of the dictation. In some institutions, nurses or technicians assisting in the operating room are also identified.

Indications, history. Here the dictator elaborates on the preoperative diagnosis and explains the reasons that led him to perform surgery on this patient and to choose the procedure and techniques used. This part of the operative report is not to be confused with the full clinical history of the patient contained elsewhere in the hospital record and perhaps dictated by someone other than the surgeon.

Clinical status, physical examination. This information is a continuation of the preceding and may appear under the same heading. The surgeon describes the patient's physical condition (including results of pertinent laboratory tests or x-rays), particularly as it has a bearing on the need for surgery and the choice of procedure. Again, this is not to be confused with the complete physical examination report contained elsewhere in the patient's record.

Operative report. The dictator's description of the actual surgical procedure may be given as a continuous narrative or may be presented under two or more of the following headings.

Anesthesia. A simple statement of the type of anesthetic used. The dictator may say simply ''general'' or ''spinal,'' knowing that detailed information about the anesthetic will be recorded by the anesthesiologist.

Position. The position of the patient on the operating table is often passed over in silence unless some special positioning is required by the nature of the procedure.

Skin preparation. Scrubbing of the skin is usually a routine procedure carried out by an assistant or technician. The surgeon may record the name of the soap or disinfectant used and any special procedures used for sterile draping.

Incision. Under this heading the surgeon records the anatomic location and orientation of the incision by which he gained access to the operative site, for example, ''right upper quadrant oblique'' or ''medial sternotomy.''

Procedure, technique. A detailed, step-by-step narrative of the operation from beginning to end. Although parts of the operative report may be quite routine, each operation varies in some details from others, and a thorough and accurate report will reflect this uniqueness. The surgeon ordinarily includes in this narrative a record of his findings and some comment on their bearing on the choice of procedure and their implications for the future health of the patient.

Grafts, implants. Any foreign objects or materials left in the patient, including grafts, artificial cardiac valves, artificial joints, orthopedic fixation devices, pacemakers, shunts, mesh, screws, wire, and cement, must be fully identified. The brand names, chemical nature, origin, sizes, shapes, adjustments or settings, and exact anatomic location of such materials are all an essential part of the record.

Closure. The repair of the incision and of any dissection or structural alterations performed during the surgery. Each layer of the body wall is closed separately, often with a different type of stitch and a different suture material for each layer. The skin may be closed with metal clips or adhesive strips.

Operative findings. When not incorporated in the operative report, this information appears under its own heading at some point in the dictation.

Supplemental and postoperative data. This part of the record supplies essential information about the patient as of the conclusion of the operation.

Drains, packs, dressings. These are devices or materials temporarily placed in or on the patient during or at the conclusion of the procedure. Since they must later be removed, recording their presence is of critical importance. Splints, casts, and other externally applied devices such as suction apparatus for evacuation of bleeding from the operative site may also be reported here.

Tourniquet time. The number of minutes during which blood flow to an extremity was shut off by a tourniquet.

Specimens, cultures. Any materials removed from the patient during surgery and intended to be submitted for laboratory study.

Sponge and needle counts. In order that no foreign material or object may be inadvertently left inside the patient, it is standard practice for sponges, needles, and certain other articles to be counted before the commencement of surgery and again just before the surgeon begins to close the wound. Usually two persons perform the counts together for greater security. The surgeon does not begin closure of the wound until the sponge and needle counts are reported correct.

Estimated blood loss. Various measures are used during an operation to monitor blood loss, including close observation of blood absorbed by sponges and measurement of blood in the trap of the suction machine.

Fluids administered. Intravenous fluids, including whole blood, administered during the procedure are sometimes recorded in the operative report. This information is also part of the anesthesia record.

Condition of patient at conclusion of operation. The surgeon reports that the patient left the operating room in satisfactory condition or, if this is not so, records any significant health problems occasioned by the surgery or anesthesia.

Complications. Under this heading the surgeon lists any unexpected and untoward consequences of the surgical procedure, such as accidental injury to healthy tissues or organs, extensive hemorrhage, or adverse reactions to anesthesia.

Postoperative plan. The surgeon's intentions regarding postoperative care, including inhalation therapy, physical therapy, graded resumption of activities, follow-up examinations, and so on.

Medical Readings

A Surgeon's View of Gastroenterology

by Thomas L. Largen, M.D., FACS

As a board-certified general surgeon in private practice for over thirty years, I have performed numerous surgical procedures. But one of my favorite subjects is gastroenterology, that branch of medical science concerned with the study of the stomach, intestines, and related structures, including the esophagus, liver, gallbladder, and pancreas.

The modern endoscope. An endoscope is a long hollow tube with a light source that can be inserted into a hollow organ to view and assess the condition of the organ. In gastroenterology, there are three categories of endoscopes: the esophagogastroscope, the sigmoidoscope, and the colonoscope.

When I was a resident in the early 1950s, only rigid endoscopes existed. The rigid esophagoscope of that era was a very dangerous instrument. It could easily perforate the esophagus, which in essence is a flimsy, thin-walled tube. Additionally, it was of little value in examining the stomach because it could not negotiate the curves and corners of the organ.

The rigid sigmoidoscope of the 1950s was about 10 inches (or 25 cm) in length, and it too had its limitations. Because it was short, it didn't allow much exposure, and because it was rigid there was the danger of perforating the lower colon.

Then in the early 1970s, Japan introduced the first fiberoptic flexible endoscope. That event alone drastically changed the direction and practice of gastroenterology. Up until 10 or 15 years ago, most GI work was performed by general surgeons. With the advent of flexible fiberoptics, medical doctors began to specialize in diagnosis, treatment, and procedures of the GI tract, and the field of gastroenterology became a specialty. Today, most endoscopes utilize state-of-the-art flexible fiberoptics.

Endoscopic diagnosis and treatment. This is an exciting time in gastroenterology practice. With the introduction of the flexible endoscope, new treatment modalities have evolved. People who present with gastrointestinal hemorrhage from either the upper GI tract (the esophagus, stomach, or duodenum) or the lower GI tract (the colon) are frequently diagnosed by means of upper and/or lower endoscopy. Bleeding sites can be controlled by application of a heat probe through the endoscope or injection of a sclerosing (hardening) agent through a long needle passed through the endoscope. Bleeding esophageal varices, a serious medical condition, are often controlled by sclerosing these dilated varicose veins through the esophagoscope.

Patients who have had strokes or other medical problems are sometimes unable to swallow or eat properly and require a temporary alternative means of obtaining nutrition. There are now techniques whereby a feeding tube can be inserted into the stomach by way of an esophagogastroscope, eliminating the need to do open surgery for this purpose. Endoscopes are also useful in removing foreign bodies from the esophagus, and occasionally from the stomach or duodenum.

Today, surgical procedures can even be performed through endoscopes. An experienced gastroenterologist can do a sphincterotomy through the scope (cutting the sphincter of Oddi, which is located in the second portion of the duodenum through which the pancreatic duct and the common bile duct enter the small intestine). Retained gallstones in the biliary ducts can be extracted using a wire basket-type catheter placed through the scope, eliminating the need for the patient to undergo an open operation.

Polypectomies (the surgical removal of outgrowths) are frequently performed to remove polyps in the stomach and colon. A wire snare is connected to an electrosurgical unit, placed through the endoscope, and the polyp is removed and the bleeding base coagulated.

Polyps are a common occurrence and may or may not be malignant.

Endoscopes are leading the way to early diagnosis and treatment of malignancies. Directed laser beams can be used through the endoscope for palliative surgery such as burning a hole through a malignant tumor in the esophagus to allow a patient to swallow. Malignancies of the stomach and colon are diagnosed much earlier, thanks to endoscopes, and this increases our chances for curing neoplasms of the entire GI tract.

Other advances. Although the use of flexible fiberoptic endoscopes dominates modern gastroenterology practice, other diagnostic modes are also used. It may come as a surprise that the value of traditional contrast media studies (upper GI series, air-contrast barium enema) rests entirely with the radiologist. It takes a dedicated, interested radiologist to produce a diagnostic exam.

Ultrasound (visualizing internal body structures by recording the reflections of ultrasonic waves) is useful in diagnosing biliary tract disease and pancreatic disease. Nuclear studies such as the DISIDA scan are helpful in identifying biliary tract involvement. There is also a nuclear scan that localizes gastrointestinal bleeding sites. Computerized tomography (CT) scans can help diagnose pancreatic and liver masses. Magnetic resonance imaging (MRI) studies are yet to be of much help in evaluating the gastrointestinal tract, although arteriography is of great help in localizing bleeding sites, and even therapeutically stopping a bleeding vessel by plugging (embolizing) the vessel with small debris, such as Gelfoam.

The use of mechanical bowel preparations and preoperative and perioperative antibiotics has markedly decreased postoperative wound infections and leaks. However, there is no substitute for good surgical technique. The gastrointestinal contents should never be allowed to spill into the wound or abdominal cavity. Gloves and instruments should be changed immediately upon completing a gastrointestinal anastomosis (sewing two ends together) and proceeding with closure of the surgical wound.

The advent of surgical staplers, originally introduced in Russia, has made gastrointestinal surgery safer, quicker, and more fun to do. Resections of various parts of the GI tract used to take two to three hours; now a resection can be accomplished in 30 to 45 minutes in most cases.

Bleeding esophageal varices. Esophageal varices (varicose veins in the esophagus) are most frequently encountered in patients with cirrhosis of the liver, and they can bleed profusely. It used to be one of the most frightening events I had to encounter because the condition was difficult to control and many patients ultimately bled to death.

Before the development of sclerosing injection procedures, treatment for bleeding esophageal varices was complicated and often ineffective. A tube containing two balloons was passed through the nose, down into the stomach. The first balloon was inflated in the stomach and pulled up rather snugly against the esophagogastric junction. The second balloon, shaped like a sausage, was blown up in the esophagus itself to tamponade the bleeding varices. The tube was held in place under tension by placing a football helmet on the patient's head and taping the tube to the helmet facemask. It looked very painful, and it was.

When the balloon procedure failed, as it often did, major surgery was required. An emergency splenorenal or portacaval shunt had to be undertaken. This is a procedure whereby the blood flow from the liver is diverted to the renal vein or the inferior vena cava, because the liver is so scarred that blood cannot flow back through it. This was a formidable procedure associated with massive blood loss and a relatively high mortality rate. Even when patients survived surgery and bleeding was stopped, many developed central nervous system problems due to high levels of ammonia in their blood and often died from liver failure.

Ulcer disease. An ulcer is simply an open sore of the mucous membrane. "Stomach ulcers" can be either gastric or duodenal. Prior to the introduction of endoscopes and H_2 antagonists (medications that block the production of gastric acid secretions), surgery was frequently carried out to treat gastric and duodenal ulcers. Because peptic ulcers are usually the result of overactive stomach secretions, treatment often included a radical subtotal gastrectomy—excision of 75 to 80% of the distal stomach to remove acid-bearing cells.

In the mid to late 1950s, it was shown through animal experimentation that hyperacidity of the stomach could be markedly reduced by simply cutting the two vagus nerves that go from the brain to the stomach. This procedure is called a vagotomy. Unfortunately, when vagus nerves are cut, the sphincter muscle at the end of the stomach becomes paralyzed and the stomach will not empty.

To counteract this problem, a surgical procedure to cause the stomach to empty was devised. It was discovered that when the pyloric sphincter is deliberately divided lengthwise and closed transversely, the stomach will empty. This procedure is called a pyloroplasty.

Some surgeons preferred to do a gastrojejunostomy, in which the stomach is sewn to the jejunum (the second portion of the small bowel).

These procedures were the mainstay treatment for peptic ulcers until the advent of Tagamet and Zantac. These two drugs are H_2 antagonists and work by halting the production of excess acid by the parietal cells of the stomach. These, along with a third drug, Pepcid, have dramatically decreased the incidence of surgery in peptic ulcer disease.

With the use of H_2 antagonists and management by a gastroenterologist, most ulcers will heal. The only reason we still operate on peptic ulcers is for perforation, obstruction due to scarring, and massive, uncontrollable hemorrhage that does not respond to heat probe or injection of epinephrine or adrenalin into the ulcer base.

Pyloric stenosis. Pyloric stenosis—severe narrowing of the lower stomach—occurs in newborns, most often the firstborn male. Symptoms occur around the fourth or fifth week of life and include projectile vomiting and an olive-sized mass in the right upper quadrant of the abdomen. Although surgical correction of the condition is imperative, the surgery itself is rather simple. The pyloric sphincter muscle is cut right down to the mucosa of the lumen of the stomach, thus effectively correcting the stenosis.

Gallstones. In the past, gallstones were traditionally classified according to their composition, and this information was then used to demonstrate the cause of the stone formation. Today this is no longer considered valid. Gallstone formation is believed to be due to an abnormality in the wall of the gallbladder itself.

Surgery on the gallbladder continues to be the most common operation done on the gastrointestinal tract. Many years ago, prior to the advent of modern anesthesia techniques, surgeons often opened the gallbladder and removed only the stones. In this way it was discovered that stones rapidly reform, and this method of treatment has been totally abandoned.

With the discovery of lithotripsy to break up kidney stones, whereby ultrasonic waves are used to crush stones so that they may be easily removed, it was thought that lithotripsy could be used to break up gallstones as well. However, the same limitations pertain to this technique as to gallbladder drugs: simple removal of the stones is not curative in nature. Gallstones always re-form. Recently, drugs have been developed to dissolve gallstones. These drugs are not effective in all cases, and even when effective, do not prevent gallstones from recurring.

The only way to cure gallstones is to remove the gallbladder totally and permanently. However, ultrasonography and lithotripsy can be successfully used in locating and removing stones in the common bile duct in patients who have already had a cholecystectomy.

Hiatus hernia. A surgery that has come a long way in the last 15 years is surgical repair of an esophageal hiatus hernia. This condition occurs when a part of the stomach protrudes up into the chest through the diaphragm. Gastric juices are then free to reflux up into the esophagus, most frequently at night when the patient is lying flat.

The patient may experience heartburn, sour eructation, or water brash. Although a physician can prescribe antacids and H_2 blocker drugs, the treatment is symptomatic and the condition is never corrected.

Before the early 1970s, repair of an esophageal hiatus hernia was a difficult surgical procedure. However, Dr. Lucius Hill from the University of Washington in Seattle devised a method of hiatal hernia repair through the abdomen that has totally changed surgical treatment of this condition. Dr. Hill noticed that the preaortic arcuate ligament just above the celiac axis runs transversely across the upper abdominal aorta, and is extremely strong. By placing sutures in this ligament and then suturing them to the esophagophrenic ligament on the lesser curvature of the stomach, he found that one could fix the esophagogastric junction below the diaphragm and re-create the acute angle of His between the esophagus and the fundus of the stomach.

Dr. Nissen of Sweden also devised an antireflux procedure in which the fundus of the stomach, which is rather floppy, is wrapped around the lower end of the intra-abdominal esophagus. The posterior wall of the fundus is sutured to the anterior wall of the fundus around the esophagus, thus forming a muscular tunnel. The result is a sphincter-like effect which prevents gastroesophageal reflux.

Patients treated with either the Nissen fundoplasty or the Hill esophageal hiatus hernia repair (usually with a modified Nissen fundoplasty) obtain excellent results and are generally symptom-free for the rest of their lives. These are relatively easy procedures, taking only 30 to 45 minutes to perform, with only four or five days of hospitalization required.

Pancreatic cancer. Cancer of the pancreas remains an extremely difficult problem and has a very high mortality rate. Probably less than 5 percent of all people with cancer of the pancreas are ever cured. As with other cancers, the pancreatic carcinoma cure rate could be improved if the diagnosis could be made earlier. Unfortunately, symptoms do not usually present until the disease is far advanced. Additionally, the pancreas is closely associated with other important structures, such as the portal vein, so that wide radical excision is usually impossible. Famous radio/TV performer Jack Benny died from pancreatic carcinoma.

Small bowel obstruction. The small bowel is loosely attached by its mesentery, a broad band of connective tissue containing its blood supply, and is free to move a considerable amount within the abdominal cavity. I like to think of it as a flimsy garden hose. As you know, when you kink a garden hose acutely, it obstructs. The small bowel does the same. If for any reason the small bowel adheres to either the abdominal wall or to another loop of small bowel and causes it to kink or bend, you have a small bowel obstruction.

I suspect this condition when a patient has an obvious small-bowel obstruction but denies previous surgery and has no incarcerated hernia or other etiologic factor. Air may be seen in the bile ducts on flat and erect abdominal x-rays, which indicates an abnormal communication between the lumen of the bile duct and biliary tree. The treatment, of course, is surgical.

Crohn's disease. Crohn's disease, also known as regional ileitis, is an inflammation of the distal small bowel. There is no known cause, and often it can lead to strictures of the distal small bowel or actual perforation and fistula formation between loops of small bowel, or even fistulas into the bladder or colon. President Dwight D. Eisenhower suffered from regional ileitis.

In the absence of complications, Crohn's disease is usually treated medically by the gastroenterologist with antibiotics and steroids. If obstruction and/or fistulas occur, the area involved is surgically excised. Unfortunately, this disease frequently recurs, whether surgically treated or not.

Appendicitis. Appendicitis is probably the best known colon disease. The appendix is a rudimentary appendage coming off the cecum. It is located in the first part of the large intestine. Appendicitis is thought by many to be a very simple disease, but there are still patients worldwide who die each year from complications of appendicitis.

Appendicitis was first described by Sir Reginald Fitz, a pathologist who lived in the 19th century. Dr. Charles McBurney subsequently became famous for describing the physical findings associated with appendicitis, including point tenderness over a specific area two-thirds of the way from the navel (umbilicus) to the right anterior hip bone (iliac crest).

To be diagnosed as having appendicitis, patients must meet at least two of the following three criteria: anorexia (loss of appetite), point tenderness over McBurney's point, and pain high on the right on rectal exam. The patient's white blood count is generally elevated, but it may not be. The temperature rarely goes above 100° in the first 24 hours.

Appendicitis generally does not perforate in less than 24 hours from the onset of symptoms. After the initial 24-hour period, the patient will likely develop gangrene and/or perforation of the appendix into the free peritoneal cavity, which is known as generalized peritonitis, or wall off into an abscess, which is called an appendiceal abscess. The appendectomy is a simple procedure in most cases; however, it can be an extremely difficult procedure if there has been perforation and abscess formation.

Colonic bleeding. Bleeding from the large intestine can be from many sources, including growths, cancer, polyps, AV (arteriovenous) malformations, and a colon condition known as telangiectasis, in which the capillaries in the wall of the colon become thinned out and start to bleed. Bleeding can also result from diverticular disease, hemorrhoids, anal fissures, and ulcers.

Colonic bleeding will generally cease with conservative medical therapy, but it often recurs, leading eventually to definitive surgery. Colon polyps can often be removed by means of the colonoscope or sigmoidoscope; however, if a polyp is broad-based or sessile in nature, it is dangerous to attempt to remove it using the scope because the bowel wall may perforate.

Ulcerative colitis. Ulcerative colitis is another inflammatory process whereby the mucosa of the colon develops ulcerations. It primarily involves the large intestine, and it can be devastating. Ulcerative colitis can sometimes perforate, leading to peritonitis. Its cause is still unknown, but it frequently develops in the third or fourth decade of life. Ulcerative colitis frequently disposes a patient to cancer of the colon. In severe cases of ulcerative colitis, surgical removal of the entire colon with a permanent colostomy is the only treatment.

Colostomy/ileostomy. A colostomy is the surgical creation of an opening between the bowel and the surface of the body. It is performed when it is impossible for feces to pass through the colon and out the anus. The patient wears a bag or pouch over the colostomy opening to contain the feces.

Having to undergo a colostomy is always a disturbing emotional experience. Sometimes colostomies are temporary in nature and can be closed electively once an infection has subsided or a fistula has healed. But many colostomies are permanent, such as in patients who have cancers of the anorectum below 8 to 10 cm from the anal verge.

Technical advances in colostomy irrigation systems, disposable colostomy bags, and new adhesives are making colostomy care easier today. In the past, patients were given a reusable bag to hold the feces. The bags were odoriferous, they leaked, irritated the skin, and in general, people were miserable. Today a colostomy doesn't have to interfere with a person's regular activities. The modern-day colostomy patient, properly instructed, is unidentifiable in the general public.

In the last 15 years or so, primarily through the work of surgeons at the Mayo Clinic, continent small-bowel pouches have been devised where an ileostomy can be emptied at the will of the patient rather than draining continuously. Surgeons have also devised new methods of creating pouches which can be anastomosed to the anal canal, thus maintaining bowel continuity and continence.

Hemorrhoids. Simply stated, hemorrhoids are varicose veins of the rectum, and they affect a large percentage of the general adult population. Hemorrhoid surgery sounds simple, but it is not always. The surgeon must take care not to injure the anal sphincter which could result in fecal incontinence.

Fistula. A fistula is an abnormal opening between two internal structures. Fistulas of the rectal canal are bothersome and are difficult to manage. Fistulas between the colon and bladder result in the sensation of passing air through the urethra, usually a consequence of diverticular disease.

Women occasionally develop fistulae between the rectum and vagina. These are difficult management problems and sometimes require diverting colostomies to completely divert the fecal stream while the fistula is repaired, followed by closure of the colostomy.

Diverticular disease. A diverticulum is a protruding pouch in the wall of the colon, a condition known as diverticulosis. Diverticulosis is often not symptomatic. Occasionally, diverticula become inflamed (a condition known as diverticulitis) and may require surgery if they bleed massively or repeatedly, when they perforate and form localized abscesses, or when they perforate into the free peritoneal cavity and cause acute generalized peritonitis. Occasionally they lead to stenosis or stricture of the colon and require surgical resection.

Laboratory Tests and Surgical Procedures

The following laboratory tests and surgical procedures may be found in gastroenterology dictation. Review these terms and their definitions.

alkaline phosphatase   An enzyme whose level in the serum is often increased in bone disease and obstructive liver disease.

ALT (alanine aminotransferase)   Formerly called *SGPT*. An enzyme whose level in the serum is elevated in hepatitis, cirrhosis, and other liver diseases.

ammonia, serum   A breakdown product of protein metabolism, increased in hepatic failure.

amylase, serum   An enzyme whose level is increased in pancreatitis and mumps.

AST (aspartate aminotransferase)   Formerly called *SGOT*. An enzyme whose level in the serum is elevated in myocardial infarction, liver disease, and other conditions.

barium swallow   See *upper GI series*.

BE (barium enema)   An x-ray that uses barium given rectally to outline the colon and rectum.

bili   Slang for *bilirubin*.

bilirubin, conjugated   Bilirubin that has been conjugated (broken down) by the liver so that it is water-soluble and can be excreted in the urine.

bilirubin, direct   Bilirubin that reacts directly with testing chemicals because it has been made water-soluble in the liver. Its level is increased in biliary obstruction.

bilirubin, indirect   Bilirubin in the serum that does not react directly with testing chemicals because it has not yet been broken down in the liver. Its level is increased in disorders that impair the function of liver cells.

bilirubin, unconjugated   Fat-soluble bilirubin that has not been broken down by the liver.

Campylobacter pylori   Older name for the organism now called *Helicobacter pylori*.

cholecystectomy   A surgical procedure to remove the gallbladder.

colonoscopy   Endoscopic procedure to view the colon using a special flexible scope.

Coloscreen   A test for occult blood in the stool.

colostomy   A surgically created opening into the colon through the abdominal wall, for evacuating the bowels.

gastroscopy   Endoscopic procedure to view the stomach using a special flexible scope.

GPT (glutamic pyruvic transaminase)   An older name for ALT (alanine transferase).

Helicobacter pylori   A gram-negative organism formerly known as *Campylobacter pylori*, which is the cause of some peptic ulcers.

Hematest   A test for occult blood in the stool.

Hemoccult II   A test for occult blood in the stool, in which stool is spread over a strip of filter paper impregnated with reagent.

laparoscopic cholecystectomy   A surgical procedure that utilizes a laparoscope and a small incision to remove the gallbladder. Known as a ''lap chole'' (ko'lee) in medical slang.

laparoscopy   Endoscopic procedure to view the inside of the abdominal cavity. Also called peritoneoscopy.

laparotomy   A surgical incision into the abdominal cavity.

LFTs (liver function tests).

O&P (ova and parasites)   Examination of stool, urine, or other material for parasites or their ova (eggs).

occult blood   Blood present in stool, urine, or other material in too small an amount to be detected by naked-eye observation, but detectable by chemical testing or microscopic examination.

SGOT (serum glutamic-oxaloacetic transaminase)   An older name for AST (aspartate aminotransferase).

SGPT (serum glutamic-pyruvic transaminase)   Older name for ALT (alanine transferase).

upper GI series with small bowel follow-through   An x-ray series that uses barium (taken orally) to outline the esophagus, stomach, and small intestine.

urobilinogen, urinary   A breakdown product of hemoglobin, increased in hemolytic anemias and liver disease.

Anatomy/Medical Terminology

Medical Terminology Matching Exercise

Complete the following matching exercise to test your knowledge of the root words, anatomic structures, symptoms, and disease processes encountered in the medical specialty of gastroenterology.

Instructions: Match each term in Column A with its definition in Column B.

Column A

A. hemorrhoid
B. diverticulum
C. -cele
D. cholelithiasis
E. polyp
F. paralytic ileus
G. entero-
H. hematochezia
I. choledocho-
J. volvulus
K. cirrhosis
L. procto-
M. postprandial
N. gastro-
O. anorexia
P. icterus
Q. ascites
R. obstipation
S. dysphagia
T. Crohn's disease
U. laparo-
V. hepatitis

Column B

_____ stones in the gallbladder
_____ twisting of segment
_____ root word meaning *anus* and *rectum*
_____ varicose vein in rectal area
_____ inflammation of ileum, causing diarrhea and fever
_____ loss of appetite
_____ inflammation of liver, caused by a virus
_____ jaundice
_____ root word meaning *stomach*
_____ difficulty swallowing
_____ fluid in the abdomen
_____ pouch in intestinal wall that can become inflamed
_____ lack of peristalsis due to an intestinal obstruction
_____ occurring after eating
_____ severe constipation
_____ suffix for *hernia*
_____ degeneration of liver cells, usually caused by alcoholism
_____ benign growth in colon, often on a stalk
_____ bright red blood in stool
_____ root word for *small intestine*
_____ root word for *common bile duct*
_____ root word for *abdomen*

Abbreviations Exercise

Instructions: Define the following common GI abbreviations. Then memorize both abbreviations and definitions to increase your speed and accuracy in transcribing gastroenterology dictation.

a.c.   _____
BE   _____
ERCP   _____
GI   _____
IBD   _____
LFTs   _____
LLQ   _____
LUQ   _____
NG (tube)   _____
n.p.o.   _____
OCG   _____
RLQ   _____
RUQ   _____
UGI series _____

Drug Matching Exercise

Instructions: Match the drug category in Column A with the trade name drugs in Column B. Note: Drug categories are used more than once.

Column A

A. laxative

B. H$_2$ blocker

C. antiemetic

D. antacid

E. antidiarrheal

F. bowel prep

Column B

_____ Tagamet
_____ Dulcolax
_____ Di-Gel
_____ Surfak
_____ Mylanta
_____ Zantac
_____ Lomotil
_____ Tigan
_____ Phillips' Milk of Magnesia
_____ Amphojel
_____ Fleet enema
_____ Pepcid
_____ Maalox
_____ Colace
_____ Compazine
_____ Imodium
_____ Ex-Lax
_____ GoLytely
_____ Cesamet

Transcription Guidelines

Capitals

1. Capitalize all letters in main headings. Subheadings are sometimes presented in all capitals in a vertical arrangement. Alternatively, only the initial letter of a subheading is capitalized.

   PHYSICAL EXAMINATION:
   VITAL SIGNS: BP 120/80, temperature normal.
   CHEST: Clear to auscultation.
   HEART: Regular rate and rhythm.

   PHYSICAL EXAMINATION:
   Vital signs: BP 120/80, temperature normal. Chest: Clear to auscultation. Heart: Regular rate and rhythm.

2. Capitalize the first word following a colon in a heading or subheading.

   DIAGNOSIS: Lung cancer, metastatic.

   SPLEEN: The spleen is enlarged.
   Spleen: Enlarged.

3. Capitalize the genus but not the species name for bacteria. When the genus is abbreviated, capitalize the one-letter abbreviation. The genus and species are correctly typeset in italics in books and journals, but it is acceptable not to italicize them in typed medical reports.

Escherichia coli	*E. coli*
Haemophilus influenzae	*H. influenzae*

4. When a genus name is made into an adjective, do not capitalize it.

Mycoplasma (genus)	mycoplasmal (adj.)
Streptococcus (genus)	streptococcal (adj.)

5. Names of viruses are not capitalized unless named for a person. Note: Herpesvirus is one word.

   herpes
   Epstein-Barr virus
   coxsackie virus

6. Capitalize titles such as M.D., R.N., CMT, CMA, ART, RRA, and academic degrees such as M.Ed., Ph.D., and so on. Doctor is correctly abbreviated as *Dr.* When transcribing a medical doctor's name, do not use both *Dr.* and *M.D.*

7. Do not capitalize the name of a physician specialist (or other specialist) or the medical specialty.

   gastroenterology, gastroenterologist
   ophthalmology, ophthalmologist
   physical therapy, physical therapist

Capitals Exercise

Instructions: Correct the capitalization errors in the following sentences.

1. Her rehabilitation can be continued on an outpatient basis by a Physical Therapist.

2. LABORATORY DATA: WHITE BLOOD COUNT 14,000.

3. The culture grew out Staphylococcus Aureus, sensitive to ampicillin.

4. Dr. John M. Smith, M.D., is an Oncologist practicing in this area.

5. This appears to be a Candidal infection, but we will wait to see if the culture shows Candida Albicans.

6. She will be seen by our Orthopedic Consultant, DR. Ortega, tomorrow.

7. The patient was very distressed when told that she was infected with Herpes.

8. AIDS patients often develop Mycoplasmal infections, particularly in the lungs.

Proofreading Skills

Proofreading Exercise

Instructions: In the paragraphs below, circle the errors. Identify misspelled and missing medical and English words and write the correct ones in the numbered spaces opposite the text.

1	PREOPERATIVE DIAGNOSES: Anal stricture.
2	
3	PROCEDURE: Resection of perianal skin
4	tags, posterior midline partial sphincterotomy,
5	anal dilatation, and Y-V anoplasty.
6	
7	The peritoneum and perianal areas were
8	prepped with Betadine and suitably drapped.
9	An anterior midline and a left posteriolateral
10	skin tag were resected, bleeding controled by
11	electrocoagulation. A half-shell retractor was
12	placed, and a partial posterier midline sphinc-
13	terotomy was carried out. Then, gently, anal
14	dilatation was carried out with one finger, two
15	fingers, and finally to three fingers. A
16	Y-shaped incision had been made begining up
17	just above the upper boarder of the anal
18	sphincter, coming down partway linearly, and
19	then going in the Y shape on each side. Some
20	scar tissue was ressected. The perianal skin
21	posteriorly was dissected away from underly-
22	ing scar tissue and sphincter, and bleeding
23	was controled by electrocoagulation. The tip
24	of this skin was then sutured to the end of the
25	Y, and mucosa-to-skin was approximated with
26	interupted 3-0 chronic sutures, turning the Y
27	into a V and effectively widening the anal
28	canal. Surgicel gauze was placed in the cannal
29	and the procedure terminated.

1. DIAGNOSIS _____
2. _____
3. _____
4. _____
5. _____
6. _____
7. _____
8. _____
9. _____
10. _____
11. _____
12. _____
13. _____
14. _____
15. _____
16. _____
17. _____
18. _____
19. _____
20. _____
21. _____
22. _____
23. _____
24. _____
25. _____
26. _____
27. _____
28. _____
29. _____

Terminology Challenge

Instructions: The following terms appear in the dictation on Tape 3A, Gastroenterology. Before beginning the medical transcription practice for Lesson 6, become familiar with the terminology below by looking up each word in a medical or English dictionary. Write out a short definition of each term.

acute abdomen series
adenopathy
ANA (antinuclear
  antibody)
AP diameter of chest
appendicitis
ASHD (arteriosclerotic
  heart disease)
auscultation
Azulfidine
barium enema
bethanechol
breath sounds
C. difficile
  (*Clostridium*)
ceruloplasmin
cholecystitis
cholelithiasis
colon
  ascending
  descending
  proximal
  sigmoid
  transverse
colonoscopy
COPD (chronic obstruc-
  tive pulmonary disease)
Crohn's disease
Demerol
diabetes mellitus
diet
  high-bulk
  low-fat
discrete
diverticulitis
diverticulosis
dysfunction
electrophoresis
epigastrium

exercise-induced asthma
fecalith
FEV1 (FEV$_1$)
forced vital capacity
gangrene
gastric contents
gastroscopy
Hemoccult card
hemorrhoids
  external
  internal
hernia
  hiatal
  indirect
  inguinal
  sliding-type hiatal
hypoactive
IV (intravenous)
ileus
induced
inflammatory bowel
  disease
intraoperative
irritable bowel syndrome
KUB x-ray
left shift (on differential
  WBC count)
liver panel
Lomotil
long-standing
maternal
Metamucil
multisystem
Mylicon
NG (nasogastric) tube
normocephalic
NSAID (nonsteroidal anti-
  inflammatory drug)
obstipated

operative cholangiogram
paralytic
paternal
pending
peptic ulcer disease
periumbilical area
prothrombin time (PT,
  pro time)
Proventil inhaler
PTT (partial thrombo-
  plastin time)
q.4h.
radiating
rebound constipation
rebound tenderness
referred tenderness
Reglan
rheumatoid factor
rhythm
right lower quadrant

sed rate (sedimentation)
serum protein
sinus bradycardia
small-bowel obstruction
spirometry
superficial tenderness
surgical clips
symptomatic
t.i.d.
Tagamet
thrombosis
tinkling bowel sounds
total serum protein
transit time
tympanic membranes
upper GI with small-
  bowel series
upper respiratory infection
Zantac

Sample Reports

Refer to the sample gastroenterology reports in Lesson 5, beginning on page 90.

Transcription Practice

After completing all the readings and exercises in Lesson 6, transcribe Tape 3A, Gastroenterology. Use both medical and English dictionaries and your Quick-Reference Word List as resource materials for finding words.

Proofread your transcribed documents carefully, listening to the dictation while you read your transcripts.

Transcribe (*NOT* retype) the same reports again without referring to your previous transcription attempt. Initially, you may need to transcribe some reports more than twice before you can produce an error-free document. Your ultimate goal is to produce an error-free document the first time.

Lesson 7. Gastroenterology

Learning Objectives

Medical

- Define common abbreviations for drug dosage abbreviations.
- Define the common abbreviations for drug dosage schedules.
- Given GI root words and suffixes, combine them to correctly match a given medical definition.
- Differentiate between various GI sound-alike terms.

Fundamentals

- Discuss the personal and professional benefits of participation in a professional association.
- Discuss the techniques of surgical anesthesia, asepsis, and hemostasis.
- List the members of the operative team, in addition to the surgeon.
- Discuss the correct use of capitals in editing medical sentences.
- Given a medical report with errors, identify and correct the errors.

Practice

- Accurately transcribe authentic physician dictation from the specialty of gastroenterology and GI surgery.

A Closer Look

Joining a Professional Association

by Ellen Drake, CMT

Joining a professional association may be the most advantageous career move you can make. Students in medical transcription, medical assisting, and medical record technology may become student members in their chosen professional association. The association for medical transcriptionists is the American Association for Medical Transcription (AAMT), which offers student memberships to those enrolled in college medical transcription programs.

AAMT offers member benefits that are usually associated with professional associations: an informative, well-respected bimonthly journal (*JAAMT*), discounts on AAMT products and meeting registration fees, and access to the professional staff in the administrative office via an 800 number. They can even help research new medical terms for you.

Since its beginning in 1978, AAMT has been influential in raising the image of medical transcriptionists (MTs) and the profession to higher levels. It has been a major player in educating employers, physicians, and the general public about the role, value, and importance of MTs as part of the medical team contributing to overall patient care. After a successful national "Write the Congress" campaign by AAMT members and national office staff in 1984, President Ronald Reagan declared a National Medical Transcriptionist Week, and it has been celebrated the third week of May every year since that time.

Since the formation of AAMT, more and more educational institutions have begun offering medical transcription training programs similar to the one you are taking. Publishing companies now recognize MTs as a profitable market and produce reference books specifically for transcriptionists.

AAMT develops and administers a certification exam which is recognized by many employers as the assurance that the certified medical transcriptionist (CMT) is a highly skilled, knowledgeable, quality-conscious individual. The CMT is required to keep up-to-date through continuing education.

One of the most valuable assets that AAMT members have is the opportunity to network. Networking, according to the *American Heritage Dictionary*, is "an informal system whereby persons having common interests or concerns assist each other, as in the *exchange of information* or the *development of professional contacts*."

Another term used today to imply the same basic idea is "connecting" or "connectivity." This term, taken from the computer realm, implies the ability to tap into a wealth of information or a variety of applications via an interwoven, connecting structure.

The structure of AAMT includes a national organization as well as state and local component associations. It is through these associations at every level that the student and the experienced MT can take advantage of AAMT's most valuable asset.

Exchange of information. Local chapters hold regularly scheduled meetings and seminars at which physicians and other allied health professionals offer transcriptionists the opportunity to increase their knowledge of various medical specialties. State and regional associations and the national association hold annual meetings, with many speakers on a variety of medical topics and professional issues. Meeting people from all over the state or nation is stimulating and exciting, and may even have an impact on your future employment. The larger associations may also offer other weekend meetings addressing needs of specific groups, such as leadership, teacher, and business conferences. These meetings provide continuing education credits for the CMT and excellent educational opportunities for all transcriptionists.

Development of professional contacts. This is the second part of the definition of networking. After working for years as an MT in a hospital, I started a medical transcription business, with my husband, a computer consultant. The only marketing we did was networking with others in AAMT. Most of my clients were either professional associates or referrals from other clients. Our business grew quickly and after only five years, we were able to sell it and go on to other things.

Other opportunities that came my way as a result of my involvement in AAMT included co-authoring the *Saunders Pharmaceutical Word Book,* consulting on other books, and editing an MT newsletter for W. B. Saunders; teaching medical transcription at a community college; and becoming director of education at Health Professions Institute.

Another important but less obvious advantage of participating in AAMT activities is the opportunity for personal growth, not just in knowledge or job advancement, but in character and personality. People who are shy and insecure can become confident leaders and excellent public speakers. Others with low self-esteem can become self-assured and sure of their worth as individuals and employees.

If you become involved in a local chapter of AAMT and join the national association, you will be welcome at chapter meetings where you will find camaraderie and encouragement. Volunteer to help at meetings. Make a point of introducing yourself to as many other MTs as possible. Seek out supervisors at the meetings and tell them you are a student and are excited about becoming a professional medical transcriptionist.

Whatever you do, don't wait until you're out looking for a job to start making contacts and make yourself known. The time is now!

For information about becoming an AAMT student member, call (800) 982-2182 or (209) 551-0883, or write to P. O. Box 576187, Modesto, CA 95357.

Faamtasies

by Judith Marshall, MA, CMT

AAMT has infinite possibilities. The connectedness that the association extends to its members spans continents. The organization had to invent itself, define its own being, sketch the outlines and then fill them in with people, people who already had two jobs—being a woman and working. AAMT called upon people for every ounce of talent and time they had to give.

Something drew us all together in 1978. What was it and to whom did it appeal? Those of you who know me will affirm that I am short-tempered, obsessive-compulsive, paranoid, hypochondriacal, argumentative, and narcissistic. Was I that way before transcription or after transcription?

When AAMT was founded, we had a holy mission, a messianic spirit that made Joan of Arc look wishy-washy. Fanatic is not too strong a word. Many of us were positively violent about AAMT and some of us were just plain crazy. I would sashay up to people at work and shove a newsletter in their face and ask, "Are you a member? If not, why not?"

When I took some information to the director of medical records in the hospital where I worked, I was about as welcome as sunlight is to a vampire. "No," he shrieked! "Get out of here with that. I have enough problems." Then I tangled with a service owner and asked him at least to give the AAMT toll-free number to the employees who kept calling me for it. "I am doing what is best for the people," he asserted, "I am paying people well, not ripping them off with dues."

Well, burnout implies that someone was hot about something, on fire about something, passionate about something, and we were. We wanted respect more than Rodney Dangerfield, we wanted recognition and we wanted to learn everything. It became a crusade and still is for many. Some of us have mellowed out. I am not as combative or foolhardy as I was, but I am more committed than ever.

Don't let me try to tell you what your reward system should be. Don't let anyone tell you. What is success to you, what is the work to you? Is it a career, is it a job? Did you wake up one morning, go into your kitchen and tug at your mother's apron and say, "Ma, I want to be a medical transcriptionist when I grow up"? Did you purposefully study and prepare for your life as a medical transcriptionist or did you wander into it? Did you think your chronic status walletus empticus would be helped by certification? Was it? Will it?

Maybe I just got tired of the stale candy on Valentine's Day that the doctors would routinely send down to Records or that tired poinsettia plant for Christmas. I never expected anyone to stuff twenty-dollar bills into my typewriter, but I did know that what we did was skilled and only we seemed to know it. I wanted *something*. I had FANTASIES of what would happen when the CMT certificates started to go up on walls:

Any doctor anywhere in any setting comes up to the MT and says, "What an incredible mind you have, I want to thank you for your exquisite work." . . . *The hospital supervisor says to the MTs, "Well, you work with it, so you will be making the final choice for the transcription equipment yourselves and I'll approve it."* . . . *The hospital tells the outside transcription service, "Turnaround time is too fast on the transcription. We can't get it on the charts fast enough. Slow down."* . . . *The doctor tells the MT, "I won't be backdating any more reports from now on or blaming my late dictation on you, saying you lost it."* FANTASIES.

When we all get together, sometimes we say we should stop transcribing for one day all over this country. No, I don't say that. I say, for one day we should transcribe everything that is said exactly as they say it. That's right. VERBATIM DAY!

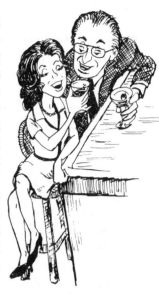

My ultimate fantasy in 1978 (I was between husbands then) was swiveling my 120-pound figure on the fanciest singles bar stool in Boston, tossing back my black lustrous silky hair and having this wonderful man come over and say, "What sign were you born under?" And I would answer, "The caduceus," and he would say, "Of course! You're a medical transcriptionist, that rewarding career filled with interesting, brilliant people. I am an orthopedic surgeon. Won't you be my suprapatellar spouse?"

Judith Marshall,
MEDICATE ME
Illus. by Cindy Stevens

Well, nothing like that happened. When I joined AAMT, I told my parents first about AAMT and my membership. My mother said, "That's nice, dear." My father said, "Why can't you just get a real job?" My best friend, Shirley, said, "Call yourself anything you like, but all you are is a typist."

The doctors weren't impressed either. One looked at my membership card and said, "CMT, or Smint, well, I certainly don't need a medical technician to do my typing." Another doctor whom I affectionately call the Doberman, chose a journal from the stack on the desk, opened it, and started to give me a spelling test. Pompous, self-righteous person that I am, I could not spell the word. It was infuriating. "Ah, ha!" he said, "You don't know everything."

Well, I never said I knew everything. But I know where to find it if I have the books.

We are back to full circle. Education. Books. Words. We wanted to know everything. That is why many of us joined and why we stay. Let's not kid ourselves about going to the library or borrowing tapes or writing summaries. The real education goes on all over this country with hundreds of doctors and nurses and physical therapists, and others, lecturing to thousands of medical transcriptionists. Touching surgical instruments, bandages, splints, handling pacemakers, watching video cassettes—that's education, that's exciting.

And best of all, yacking our heads off with each other. There is no glamour here, no bangles, beads, fern bars, Yuppie foods or fashions. Lots of information is here, controversies are here, disagreements are here, viewpoints and plain talk are here.

Should we call ourselves *transcriptionists* or *transcribers?* Does it really matter? Shall we meet in hospitals or restaurants? Shall we meet monthly, quarterly, or annually? Shall we print recipes or birth announcements in our newsletters? Should we have local, state, regional, or national representation? How can we do it, why should we do it? When and how? Should the AAMT logo be allowed on black velvet paintings or on toilet paper like the cutesy ones they sell with dollar bills on them? Should we talk about things like tax advice, salary surveys, use of combined clout—National Medical Transcriptionist Week is a good example.

This remarkable process of education is continuing. AAMT set standards in 1978. We have not only kept them, we have surpassed them. They weren't just fantasies.

Surgery and Surgical Dictation

Part 2

by John H. Dirckx, M.D.

Three cardinal features of modern surgery distinguish a surgical operation on a human patient from automotive repair: (1) Ordinarily some kind of anesthesia is administered to keep the patient from feeling pain during the operation. (2) Strict asepsis must be maintained to prevent introduction of infectious germs into the patient's body. (3) Bleeding caused by cutting tissue must be meticulously controlled. It is scarcely necessary to add, as a fourth principle, that unlike a piece of machinery, a human patient cannot be abandoned in mid-operation as ''beyond repair.'' That is, although the surgeon may find it impossible to do what he set out to do or to restore normal function, he is obliged to do his best in the circumstances and to repair his incision so as to leave the patient, if possible, at least no worse than he found him.

Surgical anesthesia may be local, by infiltration of the operative site with an anesthetic drug injected with a syringe and needle; regional (nerve block), by injection of anesthetic around a major sensory nerve supplying the operative site; spinal, by injection of the drug into the subarachnoid or epidural space of the spinal cord; or general. Whereas the first three types of anesthesia leave the patient awake, general anesthesia implies not only freedom from pain, but also unconsciousness.

Typically a patient under general anesthesia receives several drugs, some by inhalation and some by intravenous infusion. One drug may be administered to produce unconsciousness, another to produce analgesia (freedom from pain), and a third to relax skeletal muscle, particularly in abdominal surgery to facilitate adequate exposure of the operative site through the muscular abdominal wall. Inhalation anesthesia may be given by face mask but more often an endotracheal tube is used. This is a tube inserted within the patient's upper windpipe and sealed with an inflatable cuff to provide a ''closed system'' and complete control of respiratory gas exchange. Endotracheal intubation is virtually necessary when a muscle relaxant is administered, because in this situation the patient's respiratory muscles are weakened or paralyzed and the anesthesiologist must take over his breathing for him by means of a bag or respirator.

Local and regional anesthesia are used for surgery on the skin or superficial structures, and are usually administered by the surgeon himself. Spinal and general anesthesia are routinely administered by someone other than the surgeon, usually an anesthesiologist, that is, a physician specializing in the induction of surgical anesthesia.

Surgical asepsis means the rigorous exclusion of pathogenic microorganisms from parts of the patient's body rendered vulnerable to infection by surgery. Achieving and maintaining asepsis during surgery involves a number of standard procedures, including thorough disinfection of the operative suite and control of air flow through it; sterilization of all instruments, materials, drapes, and dressings used during the procedure; preparation of the patient's skin by scrubbing with surgical soap; and draping around the operative site with sterile sheets. The surgeon and all persons taking part in the operation carry out a thorough scrubbing of the hands and forearms before entering the operative suite, and put on sterile gowns and gloves before approaching the patient.

In addition, all persons entering the operative suite (anesthesiologists, x-ray technicians, aides, medical photographers, students) wear caps covering all hair, filter-type face masks to prevent transmission of disease-causing bacteria in expired air or respiratory secretions, and freshly laundered garments ("scrub suits") instead of street clothes. If the patient already has an infection, procedures are followed to prevent both the aggravation of his condition and the spread of infection to members of the operative team. All blood, secretions, and specimens are handled as if potentially infective for those coming in contact with them.

Surgical hemostasis is the control of bleeding by mechanical means. Virtually all surgical procedures cause some blood loss. In the course of a major operation, the patient may shed an amount of blood equal to his entire blood volume. Such an operation would obviously be impossible without the transfusion of several units of blood during and after the surgery. Besides the obvious danger to the patient of extensive blood loss, bleeding is a major factor contributing to the difficulty and tediousness of performing surgery. Oozing, flowing, or squirting blood obscures the operative site and must constantly be soaked up with gauze pads called "sponges" or removed from the site by application of mechanical suction. At every step of the procedure, the surgeon must be sure that hemostasis has been achieved before proceeding to the next step.

"Cut, clamp, and tie" is the basic operating program. First, make or extend an incision or dissection; second, clamp with hemostats any vessels severed in the process ("bleeders"); third, tie ligatures around the ends of the severed vessels and remove the hemostats. Alternatively, bleeding vessels may be coagulated with electric current or sealed with metal clips.

Large vessels are ordinarily ligated before being severed. Capillary oozing from a surface may be controlled with pressure or packing. During closure of the wound, the surgeon assures himself that all bleeding has been controlled at each level before proceeding to the next one, whether this takes two minutes or two hours. Postoperative hemorrhage increases pain, prolongs healing time, invites infection, threatens to disrupt surgical repairs and suture lines, and, if severe, endangers the life of the patient.

To complete this necessarily concise overview of surgery, it will be instructive to describe the operative team for a typical procedure. Besides the surgeon, there may be one or more **surgical assistants**, usually physicians but not necessarily surgeons. The first assistant for routine abdominal surgery is often the patient's family physician. Surgeons in training, medical students, nurses, and others may serve as assistants in certain circumstances.

The principal surgeon conducts the operation, makes all important decisions, and personally performs the essential procedures. Under his direction the assistant or assistants hold retractors to provide optimal exposure of the operative site, apply sponges or suction or both to keep the field clear of blood, help in clamping and ligating bleeders (a slow process with only two hands working), and perhaps close the surgical wound. For cardiac and other elaborate, highly specialized surgical procedures, there may be as many as four assistants, all with advanced surgical training. For long or complicated procedures, two or more surgical teams may work in relays.

The **scrub nurse** or **scrub technician** plays an essential role in all but the most minor procedures. (The term "scrub" refers to the fact that this member of the team, like the surgeon and assistants, performs a preliminary hand and forearm scrub and wears a sterile gown and gloves.) It is the responsibility of the scrub technician to select and sterilize all instruments, suture and ligature materials, sponges, and other articles to be used during the procedure, to arrange these on tables or stands where they will be readily available, and to hand them to the surgeon or assistants as needed.

An efficient scrub technician must have a thorough knowledge of surgical principles and techniques so as to be able to anticipate the surgeon's needs from one moment to the next and supply the requisite instruments or materials without fumbling or delay. There may be two or more scrub technicians for a procedure, one to work with each member of the operating team. An additional function of the scrub technician is to help the surgeon and assistants to don sterile gowns and gloves as they enter the operating room.

Because the scrub technician cannot handle anything unsterile, another worker, called the **circulating nurse**, **circulating technician**, or **circulator** is present in the operating room. The circulating technician assists the scrub technician by handling and opening unsterile outer wrappings or containers of sterile supplies and equipment as needed; adjusts lamps, suction machines, and other appliances; and performs a variety of other chores such as tying the (unsterile) rear tapes of the surgeon's gowns, telephoning other departments for supplies, medicines, fluids, or blood, picking these up, delivering specimens to the laboratory, taking incoming telephone messages for members of the operating team, and so forth.

The anesthesiologist is a physician who specializes in the induction of surgical anesthesia. (The term **anesthetist** is usually reserved for a nonphysician trained to administer anesthetics.) The anesthesiologist closely monitors the patient's pulse, cardiac rhythm, blood pressure, respiratory activity, and other signs, and records these data as well as all drugs given, with doses and times of administration, in an anesthetic record (partly graphic, and kept in longhand). This becomes a part of the patient's permanent record and supplements the information given by the surgeon in the operative report.

During the operation the anesthesiologist may administer various drugs to maintain as nearly normal cardiovascular function as possible and to offset adverse physiologic consequences of anesthesia or surgery. Generally the anesthesiologist places an intravenous catheter before the operation begins. This enables him to administer needed medicines rapidly and, in the event of impending shock, to give fluids, including blood, without delay. Not being "sterile," the anesthesiologist often performs many of the activities mentioned above for the circulating technician, particularly when, as often happens, one circulator is working two simultaneous operations in adjacent rooms.

Medical Readings

Pharmacology: Drug Measurement

Metric weight measurements include the kilogram, milligram, and microgram. Each of these differs by a factor of 1000.

> 1 kilogram = 1000 grams (*khilioi*, Greek, thousand)
> 1 gram = 1000 milligrams (*mille*, Latin, thousand)
> 1 milligram = 1000 micrograms
> 1 microgram = one-millionth of a gram

Drug weight measurements are not expressed in kilograms, which are more appropriately used to describe a person's weight. (Example: A 110-pound woman weighs 50 kilograms.) Extremely premature infants may be measured in grams. (Example: A 900-gram premature infant weighs just under 2 pounds.) Most drugs are measured not in grams but in milligrams and occasionally in micrograms.

The metric system includes the liquid measurements of liter and milliliter (1 liter = 1000 milliliters). Drugs are not prescribed by the liter; the milliliter (mL) is used frequently, however. For example, a common dose for the antacid Maalox is 30 mL. The Mantoux intradermal test for tuberculosis involves the injection of 0.1 mL of solution.

Common abbreviations for metric measurements are as follows.

cubic centimeter	cc
kilogram	kg
gram	g (not *gm*, now obsolete)
milligram	mg
microgram	mcg
milliliter	mL

Note: Metric abbreviations are not followed by a period. The abbreviation for grain (gr.) is followed by a period because it is from the apothecary system.

Other types of drug dosage measurements include unit, inch, drop, milliequivalent, percentage, ratio, household.

1. **Unit.** The dosages of certain drugs are never measured by the metric system but by a special designation called a unit. Some penicillins, some vitamins, and all types of insulin are measured in units. The exact value of a unit varies from drug to drug. A unit of penicillin was standardized in 1944 as 0.6 mcg of penicillin G based on its ability to cause a ring of inhibition of a certain size on a bacterial culture. Other types of penicillin are measured in milligrams. The International Unit (IU) is used to measure the fat soluble vitamins A, D, and E. Other vitamins are measured in milligrams. All forms of insulin are measured in units. The unit of insulin is defined on the weight basis of pure insulin with 28 units equaling one milligram. Insulin is manufactured in solutions with 100 units per milliliter, abbreviated as U-100.

2. **Inch.** Only one commonly prescribed drug is measured in inches, and that is nitroglycerin ointment. Special applicator papers are supplied with each tube of ointment for the purpose of accurately measuring the dose. The ointment is squeezed onto the applicator paper along the marking lines in 1/2 inch increments. The dose may range from 1/2 inch to 2 inches or more. The paper is then applied to the skin and taped.

3. **Drop.** The Latin word for *drops* is *guttae*; the abbreviation for drops is *gtt*. Eye and ear liquid medications are often prescribed in the number of drops to be given.

4. **Milliequivalent.** An equivalent is the molecular

weight of an ion divided by the number of hydrogen ions it reacts with. This number is expressed in grams. A milliequivalent (mEq) is 1/1000 of an equivalent. Doses of electrolytes, such as potassium which is an ion, are measured in milliequivalents, although their doses can also be given in milligrams.

5. **Percentage.** A percentage is one part in relationship to the whole, based on a total of 100. Thus a 10% solution would be composed of one gram of drug in 10 milliliters of solution. A 1% preparation of the steroid ointment triamcinolone (Aristocort, Kenalog), would contain l mg of drug in 100 mg of white petrolatum base.

6. **Ratio.** A ratio expresses the relationship between the concentrations of two substances together in solution. A ratio is expressed as two numbers with a colon mark between. Example: Epinephrine for intracardiac injection during resuscitation is supplied in a ratio of 1:10,000 (or one part epinephrine to 10,000 parts of solution). Epinephrine for subcutaneous injection with a local anesthetic is supplied in a ratio of 1:100,000.

Dosage schedules. Drugs are measured by the amount and the frequency of the dosage. There are a number of commonly used abbreviations which indicate the frequency of administration. These abbreviations are based on Latin words, as indicated.

Abbrev.	Latin	Medical Meaning
a.c.	*ante cibum*	before meals
ad lib.	*ad libitum*	as needed
b.i.d.	*bis in die*	twice a day
c̄	*cum*	with
h.s.	*hora somni*	at bedtime (hour of sleep)
n.p.o.	*nihil per os*	nothing by mouth
p.c.	*post cibum*	after meals
p.r.n.	*pro re nata*	as needed
q.d.	*quaque die*	every day
q.h.	*quaque hora*	every hour
q.h.s.	*quaque hora somni*	every bedtime
q.i.d.	*quater in die*	four times a day
q.o.d.	(informal usage)	every other day
s̄	*sine*	without
t.i.d.	*ter in die*	three times a day

Anatomy/Medical Terminology

GI Questions

1. Distinguish between the following GI words: diverticulum, diverticula, diverticulitis, diverticulosis.
2. Where is a peptic ulcer located?
3. Distinguish between cholelithiasis and choledocholithiasis.

Root Word and Suffix Matching Exercise

Instructions: Combine the following root words with suffixes to form words that match the definitions below. Fill in the blanks with the medical words you construct.

Root Word	Suffix
appendic(o)-	-ectomy
cholecyst-	-itis
colo-, colon(o)-	-logy
entero-	-scopy
gastro-	-stomy
laparo-	-tomy

A. inflammation of the stomach and intestines

_____

B. surgically removing the gallbladder

_____

C. using a scope to visualize the colon

_____

D. making a surgical incision into the abdomen

_____

E. using a scope to visualize the stomach

_____

F. making a new opening for the colon

_____

G. making a surgical incision into the stomach

_____

H. inflammation of the appendix

_____

I. the study of the stomach and intestines

_____

J. surgical removal of the appendix

_____

Sound-alikes Exercise

Instructions: Circle the correct term from the sound-alikes in parentheses in the following sentences.

1. There was an (acidic, ascetic, ascitic) fluid wave in the abdomen on examination.
2. The patient insisted he did not drink to excess, but he had massive (cirrhosis, psoriasis) of the liver.
3. On palpation of the abdomen over the recti muscles, it was clear that the patient had a (diaphysis, diastasis, diathesis).
4. The patient complained of constant, burning chest pain, and on gastroscopy was shown to have severe gastroesophageal (efflux, reflex, reflux).
5. On anal examination, the patient was noted to have a small tear or (fissure, fistula).
6. On bimanual exam, the patient was suspected of having a rectovaginal (fissure, fistula).
7. The colostomy procedure was considered a success, but the patient developed a colovesical (fissure, fistula).
8. The lesion was seen just beyond the hepatic (flexor, flexure).
9. The patient experienced significant pain from (fundal, fungal) pressure on the stomach.
10. The colonoscopy was performed all the way to the terminal (ileum, ilium), and the entire colon examined.
11. The (perianal, perineal) tissues were irritated, probably from the cleansing enemas prior to the procedure.
12. The baby was placed on (gavage, lavage) after it was discovered he could not swallow.
13. The (perineum, peritoneum) was entered and the bowels pushed back with a wet lap.
14. (Aural, oral) mucosa was pink and moist.
15. A brownish (mucous, mucus) discharge was oozing from the (mucous, mucus) fistula.
16. (Palpation, palpitation, papillation) of the abdomen revealed no masses.
17. The patient was placed on (parenteral, parental) feedings after the gastrectomy.
18. The colonoscope was (passed, past) beyond the hepatic (flexor, flexure), but could not be advanced (passed, past) the splenic (flexor, flexure).
19. After the abdominal hysterectomy, (perineal, perennial, peroneal, peritoneal) closure was accomplished with 0 silk.
20. The patient was placed on a (regimen, regime, regiment) of laxatives and tap water enemas in preparation for the colonoscopy.

Word Search

Instructions: Locate and circle each of the GI terms listed below. A numeral following a word indicates the number of times it can be found in the puzzle. Words are hidden horizontally, vertically, and diagonally, forwards and backwards.

```
A B D O M E N E N O T S L L A G E
N K F U H E A R T B U R N O N N P
A N E L E M I R T A N U S P O H E
L L C C M L U L A R O G M I R O R
I B E E O F I S T U L A T C E R I
G S S R R L H E R N I A S O X C T
A E H R R A I D Y S P H A G I A O
L T E Y H T H I S I S E M E A M N
L I P M O U T H T U F R E C L U I
B C A W I S I S O H R R I C H E T
L S T Q D P B N O R S R E V I L I
A A I C H O L E L I T H I A S I S
D E T M U L U C I T R E V I D B I
D B I L E Y M O T C E D N E P P A
E A S O T P A N C R E A S T O M A
R E C T U M A S T I C A T I O N O
```

anal
abdomen
anorexia
anus
appendectomy
ascites
bile
cholelithiasis
cirrhosis
Crohn
diarrhea
diverticulum
dysphagia
emesis
feces
fistula
flatus
gallbladder
gallstone
heartburn

hemorrhoid
hepatitis
hernia
ileum (2)
lip
liver
mastication
melena
mouth
obstipation
oral
pancreas
peritonitis
polyp
rectal
ruga
stoma
stool
ulcer (2)

Transcription Guidelines

Capitals

1. Do not capitalize diseases or anatomic landmarks unless they are eponyms (named for a person).

   chronic obstructive pulmonary disease
   latissimus dorsi muscle
   sphincter of Oddi
   space of Retzius

2. Do not capitalize the names of departments within a hospital.

   radiology department
   operating room
   physical therapy

3. Capitalize the trade name of a drug but not the generic name.

   Tagamet   cimetidine

4. Do not capitalize words associated with the trade name of a drug.

   Tylenol elixir
   Demerol injection

5. Capitalize the person's name that is the basis of an eponym.

   Parkinson's disease
   Bell's palsy
   Gram stain

6. When the eponym is made into an adjective, do not capitalize it.

   parkinsonian symptoms
   gram-negative bacteria

7. Capitalize a person's race, ethnic or national origin, but not skin color.

   Caucasian male   white male
   African-American male   black female
   Oriental female   Hispanic male

8. Do not capitalize words that denote categories or classifications.

   grade 2 Bruce protocol
   type IIb hyperlipidemia
   grade 1/6 systolic murmur

9. Do not capitalize the terms *gravida, para,* and the brief form *ab* (abortion).

   gravida 3, para 2, ab 1

10. The patient's allergies may be typed in all capitals within the report to make them stand out. This is particularly helpful with a drug allergy so that the patient will not be given that drug inadvertently.

    ALLERGIES to PENICILLIN and SULFA DRUGS

11. Greek letter names are not capitalized.

    alpha-chymotrypsin
    alpha-fetoprotein lab test
    beta blocker drugs
    beta-lactamase

12. Do not capitalize the names of the seasons.

    She is scheduled for follow-up in the spring.

Capitals Exercise

1. She has Cushing's Syndrome and has developed a Cushingoid facies.
2. The patient has been tried on various beta blockers, including Inderal and Lopressor Capsules.
3. This 45-year-old Black man is complaining of chest pain.
4. Heart: Positive Grade 2/6 systolic murmur.
5. His diagnosis is Diabetes mellitus, Type 2.

Proofreading Skills

Instructions: The following paragraphs taken from a discharge summary contain many typographical errors and errors of punctuation, grammar, and spelling. Circle the errors and write the correct words in the blank spaces provided.

1 HSOPITAL CUORSE: With a presumptive	1. <u>HOSPITAL COURSE</u>
2 diagnosis of acute appendicitis, rule out per-	2. _____
3 foration, the paitent was started on intravenus	3. _____
4 antibiotics in the form of Cefobid and Flagyl	4. _____
5 and taken on an emergency basis to the	5. _____
6 operating suit. At exploration his appendix	6. _____
7 was noted to be acutely inflammed and	7. _____
8 perforated. There was no absess. There was	8. _____
9 no fecalith noted. He had a moderate amount	9. _____
10 of cloudy perineal fluid. Appendectomy was	10. _____
11 performed without incident. The peritoneal	11. _____
12 cavity was not drained.	12. _____
13	13. _____
14 Cultures of peroneal fluid revealed numerous	14. _____
15 organisms including Bacteroides fragillis,	15. _____
16 psudomonas, E. coli, and fecal streptococus.	16. _____
17	17. _____
18 He was continued on intravenous antibiotics	18. _____
19 postoperatively he awakened from anesthesia	19. _____
20 with stable vital signs, and his cuorse was	20. _____
21 basically unremarkable. He remained afebrile	21. _____
22 for approximately four days; however, there	22. _____
23 were no spikes on the temperature curve, with	23. _____
24 his temperature hovering around 100-100.5°.	24. _____
25 His diet was begun on the second postopera-	25. _____
26 tive day, and he tolerated this well with no	26. _____
27 abdominal distention, nawsea, or vomiting.	27. _____
28 His adbomen remained soft. His incision re-	28. _____
29 mained clean. There were no evidence of any	29. _____
30 drainage or local inflamation. Rectal examina-	30. _____
31 tions done periodicaly revealed no tenderness.	31. _____
32 There were no fluctuance or masses felt.	32. _____

Terminology Challenge

Instructions: The following terms appear in the dictation on Tape 3B, Gastroenterology. Look up each term in a medical or English dictionary, and write out a short definition of each.

abscess
adherent
approximated
Betadine scrub and
   solution
cecum
Cefobid
clamped
copious
debris
dissection
   blunt
   finger
electrocautery
electrocoagulated
emergent
endotracheal
excised
external muscular fascia
external oblique
Flagyl
full-thickness skin graft
gutter
hemostasis
incision
inflamed
lap pad (laparotomy)

ligate, ligated
ligature
mesoappendix
necrosis
necrotic
normal saline
obliquely
omentum
operative field
perforation
peritoneal cavity
peritonealized
prepped
retrocecal
sponge and needle
   counts
supine
suture
   0 (zero, "oh")
   2-0 (two oh)
   3-0 (three oh)
   catgut
   dermal
   interrupted
   plain
   Z-type
   x 3 (times three)

Sample Reports

Review the sample gastroenterology reports in Lesson 5, beginning on page 90.

Transcription Practice

After completing all the readings and exercises in Lesson 7, transcribe Tape 3B, Gastroenterology. Use both medical and English dictionaries and your Quick-Reference Word List as resource materials for finding words.

Proofread your transcribed documents carefully, listening to the dictation while you read your transcripts.

Transcribe (*NOT* retype) the same reports again without referring to your previous transcription attempt. Initially, you may need to transcribe some reports more than twice before you can produce an error-free document. Your ultimate goal is to produce an error-free document the first time.

BLOOPERS

Incorrect	Correct
No history of tardy stools.	No history of tarry stools.
The abdomen became somewhat permanent.	The abdomen became somewhat prominent.
Oral diverticula.	Old diverticula.
Bronchoscopic exam revealed hemorrhoids.	Proctoscopic exam revealed hemorrhoids.
Rectal examination defurred.	Rectal examination deferred.

Lesson 8. Cardiology

Learning Objectives

Medical

- List cardiovascular symptoms and disease conditions that might be mentioned in the Review of Systems of a History and Physical Examination Report.
- List and describe the four basic diagnostic maneuvers used by the physician during the physical exam.
- Differentiate between the terms and origin of common heart sounds.
- List the three classes of cardiovascular drugs used to treat angina.
- Describe the path by which blood circulates in the body.
- Given a common generic cardiovascular drug, match it to its correct trade name.
- Given cardiology root words and suffixes, combine them to match a given medical definition.
- Given a category of cardiovascular drugs, indicate which drugs belong to that category.

Fundamentals

- Demonstrate the correct use of commas in punctuation of medical sentences.
- Discuss three techniques for evaluating the heart function.
- Discuss two specific vocabulary or terminology problems in cardiology transcription.
- Demonstrate the correct use of commas in punctuation of medical sentences.
- Given a medical report with errors, identify and correct the errors.

Practice

- Accurately transcribe authentic physician dictation from the specialty of cardiology.

A Closer Look

Transcribing Cardiology Dictation

by Kathleen Mors Woods

In literature and in life, the heart is always depicted as the soul of a person and is described in vivid terms. One may be called a heartbreaker, a heart throb, a sweetheart. One may be heartless, heartsick, broken-hearted, fainthearted, good-hearted, lighthearted, lion-hearted, or have a big heart, a cold heart, a hard heart, or a heart as good as gold. These glossy descriptions take on a more meaningful tone when placed in a medical context and discussion of cardiology emerges.

In the medical field, we are concerned with cardiology as the study of the heart, its functions, and its diseases, the identification of these diseases by diagnostic tests, and ultimately the correction of defects. When a newborn baby is diagnosed with a congenital heart defect, or a 16-year-old is stabbed in the chest, or a person's aorta is literally ripped out of the chest in an automobile accident (by hitting the steering wheel not wearing a seat belt), the cardiac surgeon is called upon to demonstrate a broad range of abilities in treating these patients. Transcribing reports on these procedures carries with them the excitement of a new technology, expanding every day through research and their commitment to life-saving techniques.

The various techniques cover pacemaker insertion for irregular rhythm, the automatic implantable defibrillator for sudden death, coronary artery bypass grafting for coronary (vessel) blockage, valve replacement and repair with either mechanical parts or real preserved harvested parts, to the ultimate procedure for end-stage disease—heart and heart-lung transplantation.

Cardiac evaluation. Let's start by imagining the following scenario: Your neighbor has chest pain and goes to a cardiologist. The other factors for having this chest pain (for example, kidney stones or ulcers) have been ruled out. At the cardiologist's office, an electrocardiogram is performed. Twelve leads are attached, six at the wrists and ankles (leads I, II, III, aVF, aVL, aVR), and six on the chest (V$_1$ through V$_6$).

If the patient's pain is being caused by the decrease in blood flow due to a narrowing or obstruction of an artery carrying oxygen to the heart, and if damage has been done or is occurring, this will show up on the EKG. The pain, then, is caused by an obstruction (clot) in the vessel. If this clot remains in the vessel, the vessel is occluded and the muscle of the heart (myocardium) is damaged, for the area the vessel feeds dies.

If the patient is "evolving the infarction" (having a heart attack) and admitted to a hospital in a timely fashion, several other tests are performed, including a CPK (creatine phosphokinase) curve as a measure of the infarct. CPK-MB bands are located only in the heart muscle, and blood serum levels will rise if heart cells are damaged during an infarction (but not during angina). Within the past five years, several drugs have been developed which either dissolve the clot within the vessel or work with the body's own clotting factors to dissolve it.

Another option is for the patient to have a treadmill exercise stress test and to be referred for a cardiac catheterization.

Catheterization. Cardiac catheterization was invented in 1929 by a physician named Werner Forssmann, who first tested the procedure by catheterizing his own coronary arteries. Over the years it has progressed from a simple investigative technique to a powerful diagnostic procedure.

The patient is premedicated and taken to the catheterization laboratory. A puncture is made in the groin and a catheter is fed up into the heart. If the blood supply to the legs is poor, the catheter is inserted through a brachial cutdown in the arm, a small incision in the upper part of the arm which is later sutured closed. The catheter is properly positioned and radiopaque dye injected. While the dye is being injected and coursing through the vessels, it is recorded on running 35 mm film in black and white. This is later developed and shows where the blockages are in the coronary arteries, how the valves and heart muscle are functioning, and different pressures in these arteries. This film is called a cineangiogram (like cinema), or cine ("sin-ee") for short.

Although the catheterization is quite straightforward, the terminology is technical and specialized. Terms such as *aortic gradient, LVEDP, pigtail catheter, PCWP, assumed Fick method,* and *ejection fraction* might seem quite alien. Your reference sources should include a personal word list and equipment list.

Catheters are referred to by size and name. A *7 French JL4 catheter* is translated *7 French Judkins left 4 cm curve catheter.* The word *French* refers to the French scale for sizing catheters and is often abbreviated F; thus, *7F* means *seven French.* The catheters are named for shape, size, inventor, manufacturer, or have a trade name.

Angioplasty. When your neighbor's cardiac evaluation is completed, she may be told she has blockage of only one coronary artery. One of her options at this point is to have a PTCA (percutaneous transluminal coronary angioplasty). This procedure is often done immediately following the injection of a drug such as streptokinase or urokinase to lyse (break up) the clot. It can, however, be scheduled electively.

A catheter with a tiny balloon on the 4 or 5 mm tip is placed at the site of the narrowing of the artery and the balloon is inflated by means of a hand pump, to compress or squeeze the plaque back against the artery wall and open the blood flow through the vessel.

The advantage of this procedure is that it does not involve open heart surgery. The disadvantage is that this narrowing can recur, especially in those carrying inherited (familial) diseases. An angioplasty must be done in a hospital setting that provides surgery. When an artery dissects (tears open), the patient is taken to surgery for repair of the artery.

Terminology. The cardiology transcriptionist should know the names of the coronary arteries and branches which are frequently mentioned in cardiac catheterization reports, coronary artery bypass grafting, and all the tests and procedures regarding the heart.

The major vessels are the left main coronary artery, the left anterior descending (LAD) coronary artery, the right coronary artery (RCA), and the circumflex coronary artery (circ, pronounced "serk," for short). There are branches of these that take on additions, such as the left anterior descending diagonal (LADD). Other vessels to remember are the circumflex marginal, distal branches, and the posterior descendings. The major conduits are the aorta and pulmonary artery. The valves are aortic, mitral, pulmonary, and tricuspid.

Abbreviations. Although abbreviations are frequently dictated, the transcriptionist should exercise discretion when transcribing abbreviations in medical reports. When you are required to type abbreviations, use only those abbreviations that will not be misinterpreted; if you drop one letter of an abbreviation, you change the medical meaning and location. The posterior descending artery is abbreviated PDA, which also stands for the congenital heart defect of patent ductus arteriosus. When you translate abbreviations, be sure to transcribe the correct meaning as indicated by the context of the report.

A patient with multiple occlusions may opt for open heart surgery, or coronary artery bypass graft (CABG, pronounced *cabbage)*. Open heart procedures occur in two ways—opening the chest down the middle (median sternotomy), or, less usual, spreading the ribs and entering through this area (thoracotomy). Bypasses are named for the number of vessels reconnected—single, double, triple, or whatever number.

In interpreting the dictation, the transcriptionist must become familiar with many abbreviations and eponyms. If a baby has a B-T shunt, it is the procedure named after the famous Blalock-Taussig blue baby operation first performed by those two physicians. Favalaro, Bovie, St. Jude, Carpentier-Edwards, and Bjork-Shiley are all proper names (eponyms). If an eponym is the name of one person (Johns Hopkins, Austin Flint), it is not hyphenated, and one must learn which compound terms are which.

Pediatric surgery. Pediatric surgery is exciting and ever changing. Congenital heart defects, often discovered at birth, are treated with both open and closed heart procedures. These include PDA (patent ductus arteriosus), coarc (coarctation of the aorta), VSD (ventricular septal defect), ASD (atrial septal defect), AV (arteriovenous) canal, and "tet baby," which refers to a tetralogy of Fallot repair.

In instructing new transcriptionists, I tell them when I encounter a new word in dictation and cannot verify its correct spelling, my personal preference is to attach a note to the report with a phonetic spelling of the word in question. I have found that the *sounds like* note makes it easier to later identify the correct word and fill in the blank spot in the dictation, without having to listen to half the tape to find the questionable dictation spot. For example, *dismorfick* easily turns into *dysmorphic, frenic* to *phrenic.*

Occasionally we do not realize that we are not hearing a word correctly. I remember when a certain new medical transcriptionist transcribed *patent foraminal valley* in a cardiac catheterization report. After much kidding, she was told about the defect of *patent foramen ovale.*

Medications. Other nonsurgical problems include both diseases and malfunctions. Diseases can be treated by diet and medications. The medications listed are innumerable. I like to describe the method of typing these

as though they were green beans. A green bean is a green bean, right? But there are different brand names for green beans, e.g., Del Monte and Libby. The generic name (green bean) is not capitalized; however, the trade/brand name is. Therefore, nitroglycerin is not capitalized, but Nitro-Dur is.

It is also important to recognize when a physician is dictating a category of drugs. For example, a patient is placed on nitrate therapy or antiarrhythmics; those are drug categories, not drugs, and may therefore not be listed in a drug reference. Below are listed some common categories of drugs used to treat cardiac conditions, as well as examples of each category.

Category	Generic	Brand Name
ACE inhibitor	captopril	Capoten
antiarrhythmic	lidocaine	Xylocaine
	quinidine	Quinaglute
	procainamide	Procan SR
beta blocker	propranolol	Inderal
	metoprolol	Lopressor
blood thinner	warfarin	Coumadin
	aspirin	Bayer, Ecotrin
calcium channel blocker	nifedipine	Procardia
	verapamil	Calan
cardiac glycoside	digoxin	Lanoxin
diuretic	furosemide	Lasix
nitrate	nitroglycerin	Nitro-Bid, Nitro-Dur
	isosorbide	Isordil
vasodilator	isoxsuprine	Vasodilan
vasopressor	dopamine	Intropin

A minor confusing problem for transcriptionists is references to digoxin in dictation. Patients with congestive heart failure are commonly given digoxin (Lanoxin) which comes in doses of 0.25 mg and 0.125 mg. (Note: Always place the zero before the decimal point.) Digitalis is the powdered leaf of the digitalis plant or foxglove, which is seldom used. Refined forms include digoxin (Lanoxin) and digitoxin (Crystodigin).

If a physician says the patient had a laboratory "didj level" drawn, you can translate this slang as "digitalis level" rather than digitoxin or digoxin. Digitoxin is used infrequently but can be helpful in patients with kidney failure. Digoxin is excreted unchanged by the kidneys and can build up to toxic levels if the kidneys are not functioning well. Digitoxin, however, is metabolized to an inactive form by the liver first so that it is a much safer choice for patients with kidney failure. For the majority of patients in congestive heart failure, however, digoxin is prescribed.

Another confusing term is *pro time* which stands for prothrombin time (PT); this is a measure of blood clotting factors and is measured against a control and ratio. Unusual units of measure include torr (pressure), joule (electric power), and met (treadmill scoring).

Other areas in which proper names are used are in treadmill protocols (Bruce, Naughton) and pacemakers, which are identified by company and product names, i.e., Medtronic, Pacesetter. The pacemaker is usually inserted in the cardiac catheterization laboratory but may also be inserted in a room set up to do electrophysiology studies.

Pacemakers. Pacemakers are identified by a three-letter code system, such as DDD or VVI, which need not be translated. The first letter indicates the chamber that is paced; the second letter denotes the chamber that is sensed; the third letter indicates whether the pacemaker is inhibited or triggered by the heart's own electrical activity. For example, a DDD pacemaker serves the electrical activity of both the atrium and ventricle, paces (stimulates) both the atrium and ventricle to beat, and may cause (trigger) the atrium to contract while sending no signal (inhibited) to the ventricle, depending on what natural electrical activity is occurring in the heart at that time.

Of course, as soon as you have most of the common words down, you could be introduced to the exciting new field of the AICD (automatic implantable cardioverter defibrillator). The AICD is used for patients who are candidates for what we call sudden death, which is just what it sounds like—boom, the heart stops.

In an AICD operation, a patch is placed on the heart and sewn on, with leads extending to a box (in the stomach area) which, like some types of pacemakers, can monitor the rhythm of the heart. When there is an arrhythmia (irregular rhythm), the generator box senses this, fires a jolt to the heart, and starts it back up again.

Transplants. And then, last but not least, is the exciting world of transplantation. A small, blue, and feeble baby or a once healthy adult male with end-stage heart disease—they are both living on limited time and would soon die without an organ transplant. The words used are similar to those in other cardiac surgical procedures, with the addition of the drugs used to treat immunosuppression (the body's rejection of the new organ) such as cyclosporine, azathioprine, and others.

No matter how long you have been in the field, there will always be more challenging types of operations and more words to add to your already huge list of terms. If you are fortunate, you are using a word processor with a built-in dictionary, and you can add these words to your glossary.

As a cardiology transcriptionist, you get to "know" a cardiology patient quite well through the medical history you transcribe, and you get a lot of satisfaction knowing that you are playing an essential role in a patient's return to good health.

Medical Readings

The History and Physical Examination

by John H. Dirckx, M.D.

Review of Systems: Cardiovascular. The cardiovascular system includes the heart with its covering membrane, the pericardium, and all the blood vessels of the body—arteries, arterioles, capillaries, venules, and veins. Disorders of this system can produce a remarkable diversity of symptoms, from cough to ankle swelling and from sudden blindness to sudden death.

The cardiovascular history begins with a review of past diagnoses of congenital or acquired heart murmurs, rheumatic fever, enlarged heart, coronary artery disease, heart attack, high blood pressure, varicose veins, thrombophlebitis, and treatments, past or present, prescribed for any of these. Note is made of the results of past diagnostic studies such as electrocardiograms, echocardiograms, stress testing, cardiac catheterization, and angiography, and of any surgical procedures, such as pacemaker implantation, valve repair or replacement, and coronary artery bypass graft.

Because coronary artery disease is a major cause of disability and death, any complaint of chest pain must be carefully evaluated to determine whether it represents angina pectoris, the cardinal symptom of coronary disease. A full description of chest pain includes its character, intensity, location, extent, radiation, duration, and frequency of occurrence; the effect of position, movement, breathing, and swallowing; associated symptoms such as shortness of breath, sweating, and palpitations; the effect of resting or taking medicines such as antacids or nitroglycerin; and triggering factors such as physical exertion, smoking, eating, strong emotion, or exposure to cold.

When shortness of breath is due to cardiac failure it is typically less oppressive in the upright position (orthopnea) and may occur in attacks that awaken the patient during the night (paroxysmal nocturnal dyspnea). Orthopnea is graded by the number of pillows needed to avoid respiratory distress. Wheezing, coughing, and exertional dyspnea are common to cardiac and noncardiac disorders.

Physical Examination. As with the history, the scope and character of the physical examination performed on a given patient in a given instance depend on circumstances. A Boy Scout camp physical may be rushed through in less than one minute; thorough assessment of the nervous system alone in a patient suspected of having early multiple sclerosis can take more than an hour.

The following is a fairly comprehensive list of equipment used in the performance of a physical examination.

> flashlight, head mirror, or other light source
> magnifying glass
> tape measure
> ruler
> tongue depressor
> nasal speculum or rhinoscope
> otoscope with various sizes of specula
> ophthalmoscope
> reflex hammer
> pin or pinwheel
> soft brush or cotton ball
> diascope
> clinical thermometer
> watch with second hand
> goniometer
> skin-fold caliper
> laryngeal mirror
> tuning fork
> stethoscope
> sphygmomanometer
> rubber gloves and lubricant
> vaginal speculum
> vision-testing chart

Virtually all diagnostic maneuvers employed in the physical examination are variations on four basic, classical techniques: inspection (looking), palpation (feeling), auscultation (listening), and percussion (tapping).

Inspection in medicine implies far more than just looking. A diagnostic inspection is objective, systematic, and thorough, with removal of clothing as needed, adequate lighting, and sometimes use of instruments to expose, illuminate, or magnify. The examiner correlates what he sees with visual images stored in his memory, with other physical findings, and with relevant details of the history. Inspection thus includes not only search and discovery but also recognition and interpretation.

Again, palpation goes far beyond mere prodding and pinching. The tactile sense of the trained diagnostician can detect and assess minute variations in the size, shape, and texture of organs and tissues, which he then relates to visual impressions and other elements of the history and physical examination.

Certain techniques and findings associated with palpation deserve special mention here. *Ballottement* (French, "shaking") is a technique of applying pressure intermittently to a body surface, somewhat as in bouncing a ball. By this means it is sometimes possible to detect deeply placed organs or masses that cannot otherwise be palpated. *Fluctuancy* refers to the tactile quality of confined fluid. The palpating fingers can displace this fluid and perhaps even set up waves in it, as in compressing a balloon filled with water. *Fremitus* is a sensation of rubbing or vibration felt by the palpating fingers. It can be due to friction between two structures (such as a tendon and its sheath) or to transmission of sound (such as the patient's voice) through intervening tissues. *Crepitation* or *crepitus* is a grating or crackling sound produced by feeling or manipulating a part. Fremitus and crepitus sometimes occur together and the terms are not strictly distinguished in practice.

Auscultation of internal organs is performed with a stethoscope but the technique also embraces listening to sounds produced by or in any part of the body.

Quantitative measurements play an essential role in physical diagnosis. The basic physical examination includes measurements of height, weight, temperature, cardiac rate, respiratory rate, and blood pressure, which are usually included at the beginning of the physical examination report. To an increasing extent, height and weight are recorded in metric units (centimeters and kilograms) in this country. Temperature is still generally recorded in Fahrenheit degrees, though the Celsius scale is used at a few medical centers. Temperature is taken orally except when the patient's age or condition makes the rectal route preferable.

Heart rate is recorded in beats per minute. Unless the cardiac rhythm is irregular, the examiner usually counts beats for only 15 seconds and multiplies by four. The heart rate may be counted as pulsations in a peripheral artery, most often the radial artery at the wrist (radial pulse) or as beats heard with a stethoscope placed on the chest near the cardiac apex (apical pulse). The respiratory rate, recorded as respirations per minute, is also usually determined by 15 seconds' actual observation. The examiner usually counts respirations while ostensibly doing something else (e.g., still feeling the pulse at the wrist). This is because a person who knows that his breathing is being observed finds it almost impossible to breathe at a natural rate and depth.

Blood pressure is determined in the brachial artery above the elbow with the help of a stethoscope and a sphygmomanometer. The higher of these readings is taken as the maximum pressure attained by the blood in response to a contraction of the heart (systolic pressure); the lower, the pressure to which the blood drops between contractions (diastolic pressure). By convention, these figures are reported as a fraction, with the higher number on top; e.g., 120/80, pronounced "one twenty over eighty." In certain circumstances blood pressure may be taken with the cuff applied to the thigh.

Examination of the Heart. Virtually the entire cardiac examination consists of observation of the function of the heart—the rate, regularity, and intensity of ventricular contractions, the resulting impulses imparted to the circulating blood and to the chest wall, and the sounds generated by cardiac contraction and the movement of blood. Congenital anomalies, valvular disease, arrhythmias, pericardial effusions and adhesions, ventricular dilatation and hypertrophy, congestive heart failure—all must be detected or inferred by examination of cardiac function. X-rays, cardiograms, and other noninvasive and invasive diagnostic procedures can yield more precise data about structural alterations in the heart and great vessels, but even these depend largely on assessment of cardiac function.

The anterior chest wall is inspected for pulsations and the point at which the cardiac impulse is strongest (point of maximal intensity) is found by palpation. The examiner's fingers detect not only this point but also any abnormalities associated with the heartbeat, such as a heaving of the chest wall due to unduly intense cardiac contractions, thrills due to passage of blood through abnormally narrowed valves or other orifices, and shocks from abnormally abrupt closure of valves in hypertension. Percussion can also be used to assess cardiac size and shape, although many examiners doubt the validity of this procedure.

Auscultation of the heart provides more information than any other procedure. Stethoscopes used for cardiac auscultation have two chest pieces, a narrow, cone-shaped "bell" for lower pitched sounds and a wide, flat diaphragm for higher pitched sounds. The examiner changes back and forth from one to the other as needed during the examination. He applies the stethoscope to the chest in a number of areas, following a basic routine but varying it as circumstances dictate.

Four areas of the anterior chest are designated according to the valves whose sounds are best heard there: the mitral area, the pulmonic area, the aortic area, and the tricuspid area. The subject may need to change his position, such as by leaning forward or lying on his left side, to enable the examiner to evaluate heart sounds adequately. The physician also listens for abnormal sounds: murmurs, caused by abnormal flow of blood through a valve or other orifice; clicks or snaps, caused by abnormal valve function; rubs, creaking or grating sounds caused by friction between the beating heart and an inflamed pericardium; bruits, caused by passage of blood through a narrowed artery; and others.

The normally beating heart produces two sounds in alternation, traditionally represented as *lub-dup*. The first heart sound, or S1, which is louder, deeper in pitch, and longer, results from contraction of the ventricles and closure of the mitral and tricuspid valves. For practical purposes it is considered synchronous with the beginning of systole, or ventricular contraction. The second heart sound, S2, results from closure of the aortic and pulmonic valves just after systole ends. S2 is taken as the beginning of diastole, or ventricular relaxation and refilling. The first and second heart sounds heard at specific valve areas are sometimes so designated: A1, the first heart sound at the aortic valve area; P2, the second heart sound heard at the pulmonic valve area; and so on.

Cardiac murmurs are produced by turbulence in the flow of blood passing forward through a stenotic valve, leaking back through an incompetent valve, or crossing from a place of higher to a place of lower pressure through an abnormal orifice, such as an interventricular septal defect. The diagnostician characterizes a murmur by recording its location (the point on the chest wall where it is heard best); its radiation or transmission (for example, to the carotid arteries or left axilla); its character, intensity (graded on a scale of 1 to 6; less often, 1 to 4), and duration; and its timing within the cardiac cycle. Valvular clicks and snaps are similarly characterized.

Pharmacology: Cardiovascular Drugs

Cardiac glycosides are a group of chemically related drugs, prescribed for congestive heart failure, whose molecular structure consists of chains of glucose sugars known as glycosides; hence the name *cardiac glycosides.*

In ancient times, cardiac glycosides were extracted from the dried foxglove plant (Latin name: *Digitalis*). Today, these drugs are extracted and purified or synthetically produced. The term *digitalis* refers collectively to all of the cardiac glycosides.

Digoxin is by far the most commonly prescribed cardiac glycoside. This is because it has a **shorter half-life** than the other cardiac glycosides and therefore less chance of causing toxicity. Others used less often include digitoxin and deslanoside.

Digitalis toxicity from cardiac glycosides is a serious and frequent adverse effect. Nearly one-third of patients taking a cardiac glycoside develop symptoms of digitalis toxicity because these drugs have a low therapeutic index (i.e., there is a narrow margin between the therapeutic dose and the toxic dose), and **long half-life** which is even more prolonged in elderly patients with decreased kidney function. Symptoms of toxicity may include a pulse rate below 60 beats per minute, confusion, fatigue, nausea/vomiting, diarrhea, or yellow-green halos around lights.

To prevent toxic effects, physicians order blood tests to determine the level of digitalis in the blood. These are often referred to as "dig levels" (pronounced "dij"). Symptoms from toxicity may be treated by changing the dosage to a less frequent schedule or, in severe cases, by administering digoxin immune fab (Digibind).

Antianginal drugs. The pain of angina pectoris occurs when cells of the myocardium receive insufficiently oxygenated blood to meet their needs. The drugs used to treat angina include nitrates, beta blockers, and calcium channel blockers.

Nitrates used to treat angina. As a group, nitrates act as vasodilators throughout the vascular system. The most frequently prescribed nitrate is nitroglycerin. All of the nitrates, including nitroglycerin, can be administered in several different ways:

    sublingually as a spray
    sublingually as a tablet
    transmucosally between the cheek and gum as
       a tablet
    orally as a sustained-release capsule
    transdermally as a patch
    topically as an ointment (measured in inches)
    intravenously

Beta blockers used to treat angina. Beta blockers act to decrease the heart rate which in turn decreases the need of the myocardium for oxygen; this decreases anginal pain.

Beta blockers used to treat angina include:

    atenolol (Tenormin)
    metoprolol (Lopressor)
    nadolol (Corgard)
    propranolol (Inderal)

Note: The ending *-olol* is common to generic beta blockers.

Calcium channel blockers used to treat angina. Calcium channel blockers may be used in conjunction with nitrates or beta blockers to treat angina. Calcium channel blockers relax the smooth muscle of the blood vessels to decrease arterial pressure, the pressure the heart must pump against. This decreases the heart's need for oxygen. This same action also dilates the coronary arteries and prevents coronary artery spasm which can trigger angina.

Calcium channel blockers used to treat angina include:

    diltiazem (Cardizem)
    nicardipine (Cardene)
    nifedipine (Adalat, Procardia)
    verapamil (Calan, Isoptin, Verelan)

Note: The ending *-ipine* is common to some generic calcium channel blocking drugs.

Aspirin. One tablet of aspirin daily has been shown to significantly decrease the incidence of a second heart attack because of its anticoagulant effect.

Antiarrhythmic drugs. Cardiac arrhythmias are caused by abnormalities in the normal conduction of electrical impulses from the SA node through the AV node, bundle of His, and Purkinje system in the heart.

Antiarrhythmic drugs used to treat both atrial and ventricular arrhythmias include:

    procainamide (Procan SR, Pronestyl)
    propranolol (Inderal)—a beta blocker drug
    quinidine (Cardioquin, Quinaglute)

Antiarrhythmic drugs indicated only for ventricular arrhythmias include:

    adenosine (Adenocard)
    bretylium tosylate (Bretylol)
    lidocaine (Xylocaine)
    tocainide (Tonocard)
    atenolol (Tenormin)—a beta blocker
    metoprolol (Lopressor)—a beta blocker
    nadolol (Corgard)—a beta blocker

pindolol (Visken)—a beta blocker
propranolol (Inderal)—a beta blocker
timolol (Blocadren)—a beta blocker
verapamil (Calan, Isoptin)—a calcium
    channel blocker

Antihypertensive drugs. Hypertension is a condition which manifests itself as an increase in systolic and/or diastolic blood pressure. Hypertension is caused by arteriosclerosis or kidney disease, or other diseases, or it may have no identified cause; this last type is known as essential hypertension.

Several classes of drugs are used to treat hypertension. These include diuretics, beta blockers, calcium channel blockers, ACE inhibitors, alpha receptor blockers, and vasodilators. In addition, most patients are asked to restrict the use of salt in cooking and at the table, or the physician may prescribe a low-salt diet which places a limit on total dietary sodium intake.

The treatment of hypertension follows what is known as a **step-care approach.** One antihypertensive agent, often a diuretic, is prescribed first. If a satisfactory reduction in blood pressure is not achieved, a second antihypertensive agent, such as a beta blocker, is added. Beta blockers may also be selected as the first step of treatment. Other drugs are added to the treatment regimen as necessary to achieve control of blood pressure.

Hyperlipidemia drugs. Hyperlipidemia is a general term encompassing both hypercholesterolemia (increased levels of serum cholesterol) and hypertriglyceridemia (increased levels of serum triglycerides). Hyperlipidemia is one of several well-defined risk factors for atherosclerosis; others include smoking, obesity, hypertension, stress, and sedentary life-style.

Drugs which reduce serum cholesterol levels act by causing more cholesterol to be excreted in the bile or by decreasing levels of LDL. The first two drugs are known specifically as **bile acid sequestrants**, while the other drugs are simply antihyperlipidemic agents.

cholestyramine (Cholybar, Questran)
lovastatin (Mevacor)
probucol (Lorelco)

Drugs which reduce serum triglyceride levels act by decreasing the levels of VLDL. These drugs include:

clofibrate (Atromid-S)
gemfibrozil (Lopid)

Anatomy/Medical Terminology

Fill-in Exercise: Circulation of the Blood

Instructions: The following paragraphs describe the process by which blood is circulated throughout the body. The numbered blanks correspond to the numbers in the narrative. Fill in the blanks with the correct term from the word list below.

Deoxygenated blood moves from the capillaries throughout the body to venules, to veins, and finally into the (1) before it enters the (2) of the heart.

Leaving this chamber, the blood is pumped through the (3) and into the right ventricle. From there, it goes through the pulmonary valve into the (4) that leads to the lungs. In the lungs, carbon dioxide is exchanged for (5) and the blood becomes oxygenated and bright red in color.

The oxygenated blood leaves the lungs via the (6) and enters the (7) of the heart. The valve between the left atrium and the left ventricle is known as the (8).

All heart valves have delicate (9) or leaflets that close tightly to prevent backflow of blood as the heart pumps. As the blood leaves the left ventricle, it passes through the (10) and into the (11), the largest artery in the body, to begin its journey again through the body.

1. vena cava _____
2. _____
3. _____
4. _____
5. _____
6. _____
7. _____
8. _____
9. _____
10. _____
11. _____

aorta	pulmonary artery
aortic valve	pulmonary vein
cusps	right atrium
left atrium	tricuspid valve
mitral valve	vena cava
oxygen	

Anatomy: The Circulatory System

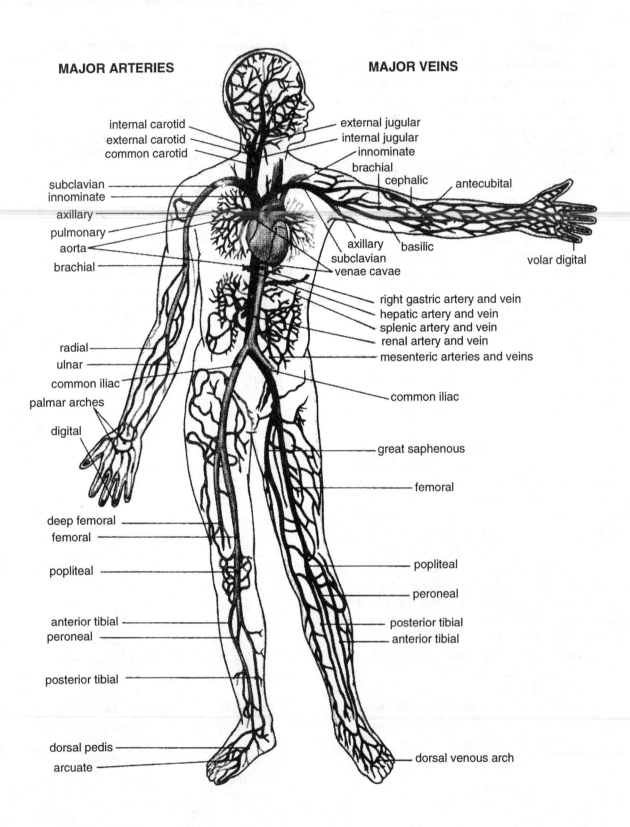

MAJOR ARTERIES

MAJOR VEINS

internal carotid
external carotid
common carotid

subclavian
innominate
axillary
pulmonary
aorta
brachial

radial
ulnar
common iliac
palmar arches
digital

deep femoral
femoral

popliteal

anterior tibial
peroneal

posterior tibial

dorsal pedis
arcuate

external jugular
internal jugular
innominate
brachial
cephalic   antecubital

axillary   basilic
subclavian
venae cavae   volar digital

right gastric artery and vein
hepatic artery and vein
splenic artery and vein
renal artery and vein
mesenteric arteries and veins

common iliac

great saphenous

femoral

popliteal

peroneal

posterior tibial
anterior tibial

dorsal venous arch

Adjective Exercise

Adjectives are formed from nouns by adding adjectival suffixes such as *-ac, -al, -ar, -ary, -eal, -ed, -ent, -iac, -ial, -ic, -ical, -ive, -lar, -oid, -ous, -tic,* and *-tous.* In addition, some adjectives have a different form entirely from the noun, which may be either Latin or Greek in origin.

Test your knowledge of adjectives by writing the adjectival form of the following cardiology words. Consult a medical dictionary to select the correct adjectival ending as necessary.

1. heart _____
2. artery _____
3. vein _____
4. atrium _____
5. ventricle _____
6. aorta _____
7. systole _____
8. myocardium _____
9. cyanosis _____
10. hypertension _____
11. aneurysm _____
12. valve _____

Drug Matching Exercise

Instructions: Match the generic name drug from Column A with its trade name in Column B.

Column A	*Column B*
A. propranolol	___ Atromid-S
B. nitroglycerin	___ Calan
C. verapamil	___ Cardizem
D. lidocaine	___ Mevacor
E. metoprolol	___ Blocadren
F. diltiazem	___ Adrenalin
G. timolol	___ Xylocaine
H. nifedipine	___ Nitrostat
I. lovastatin	___ Procardia
J. clofibrate	___ Inderal
K. epinephrine	___ Lopressor

Lay and Medical Terms

Lay Term	*Medical Term*
heart attack	myocardial infarction
high blood pressure	hypertension
hardening of the arteries	arteriosclerosis
chest pain	angina pectoris

Root Word and Suffix Matching Exercise

Instructions: Combine the following root words with suffixes to form words that match the definitions below. Fill in the blanks with the medical words that you construct.

Root Word	*Suffix*
cardio-	-plasty
endo-	-megaly
valvulo-	-ology
electro-	-gram
angio-	-ectomy
aneurysm-	-itis
phlebo-	

A. inflammation of a vein

_____

B. enlargement of the heart

_____

C. inflammation of the inner lining of the heart (Tip: Use 2 root words and 1 suffix.)

_____

D. the study of the heart

_____

E. surgical widening of a constricted valve

_____

F. record of the heart's electrical activity

_____

G. surgical widening of narrowed blood vessels

_____

H. surgical removal of an aneurysm

_____

Drug Matching Exercise

Instructions: Match the drug category in Column A with the trade name drugs in Column B. Note: Drug categories are used more than once and a drug may fit more than one category.

Column A	Column B
A. antiarrhythmic	____ Xylocaine
	____ Atromid-S
B. antihypertensive	____ Corgard
	____ Quinaglute
C. antihyperlipidemic	____ Inderal
	____ Procan SR
	____ Questran
	____ Cardizem

Drug Word Search

Instructions: Locate and circle the drugs and terms hidden in the puzzle horizontally, vertically, diagonally, forward, or backward. Numerals following a drug or term indicate the number of times it can be found in the puzzle.

```
T D R A G R O C L I D R O S I U R
B A Z X I S A L A B R M U I N K I
T E N O R M I N N L N G U R D I S
T Y T K O P B F O I A S S Y E S T
E N I A C O L Y X D V N N T R A F
N O C T B W A O I T R A E H A F A
O R L H U L G P N S C L C M L N M
R P I Y D I O C X I M D A O I A R
M A D O D L E C R B I O L L D T I
I C M T R E W C K D F M A D I K A
N E N I T N A S R E P E N E R I N
T N E M T N I O L O R T I N T E N
```

Aldomet (2)	encainide	Nitrol ointment
beta blocker	heart	Norpace
Calan (2)	HDL	Persantine
Corgard	Inderal	pill
Digibind	Isordil	Rythmol
digoxin	Lanoxin	Tenormin (2)
drug	Lasix	Tridil
DynaCirc	Lopid	Xylocaine

Commas

1. **Commas and compound sentences.** A compound sentence consists of two independent clauses joined most commonly by the conjunctions *and, but, for, or, nor*. If the two independent clauses—each a complete sentence—are short (only about five words long), a comma is not needed to separate them but may be used. If each independent clause is longer, a comma is generally used.

Before inserting a comma, check to be sure that the second part of the sentence is really an independent clause. Sometimes the second part of the sentence contains only a verb that agrees with the subject in the first part of the sentence. In that case, you do not insert a comma because a comma should never separate a subject from its verb.

Example: The patient is having chest pain, but she denies diaphoresis or dyspnea.

Explanation: Both parts of the sentence are independent clauses and contain a subject and a verb. A comma is optional because the clauses are short.

Example: The patient is having chest pain but denies diaphoresis and dyspnea.

Explanation: No comma should be used because *patient* is the subject and the sentence has a compound verb, *is having* and *denies*.

2. **Commas and adjectives in a series.** Do not put a comma between the last adjective in a series and the noun that follows it.

The patient is a 60-year-old, elderly, disoriented female.

3. When the patient's race is given, consider it to be part of the noun and not an adjective.

The patient is a 60-year-old, elderly, disoriented Caucasian female.

4. Commas can be used with adjectives according to the *a, b, and c rule* or the *a, b and c rule.* The use of the final comma before the word *and* or *or* in any list is optional.

   I have ordered a CBC, BUN, and creatinine.
   I have ordered a CBC, BUN and creatinine.

5. **Commas with *however*.** If the word *however* is in the middle of an independent clause, place commas around it.

   The patient was, however, very tired.
   The patient was very tired, however, complaining of weakness and fatigue.

6. If the word *however* separates two independent clauses, place a semicolon before *however* and a comma after it.

   The patient was very tired; however, he did not complain of weakness.

7. **Comma pairs.** Use a comma pair to set off nonessential phrases within a sentence.

   Her condition, in my opinion, is critical.

8. Use a comma pair to set off a date within a sentence, when the date is presented in the month/day/year format. When the date is presented in the day/month/year format, a comma is not needed.

   The patient is scheduled for surgery on June 15, 1993, at Valley General Hospital.

   The patient is scheduled for surgery on 15 June 1993 at Valley General Hospital.

9. Do not use a comma pair when the complete date (month, day, and year) is not given.

   She had open heart surgery in June 1989 at Valley General Hospital.

10. Omitting one of the commas in a comma pair is termed a *comma fault.*

Punctuation Exercise

   Instructions: Insert commas as appropriate in the sentences below.

1. He will be seen by social services rehabilitative medicine and by his private cardiologist.

2. His angina however will continue until he undergoes a bypass procedure in the near future.

3. This patient as far as I can see is ready for rehabilitation.

4. She was discharged on Cardizem diuretics nitroglycerin and Atromid-S.

5. The improvement if any is very slight.

6. Her CPK levels however continued to remain within the normal range.

7. He has been instructed in the use of a low-salt diet; however it is doubtful if he will comply.

8. Her symptoms included dyspnea on exertion diaphoresis and a crushing chest pain.

9. The patient is a 72-year-old Oriental female with no complaints of angina today.

10. Her hypertension is controlled with Dyazide and seems to be relatively stable.

11. The surgery was completed without complication and the patient was taken to the recovery room in satisfactory and stable condition.

12. She is scheduled for coronary artery bypass graft on September 15 1993 and she will be admitted for preoperative testing on the preceding day.

Proofreading Skills

Instructions: In the report below, circle the errors. Identify misspelled and missing medical and English words and write the correct ones in the numbered spaces opposite the text.

#	Text	#	Answer
1	PERSENT ILLNESS: This 68-year-old cauca-	1.	PRESENT
2	sian male with a history of hypertention and	2.	
3	congestive heart failure was apparently in	3.	
4	good health although he had failed to follow	4.	
5	up on his office appointments and ran out of	5.	
6	refills on probably his Lasix one week ago.	6.	
7	The pateint shortly thereafter had some slight	7.	
8	precordal chest pain which resolved. The	8.	
9	precordial chest pain returned again. The pa-	9.	
10	tient attained good relief with nitroglycerine	10.	
11	sublingual. The patient has also been on Calan	11.	
12	and Micro-K which he has continued to take.	12.	
13	He has had no chills or fever, no nuasea,	13.	
14	emmesis, or diarhea, no unusual color change.	14.	
15	He did complain of being somewhat	15.	
16	diaphorectic and dizzy with the chest pain.	16.	
17		17.	
18	FAMLY HISTRY: No familial diseeses	18.	
19	known.	19.	
20		20.	
21	PHYSICAL EXAMINATION:	21.	
22	GENERAL APPEARENCE: A slightly obese,	22.	
23	well-developed 68-year-old Caucasian male.	23.	
24	HEENT: Head symetrical. Pupils equal, react	24.	
25	to light and accomodation, no scleral icterous.	25.	
26	Ears, nose, and throat cleer. Mouth moist.	26.	
27	NECK suppel, no masses. Normal anterior	27.	
28	carotid pulsations bilaterally.	28.	
29	CHEST clear to T&A.	29.	
30	CARDIOVASCULAR: Distant heart tones, no	30.	
31	murmurs. Good peripheral pulses, including	31.	
32	dorsalis pedis.	32.	
33	ABDOMAN: Protuberent, no masses. Active	33.	
34	bowel sounds.	34.	
35		35.	
36	IMPRESSION:	36.	
37	1. Probable angina pectorus.	37.	
38	2. Rule out MI.	38.	
39	3. CHF, compensated.	39.	
40	4. Hypertension.	40.	
41	5. ASHD.	41.	

Transcription Tips

1. Unless you transcribe exclusively in a physician specialist's office, the majority of reports you will encounter will be from the three main specialties of cardiology, gastroenterology, and orthopedics. Diseases of the cardiovascular system are quite prevalent and the medical terminology is extensive. Even patients with a noncardiac chief complaint may have chronic secondary cardiovascular disorders such as arrhythmia, hypertension, or elevated cholesterol level. This is particularly true of elderly patients; thus, you should be familiar with cardiovascular terminology.

2. There are several sound-alike terms in the cardiovascular system. Memorize their meanings and select the term appropriate for a correct transcript.

   hypertension (high blood pressure)
   hypotension (low blood pressure)

   palpitation (sensation caused by irregular heart beats)
   palpation (using the hands to examine body surfaces)

   Buerger's disease (a blood vessel disease)
   Berger's disease (a kidney disorder)

3. Transcribe these slang terms correctly when encountered in dictation.

Slang	Correct Translation
"cabbage"	CABG (acronym for coronary artery bypass graft)
cath	catheterization (cardiac)
cath'd	catheterized
dig	digoxin
nitro	nitroglycerin
"romied"	ROMI (rule out myocardial infarction). Do not make a verb ("romied") of this abbreviation.
V fib	ventricular fibrillation
V tach	ventricular tachycardia

4. The heart sounds are written with a capital letter followed by a subscript number. (If your keyboard does not have subscript numbers, then type regular numbers.)

   S_1 or S1 (the first heart sound)
   S_2 or S2 (the second heart sound)
   S_3 or S3 (the third heart sound)
   S_4 or S4 (the fourth heart sound)
   A_2 or A2 (closure of the aortic valve)
   P_2 or P2 (closure of the pulmonary valve)

5. The electrocardiogram leads ("leeds") can be written with either regular or subscript numbers.

   V1 through V6 or V_1 through V_6

6. Both EKG and ECG are acceptable abbreviations for *electrocardiogram*. The *K* comes from the Greek word *kardia* (heart), and also from the German spelling, *Elektrokardiogramm*.

7. Note these difficult-to-spell cardiovascular drugs.

   Cardizem (not Cardiazem or Cardizyme)
   Combipres (only one *s*)
   Inderal (not Inderol)
   Minipress and Lopressor (two *s*'s)
   Rythmol (an antiarrhythmic drug, but note that its spelling differs from the word *rhythm*)

8. Both word roots *angio-* (Greek) and *vaso-* (Latin) mean *blood vessel*.

9. The abbreviation *AV* can mean either *arteriovenous* or *atrioventricular*. Be sure to translate it correctly based on its meaning in the sentence.

   AV fistula   arteriovenous fistula
   AV node   atrioventricular node

10. In a cardiology context, the abbreviation *AAA* and the dictated form *triple A* stand for abdominal aortic aneurysm.

Terminology Challenge

Instructions: The following terms appear in the dictated reports on Tape 4A. Before beginning the medical transcription practice for Lesson 8, become familiar with the terminology below by looking up each word in a medical or English dictionary, and write out a short definition of each term.

1700 hours
adenopathy
afebrile
aminophylline
anemia
anticoagulant
arrhythmia
atrial fibrillation
auscultation
bibasilar
Capoten
cardiac catheterization
cardiac enzyme
Cardizem
carotid pulse
CBC (complete blood count)
central venous pressure (CVP)
chemistry panel
Clinoril
Colace
congestive heart failure
Coumadin
cranial nerves II through XII
cyanosis
D5W (5% dextrose in water)
deep venous thrombosis
diaphoresis
diastolic rumble
digoxin
disoriented
dorsal
dyspneic
ejection fraction
fingerbreadths

grade 2-3/6 blowing systolic heart murmur (grade "two to three over six")
heart disease
  arteriosclerotic
  atherosclerotic
  coronary artery
  hypertensive
  valvular
hemogram
hypertension
hypotension
Inderal
infarct
inflammatory
inversion
irregularly irregular rhythm
ischemia
jugular venous distention (JVD)
kyphosis
Lanoxin
Lasix
lead ("leed")
  anterolateral
  inferior
lymphadenopathy
Metamucil
MI (myocardial infarction)
neoplasm
nitro patch
nitroglycerin
nonproductive cough
occult blood
orthopnea

p.o.
pacemaker
percussion
pitting edema
pleural effusion
PND (paroxysmal nocturnal dyspnea)
pneumonitis
potassium
psychosis
q.24h.
rales
reflexes
  deep tendon
  pathological
Restoril
S3 (heart)
S4 (heart)
sinus rhythm
sinus tachycardia
ST segment

ST wave
ST-T wave changes
sternal notch
subendocardial myocardial infarction
sublingual
substernal
T wave
Tenex
thyromegaly
tibia
TKO (to keep open)
total CPK
transdermal
treadmill stress test
unlabored
unstable angina
venogram
Voltaren
Xylocaine

Sample Reports

Sample cardiology reports appear on the following pages, illustrating a variety of formats.

Transcription Practice

After completing all the readings and exercises in Lesson 8, transcribe Tape 4A, Cardiology. Use both medical and English dictionaries and your Quick-Reference Word List as resource materials for finding words.

Proofread your transcribed documents carefully, listening to the dictation while you read your transcripts.

Transcribe (*NOT* retype) the same reports again without referring to your previous transcription attempt. Initially, you may need to transcribe some reports more than twice before you can produce an error-free document. Your ultimate goal is to produce an error-free document the first time.

HISTORY AND PHYSICAL EXAMINATION

FLINTSTONE, Betty	123456	11/17/90	B. Rubble, M.D.
Patient Name	ID Number	Date of Admission	Attending Physician

CHIEF COMPLAINT: Chest pain.

HISTORY OF PRESENT ILLNESS: This 65-year-old white female was admitted to the hospital with chest pain on the night of admission. This lasted off and on for some time, for probably several hours. It was not relieved by nitroglycerin, and because of this she presented herself to the emergency department. She also has diabetes mellitus, insulin dependent, and her sugars are sporadically in the 300 to 400 range. She has been unable to lose weight and is grossly obese.

PAST MEDICAL HISTORY: Please see old records for past medical history.

SOCIAL AND FAMILY HISTORY: See old records.

SYSTEM REVIEW: System review is essentially unchanged from the last admission. She has occasional headaches. There is some decrease in her hearing. She has cough and congestion but no pneumonia or TB. Appetite and digestion have been good, and she has not had any GI bleeding. She has no urgency, frequency, or dysuria, but she has had urinary tract infections in the past. Neuromuscular is negative. Positive history for arthritis.

PHYSICAL EXAMINATION:
VITAL SIGNS: Blood pressure is 140/80, pulse is 88 and regular, respirations 16 and regular.
GENERAL: This is a well-developed, obese female complaining of chest pain and shortness of breath.
HEENT: Head is normocephalic. She has bilateral arcus senilis and compensated edentulism.
NECK: Neck is supple, no bruits noted.
BREASTS: Breasts are without masses.
LUNGS: Lungs reveal scattered wheezes and basilar rales.
HEART: Heart reveals a regular sinus rhythm. She has a soft apical murmur.
ABDOMEN: Abdomen is 4+ protuberant. No masses were felt.
EXTREMITIES: Unremarkable with the exception of 1+ edema. Peripheral pulses are diminished but present.
NEUROLOGIC: Reflexes are equal and active. Neurologic is physiologic.

IMPRESSION:
1. Arteriosclerotic heart disease with chest pain and congestive heart failure.
   Rule out myocardial infarction.
2. Diabetes mellitus.
3. Exogenous obesity.
4. Degenerative osteoarthritis.

BARNEY RUBBLE, M.D.

BR:hpi
D&T: 11/17/90

JOSEPH SCOTT POWELL

#092796

Date of Consultation: 6/25/92

Attending Physician: Edward X. Hale, M.D.

CONSULTATION REPORT

The patient is seen in consultation because of chest pain and cardiac irregularity.

The patient tells me that about 10 years ago he had a severe episode of chest pain and was hospitalized for a heart attack.

About three days ago, he started having more shortness of breath. He also began having chest pains plus nausea and vomiting. His breathing was quite difficult, and so he came in to the emergency department, was found to be in congestive heart failure with cardiac irregularity, and was admitted to the hospital for further care.

The rest of his history can be obtained from his previous record.

On physical examination the patient does appear older than his stated age of 69 by at least five years. His blood pressure is 186/80, his pulse is 100 to 178, and he has runs of paroxysmal atrial tachycardia (PAT), frequent premature ventricular contractions, and he has had a couple of short runs of ventricular tachycardia. During one of his runs of PAT, I gave him 5 mg of verapamil intravenously, and this reduced the rate dramatically. His neck veins are distended. He has moist rales over both lungs. The heart is at the midclavicular line in the fifth interspace, and there is a systolic murmur at the apex. His abdomen is soft. No masses can be felt. He has 2+ edema in the lower extremities. Both of his knees have bruises from a previous fall. I did not do a rectal exam because of his respiratory difficulty.

It is my impression that he has a combination of arteriosclerotic and hypertensive cardiovascular disease with mild cardiomegaly, probably left ventricular hypertrophy, and congestive heart failure with functional classification of III. He also has pulmonary emphysema secondary to his smoking, with chronic obstructive pulmonary disease.

I have taken the liberty to discontinue the Theo-Dur for the present because I do not want to cause more cardiac irritability, and we will continue with the Calan, the diuretic, a low dose of Xylocaine, and we may have to go back to digoxin, but I would rather wait for a time in view of his ventricular ectopic beats.

Thank you for allowing me to see this patient, and I shall be glad to follow him with you.

RICHARD BESSERMAN, M.D.

RB:hpi
d&t:6/25/92

CARRIE CRABBE   #012465   Date of Visit: 4/13/92   Attending: F. O. Paws, M.D.

EMERGENCY DEPARTMENT NOTE

The patient is a 19-year-old white female who has a rather long and complicated medical history. Since 16 years of age, the patient has had chronic fatigue, extreme exercise intolerance, episodes of anorexia nervosa, and recurrent syncopal attacks. She is not able to walk up a flight of stairs or walk more than one block because of fatigue and dyspnea with exertion.

The patient was noted to have sinus bradycardia with heart rates in the 40s at times. She had an echocardiogram which showed mitral valve prolapse. She had a treadmill exercise test at which time she was able to go into stage 3 and achieved a maximum heart rate of 185 per minute. The test was remarkable for a rather flat blood pressure response with systolic BP 114 at rest and into the exercise, with no appropriate increase during the exercise test. In addition the patient developed a prolonged PR interval of 0.34, with some blocked APCs during the recovery phase of the exercise. She had evidence of both sinus node dysfunction and AV nodal disease.

IMPRESSION:

1. Recurrent syncopal episode of unknown etiology. Patient does not have significant postural hypotension on examination. Patient has a history of sick sinus dysfunction. It is possible that the patient has a significant bradyarrhythmia precipitating syncopal episodes.

2. Possible sinus node dysfunction.

_____

I. M. PHITT, M.D.

IMP:hpi
d&t: 4/13/92

RANDY ANDREWS

#100465

Admitted: 6/3/92

Discharged: 6/6/92

DISCHARGE SUMMARY

ADMISSION DIAGNOSIS:
1. Left carotid artery stenosis with ulceration and previous left hemispheric cerebrovascular accident (CVA).
2. Arteriosclerotic peripheral vascular disease with aortoiliac stenosis.

OPERATIVE PROCEDURE: Left carotid endarterectomy.

COMPLICATIONS: None.

CONDITION ON DISCHARGE: Improved.

HISTORY AND PHYSICAL FINDINGS: The patient is a 62-year-old male who 10 weeks ago had a hemispheric neurologic event with marked weakness in his right arm and some speech difficulty. He has been worked up with a CT that revealed no tumor, infarct, or hemorrhage. He subsequently had Doppler studies that were suggestive of stenosis, and eventually had arteriograms that revealed about a 70% stenosis with a very significant deep ulcer. The patient had been on aspirin and Persantine. Ergometric studies did not reveal any significant cardiac ischemia. The patient is also known to have chronic aortoiliac occlusive disease with significant claudication, but no rest pain.

After discussion regarding therapeutic options with the patient and his wife, including the multiple major complications of operative versus nonoperative management, he elected to proceed with a carotid endarterectomy. This was accomplished on the day of admission, and it should be noted that the patient did have a recent hemorrhage under the plaque with a very shaggy ulcer in the left internal carotid.

The patient had an uneventful operative procedure, and his postoperative course has been equally benign. He is being discharged home on the morning of his third postoperative day ambulatory. Wound is clean and no sign of any hematoma. He neurologically remains stable. He is to continue his aspirin and Persantine as preoperatively and will be followed in the office.

RICHARD BESSERMAN, M.D.

RB:hpi
d: 6/9/92
t: 6/10/92

JOSE GARCIA

#112538

DATE OF PROCEDURE: 5/25/92

OPERATIVE REPORT

PREOPERATIVE DIAGNOSIS: Presyncope with intermittent junctional bradycardia.

POSTOPERATIVE DIAGNOSIS: Same.

OPERATION: Dual-chamber DDD transvenous pacemaker placement.

PACEMAKER GENERATOR: Pacesetter Model 2010T.

SETTINGS:
Bipolar leads: Atrial pulse width 0.6 msec. Sensitivity 1 mv. Pulse amplitude 4 volts.
    Refractory period 275 msec.
Ventricular bipolar lead: Pulse width 0.6 msec. Sensitivity 2 mv. Pulse amplitude 4 volts, and
    refractory period 250 msec.
Pacemaker mode: DDD. Rate: 70 pulses per minute. AV delay: 155 msec.
Lead threshold: Atrial lead model #P452PBV. Threshold 0.45 volts at 0.6 milliamps. Pulse
    width 0.6 msec. P wave amplitude 3 mv. Lead impedance 490 ohms.
Ventricular lead: Bipolar lead model #10167. Threshold 0.7 volts with 0.8 milliamps at pulse
    width of 0.6 msec. R wave amplitude 14.5 mv. Lead impedance 750 ohms.

OPERATION: The patient was prepped and draped in the usual manner. Using sedation and
1% Xylocaine anesthesia, an infraclavicular incision was made. The pocket was carried down
to the fascia and placed subfascially. Then the subclavian vein was located with a needle and a
guide wire placed into the vein. Two introducers were placed over this wire, and the atrial and
ventricular lead placed into the superior vena cava. Then the atrial lead was put into place and
the leads screwed in. Then the ventricular lead was placed in the ventricular apex.

Thresholds were measured as obtained and were found to be quite adequate. The lead was
checked for length on fluoroscopy and then attached into the pocket around a collar with a 2-0
silk suture. Then the leads and generator were connected together and the pacemaker placed into the pocket. Hemostasis appeared to be good. The fascia was closed with interrupted 2-0
Vicryl and the subcutaneous tissue closed with running 3-0 Vicryl sutures. Skin was closed
with a 4-0 Vicryl subcuticular stitch. The patient was taken to the recovery room in satisfactory
condition.

RICHARD BESSERMAN, M.D.

RB:hpi
d&t: 5/25/92

JOE BLEAUX

#102732

Date: 6/25/93

ELECTROCARDIOGRAM

ATRIAL RATE: 100
PR INTERVAL: Variable
VENTRICULAR RATE: 80

The ST segments are sagging in leads I, II, aVL, V5, and V6, and are slightly depressed in V2–V4. The rhythm is Wenckebach. There is second-degree heart block. The T waves are low in leads I, aVL, V5, and V6.

IMPRESSION:
1. Second-degree heart block (Wenckebach).
2. Nonspecific ST segment and T wave changes.
3. There is a significant change since the last electrocardiogram.

_____

RICHARD BESSERMAN, M.D.

RB:hpi
d&t:6/25/93

Lesson 9. Cardiology

Learning Objectives

Medical

- Describe the causes of and treatments for common cardiovascular diseases.
- List and briefly explain various invasive and noninvasive cardiac diagnostic procedures.
- Discuss the purpose and technique involved in performing common cardiovascular laboratory tests and surgical procedures.
- Given a cross-section illustration of the heart, memorize the anatomic structures.
- Given a cardiovascular root word, symptom, or disease, match it to its correct medical definition.
- Define common cardiovascular abbreviations.

Fundamentals

- Discuss these aspects of confidentiality of the healthcare record: ownership, release of contents, personal knowledge of the contents, confidentiality agreements.
- Discuss the correct use of commas in punctuating medical sentences.
- Given a medical report with errors, identify and correct the errors.

Practice

- Accurately transcribe authentic physician dictation from the specialty of cardiology.

A Closer Look

Confidentiality and the Patient Healthcare Record

by Linda Campbell, CMT

The American Association for Medical Transcription stresses the importance of confidentiality in medical transcription in its Code of Ethics (Revised, 1987). AAMT members pledge to "protect the privacy and confidentiality of the individual medical record to avoid disclosure of personally identifiable medical and social information and professional medical judgments."

A transcribed medical report or patient healthcare record is a permanent legal document owned by the institution in which care was given or by the physician in whose office the patient was treated. The medical transcriptionist is responsible for accurately transcribing the physician's dictation and for maintaining the confidentiality of the information transcribed or accessed in the course of the work.

The contents of the medical record cannot be disclosed, even with an official request, except with the express written permission of the patient.

Knowledge obtained from transcribing a report should not be discussed with co-workers (even another medical transcriptionist) and must never be related to anyone outside the office. Even if the patient in the report is a relative or friend or a famous person, the details of every report must remain absolutely confidential. You must not even acknowledge that you know that that person is ill or has been treated.

In addition, drafts of reports that are not placed on the patient's chart must be shredded before being discarded. Other healthcare professionals must maintain confidentiality of the medical record as well, except in some cases where law mandates that cases of child abuse and certain communicable diseases be reported to the relevant authorities. However, it is the physician's responsibility—not the medical transcriptionist's—to report such information to the authorities.

Because confidentiality is a critical issue, your employer will inform you of the facility's policy about patient confidentiality. The employer may also require you to sign a confidentiality statement similar to the sample provided below, and will inform you of the penalties for violating patient confidentiality. In most facilities a breach of patient confidentiality is grounds for immediate dismissal from the job.

Confidentiality Agreement

This agreement is entered into by _____

_____

(hereinafter known as Employee) and _____

_____

(hereinafter known as Facility).

Employee understands that, in the performance of duties as a medical transcriptionist, all patient and client information is to be held in strictest confidence, including but not limited to the transcription of medical documents.

Employee recognizes that the disclosure of such information shall result in immediate dismissal from Facility.

Employee also acknowledges that any such violation may give rise to irreparable damage to Facility, and that Facility and any injured party may seek legal remedies against Employee.

This Agreement is entered into on (date)

_____ .

_____
Employee Signature

_____
Witness Signature

Call Me Madam

by Judith Marshall, MA, CMT

Those twenty dwarves turning handstands on the carpet of my mind must be medical transcriptionists. With the temperature at minus 29 degrees I am getting a little bugsy myself and more than hyperalert at the computer. Is the content of the medical dictation changing for the worse or am I just suffering contact dermatitis from Tide in those new little boxes?

There is an increase in the use of first names, not just in psychiatric summaries but in all specialties. A 71-year-old female enters the hospital for "rule out myocardial infarction" and the doctor tells us "Fiona" did this and that. If Fiona is from a nursing home, the chances increase dramatically that her surname will be amputated. The older a male patient becomes, the more likely is he to be called by his first name.

If a patient is admitted for drug or alcohol detoxification or any AIDS-related reason, the use of first names increases. I don't think it is a matter of confidentiality. I think it is a matter of doctors doing, pardon me George, "the power thing."

For the past thirty years, I have been listening to the Ob-Gyn doctors and one has to give them an A in consistency. They are still patronizing as heck, though they are much more democratic now and have progressed beyond the "little mothers." More women are practicing in obstetrics and gynecology but, unfortunately, have developed a style of "manly" dictation, i.e., using the patient's first name. All those nurse-midwives fought so hard in so many places for the right to be part of the hospital medical team. Then they dictate using the woman's first name, and oy, we are up to our ankles in girl stuff.

Am I the only sentinel? Are there other "first name police" out there? Weren't we trained never to transcribe the patient's name in the body of a report? Not for anyone, not even for babies and children. Is this a question of form, content, ethics, manners, or, heaven help us, total quality? Does AAMT or AHIMA think about these things?

In the McDonaldization of American medical language as practiced in dictating summaries, there seems to be less consideration, kindness and, yes, morality when dealing with human suffering. What, in person, can be a ploy to ameliorate the dehumanizing technological aspect of medical care becomes, on paper, plain crass.

In routine long-term transcription for a sixtyish gentleman internist, I dutifully type his "chronic anxiety-depression syndrome" diagnosis for all his female patients over forty. Since the women never see the reports, I suppose they never know. The transcription supervisor told me he appeared on Valentine's Day morning and asked her why she wasn't wearing red. "I like to see all of my girls in red today."

After the Clarence Thomas/Anita Hill brouhaha, why should I get my pantyhose in a twist over the use of first names in medical reports? Because what I am talking about is basic human dignity. Because when formal hospital documents become chatty and palsy-walsy and careless and sloppy, it worries me. And when a patient is bare-bottomed, poked, prodded, sedated, and confused, that is especially when he needs to be a Mister. Not just Joe. A woman in diapers or bleeding through her clothes or being examined status post mastectomy needs to be a Missus. Not just Kathy.

Last week I visited a friend who had cardiac surgery in a major Boston teaching hospital. He handed me his discharge summary. It was printed all in caps, with abbreviations from the diagnoses to the last sentence. "THE PT. WAS AD. TO THE HOS." The lengthy discharge diagnoses were all abbreviated. Hello, Joint Commission?

I called a woman in the biz who knows the area. She said the hospital was encouraging the residents to sit at the screen and peck out their summaries and paying them a couple of bucks to do it. "All they want is the record, Judith," she said. "Never mind anything else."

Next time you visit your doctor, see how the secretaries and nurses address you. If it is by your first name, correct them. Then correct the doctor. It is a short hip-hop from name to attitude.

Medical Readings

A Cardiologist's View

Part 1

by Michael J. O'Donnell, M.D.

Cardiology and cardiovascular surgery are both concerned with the diagnosis and treatment of diseases of the heart, great vessels, and peripheral circulation. The difference between cardiologists and cardiovascular surgeons lies in the methods used to treat these diseases.

The cardiologist is, by training, an internist who specializes in the diagnosis and medical treatment of cardiovascular disease. The cardiac surgeon specializes in the surgical treatment of cardiovascular disease. In no other area of medicine does an internist work so closely with a surgeon as in the management of cardiovascular disease.

Cardiologists must rely on their cardiovascular surgeon colleagues when surgical intervention is needed in the treatment of their patients. Similarly, cardiovascular surgeons rely on their cardiologist colleagues for the majority of their case referrals. The cardiologist and cardiovascular surgeon collaborate during a surgical procedure if the patient develops hemodynamic instability or refractory cardiac arrhythmia, and also during the postoperative period in the routine management of the cardiac surgery patient. Thus there is considerable overlap between the two specialties.

The cardiology patient. Patients with *myocardial ischemia* (inadequate blood supply to the heart) are those most frequently seen by both cardiologists and cardiovascular surgeons. Myocardial ischemia is usually caused by arteriosclerosis, or hardening of the arteries. These patients are seen initially by a cardiologist for evaluation; those who are found to have extensive disease may be referred to a cardiovascular surgeon for a coronary artery bypass procedure.

The next largest group of patients seen by cardiologists are those who suffer from varying degrees of *congestive heart failure,* where the heart's pumping capability is impaired. This condition may develop as a result of coronary artery disease, valvular heart disease, or other abnormal processes, some of which may not be identifiable. These patients are generally not surgical candidates and therefore are cared for almost exclusively by cardiologists.

The third largest group of patients seen by both the cardiologist and the cardiovascular surgeon comprises those with *valvular heart disease,* either congenital or acquired. Congenital valvular disease refers to a structural malformation of one or more cardiac valves that is present at birth and that eventually leads to cardiac dysfunction requiring evaluation and treatment. In the majority of patients with valvular disease, the condition is acquired; that is, the patient is born with structurally normal heart valves but then develops valvular abnormalities as a result of acquired disease.

Another common cardiologic condition is *arrhythmia,* a disturbance of the heart rhythm. Arrhythmias are classified as either supraventricular or ventricular, depending on their site of origin. Generally they are treated medically but in selected cases surgical intervention may be warranted.

Numerous other conditions are treated by both cardiologists and cardiovascular surgeons, but taken together they represent only a small portion of cardiologic or cardiovascular surgical practice.

The proportion of cardiac surgical patients in a cardiologist's practice depends largely on where the cardiologist practices. A cardiologist practicing in a rural setting where there is no cardiovascular surgeon would have no surgical patients under his care. A cardiologist working in a teaching hospital or large regional or metropolitan medical center, whether a private or university hospital, might have as many as 50% surgical patients in his practice.

Cardiac patients vary widely in age. The youngest patient seen by a cardiologist or cardiovascular surgeon might be a newborn infant with a severe heart defect requiring surgery within the first few hours of life. At the other extreme are patients in the final years of life. As a general rule, the older the patient, the less likely is surgical intervention to be indicated.

Cardiovascular disease. Cardiovascular disease continues to be the most serious threat to life and health in the United States. One in every three men in this country can expect to develop some major cardiovascular disease before reaching the age of 60. The odds for women are approximately 1 in 10, although these odds continue to rise as more women develop the same risk factors as men. Coronary disease is the major cause of death after the age of 40 in men and after the age of 50 in women. Approximately 19% of the U.S. population have heart disease or hypertension (high blood pressure), causing limitation in activity. The most common cardiovascular diseases are hypertension and arteriosclerosis-related diseases (which include coronary heart disease, cerebrovascular disease, and peripheral vascular disease). Cardiovascular disease accounts for half of all deaths in the U.S. Of these, 70% are related to cardiovascular disease, while 16% are related to stroke. Coronary heart disease causes approximately 800,000 new heart attacks each year and an additional 450,000 recurrent heart attacks.

The presenting complaint for coronary disease in women is most likely to be angina pectoris, whereas in men it is most likely to be myocardial infarction (heart attack) or sudden death. Therefore, only 20% of heart attacks are preceded by long-standing angina pectoris. Unrecognized myocardial infarctions are common, accounting for approximately 20% of all heart attacks. One-half of these are silent and the remaining half are atypical in that neither the patient nor the physician considers the possibility of a myocardial infarction. Roughly two-thirds of patients who experience a myocardial infarction do not make a complete recovery. However, 88% of those patients under the age of 65 are able to return to their usual occupations. Within approximately five years after initial myocardial infarction, 13% of the men and almost 40% of the women develop a second myocardial infarction. The mortality rate is 30% for the initial myocardial infarction and 50% for recurrent myocardial infarction. The ten-year survival rate is 50% for men and 30% for women.

Hypertension. Hypertension is by far the most prevalent cardiovascular disease and is one of the most significant risk factors for cardiovascular disease and death. Hypertension is defined as blood pressures of 140/90 mmHg or greater. The prevalence of hypertension is approximately 30% for persons between 25 and 75 years of age. The prevalence increases with age, and is highest among blacks and the elderly. Awareness of hypertension has markedly increased. Malignant hypertension as a cause of death is becoming a rarity. Hypertension disease mortality is largely due to arteriosclerotic sequelae or complications, such as coronary disease, stroke, and cardiac failure.

Stroke. The most common variety of stroke seen by a cardiologist is the atherothrombotic brain infarction (blocking circulation to the brain), which accounts for approximately 59% of all strokes. The next most common is cerebral embolus (blood clot to brain) (14%), followed by subarachnoid hemorrhage (9%), and intracerebral hemorrhage (5%). The chances of having a stroke before age 70 are approximately 1 in 20 for either sex. Unlike hypertension and other arteriosclerosis-related diseases, there is no clear-cut male predominance in stroke incidence. Stroke remains the third most frequent cause of death, behind heart disease and cancer.

Heart failure. Heart failure is a condition that develops after the myocardium has exhausted all its reserve and compensatory mechanisms. Once overt signs of heart failure occur, 50% of all patients will die within five years despite aggressive medical management. The etiology (cause) of cardiac failure may be hypertension, ischemic myocardial disease, or congenital or acquired valvular disease. The dominant cause is hypertension, which precedes failure in approximately 75% of cases. Coronary heart disease, generally accompanied by hypertension, is responsible in 39% of cases. Despite modern intervention for cardiac failure, the prognosis remains grim.

Cardiac arrhythmia. An arrhythmia (abnormal heartbeat) results from some disturbance in the formation or transmission of the cardiac impulse. It may be a manifestation of any of the major forms of heart disease and is an important source of mortality. Many such deaths occur suddenly and without warning. Cardiac arrhythmia and congestive failure are critical developments common to the course of most types of severe heart disease.

Valvular heart disease. One cause of acquired valvular disease is rheumatic fever. Rheumatic heart disease may cause degenerative valvular disease as well as mitral valve prolapse. Rheumatic fever or rheumatic heart disease in the U.S. has significantly decreased in recent years because of the use of antibiotics in the treatment of streptococcal infections. However, the disease still occurs in disadvantaged areas such as inner cities and remote rural areas.

The end result of rheumatic valvular disease is disruption of normal valvular tissue and subsequent calcification (calcium deposits) and stenosis (narrowing). The mitral valve is nearly always involved and in many instances the aortic valve is affected as well. Once the stenosis becomes critical, the patient will need either surgical replacement of the valve or nonsurgical treatment by balloon valvuloplasty.

Other forms of acquired valvular disease can also lead to valvular stenosis. Degeneration of a valve can result in valvular insufficiency rather than stenosis. The most common presentation for patients with either stenosis or insufficiency is progressive dyspnea (difficulty breathing) on exertion with easy fatigability. The patient may also begin to experience chest discomfort unrelated to any coexisting coronary artery disease and myocardial ischemia.

Congenital heart disease. Congenital heart disease is generally seen by pediatric rather than adult cardiologists or cardiovascular surgeons. The types and presentations of congenital heart disease can be somewhat complex and their diagnosis and surgical management can be equally complex. Therefore, it remains a subspecialty area within the field of cardiology and cardiovascular surgery.

Structural abnormalities of the heart or intrathoracic great vessels seem to affect 8 to 10 of every 1,000 newborns in the U.S. Approximately one of these 1,000 live newborns has a congenital cardiac defect that cannot be managed medically or surgically. The incidence of most congenital heart diseases has remained stable for many years. Rubella vaccine has reduced rubella-caused congenital heart disease, and congenital heart defects associated with Down syndrome are less common because older women are having fewer babies. There still remains a lack of knowledge of the cause of most congenital heart disease, although it has been shown that alcohol and some prescription drugs can cause cardiac defects. The majority of congenital heart defects, however, probably result from complex genetic-environmental causes not presently understood.

Pulmonary thromboembolism. A final disease entity seen by both the cardiologist and the cardiovascular surgeon is pulmonary thromboembolism. This occurs when an embolus (usually a clot from the deep veins in the pelvic cavity or lower extremities) dislodges and travels along with the normal blood return to the right heart. As the right heart supplies blood to the pulmonary vasculature, the embolus lodges within the lung circulation.

Pulmonary thromboembolism is the most common lethal pulmonary disease. If left untreated, recurrent episodes are likely, and more than 25% of these will be fatal. Most fatalities occur within one hour of the onset of symptoms, and sudden death due to pulmonary embolism can be confused with sudden coronary death. Predisposing factors include chronic pulmonary disease, malignancy, estrogen therapy, orthopedic trauma, immobilization, recent operative procedures, obesity, pregnancy, and blood disorders.

Diagnostic studies, invasive and noninvasive. Highly specialized radiologic and other diagnostic technologies probably find more application in the practice of cardiology than in any other subspecialty.

Electrocardiography. The standard evaluative tool of the cardiologist is the electrocardiogram (EKG), which measures the electrical impulses generated by the heart. With the standard 12-lead EKG it is possible to diagnose myocardial infarction (past or present), ischemic heart disease, left ventricular hypertrophy (enlargement), hypertensive heart disease, cardiac dysrhythmias, and other cardiac maladies. Advanced techniques based on the EKG include 24-hour Holter monitoring, stress electrocardiography, and signal-averaged electrocardiography.

Vectorcardiography. Vectorcardiography assesses the direction of the heart's electrical activity, either in sum or at a particular instant. With each cardiac cycle the electrical activity travels through the heart in a loop, a configuration that may be altered in predictable fashion by various kinds of heart disease.

Electrophysiologic studies. All of the electrical studies mentioned above are noninvasive; that is, no catheters are inserted into the heart. One technique that does require invasive technique is the electrophysiologic study. This is a procedure in which a sensing and stimulating electrode is placed via catheter in various positions within the heart, particularly the right chambers. In this way the electrical activity of the heart can be measured from an internal rather than an external observation point.

Additionally, the heart may be stimulated through these catheters in order to assess whether the patient is susceptible to ventricular tachycardia or other ventricular or atrial arrhythmias. If susceptibility to these rhythm disturbances is found, various antiarrhythmic drugs may be tried and repeat stimulations used to assess the efficacy of the drug regimen.

Ultrasound. Nonelectrical techniques for diagnosis of cardiac disease include ultrasound, radioisotopes (radioactive substances), and x-rays. Cardiac ultrasound is better known as echocardiography and cardiac Doppler evaluation. In these techniques, ultrasound waves directed at the cardiac chambers and valves are reflected into the receiving portion of the transducer, amplified, and projected onto a screen. This allows for real-time evaluation of cardiac function. Doppler study is a procedure in which the ultrasound waves are reflected by moving red blood cells, so that velocities can be measured through the cardiac valves and chambers. This is an extremely useful tool for measuring and assessing valvular stenosis, insufficiency, and structural defects such as atrial septal or ventricular septal defects.

Nuclear cardiology. Nuclear cardiology is a fast-growing field in which radioisotopes are employed in various ways, including thallium scans, multi-gated blood pool analysis (MUGA), and positron emission scanning. In all of these radionuclear techniques, radioisotopes given intravenously are picked up and quantified by scanning the chest cavity, with particular attention to the heart. These tests can provide data on the perfusion, function, and physiologic demands of the myocardium.

Radiology. The use of diagnostic x-rays in cardiology includes routine chest x-ray, fluoroscopy, and CT scanning. The most recent advance in this field is ultrafast CT scanning, which is being developed largely at the University of Illinois Medical Center. The ultrafast CT scan provides estimates of blood flow through cardiac chambers and coronary arteries or coronary artery bypass grafts. This useful tool, though still in its infancy, may make it possible to estimate the degree of severity of coronary artery disease without invasive measures.

Another recent advance in the field of cardiac radiology is magnetic resonance imaging (MRI). The advantage of MRI is its ability to visualize with great clarity the soft tissues of the body. This technique makes possible a structural assessment of cardiac chambers and valves as well as estimation of blood flow. This is another noninvasive procedure that holds great promise for accurate evaluation of coronary artery disease and other cardiac pathology.

Cardiac catheterization. This is an invasive technique that requires the introduction of a diagnostic catheter through a peripheral vessel, under fluoroscopic guidance, into the various cardiac chambers. By this means, pressure readings can be taken directly from a variety of sites. Placement of the catheter in the coronary ostia (openings) and injection of contrast medium permits radiographic visualization and recording of the coronary blood flow on motion picture film (coronary cineangiography).

The purpose of all of these cardiac diagnostic studies is to strive to treat the patient medically. In about half of the patients, however, an invasive therapy will be indicated. This may include coronary artery angioplasty, balloon valvuloplasty, or cardiac surgery either with coronary artery bypass grafting or repair or replacement of a valve.

Laboratory Tests and Surgical Procedures

anisocytosis Unusually wide variation in the size of cells, particularly red blood cells.

arteriosclerosis Hardening of the arteries (*sclero-*, "hardening"). Arteriosclerosis refers to a group of diseases including atherosclerosis, but in practice many physicians use arteriosclerosis and atherosclerosis interchangeably. See *atherosclerosis*.

atherosclerosis (*athero*, "yellow, fatty degeneration," *sclero*, "hardening," *osis*, "abnormal condition" Abnormal condition of hardening of the arteries due to plaque caused by yellow, fatty degeneration. See *arteriosclerosis*.

band forms, bands Immature neutrophils whose nuclei appear as bands, in contrast to mature neutrophils, whose nuclei are segmented or lobed.

basos An acceptable brief form for *basophils*.

blast forms, blasts Very immature cells, particularly leukocytes, not normally found in peripheral blood but present in acute leukemia.

bleeding time The number of minutes it takes for a small incision in the skin, made with a lancet, to stop bleeding. Either the Duke method (puncture of the earlobe) or the Ivy method (puncture of the forearm) may be used.

blood type A genetically determined and permanent characteristic of a person's red blood cells, based on the presence of certain antigens. Two blood type systems of clinical importance are the ABO (comprising types A, B, AB, and O) and the Rh (comprising Rh-positive and Rh-negative). Blood for transfusion must be typed and then crossmatched (experimentally combined) with the prospective recipient's blood to avoid reactions due to incompatibility of bloods. Other red cell antigens not used for type and crossmatching include Duffy, Kell, Kidd, and Lewis. These are often used when blood typing is used as evidence of nonpaternity.

burr cell An abnormal red blood cell with a jagged contour.

cardiac catheterization A procedure that involves passing a flexible catheter through the femoral artery and into the heart to measure pressures within the heart's chambers. Dye is then injected to show patency or obstruction of the coronary arteries.

CBC (complete blood count).

cholesterol, serum A lipid (fatty) material formed in the liver and transported in the blood, which serves as a building block for various hormones and other substances. Elevation of serum cholesterol, which is usually due to an inherited disturbance of lipid metabolism, is associated with increased risk of atherosclerosis. See *HDL, LDL, VLDL*.

clotting factors See *factors, blood clotting*.

clotting time The time needed for a clot to form in a tube of freshly drawn blood under standard conditions. The Lee-White method is the one most often used.

coags Slang term for *coagulation studies*.

complete blood count (CBC) A group of blood tests including counts of red blood cells, white blood cells, and platelets; a differential count of the various types of white blood cells; and a determination of hemoglobin and hematocrit.

coronary artery bypass graft (CABG)—surgical procedure done to bypass one or more occluded coronary arteries by using a vein graft from the leg.

CPK (creatine phosphokinase) A serum enzyme that can be chemically distinguished into three isoenzymes or fractions: the MB isoenzyme, elevated in myocardial infarction; the MM isoenzyme, elevated in cerebral infarction; and the BB isoenzyme, sometimes elevated in uremia and other conditions. When separated in the laboratory by electrophoresis, these isoenzymes appear as distinct bands in a visual display. Hence the expression *MB band* is roughly synonymous with *MB isoenzyme*. Do not confuse *creatine* with *creatinine*.

CPR (cardiopulmonary resuscitation) The use of external compression of the heart coupled with breathing techniques to revive a victim whose heart and respirations have stopped.

crit Slang term for *hematocrit*.

diff Slang term for *differential count of white blood cells*.

differential white blood cell count A determination of the relative numbers of the six types of white blood cells normally found in peripheral blood. When the count is performed visually, a technician observes 100 white blood cells in a stained smear of whole blood and reports the number of each cell type found as a percent. The differential count can also be done electronically. The six types of white blood cells are segmented neutrophils (PMNs or segs), band neutrophils (bands, representing the immature form), eosinophils (eos), basophils (basos), lymphocytes (lymphs), and monocytes (monos).

Duke bleeding time See *bleeding time*.

ECG, EKG (electrocardiogram) A tracing of the electrical activity of the heart. An EKG traces the conduction of the electrical impulse generated by

ECG, EKG (electrocardiogram) *(cont.)*
the SA node as it travels through the atria (P wave on the EKG) and through the ventricles (QRS complex on the EKG). Then, during the recovery period as the heart prepares to contract again, the T wave is evident on the EKG. As this electrical impulse travels through the heart, it can be detected on the skin by EKG electrodes.

The basic EKG records 12 leads. Three peripheral electrodes are placed: on the right arm, left arm, and left leg. Six other electrodes are placed at precise locations on the chest around the heart area. The EKG technician can change from one lead to the next by using a dial on the EKG machine. Leads I, II, and III (the so-called limb leads or bipolar leads) are obtained by simultaneously recording the electrical activity from the extremities. By combining the input from two of these three electrodes, the EKG machine generates a tracing for lead I (right arm and left arm), lead II (right arm and left leg), and lead III (left arm and left leg). The next three leads are called augmented leads because they increase or augment the amplitude or size of the tracing by 50%. The augmented leads are aVR (augmented voltage, right arm), aVL (augmented voltage, left arm), and aVF (augmented voltage, left foot).

The remaining six leads necessary to complete the 12-lead EKG are known as the precordial or chest leads. These electrodes are placed on the chest and are designated by a *V*. Lead V1 is positioned over the fourth intercostal space at the right sternal border and records the electrical activity of the right ventricle. Lead V2 is positioned over the fourth intercostal space at the left sternal border and records the electrical activity of the right ventricle. Lead V3 is positioned midway between V2 and V4 and records the electrical activity of the left ventricle. Lead V4 is positioned over the fifth intercostal space at the midclavicular line and records the electrical activity of the left ventricle. Lead V5 is positioned over the fifth intercostal space at the anterior axillary line and records the electrical activity of the left ventricle. Lead V6 is positioned over the fifth intercostal space at the midaxillary line and records the electrical activity of the left ventricle. Each of the 12 leads gives a different picture of the electrical conduction of the heart.

echocardiogram   An ultrasound procedure that uses sound waves to show the structure and motion of the heart.

electrolytes, serum   Chemical substances present in the blood in the form of negatively or positively charged ions. The principal electrolytes of the blood are sodium, potassium, chloride, and bicarbonate.

eos   Brief form for *eosinophils.*

erythrocyte   A mature red blood cell. Compare *reticulocyte.*

exercise stress test   Test during which the patient exercises on a treadmill to stress the heart and reproduce symptoms of angina and EKG changes.

factors, blood clotting   Substances present in the blood that participate in the clotting process.

Factor I	fibrinogen
Factor II	prothrombin
Factor III	tissue thromboplastin
Factor IV	calcium
Factor V	labile factor (proaccelerin)
Factor VI	rapidly destroyed by thrombin; cannot be identified by its activity in serum
Factor VII	stable factor (proconvertin)
Factor VIII	antihemophilic globulin (AHG)
Factor IX	Christmas factor
Factor X	Stuart-Prower factor (not Power)
Factor XI	plasma thromboplastin antecedent
Factor XII	Hageman factor
Factor XIII	fibrin-stabilizing factor

granulocytes   White blood cells with conspicuous cytoplasmic granules. According to the staining properties of these granules, the cells are classified as neutrophils, eosinophils, and basophils.

H&H   A slang abbreviation for *hemoglobin and hematocrit.* The hemoglobin level is usually dictated first.

Hct, HCT (hematocrit).

HDL (high-density lipoproteins).

hematocrit (Hct, HCT)   The percentage of a blood sample that consists of cells. The sample is spun in a centrifuge, which quickly drives all the cells to the bottom of the tube. The length of the column of cells is expressed as a percent of the total length of the specimen. Red and white blood cells and platelets are all included, but red blood cells far outnumber the other formed elements.

hematocrit, central   A hematocrit value determined by using a blood sample drawn from a central line catheter.

hemoglobin (Hgb)   The oxygen-carrying complex of iron and protein in red blood cells. The hemoglobin level is reduced in anemia.

hemoglobin A_1   Normal adult hemoglobin.

hemoglobin F   Normal fetal hemoglobin, found also in adults with certain forms of anemia and leukemia.

hemoglobin S   The abnormal hemoglobin found in the red blood cells of persons with sickle cell anemia.

Hgb, HGB (hemoglobin).

high-density lipoprotein (HDL)   Lipid-carrying serum proteins associated with a relatively low risk of cholesterol deposition in arteries.

Holter monitoring   A continuously recorded EKG as monitored by a portable EKG machine worn by the patient. This procedure is done on an outpatient basis for 24 hours to detect arrhythmias.

IgA (immunoglobulin A).

IgD (immunoglobulin D).

IgE (immunoglobulin E).

IgG (immunoglobulin G).

IgM (immunoglobulin M).

immunoglobulins   Serum proteins that act as antibodies, also known as gamma globulins. They are divided into five classes: IgA, IgD, IgE, IgG (by far the most abundant), and IgM.

isoenzyme   Any of a group of enzymes having similar chemical effects but differing in structure and often arising from different sources in the body. See *CPK, LDH.*

Ivy bleeding time   See *bleeding time.*

lactic dehydrogenase   See *LDH.*

LDH (lactic dehydrogenase)   An isoenzyme. LDH_1 is found in heart muscle; levels are increased after myocardial infarction. LDH_2 is normally found in higher amounts in the serum than is LDH_1. When the level of LDH_1 surpasses that of LDH_2, this is called a "flipped LDH."

LDL (low-density lipoprotein).

Lee-White clotting time   See *clotting time.*

left shift   See *shift to the left.*

leukocytes   White blood cells. Six types of white blood cells are normally found in the circulating blood: band (immature) neutrophils, segmented (mature) neutrophils, eosinophils, basophils, lymphocytes, and monocytes.

lipoproteins, serum   Serum proteins that bind and transport lipid materials including cholesterol.

low-density lipoproteins (LDL)   Lipid-carrying serum proteins associated with a relatively high risk of cholesterol deposition in arteries.

lymphocyte, B (B cell)   A type of lymphocyte that forms antibodies.

lymphocyte T (T cell)   A type of lymphocyte that is involved in cellular immunity. Subtypes (killer, suppressor, helper T cells) are named according to their functions.

lytes   Slang term for *electrolytes.*

MB bands   See *CPK (creatine phosphokinase).*

MCH (mean corpuscular hemoglobin)   The mean (average) weight of hemoglobin per red blood cell, calculated from the hemoglobin level and the red blood cell count.

MCHC (mean corpuscular hemoglobin concentration)   The mean (average) concentration of hemoglobin in red blood cells, calculated from the hemoglobin level and the hematocrit.

MCV (mean corpuscular volume)   The mean (average) volume of a red blood cell, calculated from the hematocrit and the red blood cell count.

microhematocrit   A hematocrit measurement performed on a small specimen of blood obtained by fingerstick and centrifuged in a capillary tube.

monos   An acceptable brief form for *monocytes.* Do not confuse with *mono*, a slang term for infectious mononucleosis.

MUGA scan   Radiology procedure in which a radioactive isotope is injected into the arteries with a subsequent scan showing uptake of the isotope by the heart. These radioactive emissions are electronically collected and analyzed by computer, resulting in a series of successive images all taken at the same point in the cardiac cycle. This test is used to assess heart size, shape, and function. *MUGA* stands for *multiple gated acquisition.*

myelocytes   White blood cells formed in bone marrow: neutrophils, basophils, eosinophils, and monocytes.

neutrophil, segmented   A mature neutrophil with a segmented or lobulated nucleus. Acceptable brief forms include *segs.* Also called *polymorphonuclear leukocytes* or *polys.* See *bands, stabs.*

ovalocytosis   An abnormal oval shape of red blood cells, seen in various congenital disorders of red blood cell formation including elliptocytosis.

partial thromboplastin time (PTT)   The time required for a clot to form in blood treated with certain reagents. Abnormal prolongation of this time occurs in deficiency of various coagulation factors and after treatment with heparin.

percutaneous transluminal angioplasty   Procedure used to dilate an occluded artery, usually a coronary artery, by passing a catheter (with a deflated balloon section) to the site of the occlusion and inflating the balloon to compress the obstruction and enlarge the lumen of the vessel.

platelets Noncellular formed elements in circulating blood, produced in bone marrow and active in blood coagulation. Also called *thrombocytes*.

PMNs (polymorphonuclear leukocytes).

poikilocytosis An abnormally wide variation in the shapes of red blood cells, as seen in a stained smear.

polymorphonuclear leukocytes (PMNs or polys) White blood cells with segmented or lobulated nuclei. An acceptable brief form is *polys*. The term is often used synonymously with *neutrophils,* although eosinophils and basophils are also polymorphonuclear leukocytes.

polys An acceptable brief form for *polymorphonuclear leukocytes*.

prothrombin time (pro time, PT) The time required for a clot to form in blood treated with certain reagents. The result may be reported as both a time (in seconds) and a percent of normal prothrombin activity as detected by the same test in a control. The prothrombin time is prolonged in deficiency of certain coagulation factors and after treatment with heparin or coumarin anticoagulants.

pro time, PT (prothrombin time).

PT/PTT (prothrombin time and partial thromboplastin time).

RBCs (red blood cells).

red blood cell count The number of red blood cells per cubic millimeter (cu mm or mm^3) of blood, as counted by a technician using a microscope or by an electronic cell counter. The count may be reported either as a simple numeral (e.g., 5,300,000/cu mm) or as the product of a number less than ten and 10^6 (e.g., 5.3 x 10^6). The count may be dictated simply as 5.3 and may be so transcribed or may be expanded to 5,300,000.

red blood cells (RBCs) The most numerous cells of the blood, which carry oxygen from the lungs to the tissues, and carbon dioxide from the tissues to the lungs.

red blood cells, nucleated Immature red blood cells, released from the bone marrow before disappearance of their nuclei. Mature RBCs have no nuclei.

red blood cell indices Measures of the volume and hemoglobin content of red blood cells, derived by calculation from the hemoglobin, hematocrit, and red blood cell count. The red cell indices are the mean corpuscular volume (MCV), mean corpuscular hemoglobin (MCH), and mean corpuscular hemoglobin concentration (MCHC).

reticulocyte An immature red blood cell whose cytoplasm contains an irregular network of degenerating nuclear material. An increase in the number of reticulocytes indicates increased red blood cell production in response to blood loss or hemolysis.

segs An acceptable brief form for *segmented neutrophils*.

shift to the left An increase in the relative number of immature neutrophils, as detected in a differential white blood count. The various types of cells were formerly recorded on forms arranged in columns, the more immature neutrophils being recorded at the extreme left of the form.

sickle cell An abnormal red blood cell, found in persons with sickle cell anemia, which assumes a sickle or crescent shape at reduced oxygen levels.

sickling An abnormal sickle or crescent shape observed in red blood cells on a blood smear.

spherocytosis Abnormal spherical shape of red blood cells as noted in a stained smear of whole blood on microscopic examination.

stabs Another name for bands (immature neutrophils). The German word *Stab* means "staff" or "rod," referring to the unsegmented nucleus of an immature neutrophil.

target cell An abnormal red blood cell with a bull's-eye appearance due to flattening of the cell with a prominent spot of hemoglobin in the center.

thrombocytes See *platelets*.

treadmill stress test See *exercise stress test*.

triglycerides, serum The level of fat in the serum, usually measured in the fasting state.

12-lead EKG See *electrocardiogram*.

VLDL (very low-density lipoproteins).

white blood cells (WBCs) See *leukocytes*.

white blood cell count (white cell count, white count) The number of white blood cells per cubic millimeter (cu mm) of blood, as counted by a technician using a microscope or by an electronic cell counter. The count may be reported as either a simple numeral (e.g., 7,200/cu mm) or as the product of a small number and 10^3 (e.g., 7.2 x 10^3). In the latter case, the report may be dictated simply as 7.2 and may be so transcribed or may be expanded to 7,200.

Anatomy/Medical Terminology

Anatomy: The Cardiovascular System; The Conduction System

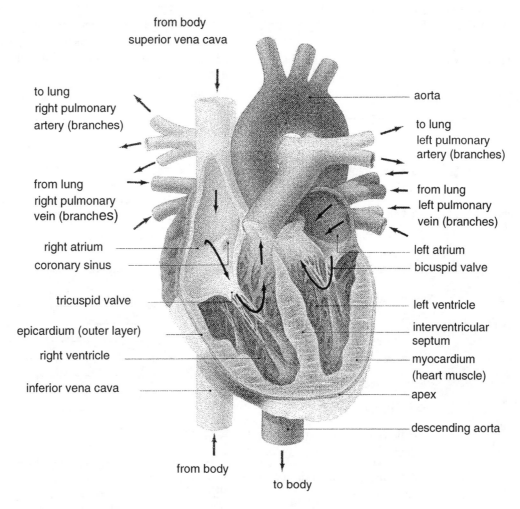

from body
superior vena cava

aorta

to lung
right pulmonary
artery (branches)

to lung
left pulmonary
artery (branches)

from lung
right pulmonary
vein (branches)

from lung
left pulmonary
vein (branches)

right atrium

left atrium

coronary sinus

bicuspid valve

tricuspid valve

left ventricle

epicardium (outer layer)

interventricular
septum

right ventricle

myocardium
(heart muscle)

inferior vena cava

apex

descending aorta

from body

to body

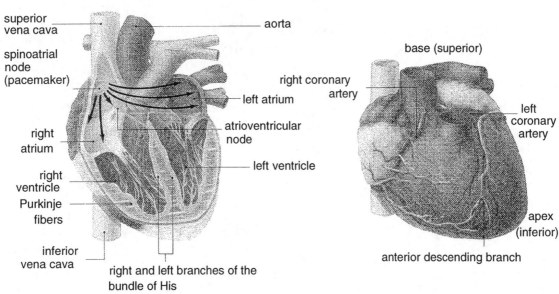

superior
vena cava

aorta

base (superior)

spinoatrial
node
(pacemaker)

right coronary
artery

left
coronary
artery

left atrium

right
atrium

atrioventricular
node

left ventricle

right
ventricle

Purkinje
fibers

apex
(inferior)

inferior
vena cava

anterior descending branch

right and left branches of the
bundle of His

Medical Terminology Matching Exercise

Complete the following matching exercise to test your knowledge of the word roots, anatomic structures, symptoms, and disease processes encountered in the medical specialty of cardiology.

Instructions: Match the term in Column A with its definition in Column B.

Column A   *Column B*

A. sphygmo-   _____ blood vessel
   manometer
                    _____ irregular heartbeat
B. pericardium
                    _____ vein
C. angio-
                    _____ extremely rapid, ineffective
D. arrhythmia   heartbeat

E. coronary   _____ leg pain on exercise due to
   arteries   blockage of arteries

F. -megaly   _____ supply heart muscle with
                         oxygenated blood
G. heart-lung
   machine   _____ membranous sac around the
                         heart
H. aneurysm
                    _____ used to measure blood
I. athero-   pressure

J. claudication   _____ enlargement of

K. phlebo-   _____ fatty plaque

L. ventricular   _____ circulates blood during heart
   fibrillation   surgery

                    _____ ballooning of part of artery
                         wall

Abbreviations Exercise

Common abbreviations may be transcribed as dictated in the body of a report. Uncommon abbreviations must be spelled out, with the abbreviation appearing in parentheses after the translation. All abbreviations (except laboratory test names) must be spelled out in the Diagnosis or Impression section of any report.

Instructions: Define the following cardiology abbreviations. Then memorize both abbreviations and definitions to increase your speed and accuracy in transcribing dictation from cardiology.

AAA _____

ASCVD _____

AV _____

AV _____

BP _____

CABG _____

CAD _____

CCU _____

CHF _____

CPR _____

DOE _____

DVT _____

JVD _____

LVH _____

MI _____

NSR _____

PAC _____

PDA _____

PMI _____

PND _____

PTCA _____

PVC _____

ROMI _____

SBE _____

SOB _____

VSD _____

Transcription Guidelines

Commas

1. **Commas and titles.** Use a comma pair to set off a degree or title.

   Pamela Bensen, M.D., has agreed to see the patient in the emergency department.

   Pamela K. Wear, RRA, and Vera Pyle, CMT, presented a seminar on confidentiality of medical records.

2. **Commas and appositives.** Use a comma pair with an appositive if it provides information that is not essential to understanding the meaning of the sentence. (Note: An appositive is a phrase that immediately follows another word to identify or explain it.) If the appositive provides information that is essential to understanding the meaning of the sentence, do not use commas.

   Dr. Michael J. O'Donnell, the head of the department of cardiology, will provide us with a detailed follow-up evaluation on this patient.

   My patient Ima N. Payne has asked me to write this letter to inquire about insurance coverage of this surgical procedure.

3. **Commas and diagnoses.** Use a comma when the disease entity or condition is followed by its location in the body or when the term is followed by an adjective describing it.

   Deep venous thrombosis, right leg.
   Claudication, two-block.

4. **Commas and introductory phrases and clauses.** Use a comma to separate an introductory adverbial clause or prepositional phrase from the main independent clause of the sentence. If the introductory phrase or clause is short (less than five words), you may omit the comma if the meaning is clear.

   When he experiences his typical chest pain, he always takes nitroglycerin sublingually.

   On this occasion the patient is pleasant and cheerful.

5. **Commas and semicolons.** Use a comma to separate internal elements in sections that are already separated by semicolons.

   Heart: Regular rate and rhythm; no murmur, gallop, or rub; S1 and S2 normal.

Punctuation Exercise

Instructions: Insert appropriate punctuation in the sentences below.

1. Joseph Renwald M.D. a famous cardiologist will be speaking at our next AAMT meeting.

2. The patient needs to take the following medications: Lasix a diuretic Inderal for hypertension lidocaine for arrhythmias and Mevacor for his hypercholesterolemia.

3. Air was aspirated from the left ventricle and the aorta and the cross-clamp removed.

4. After surgery he will be taken to the CCU.

5. DISCHARGE DIAGNOSIS: Angina pectoris disabling and unstable.

6. When he experiences the chest pain he states he is able to get relief with two sublingual nitroglycerin.

7. My patient Yolanda Jones is scheduled for surgery tomorrow.

8. Please forward the patient's records to Ruth Crenshaw the manager at Imperial Insurance Company who will process her claim.

Proofreading Skills

Instructions: In the paragraphs below, circle the errors. Identify misspelled and missing medical and English words and write the correct ones in the numbered spaces opposite the text.

1	CHEIF COMPLAINT: "My heart misses
2	beets."
3	
4	HISTRY OF PRSENT ILLNES: This 37-year-
5	old mail plumber reports a two-year histry of
6	palpations occurring approximately once a
7	week at random times with no reference to
8	phyiscal activity meels or emotional state.
9	These spells are of sudden onset and breif
10	duration and not associated with pane dyspnea
11	or alteration of conscientiousness. Palpitations
12	consist of a sensation of skiping or missing
13	or, as he puts it, "like an engine not firing on
14	all cylinders."
15	
16	PHSYICAL EXAMNATION: This is a nor-
17	mally develloped and nourished hispanic male,
18	well-oriented coopertive and in no distress.
19	Head: Normal cephalic. Pupil are equal and
20	react to light and accomodation. ENT:
21	Unremarkable. Carotid pulses are bilateraly
22	equal. No bruits can be auscultated. The
23	thorax is symetrical with no increase of AP
24	diameter, and respiration are full and
25	unlabored. Lung fields clear to precussion and
26	auscultation.
27	
28	Cardiac palpitation reveals no precordal
29	shocks or thrills. The point of maximal inten-
30	sity lies in the fifth intraspace well within the
31	midclavicular line. On auscultation there are a
32	moderate sinus arhythmia, no murmurs clicks
33	or fiction rubs. Physilogic splitting of S2 is
34	noted. Radial, femoral, and posterior tibial
35	pulses is full and symetrical.
36	
37	Twelve-leed EKG documents sinus arrythmia
38	with no evidence of prexcitation, and a PR in-
39	terval of 0.18 with a rate of 88. Electrical ac-
40	cess is between 45 and 60°. No Q waves, ST
41	changes, or T wave inversion.

1. CHIEF _____
2. _____
3. _____
4. _____
5. _____
6. _____
7. _____
8. _____
9. _____
10. _____
11. _____
12. _____
13. _____
14. _____
15. _____
16. _____
17. _____
18. _____
19. _____
20. _____
21. _____
22. _____
23. _____
24. _____
25. _____
26. _____
27. _____
28. _____
29. _____
30. _____
31. _____
32. _____
33. _____
34. _____
35. _____
36. _____
37. _____
38. _____
39. _____
40. _____
41. _____

Terminology Challenge

Instructions: The following terms appear in the dictation on Tape 4B. Before beginning the medical transcription practice for Lesson 9, become familiar with the terminology below by looking up each word in a medical or English dictionary, and write out a short definition of each term.

ADA diet
angiography
anoxic
antianginal
arrhythmia
Atarax
atropine
AV (atrioventricular)
  block
balloon angioplasty
bradycardia
bundle branch block
bypass surgery
CABG (coronary artery
  bypass graft)
Capoten
captopril
cardiac arrest
cardiomegaly
cardioverted
CHF (congestive heart
  failure)
congestive cardio-
  myopathy
CPK enzyme
CPR (cardiopulmonary
  resuscitation)
CVA (cerebrovascular
  accident)
Dalmane
DC countershock
differential (on CBC)
dipyridamole
dysfunction
ectopy
encephalopathy
epinephrine

ET (endotracheal) tube
exudate
flat line EKG
friction rub
fundi
grade 2 hypertensive
  change
hemiparesis
hemodynamic
hypercholesterolemia
idioventricular rhythm
inferolateral
interstitial pulmonary
  edema
Isordil
joule
LDH
lead III on EKG
lidocaine
MB fraction
Micro-K
midsystole
MM fraction
nitroglycerin SL
NPH insulin
O2, O_2
P wave
pacemaker failure to
  capture
pCO2, pCO_2
perfusion
pericardial
Persantine
pH
platelets
pO2, pO_2
Procardia

PT (prothrombin time)
PTT (partial thrombo-
  plastin time)
q.h.s.
quinidine
regimen
regular insulin
resumption
resuscitation
reversible ischemia
SMAC panel
subtherapeutic
Swan-Ganz catheter
syncope
Synthroid

t.i.d.
telemetry
thallium treadmill stress
  test
third-degree complete
  heart block
thoracotomy
toxic digoxin level
triglycerides
type II diabetes mellitus
vein harvesting
ventricular fibrillation
ventricular tachycardia
vibratory sense
wide-complexed rhythm

Transcription Practice

After completing all the readings and exercises in Lesson 9, transcribe Tape 4B, Cardiology. Use both medical and English dictionaries and your Quick-Reference Word List as resource materials for finding words.

Proofread your transcribed documents carefully, listening to the dictation while you read your transcripts.

Transcribe (*NOT* retype) the same reports again without referring to your previous transcription attempt. Initially, you may need to transcribe some reports more than twice before you can produce an error-free document. Your ultimate goal is to produce an error-free document the first time.

Learning Objectives

Medical

- Describe the use of pacemakers, defibrillators, cardiac catheters, stents, and lasers.
- Describe the action of common emergency drugs.
- Differentiate between various cardiovascular sound-alike terms.

Fundamentals

- Discuss the proper use and abuse of authority.
- Demonstrate the correct use of commas in punctuating medical sentences.
- Demonstrate correct subject-verb agreement in editing medical sentences.

Practice

- Accurately transcribe authentic physician dictation from the specialty of cardiology.

A Closer Look

The God–Doctor Syndrome

by Judith Marshall, MA, CMT

Understanding the language of medicine and having the ability to interpret that language is a hallmark of the medical transcription profession.

Many doctors find it incomprehensible that someone not an M.D. or an R.N. can speak their language. They sometimes resent the intrusion into their secret and mystifying world of arcane goings-on. When my husband had emergency eye surgery, I wasn't there. The surgeon called me at work to explain what happened. As doctors often do when explaining things to lay persons, he raised his voice as if I were deaf. People tend to do this with foreigners as well.

"Well, Mrs. Marshall, think of the eye as a globe and—"

"Let's cut the babytalk, doctor. What happened and tell me in medical terms. The local doctor said he went blind in one eye."

"Are you a nurse?" he bristled.

"No, I'm a medical transcriptionist."

"That's nice. We're always looking for good typists; maybe I can throw some work your way. Now, where was I? Oh, yes, think of the eye as a globe, Mrs. Marshall."

Now that I know who I am, I wonder who doctors are. Are they people, too, or have they become technicians? Have the intelligent, well-educated scholarly sorts given way to the number-chanters, whose reports are speckled with laboratory data and little else?

Why are some doctors so arrogant, so overbearing, so maddeningly patronizing, so insensitive, so macho, so chauvinistic, so brusque? Other people say hello. They say, "Kiss my ring, you peasant." Why can't they tell the difference between IN and ON, **in** the month of May, **on** September 1. Why do they slur over

158

the words they don't understand and make up words and think no one will know the difference? "The GU exam was normal on this circumscribed male." "The lungs were clear to auscultation and precision." Yes, the same words over and over again on many different histories and physicals. Yes, these are American doctors.

So how did doctors get their particular highfallutin' view of themselves? Was it just the higher income or was it something else?

I know how they got that way. I figured it out. We made them what they are. We waited in their offices for hours, smiling weakly and not even asking what the delay was about. Where they really in surgery? The man is a dermatologist, for heaven's sake. Why does one patient say he has the 10:30 appointment, and four others also say they have the 10:30 appointment?

Doctors' offices are just like the airlines. I call and ask if things are running on time; "oh, yes, of course." I get there and there is a two-hour delay. Peter Gott, a physician I adore, writes about this problem in his book, *No House Calls.* "The doctor keeps people waiting because he is so disorganized that he has overscheduled himself. He is hungry to keep his office filled. . . ." I understand Dr. Gott's colleagues do not adore him.

Patients who endure unpleasantness have problems with authority figures. I, however, am free of these problems. Having spent my formative years in the clutches of nuns, right through the first year of college, and having spent four years in a convent school where the road to hell was paved with patent leather shoes and pearls and where I learned Latin the old-fashioned way—through stark terror—I have no problems with authority figures. I learned that the priests were coddled, obeyed, respected, and the center of the whole shebang. I came out of it unscathed. Of course I did. When the pastor of St. Joseph's swings through the bingo hall on Tuesday nights to greet the players, I automatically stand up, duck my head, and chant, "Good evening, Fawtherrrrr."

The same with doctors. I went to work in a hospital at the tender age of 14 and was told that the doctors were to be coddled, obeyed, respected, and were, of course, the center of the whole shebang. "But," I stammered, "I thought the hospitals were for the patients." The kitchen crew laughed about that one for hours, but they forgave my naiveté. I was just a kid.

I poke fun at physicians. I tease them, satirize them, draw grotesque caricatures of them and, in general, talk like a tough little cookie. But when one of those white-coated men or women approaches me, I am mesmerized. I rise and say, "Good morning, Doctor. How would you like your coffee, sir, uh, ma'am?" I become irritatingly deferential and reverential. My body starts shrinking in height and I have to restrain myself from genuflecting. They call me Judy and I try, I really try, to call them by their first name. For crying out loud, it is someone 23 years old. But all that comes out is "Doctor."

Let me give you an example of how authority works and the immense power we confer upon doctors. It was the summer of 1976. My brother had come up from the Cape to our premier hospital. He had a beard, shorts, sandals, and a scruffy appearance. It was a hazy, sultry Sunday. Paul also had a fever of 102°, intense abdominal pain localized in the right lower quadrant, and intractable vomiting. The genius of an intern who saw him just declared Paul a drug addict and sent him home. I was alone in my apartment when Paul called. "I am dying," he said. "Help me." I ran to his apartment in a cotton shift and bedroom slippers. After looking at him for a minute, I decided his assessment was correct. Some mysterious calm came over me and I called the emergency department of the same hospital which had so inelegantly tossed him out.

"This is Doctor Green from Children's Hospital. Some idiot just discharged my brother when it is clear to me he has acute appendicitis. What was his white count anyway? Wait until I find out who did this. And make it snappy." The nurse was quick to tell me the count was 19,000 with a left shift. The speed with which she answered indicated that the chart was right by the telephone. It was still there when I got Paul back to the emergency department. I had to bribe the taxi driver with a twenty because he said he would not take sick people in his taxi. Besides waving the twenty at him, I waved an emesis basin they had given Paul and told him authoritatively I was a doctor. No makeup, hair in rollers, miserable cheap clothing—but this guy believed me.

When we arrived in the emergency department it was as if the waters of the Red Sea were parting for the sister-doctor of the poor sick patient. Thirty minutes later Paul was in the operating room. They even handed me the chart. The intern who had discharged Paul mysteriously disappeared. The medical record, I might add, was also altered, with both "drug addiction" and the doctor's name being whited out.

I waited outside the operating room for a very long time. There was no one in Boston to call. There was no one at home in Cleveland. The thought occurred to me that I couldn't keep up the masquerade as a doctor much longer, especially if the resident started asking questions. I need not have worried. The surgeon came out, wearing wooden clogs and a flowered surgical cap, a soaking wet Esther Williams type just out of the pool.

"It was bad, but your brother is alive and he will recover."

I forgot everything except that this man was a genius. He had saved my brother's life and I wanted to throw my arms around his feet and strew his path with roses.

And that's how authority works. It is conferred and it is often misused or misperceived, but as long as doctors can cure and cut and heal and help in a mystical way, we are going to worship them.

Well, maybe a little bit.

Medical Readings

A Cardiologist's View

Part 2

by Michael J. O'Donnell, M.D.

Cardiovascular surgery. The simplest cardiovascular surgical procedure is carotid endarterectomy. This involves opening up a segment of the internal carotid artery that has become obstructed by atherosclerotic disease, causing intermittent neurologic problems. In this procedure, the diseased portion of the artery is exposed via a surgical incision in the lateral aspect of the neck. Once the carotid artery is exposed, it is clamped above and below the obstruction. Then an incision is made into the vessel and the atherosclerotic material is peeled away. The incision in the vessel is sutured, the clamps are removed, and the skin is sewn closed. During this procedure, the patient is under general anesthesia but does not require the use of a heart-lung bypass machine.

The most difficult kind of cardiac surgery is repair of congenital heart defects in the infant. The surgery is technically difficult, as extensive cardiac remodeling must often be done to correct these complex abnormalities. The best example of an involved procedure in regular use would be the Mustard operation to correct tetralogy of Fallot (pulmonary stenosis, ventricular

septal defect, dextroposition of the aorta, and right ventricular hypertrophy). In addition, the smallness of the patient contributes to the difficulty encountered in performing the surgery.

Cardiopulmonary bypass. The purpose of the heart-lung bypass machine is to take over the patient's cardiac and pulmonary function while surgery is being performed on the heart. The machine includes a pumping mechanism to maintain blood pressure and circulation to vital organs. In addition, the machine functions as an oxygenator since the lungs are bypassed once the patient's heart is placed in cardiac arrest. Oxygen taken from the hospital's oxygen supply lines diffuses across a bubble oxygenator which comes in contact with the patient's blood as it passes through the cardiopulmonary bypass machine. During this time, the patient's red blood cells derive adequate oxygen from the machine even though the lungs are not functioning. Thus the surgeon can perform an intricate procedure on a nonbeating heart without jeopardizing the patient's vital organs.

Cardiac rehabilitation. Cardiac rehabilitation is an integral part of the field of cardiology. A patient who has sustained a myocardial infarction, developed congestive failure, or undergone cardiac surgery is generally placed in a cardiac rehabilitation program to provide for a controlled increase in heart function and tone. Such a program generally consists of three phases.

Phase 1 is performed in the hospital after the patient is released from the intensive care unit. This initially involves bedside exercises and then progresses to walking for gradually increasing distances and periods. After discharge, cardiac surgery patients are usually given one to two weeks to continue their recuperation and phase 1 cardiac exercises at home. They are then seen in the office by a cardiologist and an evaluation is made regarding advancement to phase 2 cardiac rehabilitation.

Phase 2 consists of an 8- to 12-week course in which the patient reports to a cardiac rehabilitation center on a twice-weekly basis. The patient performs progressive cardiac exercises that are primarily aerobic, such as bicycle, treadmill, and arm wheel exercises. During these sessions, the patient's heart rate and blood pressure are continually monitored. The patient also is educated on life-style changes that are required for improvement in cardiopulmonary status, such as diet, stress management, and behavior modification in those patients who must stop smoking or discontinue other high-risk behavior.

Finally, phase 3 cardiac rehabilitation is given to

those patients who wish to continue on a more strenuous program following successful completion of the phase 2 program.

Other cardiac diseases. Other cardiac patients include those with anomalous (abnormal) coronary arteries that do not originate from their usual positions in the aortic root. These are always a joy to find during a cardiac catheterization, and test a cardiologist's memory as to the innumerable types and purposes of catheters that are available. Even more unusual cases are those involving unsuspected congenital defects, such as coarctation of the aorta or supravalvular or subvalvular aortic stenosis.

I distinctly remember one such case in which a young woman with Down syndrome was brought into the hospital by her aunt for evaluation. After completing my history-taking from the aunt and briefly questioning the patient, I proceeded to examine her and found that she was deathly afraid of me and my stethoscope. I did my best to console her and assure her that nothing I was going to do would hurt her. She quickly became a trusting friend and returned to the happy state typical of Down syndrome patients. The exam confirmed the diagnosis of Williams syndrome and supravalvular aortic stenosis. Williams syndrome, transmitted generally as an autosomal dominant trait, is characterized by the triad of mental retardation, elfin facies, and supravalvular aortic stenosis.

To document the severity of her supravalvular aortic stenosis, cardiac catheterization was performed. Prior to the catheterization, my new-found friend had many innocent questions as to what exactly the procedure involved. Although I am sure she had little technical understanding of what she was about to undergo, she looked at me with complete trust and said that as long as she knew that I would not hurt her she would proceed with the test—only after giving me a hug and a kiss prior to going to the cardiac catheterization laboratory.

At the time of her catheterization, she was found to have severe supravalvular aortic stenosis. It was a technical challenge to cannulate her coronary arteries because the supravalvular aortic stenosis, consisting of a ridge of fibrous tissue just distal to the level of the coronary ostia, overlapped the ostium of the left main coronary artery. This was causing her myocardial ischemia. She underwent successful surgical repair. In my daily visits to her after surgery, I would always see a trusting and happy face and would be rewarded with a hug and a kiss that sent me on the rest of my rounds, ready to face the challenges of another day.

Cardiology and related disciplines. The relationship between the cardiologist and other specialists is one of daily interaction. A great many patients with cardiovascular disease have other medical illnesses as well, which require evaluation and treatment by other medical specialists. In particular, specialists in pulmonary disease, nephrology, and gastroenterology are commonly consulted to aid in the treatment of cardiac patients.

Pulmonology. Many patients have developed cardiac disease because of a heavy smoking history. A large proportion of them go on to develop chronic obstructive lung disease. Many of these patients have difficulty in being weaned from the ventilator in the postoperative period. The assistance of a pulmonologist in these circumstances can be invaluable.

Nephrology. The atherosclerotic process that results in coronary artery disease may also result in other vascular diseases, including peripheral vascular and renal vascular disease. Hence many cardiac patients have renal insufficiency (kidney failure), on either an acute or chronic basis. The medical support of a nephrologist in the treatment of such renal disorders can be crucial.

Gastroenterology. Many cardiology patients are found to be anemic, and the etiology of the anemia frequently turns out to be chronic GI blood loss. Thus many patients are seen in consultation by a gastroenterologist to find the source for their anemia.

New developments in cardiology. Cardiology is by far the fastest growing medical field in terms of technical developments.

Cardiac drugs. The various new classes of drugs for control of angina pectoris, and treatment of patients with congestive failure and arrhythmias, are too numerous to list here. It would be a conservative estimate that, on the average, 15 to 25 new cardiac drugs are brought out each year. New classes of cardiac drugs are becoming more and more specific in their therapeutic effects and more free of unwanted side effects.

Heart transplant. Developments in the area of cardiac transplantation are currently centered on the production of new immunosuppressive drugs. The most common medical problem encountered in the treatment of cardiac transplant patients is rejection of the transplanted heart. Therefore, most investigative efforts are focused on development of newer classes of immunosuppressive agents that are specific for preventing rejection of the newly transplanted heart but do not suppress the patient's host defenses against life-threatening infections.

Pacemakers. New developments are occurring almost daily in the refinement of cardiac pacemakers. Pacemakers that can respond to the patient's metabolic work demands, as a normal heart would, are currently being evaluated. These ingenious devices are able to maintain variable heart rates depending on the body's demands in skeletal muscle activity, changes in core temperature, and changes in overall blood flow.

Defibrillators. Patients who have ventricular arrhythmias that do not respond to medical treatment are now given new hope with the development of automatic implantable cardiac defibrillators. These devices have electric pads that are secured to the surface of the heart and sense its electrical activity. When a sustained ventricular arrhythmia is detected, the device delivers a low-voltage shock directly to the heart to restore a normal rhythm. Although the patient is able to sense this small electrical discharge, this is a small price to pay, in view of the fact that the odds are against surviving a cardiac arrest occurring outside the hospital.

Catheters. In the treatment of intracardiac arterial disease, there has been rapid development in the technology of catheters, balloons, and guide wires. Research has been primarily directed towards newer materials to provide increased strength, decreased bulk, and smoother tracking over the guide wire. These changes allow more complex coronary angioplasty to be undertaken with a decreased risk of complications and restenosis.

Stents. A stent is a permanent intravascular device that can be inserted at the time of coronary angioplasty when acute closure of a vessel occurs. Introduced into the occluded area and then expanded, the stent provides a supporting framework to support and keep the vessel open. Stents may also be employed in patients who have had what is termed a chronic restenosis. These patients have undergone repeated angioplasty procedures for the same coronary artery lesion, which continues to reappear despite multiple dilatations. The stent may be inserted immediately after balloon dilatation to form a supporting framework that will not allow the vessel to restenose.

Lasers. There is continuing research in the area of laser ablation (eradication and removal with a laser) of coronary artery lesions. Various kinds of laser systems are under development. These include laser catheters that have a metal cap tip in which laser energy is used to heat the cap to extremely high temperatures so that it can melt through atheromatous lesions.

Other catheter systems have what is termed direct laser energy emerging from the catheter tip to cut a channel through the atheromatous lesion. These catheters are currently able to reestablish only a small channel through an otherwise totally or subtotally occluded atheromatous lesion. After this procedure, a balloon catheter is advanced through the new channel and balloon angioplasty is performed to make a larger channel for blood flow.

Another type of laser system that is currently under development is a laser balloon, which is essentially an angioplasty dilatation catheter with the capability of diffusing laser energy through the internal balloon surface outward to the endothelium of the coronary artery in contact with the balloon.

Other devices. Mechanical ablation devices consist of either drill bits or coring tools that are placed into an artery with an atheromatous lesion. The drill, spinning at rates as high as 200,000 rpm, pulverizes the atheromatous lesion. The other device cores or shaves the lesion with a blade. These devices are expected to prove more effective than balloon angioplasty in the treatment of atheromatous lesions, since they remove the lesion instead of just splitting or breaking it apart as in balloon angioplasty.

All of these investigational devices are still under development, and research is in progress to determine which of them will live up to expectations.

The future of cardiology. Over the past ten years, rapid developments in cardiology have made it so broad and complex a field that it is difficult for one person to keep current and retain a sufficient level of skill in all areas. Therefore, various divisions within the subspecialty of cardiology are emerging.

Nuclear cardiology, for example, with advances in radioisotopes and computer-assisted imaging equipment, has expanded to the point where additional training must be obtained to achieve full competence. The rapid development of technology in the treatment of atheromatous lesions has probably outpaced all other areas in the field of medicine. Fellowships in interventional cardiology have therefore been developed to concentrate careers in this area.

Other highly specialized areas include echocardiography and Doppler evaluation of the heart. Nontechnical areas include those of preventive cardiology, hypertension, and treatment of lipid disorders. In all these areas, new developments have emerged that demand specialized study and narrowing of the scope of practice. As the years pass we will see more and more subdivision within the specialty of cardiology.

Being a cardiologist is very rewarding. Patients who are chronically or acutely ill come to us for help, and after assessing and evaluating, we are usually able to help them. Whatever their illness, they usually notice a significant improvement after treatment and are able to enjoy life to a fuller extent. I cannot tell you what a pleasant experience it is to see patients in the office after they have had a recent hospitalization for a cardiac illness, and to have them tell me how much better they feel and what a change it has made in their life.

Positive results cannot be expected in every patient treated, as some do have terminal illness. However, those who respond to treatment make up for the long work hours both during the day and during the night. The rewards of being a cardiologist or a cardiac surgeon are particularly great when we achieve the occasional dramatic result.

The best example of a dramatic recovery would be a patient who presents to the emergency department with an acute myocardial infarction complicated by cardiogenic shock. The mortality rate for such patients is exceedingly high; however, with rapid intervention and today's technology, many of these patients can be saved. I can tell you of no greater reward than to see these patients walk out of the hospital 7 to 10 days after their initial event, to go home and return to a normal life with no significant limitations of lifestyle.

Cardiology is an exciting, rapidly expanding field, and one of which I am proud to be a part.

Pharmacology: Emergency Drugs

When a patient's cardiac or respiratory function decreases, a life-threatening condition exists. This decrease in function may be due to a variety of causes such as myocardial infarction, ventricular fibrillation, respiratory failure, or drug overdose. When a patient experiences cardiac and respiratory arrest, there is a cessation of spontaneous respirations with either absence of the heart beat (asystole) or the presence of such severe arrhythmias as to negate cardiac output. Unless these life- threatening problems can be corrected within a matter of minutes, carbon dioxide (pCO_2) and lactic acid levels in the blood will rise rapidly, the blood pH will become more acidic, and cell metabolism in the vital organs will slowly come to a halt; the patient will die.

Basic life support measures as performed in cardiopulmonary resuscitation (CPR) involve mechanically circulating the blood and inflating the lungs. Advanced cardiac life support (ACLS) also includes the use of drug

therapy. The type of emergency drug selected is based on the patient's symptoms. Drugs are used to maintain heart rate and blood pressure and to correct serum pH imbalances. Intravenous lines are inserted to provide access for drug administration. A **crash cart** containing all necessary emergency drugs and resuscitative equipment (including defibrillator paddles) is available in every patient area in the hospital.

The following routes of administration are used for emergency drugs.

intravenous Drugs are given by intravenous push or **bolus** to produce a maximum drug effect in the shortest period of time. Following successful resuscitation, continuous I.V. drip infusion is then used. The intravenous route is by far the most common way of administering emergency drugs.

endotracheal An alternative route to intravenous is endotracheal. Drugs are administered by injecting the solution into the endotracheal tube that is used to ventilate the patient. As the lungs are mechanically ventilated, the drug solution is rapidly absorbed by the lung tissue into the pulmonary capillary network. Therapeutic serum drug levels can be attained that equal those of intravenous administration; however, only certain drugs can be administered endotracheally. These drugs include epinephrine (Adrenalin), atropine, lidocaine (Xylocaine), verapamil (Calan), bretylium, and naloxone (Narcan). Note: Narcan is a narcotic antagonist given only to patients with suspected narcotic overdose.

intracardiac This route is not frequently used but can be valuable when other routes have failed to produce a therapeutic result. This route carries with it the risk of pneumothorax, cardiac tamponade, or coronary artery laceration if the injection is not properly placed into the left ventricular chamber. Only epinephrine (Adrenalin) and atropine are given by this route.

For emergency purposes, all other routes of administration result in too slow an absorption rate for the drug to produce therapeutic results before the patient dies.

Drugs commonly given during emergency resuscitation include epinephrine (Adrenalin), lidocaine (Xylocaine), atropine, sodium bicarbonate, calcium chloride, and vasopressors.

Epinephrine. Epinephrine (Adrenalin) normally is produced in the body and released by the action of the sympathetic nervous system. The body's response physiologically to epinephrine involves:

- Constriction of blood vessels due to stimulation of alpha receptors. This raises the blood pressure.
- Increased heart rate and cardiac output due to stimulation of beta$_1$ receptors in the heart muscle.
- Relaxation of bronchial smooth muscle resulting in bronchodilation, due to stimulation of beta$_2$ receptors.

During a cardiac arrest, epinephrine (Adrenalin) is used to increase the rate and force with which the heart beats. It is not useful for correcting cardiac arrhythmias. However, if the heart is in ventricular fibrillation, epinephrine (Adrenalin) makes the myocardium more responsive to the use of a defibrillator to restore normal rhythm. If the heart has completely stopped beating (asystole), epinephrine (Adrenalin) can actually stimulate contractions of the myocardium. It also constricts the blood vessels and raises the blood pressure. Thus, while epinephrine (Adrenalin) stimulates the heart to beat, it also helps to maintain perfusion to the heart and brain to improve the chances for a successful resuscitative effort.

Lidocaine. Lidocaine (Xylocaine) is indicated for the management of life-threatening ventricular fibrillation, and is the drug of choice in resuscitative efforts for patients with this problem. It has no therapeutic effect if the heart is in asystole.

Atropine. Atropine blocks the action of acetylcholine released from the vagus nerve. The vagus nerve is part of the parasympathetic nervous system with branches that innervate the myocardium at the SA and AV nodes. When acetylcholine is released, the heart rate slows. Atropine blocks that action and is used specifically to treat bradycardia.

Sodium bicarbonate. During cardiac and respiratory arrest, the blood pH decreases rapidly as waste products accumulate in the blood. In this environment of severe acidosis, all types of emergency drug therapy lose their effectiveness. Sodium bicarbonate corrects the acidosis and returns the blood pH to within normal range. There is some controversy, however, as to the true effectiveness of sodium bicarbonate. Some studies suggest it may actually increase acidosis through a chemical reaction which releases more CO_2 into the blood.

Calcium chloride. Calcium chloride can stimulate the myocardium to contract more forcefully and may even stimulate a contraction when the heart is in asystole and has failed to respond to epinephrine.

Vasopressors. Drugs in this class are used to increase blood pressure, and treatment with them is begun after the patient has been resuscitated. They are given by I.V. drip. All of these drugs stimulate beta$_1$ receptors to increase the heart rate; they also stimulate alpha receptors in the blood vessels to produce vasoconstriction and raise the blood pressure. This class of drugs includes:

> dobutamine (Dobutrex)
> dopamine (Intropin)
> isoproterenol (Isuprel)
> norepinephrine (Levophed)

Vasopressors also have the desirable effect of maintaining blood flow to the kidneys so that kidney ischemia from hypotension does not later result in renal failure which would complicate an otherwise successful resuscitative effort.

Anatomy/Medical Terminology

Cardiology Questions

1. Describe the difference between *atherosclerosis* and *arteriosclerosis*.

2. How would you correctly transcribe this sentence?

   The patient had a "cabbage" performed in 1983 with no sequelae.

3. Oxygenated blood enters the heart from the lungs via what vessel?

4. Blood flows from the heart to the rest of the body through what vessel?

Anatomy: Blood Supply to the Heart; Blood Flow Through the Heart

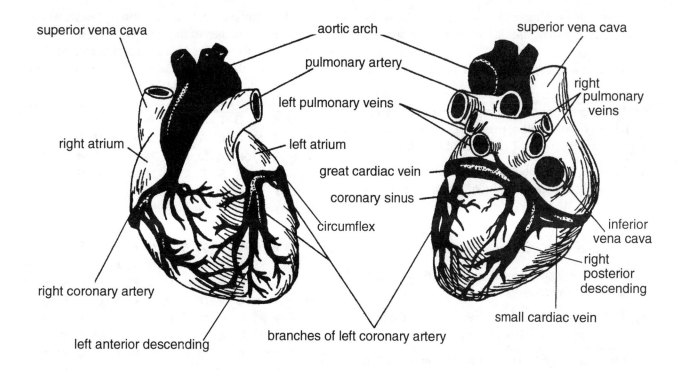

superior vena cava

aortic arch

pulmonary artery

left pulmonary veins

right atrium

left atrium

great cardiac vein

coronary sinus

circumflex

right coronary artery

left anterior descending

branches of left coronary artery

superior vena cava

right pulmonary veins

inferior vena cava

right posterior descending

small cardiac vein

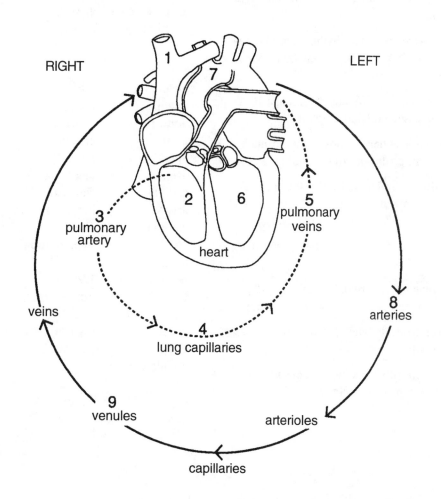

RIGHT

LEFT

1

7

3
pulmonary
artery

2

6

5
pulmonary
veins

heart

veins

4
lung capillaries

8
arteries

9
venules

arterioles

capillaries

Sound-alikes Exercise

Instructions: Circle the correct term from the sound-alikes in parentheses in the following sentences.

1. (Cor, Core, Corps): The heart was not enlarged.

2. The cardiac catheterization showed that although there were obstructed major vessels, there was sufficient (recanalization, recannulation) that medical therapy rather than bypass could be tried.

3. After the first angioplasty, the patient's vessel restenosed, so a (recanalization, recannulation) was done.

4. The echocardiogram showed the patient's (ejection, injection) fraction to be acceptable.

5. The vessel (loops, loupes) were pulled up (taught, taut), and the aneurysm tied off.

6. (Canalization, Cannulation) was done via the femoral artery with a JL4 guiding catheter.

7. An (osteal, ostial) lesion was noted near the takeoff of the posterior descending artery from the right coronary artery.

8. The EKG showed irregular rhythm, and the patient complained of (palpations, palpitations, papillations).

9. The patient was having difficulty breathing and experienced (perfuse, profuse) diaphoresis.

10. The angiogram was nondiagnostic due to inadequate (perfusion, profusion) of dye into the aorta.

11. There was diffuse inflammation of the (pericardium, precordium) and severe congestive heart failure.

12. The patient complains of (pericardial, precordial) chest pain.

13. Prior to coronary artery bypass grafting, the patient was put on intra-aortic balloon (pump, sump).

14. A (pump, sump) drain was placed in the thorax and the chest closed.

15. The (chordae, chordee) tendineae of the atrioventricular valve cusp were severed.

Word Search

Instructions: Locate and circle the cardiology terms hidden in the puzzle horizontally, vertically, and diagonally, forward and backward. A numeral following a term in the word list indicates the number of times it can be found in the puzzle.

```
D O E L O T S Y S A O L A R T I M
A P E R I C A R D I U M U G A A Y
V N L I E V L A V M H T Y H R R O
E E G A R E T L O H A A A G E R C
V C I I I M N L O T M O O T K E A
L V H N N R U I E Y E I R R G S R
A P I F R A T P V H D A T S T T D
V E N A C A V A Q R E C A B G A I
V S C R M Y O C A R D I U M S T U
E L I C P S U C L A N E U R Y S M
N U T T U V O V P D O O L B S U U
T P R C I R C U L A T I O N T N I
R N O I T A T I P L A P I P O I R
I C A C R R M Y D P W E E V L S T
C R E K A M E C A P V S A P E X A
L L P E E N O I T A L L I R B I F
E C H O H Y P E R T E N S I O N N
```

aneurysm	CPK	palpitation
angina	cusp	PDA
aorta (2)	DOE	pericardium
aortic	edema	plaque
apex	EKG	pulse
arrest	electrocardiogram	PVC
arrhythmia	fibrillation	QRS
artery	heart (2)	rhythm
asystole	Holter	septum
atrial	hypertension	sinus
atrium	infarct	systole
blood	LVH	valve
CABG	mitral	vein (3)
capillary	MUGA	veins
CCU	myocardium (2)	vena cava
CHF	pacemaker	ventricle
circulation		

Transcription Guidelines

1. **Subject–verb agreement.** The subject of a sentence (a noun or pronoun) must agree in number with its verb. A singular subject must be matched with a singular verb, a plural subject with a plural verb. Subject-verb agreement errors occur frequently in medical dictation, and it is the medical transcriptionist's responsibility to correct such errors.

   The first steps in assuring subject-verb agreement are to analyze the sentence, identify the subject of the sentence, and decide if the subject is singular or plural. Then check to see that the verb agrees with the subject.

   If dictated:
   The **edema** in both legs **have** not yet responded to diuretics.

   Transcribe:
   The **edema** in both legs **has** not yet responded to diuretics.

   Note: The word *legs* is part of the prepositional phrase intervening between the subject and the verb.

2. When a compound subject is present, select the noun that is closest to the verb and make them agree in number.

   Example: No definite adenopathy or masses were felt.

3. **Commas.** The comma is probably one of the most misused punctuation marks in written language. Misuse includes inserting too many commas, too few, or using them inappropriately so that the meaning of a sentence is unclear, or, worse, misconstrued. In medicine, this can have serious consequences by affecting or changing medical meaning.

   In the following example, notice how the missing comma in the first sentence alters the interpretation.

   Incorrect: This 51-year-old alcoholic male was found in a confused and disoriented state, lying on the floor by his girlfriend.

   Correct: This 52-year-old alcoholic male was found in a confused and disoriented state, lying on the floor, by his girlfriend.

   In the first statement, the meaning conveyed is that the man was found on the floor next to his friend. When correctly punctuated, it is clear that the man's friend found him lying on the floor.

4. The following statements demonstrate an alteration in medical meaning when the comma is used in the wrong place or not used at all.

   Incorrect: Air was aspirated from the left ventricle, and the aorta and the cross-clamp removed. (Incorrect because the aorta is not removed, of course.)

   Correct: Air was aspirated from the left ventricle and the aorta, and the cross-clamp removed.

   Incorrect: There was pain in the femur with a positive McMurray maneuver to suggest an O'Donoghue's triad.

   Correct: There was pain in the femur, with a positive McMurray maneuver to suggest an O'Donoghue's triad. (The pain was not caused by the McMurray maneuver.)

5. In the following example, misplaced commas convey an anatomic inaccuracy.

   Incorrect: In diverticulitis the bowel may narrow down, where the pockets are causing lower abdominal pain, diarrhea, and constipation. (Incorrect because the pockets are not causing the symptoms; the narrowing down is.)

   Correct: In diverticulitis, the bowel may narrow down where the pockets are, causing lower abdominal pain, diarrhea, and constipation.

6. Which of the following statements is correctly punctuated?

A: The stomach and duodenum which usually lie in the left upper abdomen and epigastrium are rarely felt unless they are involved with large tumors.

B: The stomach and duodenum, which usually lie in the left upper abdomen, and epigastrium are rarely felt unless they are involved with large tumors.

C: The stomach and duodenum, which usually lie in the left upper abdomen and epigastrium, are rarely felt unless they are involved with large tumors.

D: The stomach and duodenum which usually lie in the left upper abdomen, and epigastrium are rarely felt, unless they are involved with large tumors.

Choice A is acceptable, but choice C is easier to understand. Choices B and D are incorrect because the epigastrium is not felt; it is a region of the upper middle part of the abdomen, not an organ like the stomach or duodenum.

7. Although a comma is not necessary in the following statement, it enhances readability:

She was sedated with Haldol, and then was kept on Pamelor and Mellaril which she had been started on a few days prior to admission.

TIP: If in doubt, read the statement aloud. Where natural pauses occur orally, commas are probably appropriate.

Subject-Verb Agreement Exercise

Instructions: Circle either the singular or plural form of the verb in parentheses to demonstrate correct subject-verb agreement.

1. No evidence of congestive heart failure and edema (is, are) seen on chest x-ray.

2. The occlusions in the region of the left anterior descending artery (appears, appear) to be significant.

3. We have no way of telling what the exact relationship of his pathology to his symptoms (is, are).

4. There (is, are) minimal episodes of arrhythmia seen on the EKG.

5. No episodes of angina (was, were) noted by the patient.

6. The age and sex of a patient (cause, causes) variation in the normal range of laboratory values.

7. Finger-to-nose test and heel-to-shin test (is, are) normal.

8. Inspection of the upper extremities (show, shows) some scattered small abrasions over the dorsal aspects of the hands.

9. No evidence of mucosal ulcerations or polypoid filling defects (was, were) seen.

10. Some hypertrophy of the facet joints (is, are) noted at this level.

11. A moderate exudate of polymorphonuclear leukocytes (is, are) seen.

12. Acute blood clot and old organized and degenerate blood clot (is, are) observed.

13. His BUN was within normal limits, as (was, were) his sodium and potassium.

14. No fecalith or perforations (is, are) identified.

15. Cardiac and respiratory compensation (was, were) used.

Transcription Tips

A professional medical transcriptionist always strives to transcribe a report completely, without leaving blanks, by thoroughly utilizing reference books and other resources to research words. However, even experienced transcriptionists know that it is nearly impossible to complete a day's work of difficult and challenging dictation without leaving at least one blank. Leaving a blank, when one has exhausted all resources to find the correct information, does not reflect negatively on the transcriptionist.

Sometimes, in an effort to hide what they consider a failing on their part, some transcriptionists will make up words to fill in dictation that is garbled or unclear. This is termed "creative" transcription, an undesirable and unethical solution to the problem.

When you encounter difficult passages or garbled words in dictation, you should research carefully and, if you still cannot transcribe a word or phrase, do not be afraid to leave a blank with a note to the dictator, stating what the word sounded like; the dictator will fill in the blank correctly before signing the report.

The following **humorous** response to the dilemmas of a transcriptionist is provided here just for fun.

Advice to Transcriptionists

by Shirley U. Jezt

There are questions continually bandied about among transcriptionists in this office. I do not complain, but I have noticed a certain reluctance to solicit my opinion in these debates. I am conscious that this is doubtless due to others holding me in awe. Therefore, I have decided to write up some of my opinions in the interest of sharing them with my less experienced and reticent co-workers and making them as successful as possible—who knows? perhaps even approaching my position of high esteem.

First and foremost, one must learn to take control. I have watched with disgust while a transcriptionist turns to someone beside her and actually confesses, "I can't hear this word." Well, my dear, you're going about this all wrong. The solution is simple and quick: just type *something*. Why else did you spend time and money on a medical terminology class if not to have a word to stick in when you need one? This is not only faster and more painless than fretting over the dictation, but also keeps you from having to confess to someone else that you can't hear and can't understand (you'll never advance that way). Let's face it; that's one of the beauties of this job: once you erase the cassette, you can swear it was dictated exactly that way and who can prove it wasn't?

And while I'm on the subject of creativity in the workplace, let me deplore the repetitive nature of most reports I see. Those physical exams could have been rubber-stamped instead of transcribed. Let's see a bit more personality here. I type "no murmurs, rubs or gallops" only once a day. After that I try to vary the monotony with a little PVC here and an old MI there. Use discretion, though—that goes without saying. I've had some bad experiences with horrid, rude doctors whose scientific minds can't appreciate a little creativity. So for goodness sake, be sure to go easy on the ones who proofread their reports before signing.

Now a few phrases of tested reliability to use with an interfering co-worker (we all know people like that) or a picky boss:

1. "I didn't know that." This can be used often, so long as you don't use it twice to cover the same little slip.

2. "That's what it sounded like." This is especially useful if you imply that you played the dictation out loud and got others to agree with you.

3. And if the evidence is heavily against you: "Yes, I *thought* it was odd, but that's what it sounded like." This way you show that you were intelligent enough to anticipate the problem.

4. "I saw it that way somewhere." This will sometimes work only if you can actually produce a fourth-rate source of some kind.

5. "Jane told me that was right." Needless to say, this should be restricted to people like Jane who work in another department.

6. "I was going to correct that, but I forgot." Yes, this does confess to a little memory lapse, but at least you disarm them with your quickness. You saw the mistake even before they did.

7. "That's how Dr. X spelled it." I've rarely seen this one fail. I've tried expanding it to "That was Dr. X's syntax," but this hasn't been quite as successful.

8. "Oh, that's just a typo." This will cover many a misspelling.

9. And if they've got you dead to rights: "Well, I'm not a *perfect* proofreader. Who is?" This at least makes them look finicky and unfair and tends to shift the blame away from yourself.

Terminology Challenge

Instructions: The following terms appear in the dictation on Tape 5A. Before beginning the medical transcription practice for Lesson 10, become familiar with the terminology below by looking up each word in a medical or English dictionary. Write out a short definition of each term.

a.c.
akinesis
anastomosis
Ancef
angiodysplasia
aortic root
apical aneurysm
arteriotomy
artery
  left anterior descending
    (LAD)
  left circumflex coronary
  left internal mammary
  main circumflex
    coronary
  posterior descending
    coronary
  right coronary (RCA)
atrial rate
axis deviation
Betadine
branch (of artery)
  diagonal
  first obtuse marginal
  second obtuse marginal
cannulated
Carafate
cardioplegia solution
cardiopulmonary bypass
chronic lead placement
Clonidine
Colace
collateral flow
conduit
CPI Astra bipolar
  generator
crescendo angina pectoris
cross-clamped
decannulation
Dexon

end-to-side anastomosis
enucleated
exertional angina
ferrous sulfate
g (gram)
graft occlusive disease
h.s.
high-grade lesion
hypokinesis
instilled
intimal hyperplasia
Kefzol
lead aVF
lead aVL
lead I
lead II
lead III
lead V1
lead V2
lead V3
lead V4
lead V6
lesion
median sternotomy
  incision
mitral valve
monitoring lines
myocardial hypothermia
Nitro-Dur II
occluded graft
pacemaker capture
pacemaker generator
pacemaker leads
pacemaker resistance
pacemaker sensitivity
paroxysmal supraven-
  tricular tachycardia
patent
plaque
pleural space

PR interval
premature ventricular beat
pulmonary artery vent
pulsatile perfusion
Q wave
QRS
Quinaglute
reciprocal change on
  ECG
retracted
revascularization
  procedure
right atrium
saline
saphenous vein graft
selective coronary
  arteriogram
side-biting clamp
Silastic tapes

stenosis
supravalvular aortogram
suture
  3-0 ("three oh" or
    "three zero")
  4-0
  6-0
  7-0
  Dexon
  Prolene
  Vicryl
systemic hypertension
tube
  right-angle
  straight chest
ventricular rate
ventriculogram
watt-second shock
Zantac

Transcription Practice

After completing all the readings and exercises in Lesson 10, transcribe Tape 5A, Cardiology. Use both medical and English dictionaries and your Quick-Reference Word List as resource materials for finding words.

Proofread your transcribed documents carefully, listening to the dictation while you read your transcripts.

Transcribe (*NOT* retype) the same reports again without referring to your previous transcription attempt. Initially, you may need to transcribe some reports more than twice before you can produce an error-free document. Your ultimate goal is to produce an error-free document the first time.

Learning Objectives

Medical

- List common pulmonary symptoms and diseases mentioned in the Physical Examination section of the H&P.
- Describe the action of these classes of pulmonary drugs: bronchodilators, corticosteroids.
- Discuss the purpose and technique involved in performing common pulmonary laboratory tests and surgical procedures.
- Given a pulmonary root word, symptom, or disease, match it to its correct medical definition.
- Given a cross-section illustration of the respiratory system, memorize the anatomic structures.
- Define common pulmonary abbreviations.
- Construct the adjectival form of common pulmonary terms.

Fundamentals

- Discuss the correct use of semicolons and colons in punctuating medical sentences.
- Given a medical report with errors, identify and correct the errors.

Practice

- Accurately transcribe authentic physician dictation from the specialty of pulmonary medicine.

A Closer Look

Confessions of an Addict

by Judith Marshall, MA, CMT

I grew up in Cleveland under the shadow of the great steel mills. I thought the color of the sky was orange and the natural quality of air was acrid. I would wake up and hear the birds coughing. I thought all mothers and fathers, aunts and uncles, and grandparents came with cigarettes in their mouths and lived in a cloud of smoke. At age 14 I got a work permit and somehow it seemed natural that I began smoking in the basement of a hospital, desperately trying to appear sophisticated and grown up.

Over 30 years ago I began my smoking career and, oh, how I loved it. Cigarettes were my best friend, my pal, my lover, my source of strength, my comfort, delight, reward, and badge of elegance. Cigarettes were then socially acceptable and medically benign.

Smoking and medical transcription were natural together. As soon as I could bounce a *Dorland's* on my knee, I realized that I was born to smoke and to transcribe, preferably at the same time. I perfected a system of drinking coffee in the morning and cola in the afternoons along with the two packs (and later three) of cigarettes a day. My system was so full of caffeine and nicotine it was no wonder I typed two thousand words a minute.

I blamed my near-constant headaches on the dumb doctors who didn't know how to dictate. The cough and shortness of breath were more insidious in onset, and I found I could blame those on something other than cigarettes as well. All of us working in the hospital basement smoked all day long and so did the doctors. The dictation room was like Brigadoon, wafting in and out of a fog.

Each new voice on the tape called for another cigarette. Each tape completed, another cigarette. Every break in the cafeteria demanded a cigarette. There were ashes in my typewriter, in my hair, and in my shoes. I remember a little soft brush I kept in my desk so I could whisk the work before I turned it in.

My excuse was that I smoked to keep my weight down. Then one day I took a cigarette, sat in front of a mirror and smoked it. In the mirror I saw A FAT SMOKER.

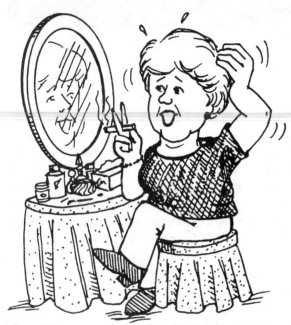

Judith Marshall, MEDICATE ME
Illustrated by Cindy Stevens

Then began the desperate search for a painless way to quit. I began asking doctors how they quit smoking. The younger ones had never started, they were quick to tell me. The older ones stressed a beatific attitude I came to despise. "Oh," they said nonchalantly, "I just threw them out the car window one day and that was that, fifteen years ago." Litterbugs! The weaker of that group took up gumballs, chocolates, mints, or chewing gum. The stronger took up scalpels. I don't trust anyone who is not addicted to **something**.

Hypnotism appealed to me, but its fascination was short-lived. It frightened me more than cigarettes. I was positive that once I went under, other more virulent habits would surface—I would begin eating chalk or running amok wearing banana leaves (and probably rolling them up and smoking them as well).

The bookstore was no help. There were hundreds of books on dieting but none on how to quit smoking. I discovered the powerful tobacco industry had its tendrils everywhere. I turned to popular magazines. They just made me want to smoke more. All those slender, beige, beautiful people. They were rich, well-dressed,

laughing, carefree people partying on rooftops on a gorgeous summer evening. No one looked over thirty.

I couldn't relate to the strong and handsome cowboys or sailors but I did begin to collect other ads. I bought white satin pajamas and a white satin dog. I wanted that satin moment. I wanted to go a long way, baby. I wanted flowers decorating my cigarettes and a butterfly tattoo on my ankle. My favorite was the ballerina ad. She was young, slim, beautiful, and slightly damp from all those pliés. She was relaxing in the dance studio, lighting up. The message was that she could function and exercise without trouble breathing.

I went to work out at the gym and it was Cardiac City. Obviously it was my fault, not the cigarettes.

Remarkable creature that I am, I can play bingo, crochet, talk, and smoke, simultaneously. So I began to choose the workplace with an eye towards the comfort and ease with which I could smoke. I shifted from hospital to doctor's office to transcription service in a ceaseless hunt for the ashtray.

I began to scour the charts looking for patients with lung cancer who had never smoked. This gave me immeasurable feelings of security. Conversely, I delighted in patients whose summaries indicated that they lived to an old age despite eighty pack years. I mentally logged this as more proof that I too could escape. Everyone has an Uncle Joe who beats the odds, smokes four packs a day, drinks a fifth of bourbon a day, and lives to ninety-five. It helps us rationalize our habits. From my vantage point in transcription I adopted literally hundreds of Uncle Joes. It was very consoling.

Professional meetings were more appealing to me if they were dinner or luncheon meetings. I could smoke with impunity in the restaurant. And the Scotch with the cigarettes wasn't bad either. My major concern while flying out to the national meeting in Denver in 1982 was whether the altitude would affect my smoking habit and make it less enjoyable. (It certainly did.) I was furious at that meeting because some of the morning session rooms did not have coffee, only ice water. Only a smoker can appreciate how welcome hot coffee is with a cigarette in the morning and how repulsive ice water.

What new trade would I have to learn if I quit smoking? I was positive I could not transcribe without smoking. I became angry with doctors. I wanted answers from them. "The patient was placed on a 1200-calorie ADA diet, advised to exercise and quit smoking." Pompous, unfeeling clucks. What did they know about it? I could hear the disgust in the doctors' voices as they related in the course of the discharge summary that the patient, having sustained a moderate myocardial infarction and having undergone CABG, resumed smoking upon discharge.

The answer never did come from the doctors. The postman delivered it. In the summer of 1983 an innocent-appearing postcard addressed to Occupant fluttered into my mailbox. It promised a free, introductory stop-smoking session. It promised to unhook me forever from the habit of coffee-cola-cigarettes, practically painlessly. I told the counselor that if they could do all of that, I was the Queen of Rumania.

Everyone calls me Your Majesty now. I quit smoking July 29, 1983. After five weeks of participation in a group, doing all my homework, using a method of gradual withdrawal and behavior modification, I graduated.

On a steaming hot Friday I put out that last cigarette and, like any rational intelligent adult, headed for the kitchen. I defrosted everything in the freezer and as soon as it was cooked, I ate it. Then I began working on the larger freezer in the basement. If I had had a microwave oven instead of having to wait, I would have cleaned out our entire year's supply of codfish balls.

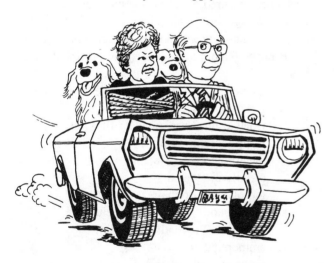

Judith Marshall, MEDICATE ME
Illustrated by Cindy Stevens

Finally I asked my husband to chain me inside the car, pack a suitcase for the dogs, and drive us to the Maine coast so I could sit on the rocks and breathe (without smoking or eating). I calmed down.

Our stop-smoking program recommended saving the money spent on cigarettes and putting it in a glass jar, then buying oneself a present. So far we have a new complete set of English bone china. Next is a trip to England!

The History and Physical Examination

by John H. Dirckx, M.D.

Examination of the Thorax, Breasts, and Axillae. The physician observes the configuration of the chest walls, breathing movements, the skin, and the breasts before turning his attention to the internal organs of the thorax.

The development and symmetry of the thorax are noted. Congenital deformities and injuries or diseases of the ribs or spine can alter the shape of the thorax. In pulmonary emphysema the anteroposterior diameter of the chest is often increased so that the rib cage approaches a cylindrical shape (barrel chest). Unless the subject is thin, the examiner will need to find some of the bony landmarks of the chest wall by palpation.

Movements of the chest wall associated with breathing can be influenced by a number of factors, including, of course, the rate and rhythm of breathing itself. A patient with severe dyspnea may use muscles of the neck and upper chest to enhance lung filling that are not normally involved in breathing (accessory muscles of respiration).

Examination of the Lungs. Evaluation of the lungs is performed almost entirely by the techniques of auscultation and percussion. The passage of air into and out of the lungs during normal respiration produces a characteristic sequence of sounds, as heard with the stethoscope through the chest wall. Structural changes in the breathing apparatus due to disease or injury cause predictable changes in the quality and loudness of the breath sounds and can induce abnormal sounds as well. The subject is instructed to breathe somewhat more deeply than normal with his mouth open (to avoid extraneous sounds caused by the passage of air through the nose) while the examiner listens at specific places on the front and back of the chest. Ordinarily the diaphragm chest piece of the stethoscope is preferred for this purpose.

Normal inspiration and expiration yield a faint sighing or whispering sound called vesicular breathing. This sound might be compared to that of a steady, gentle breeze passing through and stirring the leaves of a tree. The inspiratory phase of vesicular breathing is slightly longer than the expiratory phase, and slightly louder.

The expiratory phase may be inaudible. When the two phases of respiration are about equal in intensity, one speaks of bronchovesicular breathing. When the expiratory phase is louder, the term bronchial (or tubular) breathing is applied.

Certain abnormal conditions can superimpose abnormal sounds (rhonchi, rales, or rubs) on the basic inspiratory-expiratory breath sounds. A rhonchus is a continuous sound such as is made by a whistle or horn. A rale is irregular and discontinuous, like bubbling fluid, crackling paper, or popping corn.

Rhonchi result from narrowing of bronchiolar passages by bronchospasm (in asthma), swelling, thickened secretions, or tumor. Rhonchi vary widely in pitch and intensity. In asthma, rhonchi of many different pitches may be heard together. Rales are due to passage of air through fluid—mucus, pus, edema fluid, or blood—or to sudden expansion of small air passage that have been plugged or sealed by mucus.

A pleural friction rub is a creaking, grating, or rubbing sound caused by friction between inflamed pleural surfaces during breathing. Sometimes it resembles the sound of a creaking shoe, sometimes the sound of two tree branches rubbing together in the wind.

Reduction or absence of breath sounds over a part of the chest wall can result from any of several conditions—collapse of lung tissue (atelectasis), consolidation of lung tissue due to pneumonia, presence in the pleural space of air (pneumothorax), blood (hemothorax), pus (empyema), or fluid (hydrothorax, pleural effusion), and tumor.

Percussion of the chest, though a valuable diagnostic procedure, has been largely supplanted by x-rays. This procedure is based on the fact that structural alterations within the thorax change the behavior of sound waves produced by tapping the chest.

In the standard percussion technique, called mediate percussion, the examiner places the palm of his hand with outspread fingers against the subject's chest and taps the back of his middle finger smartly with the flexed tip of his other middle finger.

The percussion note over normal lung tissue is described as resonant. In atelectasis, consolidation, or pleural effusion the note is dull or even flat; in pneumothorax or emphysema it may be hyperresonant or even tympanitic (drumlike). Percussion can be used to find the levels of the right and left hemidiaphragms in inspiration and expiration and to trace the left border of an enlarged heart.

Pharmacology: Pulmonary Drugs

Respiratory diseases such as asthma, chronic obstructive pulmonary disease (COPD), and emphysema require medication to treat chronic and acute symptoms as well as prevent acute attacks. Aside from the antibiotics used to treat respiratory infections, there are two main classes of drugs prescribed to treat pulmonary diseases. These include bronchodilators and corticosteroids. The drugs used to treat tuberculosis will also be discussed.

Bronchodilators. Bronchodilators relax the smooth muscle that surrounds the bronchi, thereby increasing air flow. This dilatation of the bronchi is due either to stimulation of beta$_2$ receptors in the smooth muscle of the bronchi, the release of epinephrine which itself stimulates beta$_2$ receptors, or to inhibition of acetylcholine at cholinergic receptor sites in the smooth muscle.

Some bronchodilators are given orally; some are given intravenously; some are prescribed as a solution in a dispenser (inhaler) with a special mouthpiece. The dispenser nebulizes the medicine and automatically injects a premeasured dose into the lungs as the patient inhales through the mouth. The prescribed dosage for these **metered-dose inhalers** is in numbers of puffs.

Bronchodilators administered through inhalers include:

>   albuterol (Proventil, Ventolin)
>   ipratropium (Atrovent)
>   isoetharine (Bronkometer, Bronkosol)
>   isoproterenol (Isuprel)
>   metaproterenol (Alupent)
>   pirbuterol (Maxair)
>   terbutaline (Brethaire)

Bronchodilators given orally include:
>   albuterol (Proventil, Ventolin)
>   aminophylline
>   isoproterenol (Isuprel)
>   metaproterenol (Alupent)
>   theophylline (Slo-Phyllin Gyrocaps,
>   Theo-Dur Sprinkle)

Combination products. The following oral drugs combine two different bronchodilators and other ingredients.

>   Bronkaid (theophylline and ephedrine and
>   guaifenesin [an expectorant])
>   Marax (theophylline and ephedrine and
>   hydroxyzine [Vistaril]–an antianxiety drug
>   used to counteract the stimulant effects of
>   ephedrine)

Primatene (theophylline and ephedrine)

Tedral (theophylline and ephedrine and phenobarbital [a sedative to counteract the effects of ephedrine])

Corticosteroids. Corticosteroids reduce inflammation and tissue edema. They cannot provide bronchodilation and so are always used in conjunction with the bronchodilators described previously. Their use is prophylactic, and they are not effective during acute attacks of bronchospasm. These drugs are given by inhaler, and the dosage is prescribed as a number of puffs.

beclomethasone (Beclovent, Vanceril)

dexamethasone (Decadron Respihaler)

flunisolide (AeroBid)

triamcinolone (Azmacort)

Antituberculosis drugs. Tuberculosis is caused by *Mycobacterium tuberculosis,* a gram-positive rod which is resistant to antibiotics that are usually effective against gram-positive bacteria. Continuous therapy with some combination of the antituberculosis drugs listed below is usually necessary to complete treatment.

ethambutol (Myambutol)

isoniazid (INH)

rifampin

Laboratory Tests and Surgical Procedures

ABGs (arterial blood gases).

acid-fast bacilli (AFB)   Bacilli that, once stained with a fluorochrome dye, are not decolorized by acid-alcohol. The only acid-fast bacilli of clinical significance are organisms of the genus *Mycobacterium,* which cause tuberculosis and leprosy.

acid-fast stain   A staining procedure in which sputum, tissue, or other material is exposed to fluorochrome dye and then washed with acid-alcohol. Organisms of the genus *Mycobacterium* and some others retain the dye and are said to be acid-fast.

AFB (acid-fast bacilli).

agglutinins, cold   Antibodies formed by persons with mycoplasmal pneumonia, which cause red blood cells to clump when chilled but not at room or body temperature.

agglutinins, febrile   A group of antibody tests, each for a specific febrile (fever-causing) infectious disease, used as a screening procedure in patients with fever of unknown origin (FUO).

arterial blood gases (ABGs)   So-called because they are usually measured in a specimen of blood drawn from an artery. See *blood gases.*

base excess   See *blood gases.*

bicarbonate   An electrolyte; a negatively charged ion found in the serum. Measured during arterial blood gas test.

blood gases   Oxygen and carbon dioxide, the principal gases dissolved in the blood. Sometimes called arterial blood gases because they are usually measured in a specimen of blood drawn from an artery. Blood gas measurements include partial pressures of oxygen (PO_2) and of carbon dioxide (PCO_2) and oxygen saturation. From these data and the serum pH, it is possible to calculate the bicarbonate level. Alternatively, the base excess may be reported as the variation from a neutral blood pH.

bronchoscopy   Procedure to visualize the bronchi by means of an endoscope.

cardiopulmonary resuscitation (CPR)   The use of external compression of the heart coupled with breathing techniques to revive a victim whose heart and respirations have stopped.

chest x-ray (CXR)   X-rays of the chest are taken to assess the clarity of the lung fields. Milky or opaque shadows in the lung fields can denote edema or mucus secretions. An AP (anterior-posterior) film shows the lungs as the x-rays pass from the front of the body (anterior) to the back (posterior). A PA (posterior-anterior) film shows the lungs as the x-rays pass from the back of the body to the front.

CO_2 (carbon dioxide)   When measured in arterial blood, carbon dioxide is reported as a partial pressure (PCO_2).

CPR (cardiopulmonary resuscitation).

CXR (chest x-ray).

electrolytes, sweat   Sodium and chloride ions in the sweat, increased in persons with cystic fibrosis.

FEV_1, FEV1 (forced expiratory volume in one second).   The amount of air that can be forcefully exhaled in one second following maximum inspiration.

FiO2, FiO_2 (fractional inspired oxygen, or inspired flow of oxygen).   Note: Lowercase *i.*

FUO (fever of unknown origin).

FVC (forced vital capacity).   The total amount of air that can be exhaled forcefully following maximum inspiration.

Haemophilus influenzae (*H. influenzae*)   A gram-negative organism that causes respiratory and ear infections and is also an important cause of meningitis in children. *H. flu* is a slang term.

HCO_3^-, HCO3$^-$ (bicarbonate ion).

IMV (intermittent mandatory ventilation)   Usually followed by a number, e.g., IMV of 5.

Mantoux test   Skin test for tuberculosis (TB). A needle is inserted intradermally, and a small amount of purified protein derivative (PPD) from the bacterium *Mycobacterium tuberculosis* is inserted under the skin. A Mantoux test is a definitive test and is usually done to confirm a previously positive tine test. A positive reaction means the patient has or has had tuberculosis.

O_2, O2 (molecular oxygen)   When measured in arterial blood, oxygen is reported as a partial pressure (PaO_2).

O_2 saturation   The amount of oxygen being carried by the hemoglobin, compared to the amount that could be carried, and expressed as a percent (100% being total saturation).

$PaCO_2$, PCO_2   Partial pressure of carbon dioxide, CO_2, dissolved in the blood.

PaO_2, PO_2   Partial pressure of oxygen, O_2, dissolved in the blood.

PCP (*Pneumocystis carinii*).

PEEP (positive end-expiratory pressure)   Usually followed by a number, e.g., PEEP of 6.

PFTs (pulmonary function tests).

pH   A measure of the acidity or alkalinity of a substance. A pH of 7.0 indicates neutrality. Numbers above 7.0 indicate alkalinity, numbers below indicate acidity. The *p* is always a lowercase letter. When the term *pH* begins a sentence, insert the word *The* before it.

Pneumocystis carinii (PCP)   A parasite that causes pneumonia in children and in AIDS patients.

PPD test   See *tine test.*

tine test   Skin test for tuberculosis. A multiple-puncture device is used to pierce the skin and insert a small amount of purified protein derivative (PPD) from the bacterium *Mycobacterium tuberculosis.* A positive reaction is confirmed by doing a Mantoux test. The four small blades used to puncture the skin are called tines because they resemble the tips or tines of a fork.

torr   A unit of pressure equal to one millimeter of mercury, used to record partial pressures of arterial blood gases.

V/Q scan (ventilation/perfusion scan, V/Q scan)   (The *Q* stands for quotient.) A test of lung perfusion and ventilation by means of scanning for radioisotope uptake by lung tissues. Areas of poor blood flow and poor ventilation within the lungs due to emphysema, edema, or other disease conditions do not concentrate the radioisotope, and this shows when a scan of the area is done.

Anatomy/Medical Terminology

Medical Terminology Matching Exercise

Complete the following matching exercise to test your knowledge of the word roots, anatomic structures, symptoms, and disease processes encountered in the medical specialty of pulmonary medicine.

Instructions: Match the term in Column A with its definition in Column B.

Column A	*Column B*
A. cyanosis	_____ smallest branches of bronchi
B. epiglottis	_____ crackling sounds on inspiration
C. bronchioles	
	_____ diaphragm
D. asthma	
	_____ uppermost area of lung
E. alveolus	
	_____ depression on side of lung where blood vessels enter
F. -pnea	
G. pleura	_____ mucus coughed up
H. lobe	_____ genetic disorder causing thick mucus secretions
I. atelectasis	
	_____ bluish discoloration of skin
J. hilum	
	_____ breathing
K. phreno-	
	_____ collapsed lung
L. apex	
	_____ membrane around lungs
M. cystic fibrosis	
	_____ air sac where gas exchange takes place
N. rales	
O. sputum	_____ closes opening to larynx
	_____ spasm of bronchi
	_____ division of lung

Anatomy: The Respiratory System

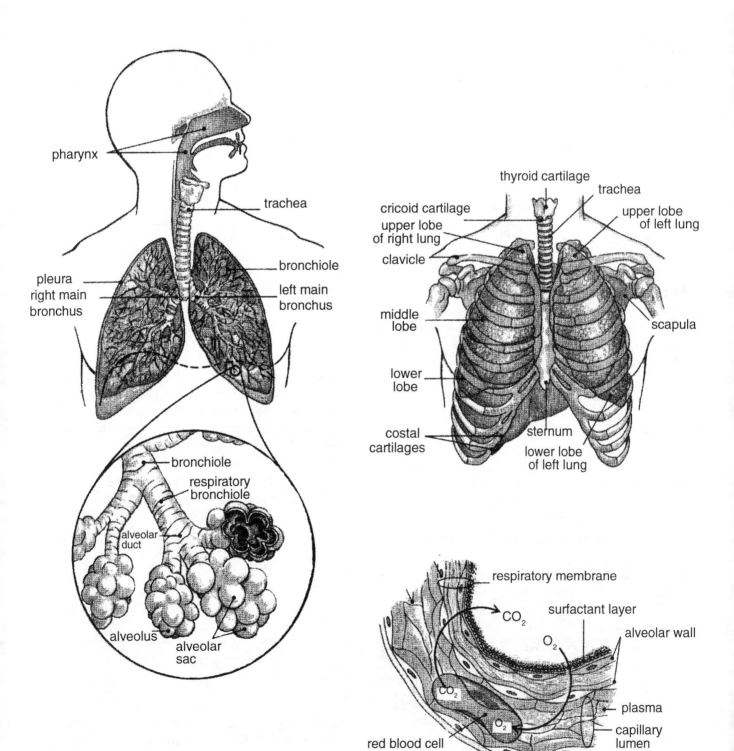

pharynx

trachea

bronchiole

pleura
right main
bronchus

left main
bronchus

bronchiole

respiratory
bronchiole

alveolar
duct

alveolus

alveolar
sac

thyroid cartilage

trachea

cricoid cartilage

upper lobe
of right lung

upper lobe
of left lung

clavicle

middle
lobe

scapula

lower
lobe

costal
cartilages

sternum

lower lobe
of left lung

respiratory membrane

surfactant layer

CO_2

O_2

alveolar wall

CO_2

O_2

plasma

capillary
lumen

red blood cell

Abbreviations Exercise

Common abbreviations may be transcribed as dictated in the body of a report. Uncommon abbreviations must be spelled out, with the abbreviation appearing in parentheses after the translation. All abbreviations (except laboratory test names) must be spelled out in the Diagnosis or Impression section of any report.

Instructions: Define the following pulmonary medicine abbreviations. Then memorize both abbreviations and definitions to increase your speed and accuracy in transcribing pulmonary medicine dictation.

A&P _____
ABG _____
AFB _____
ARDS _____
COPD _____
CXR _____
DOE _____
ET tube _____
FEV₁ _____
FVC _____
LLL _____
LUL _____
PFTs _____
PPD _____
RAD _____
RDS _____
RLL _____
RUL _____
SOB _____
URI _____

Descriptive Terms in Pulmonary Medicine

1. A **cough** may be described as brassy, bubbling, croupy, hacking, harsh, hollow, loose, metallic, nonproductive, productive, rasping, rattling, or wracking.

2. **Sputum** may be described as blood-streaked, foul-tasting, frothy, gelatinous, green, purulent, putrid, ropy, rusty, viscid, viscous, watery, or yellow.

3. **Rales** may be described as bibasilar, bubbling, coarse, crackling, crepitant, moist, post-tussive, or sticky.

4. **Rhonchi** may be described as coarse, high-pitched, humming, low-pitched, musical, post-tussive, sibilant, sonorous, or whistling.

Adjective Exercise

Adjectives are formed from nouns by adding adjectival suffixes such as -ac, -al, -ar, -ary, -atic, -eal, -ed, -ent, -iac, -ial, -ic, -ical, -lar, -oid, -ous, -tic, and -tous. In addition, some adjectives have a different form entirely from the noun, which may be either Latin or Greek in origin.

Instructions: Test your knowledge of adjectives by writing the adjectival form of the following pulmonary medicine words.

1. lung _____
2. bronchus _____
3. hilum _____
4. alveolus _____
5. diaphragm _____
6. pleura _____
7. cyanosis _____
8. trachea _____
9. dyspnea _____
10. emphysema _____

Drug Word Search

Instructions: Locate and circle the pulmonary medicine terms hidden in the puzzle horizontally, vertically, and diagonally, forward and backward. A numeral following a term in the word list indicates the number of times it can be found in the puzzle.

```
E  P  I  N  E  P  H  R  I  N  E  T  F
X  A  R  A  M  A  R  A  X  T  R  E  R
O  Z  E  D  U  A  E  R  O  B  I  D  E
S  M  B  R  C  M  X  U  L  K  F  R  K
U  A  V  U  O  R  S  A  V  N  A  A  D
R  C  T  G  M  B  R  G  I  J  D  L  I
F  O  H  D  Y  O  I  N  N  R  I  E  N
L  R  E  G  S  G  H  D  H  U  N  R  U
A  T  O  P  T  A  S  G  N  U  L  P  S
T  Y  D  A  L  U  P  E  N  T  H  U  E
N  V  U  E  A  T  N  A  V  R  U  S  N
I  P  R  O  V  E  N  T  I  L  J  I  P
```

AeroBid (2)	Exosurf	lungs (2)	Proventil
Alupent	INH	Marax (2)	Rifadin
Azmacort	inhaler	Maxair	Survanta
drug	Intal	Mucomyst	Tedral
epinephrine	Isuprel	oral	Theo-Dur

Transcription Guidelines

Semicolons and Colons

1. **Semicolons and independent clauses.** Use a semicolon to separate two independent clauses that are not joined by a conjunction such as *and, but, for, or, nor*, but are related in meaning. In this case the semicolon is taking the place of a period.

   Lungs are clear to auscultation; no rales or rhonchi are present.

2. **Semicolon with *however*.** If the word *however* separates two independent clauses, place a semicolon before *however* and a comma after it.

   The patient was very tired; however, he did not complain of weakness.

3. **Semicolons and commas.** Use a semicolon to separate main sections when the separate internal elements are already separated by commas.

   Heart: Regular rate and rhythm; no murmur, gallop, or rub; S1 and S2 normal.

4. **Colons and headings.** Use a colon after a heading, followed by a space.

   CHIEF COMPLAINT: Left-sided paralysis.

5. **Colons and lists.** When a complete sentence ends with the words *as follows* or *the following,* use a colon and then continue with the list or series that follows.

   His symptoms include all of the following: dyspnea on exertion, fatigue, and productive cough.

6. Do not use a colon between a verb and a list that follows.

   His symptoms include exertion, fatigue, and productive cough.

7. **Colons and ratios.** Use a colon to express a ratio (a mathematical expression showing the relationship of one part to another). Xylocaine 1:100,000 indicates that there is one part Xylocaine to 100,000 parts solution (normal saline in this case).

8. **Colons and time.** Use a colon to express hours and minutes, but do not use a colon with military time.

   The patient was admitted to the emergency department at 2:20 a.m.

   The patient was admitted at 1420.

Punctuation Exercise

Instructions: Identify errors in punctuation and capitalization in the following sentences, and correct them.

1. Vital signs Temperature 98.5 degrees decreased from yesterday pulse 86 respirations 14

2. The patient related numerous operations to include the following bronchoscopy appendectomy and tonsillectomy

3. The patient's complaints were nausea vomiting abdominal tenderness and weakness

4. The patient was admitted at 0400 and discharged the same day at 1500

5. His respirations remain labored however he continues to produce copious amounts of sputum

6. Palpation of the feet revealed no pulses present in the dorsalis pedis artery however the perfusion in the feet postoperatively appeared clinically better with some return of capillary refill and slight but significant warming of skin temperatures.

7. Cross-clamp time was 1 hour and 18 minutes cardiopulmonary bypass time 2 hours and 10 minutes lowest esophageal temperature was 24° C.

Proofreading Skills

Instructions: In the report below, circle the errors. Identify misspelled and missing medical and English words and incorrect punctuation, and write the correct words and punctuation in the numbered spaces opposite the text.

1	DISCHRAGE DIAGNOSES:
2	1. Right lower lobe pnewmonia.
3	2. COPD.
4	3. History of CHF.
5	4. Atrial arhythmia.
6	
7	ADMITTING H&P FINDINGS:
8	The patient is an 82-year-old hispanic male
9	who had increasing shortness of breathe and
10	weekness and weight lost and anorexia for
11	two or three days prior to admission. There
12	had been evidently no change in her medica-
13	tions. Phisical exam revealed temp to be 100°
14	pulse was 88. Coronary: regular rate and
15	rhythm. Lungs clear. Extremties without
16	edema.
17	
18	LAB ON ADMISSION: CBC white count
19	19,800 with 73 polys 15 bands 12 lymphs.
20	Hematocrit 39.8. Lytes were within normal
21	limmits. Chest xray showed some bluring of
22	the right costophrenick angel consistant with a
23	right lower lobe pneumonia. Further lab
24	showed a digoxin level of 1.2, theophylline
25	level of 30.4, quinidine level of 6.0.
26	
27	HOSPITAL COARSE: The patient was admit-
28	ted to the medicall floor. The theophylline
29	was witheld until levels droped into the
30	theraputic range. Quinidine was discontinued,
31	and the patient was changed to Verapamil. He
32	was noted to have occasional PVCs and
33	PACs. Subsequently he was noted to occa-
34	sionally have multifocal atrail tackycardia with
35	aberrency versus ocasional PVCs. LDH isoen-
36	zimes failed to show any evidence of myocor-
37	dial infartion. Serial cardiograms showed no
38	acute changes. Follow up chest x ray the day
39	before discharge faled to show any improve-
40	ment from admission, but the patient's clinical
41	status had improved to the point that dischrge
42	was felt to be safe.

1. DISCHARGE _____
2. _____
3. _____
4. _____
5. _____
6. _____
7. _____
8. _____
9. _____
10. _____
11. _____
12. _____
13. _____
14. _____
15. _____
16. _____
17. _____
18. _____
19. _____
20. _____
21. _____
22. _____
23. _____
24. _____
25. _____
26. _____
27. _____
28. _____
29. _____
30. _____
31. _____
32. _____
33. _____
34. _____
35. _____
36. _____
37. _____
38. _____
39. _____
40. _____
41. _____
42. _____

Transcription Tips

1. Memorize difficult-to-spell pulmonary terms:

   larynx (*not* larnyx)
   pharynx (*not* pharnyx)
   phlegm (starts with *ph*, has silent *g*—"flem")
   pneumonia (silent *p*)
   xiphoid (the initial *x* has a *z* sound)

2. The respiratory term *alveolar* refers to the alveoli in the lungs. *Alveolar* is also used to describe a ridge in the oral cavity and will be heard in dictation of the ears, nose, and throat.

3. Note the correct format for these terms relating to the patient's smoking history:

   a 50-pack-year history of smoking (meaning a pack a day for 50 years, or 2 packs a day for 25 years, etc.)
   smokes 2½ packs a day

4. Translate the slang term *trach* (tracheostomy) when it appears in dictation.

5. The unusual phrase *pulmonary toilet* refers to various measures such as postural drainage, percussion, and hydration to clear secretions from the respiratory tract.

6. Do not confuse *perfusion* (the amount of blood reaching a tissue) and *profusion* (present in abundance).

Terminology Challenge

Instructions: The following terms appear in the dictation on Tape 5B. Before beginning the medical transcription practice for Lesson 11, become familiar with the terminology below by looking up each word in a medical or English dictionary. Write out a short definition of each term.

1-second forced expiratory volume (FEV_1, FEV1)
22-gauge needle
A2
accessory respiratory muscles
adrenals
AFB (acid-fast bacilli)
Aldoril
Alupent
anteroposterior diameter
asbestos
bronchial brushings and washings
brochoscopy
bronchospasm
bronchovesicular breath sounds
Bronkometer
carbon black
cardiomegaly
carina
cautery
cavitary mass
coarse rhonchi
consolidative change (on chest x-ray)
cor
CT scan
cytology
diaphoresis
dyspnea
end-inspiratory wheeze
endobronchial
equivocal
expiratory
extrinsic
exudative
FEF_{25-75}, FEF25-75

fiberoptic
fibrosis
fine-needle aspiration
first tracheal ring
friable
FVC (forced vital capacity)
Gram stain
hilar
hyperreactivity
IgE antibody
Inderal
infiltrate
ligating
lobes of lung
longitudinally
main stem bronchi
main stem carina
mediastinum
metastasis, metastases
methacholine challenge
mucoid
nebulizer
nonproductive cough
noxious inhalants
orifice
P2
Panel A
percussion note
perfusion
pleural effusion
pleural friction rub
productive cough
promethazine
pulmonary function studies
radioallergosorbent test (RAST)
radiographs
reactive airway disease

Terminology Challenge *(cont.)*

refractory
respiratory excursions
serosanguineous
sibilant
small-cell carcinoma
SOB (shortness of breath)
space-occupying lesion
strap muscles
suprasternal notch
suture
    1-0 ("one-oh,"
     "one-zero")
  silk
tetracycline

Theo-Dur
thoracentesis
thorax
TDI (toluene di-isocya-
    nate)
tracheal hook
tracheostomy tube
tracheotomy
transverse
Vanceril
ventilatory and perfusion
    lung scan
vital capacity
well-differentiated lesion

Transcription Practice

After completing all the readings and exercises in Lesson 11, transcribe Tape 5B, Pulmonary Medicine. Use both medical and English dictionaries and your Quick-Reference Word List as resource materials for finding words.

Proofread your transcribed documents carefully, listening to the dictation while you read your transcripts.

Transcribe (*NOT* retype) the same reports again without referring to your previous transcription attempt. Initially, you may need to transcribe some reports more than twice before you can produce an error-free document. Your ultimate goal is to produce an error-free document the first time.

Sample Reports

Sample pulmonary medicine reports appear on the following pages, illustrating a variety of formats.

BLOOPERS

Incorrect	Correct
The patient complains of perineal asthma.	The patient complains of perennial asthma.
Atelectasis due to inspissated bugs.	Atelectasis due to inspissated plugs.
Pain in the chest aggravated by defreezing.	Pain in the chest aggravated by deep breathing.
Increasingly steep breath.	Increasingly deep breathing.

WILLIAM NEAL   #101091   DATE: 01/02/92   Attending: A. RODRIGUEZ, M.D.

PULMONARY MEDICINE CONSULTATION

This is a 32-year-old white male, lifelong nonsmoker, referred to me. He complains of a less than two-week history of dry cough associated with dull substernal discomfort and dyspnea particularly on exertion. Otherwise, he has been remarkably free of any other associated symptoms. In particular he denies any preceding cold or flu or allergic exposure. He denies any associated fevers, chills, sweats, or weight loss.

He admits to having childhood asthma, but felt he grew out of this by the time he was a teenager. He has traveled extensively outside the U.S., including travel to the California deserts and Central Valley. He has not had pneumonia vaccine. He had a TB skin test ten years ago and a flu vaccine three years ago.

PAST MEDICAL HISTORY is remarkably negative.

PHYSICAL EXAM: Blood pressure 140/80, pulse 85, respiratory rate 22, temperature 99.3. Chest exam is completely normal, with no rales, wheezes, rhonchi, or rubs. Even on forced exhalation, there was no cough or prolongation. Cardiac exam showed a regular rate and rhythm with no murmur or gallop.

LABORATORY DATA: PA chest x-ray is striking for a new interstitial infiltrate seen in both midlung zones with some shagging of the cardiac borders, indicating involvement of the lingula and right middle lobe. Surprisingly, the lowest part of the lung fields and the apices appear to be spared.

Spirometry before and after bronchodilator performed in my office shows a vital capacity of 3.79 or 69% after an 11% improvement with bronchodilator. FEV1 achieves 3.24 liters or 72% of predicted after 12% improvement with bronchodilator. FEV1/FVC ratio was mildly increased at 85 instead of predicted 82.

ASSESSMENT AND PLAN: Differential diagnosis includes the following:
1. Hypersensitivity pneumonitis.
2. Mycoplasmal pneumonia.
3. Less likely candidates appear to be Wegener's granulomatosis, Goodpasture's syndrome, sarcoidosis, alveolar proteinosis, and allergic bronchopulmonary aspergillosis.

RECOMMENDATIONS:
1. CBC with differential, chem-20, Wintrobe sed rate, angiotensin converting enzyme, urinalysis, and mycoplasmal titers.
2. Full pulmonary function tests within two weeks.
3. Vibramycin 100 mg q.d. for 14 days.

If he still has significant symptoms and restriction on PFTs within two weeks, he will have to be evaluated for one of the more chronic diagnoses, which may ultimately require open lung biopsy. Otherwise, we should hope that within two weeks the patient will be improved and his x-ray will have cleared.

EDWARD X. HALE, M.D.

EXH:hpi
d&t: 01/02/92

CHART NOTE

SARAH ANNA RATLEY   12/12/92

Symptoms of recurrent episodes of coughing and wheezing. She has never had a hospitalization, but her major symptom of asthma requires daily therapy with inhaled bronchodilator. She
is much better using a Pulmo-Aide with inhalations of Alupent and atropine and Intal than she
is in using the hand-held nebulizers. First, atropine is not available for the metered-dose
inhalers, and secondly, the medication as delivered by the Pulmo-Aide is much more effective
because of a better delivery system. I had prescribed this some time ago and believe that she
will continue to need this on a permanent basis.

EXH:hpi

CHART NOTE

RITA GOLDEN   12/12/92

The patient was seen in my office for skin testing, and all of her skin tests have turned out to
be negative. It is my impression, therefore, that she has intrinsic asthma. I have seen her for
several visits. Since her last visit to my office, I attempted to get her off steroids, but she
prefers the use of long-term, every-other-day prednisone in an attempt to decrease her costs for
other medications. She understands all of the risks of steroids, and I am reluctantly agreeable to
go along with this. At the present time she is taking Theo-Dur 750 mg per day, Ventolin 2 mg
t.i.d., prednisone 10 mg every other day, Azmacort, and Vancenase, and I have recently added
IsoClor b.i.d.

_____
EDWARD X. HALE, M.D.

EXH:hpi

LESLIE HALL   #082741   06/25/93   Attending: J. Smith, M.D.

EMERGENCY DEPARTMENT REPORT

HISTORY OF PRESENT ILLNESS: The patient is a one-year-old female that has been congested for several days. The child has sounded hoarse, has had a croupy cough, and was seen by Dr. Smith two days ago. Since that time, she has been on Alupent breathing treatments via machine, amoxicillin, Ventolin, cough syrup, and Slo-bid 100 mg b.i.d., but is not improving. Today the child is not taking food or fluids, has been unable to rest, and has been struggling in her respirations.

PHYSICAL EXAM showed an alert child in moderate respiratory distress.
VITAL SIGNS: Respiratory rate was 40, pulse 120, temperature 99.6.
HEENT within normal limits.
NECK: Positive for mild to moderate stridor.
CHEST showed a diffuse inspiratory and expiratory wheezing. No rales were noted.
HEART: Regular rhythm without murmur, gallop, or rub.
ABDOMEN: Soft, nontender; bowel sounds normal.
EXTREMITIES within normal limits.

In viewing the chest wall, the patient had subcostal and intercostal retractions. The child was sent for a PA and lateral chest x-ray to rule out pneumonia. No pneumonia was seen on the films. It was agreed to admit the patient to the pediatric unit for placement in a croup tent with respiratory therapy treatments q.3h. The child was also placed on Decadron besides the amoxicillin and continuation of the Slo-bid.

EMERGENCY DEPARTMENT DIAGNOSIS:
1. Acute laryngotracheal bronchitis.
2. Bronchial asthma.

_____

S. ALDARONDO, M.D.

SA:hpi
d&t:6/25/93

Name: GEORGE HOWARD   Date: 01/02/93

Procedure: FIBEROPTIC BRONCHOSCOPY

Bronchoscopist: HANS GRABGELD, M.D.

Indications: WORSENING PULMONARY INFILTRATES IN A FEBRILE PATIENT,
UNKNOWN ETIOLOGY, RULE OUT RESISTANT NOSOCOMIAL
PNEUMONIA

Premedication: Versed 1 mg IV

Anesthesia: 1% topical Xylocaine, total of 30 cc

Instrument: OLYMPUS BFP10 BRONCHOSCOPE

PROCEDURE: After informed consent was obtained from the patient's mother and appropriate premedication, the bronchoscope was inserted directly through the tracheostomy tube while the patient contined to receive oxygen supplementation. The lower trachea and tracheobronchial tree were then fully examined in this fashion. There was very severe, intense tracheobronchitis noted with very friable mucosa. Patchy areas of denudation of the mucosa were also noted, particularly along the right lateral wall. The main carina was sharp and in the midline. The right and left bronchial trees showed the same diffuse erythematous changes, but no purulence and no endobronchial abnormalities. Bronchial washings were obtained from throughout the tracheobronchial tree and submitted for Gram stain, routine acid-fast bacilli, fungal smears and cultures, and cytologic review. The instrument was then removed, and the procedure terminated. No complications were encountered.

DIAGNOSTIC IMPRESSION: SEVERE TRACHEOBRONCHITIS.

HG:hpi   **PROCEDURE REPORT**   HANS GRABGELD, M.D.
D: 01/02/93
T: 01/02/93

                                                HOWARD, GEORGE

            PARADISE HOSPITAL   ROOM 301-B
            Paradise Valley, Arizona   MPI 24-99-71

Lesson 12. Endocrinology

Learning Objectives

Medical

- Describe areas examined or inspected by the physician in the General Appearance section of the H&P.
- Describe the function and location of five endocrine glands.
- Describe how insulin and antidiabetic pills differ in their therapeutic action in reating diabetes mellitus.
- Discuss the purpose and technique involved in performing common endocrine laboratory tests and surgical procedures.
- Given an endocrine root word, symptom, or disease, match it to its correct medical definition.
- Given a cross-section illustrating the endocrine system, memorize the anatomic structures.
- Define common endocrine abbreviations.

Fundamentals

- Demonstrate the correct use of numbers in editing medical sentences.
- Given a medical report with errors, identify and correct the errors.

Practice

- Accurately transcribe authentic physician dictation from the specialty of endocrinology.

A Closer Look

Fat Chance

by Judith Marshall, MA, CMT

It really all started the night my husband put his arm around me and told me I was as cute as a baby Clydesdale. Then he reminisced about his youth and romantic adventures, recalling fondly that he loved going out with big women because "fat women are so grateful." I had another male saboteur on my hands. The myth had caught up with me. I had been brought up to believe that men would take care of me. First my father, then husband, and always and forever, the doctor.

My health was in my doctor's hands through pregnancy ("Now you can eat for two!"); minor health complaints ("If you are tired and can't sleep, have some Valium, take up bridge, do volunteer work; dye your hair, buy a new dress, stop dwelling on yourself"); and menopause ("Menopause is a consideration but don't worry. In a few years you'll dry up and that will be that!").

It must have been a neurotic need for punishment which drew me back to him for help with weight control. He listened to me intently and solicitously patted my hand. His voice sounded like dry leaves scraping against a sidewalk. "Diet and exercise, my dear. What is it you, ah, do for a living?" I reminded him that I work full time as a medical transcriptionist. He gave me that constipated smile of his and nodded sagely. "Yes, I have a young girl who does my work for me at home. A mother, you know. Has the child in the playpen beside her. It's wonderful. She's managed to learn all **my** words."

As I sat there, I knew I made him uncomfortable. To him I represented failure. There was nothing he could bandage, splint, or remove surgically (never mind suction lipectomy). Worse, I was a medical transcriptionist who knew the lingo and wanted answers. There were no pills, no ointments to be dispensed. He had nothing to offer except his contempt.

The last I heard they had already built the great railroads out West so I couldn't join a labor gang. I had a career anyway, one which burned about 250 calories a day if I counted picking up *Gray's Anatomy*, several brisk hikes to the copy machine, and rifling through the *PDR*. I was no longer just an endomorph. I *WAS* Jaba the Hutt. My fat cells were indestructible, like cockroaches constantly evolving to meet any chemical challenge to their extinction, and surviving, always surviving.

Why couldn't I lose weight on 1000 calories a day? Why was I so ravenously hungry? Why, after forty, was it so hard to lose even a pound and why were my hips pulling downward to my ankles? Should I take up smoking again? I lost time, I lost money, I lost my temper, I lost my nerve, I lost face, and I even lost teeth. Why couldn't I lose weight?

I had so many risk factors I should have been dead at thirty-five. Time was running out. I had just sustained an eight-pound gain on a weekend in Cleveland (Slovenian-style pork roast and Rudy's fresh kielbasa with homemade dumplings). My porcine proportions yearned for a glimpse of the physiology of anorexia nervosa and bulimia. I would no longer be called the Sow City Wrangler at the square dances on Thursday night. I would take the fat out of femme fatale.

If the medicine man had failed me, I would hot-foot it to the best qualified female internist in Boston. This physician would understand my problems. She would be a nutritional Whiz Kid, a Phi Beta Kappa of calories. With great trepidation and after pinning my clothes together (the buttons had popped), I visited the doctor. Her tiny frame was sheathed in a size six designer dress in a bold brown check, and she wore a heavy, expensive gold chunky bracelet around her neck. She was about thirty years old. After a thorough review, examination, and blood work, she peered at me across the desk and said, "You simply follow this 1200-calorie diet and stop noshing between meals. See you in six months and you should be ten pounds lighter by then." She looked pointedly at her watch.

Lordy, lordy, nothing had changed. The lard continued to expand. I began to transcribe frenetically. I never could eat and type at the same time. Besides, we are not allowed food in the work area, so I worked a lot of overtime. The diet the doctor had given me was preprinted and not realistic—unless you had someone to do the food shopping, then prepare all the meals three times a day plus snacks, then lock it all up in the garage for the night. The doctors' battle to fight obesity is so monumentally time-consuming and frustrating, no wonder they just hand out a form diet.

Obesity, of course, is a uniquely female problem in a world that took centuries to recognize premenstrual syndrome. (Now it's trendy. We have a PMS clinic in the neighborhood, for heaven's sake.) I insinuated myself into a cluster of doctors at a cocktail party and whispered, "Female, fat, and forty," just to see them recoil in horror.

I had been told by doctors that I had no will power, that I was secretly bingeing. My one experience with diet pills led me to try to fly by jumping off the Massachusetts General Hospital. Reading diet books took no fat off me but padded the wallets of the authors. Watching Jane Fonda's exercise tape sunk me into a deep depression.

The language of food, cookbooks, and restaurant critic columns holds more prurient interest for me than pornography. I could even salivate over a well-written history, the doctor recounting the patient's daily dietary habits. My transcription, however, was suffering. I typed that the patient with pneumonia had "congested lunches" and that an asthmatic patient was to be "weighed off from steroids on a tapering basis."

Desperate and disgusted, seeking supernatural cures, I waddled into a weight loss clinic. They listened to me as if the most important thing in the world was my weight problem. Without pills, shots, packaged foods, or gimmicks, I am on a 500-calorie diet. I am walking three miles a day and dancing six hours a week. Richard Simmons, eat your heart out. A program of behavior modification and fat restriction gave me a lipid profile and a blood pressure reminiscent of my salad days.

It's not perfect. I hate going there five days a week. The nurses are all gorgeous, tall and willowy. The closest any of them ever came to cholesterol was walking through a field of buttercups. They keep meticulous records. "Going fishing again? Watch yourself. You always tend to drink beer when you go fishing." Some of them don't have to say anything to make me feel guilty. They just stand there, looking like my mother. But this time I am paying for feeling guilty. Mother did it for nothing.

My doctor thinks the clinic is owned and run by charlatans, that the program is unhealthy, that the weight loss is too fast. My doctor warned me that when I finish this ridiculous and dangerous program, I will put every single pound back on and then some.

Fat chance, doc.

Whining and Dining

by Judith Marshall, MA, CMT

About five years ago, I wrote a column entitled "Fat Chance" in which I was truly obnoxious, hooting about a spectacular weight loss achievement. I was convinced I would never gain any of it back.

Pass the humble pie. As soon as I quit starving and square dancing, it was do-si-do into old bad habits. All of my recipes were marked, "Serves six, or two if they are Marshalls." If my professional organization charged people like me by the pound, there would be no dues increase. They could add a wing onto their building. But how could someone as smart as me evidently not know how to eat?

LOW FAT DIET AND EXERCISE is the answer to permanent weight control. Why are we spending millions of dollars in the diet industry? I have paid people to starve me, brainwash me, exercise me, puncture me, humiliate me, and weigh and measure me like a piece of pork (they probably thought so, too). And that was just the diet merchants, not the gyms and salons. I bought an exercise bike that tells me my pulse, blood pressure, rate of speed, and even croaks encouragement in a hoarse staccato computer voice—you can do it, you can do it, you can do it.

I have done it. I keep doing it. Veterans of fat wars have chomped through it all. Lose 70, put back 50, lose 50, put back 90. If the equation is fat equals stupid, take me to the head of the class. How easy to rationalize that large sizes are okay but my tired frame with small bones was never meant to carry more than 120 pounds. Once again, in my new environment in the Northeast Kingdom, I searched for thinness.

Overeaters Anonymous was too religious for me, an amorphous cosmic pantheism. The pressure of self-disclosure was too great. In Vermont, where the cows outnumber the people, can anyone be anonymous?

After the OA meeting, a woman turned to me and asked, "What was your name again? I would hate to be telling all this personal stuff to someone I didn't know."

Weight Watchers, it seemed to me, spent all their time shopping for food, weighing, measuring, discussing, eating and counting, filling out forms, and having a whale of a good time. How much money do they spend on gorgeous television commercials to sell food—and does the corporation really care if people lose weight or if people buy their prepackaged food?

My twin devils are time and boredom. The only thing left in my narrow vision was Optifast. And the only thing narrow about me was my vision. An enormous weight loss in three months of fasting, and the team approach (physician, psychologist, and dietitian) were all very appealing. The cost was nearly $3000 and cleverly charged in upside-down pyramid fashion. I lasted five weeks.

The team members were all young and very thin. They were extremely maternalistic with the women and deferential to the men. It was truly difficult not to laugh when they passed out official-looking wallet cards with a red cross symbol, saying that if we fainted with hunger in an airport, we were somehow to produce this card and be revived by three ounces of lean chicken. The silly talk and har-de-har-har joviality were at first annoying, then depressing. One man suggested the first night we all go down to one of those places that serves all you can eat and pig out, as he delicately put it, and wouldn't that give the waitresses a fit to see us all coming.

If the others thought fat grams arrived via Western Union or varicella was a pasta, I didn't stick around long enough to know. I was surprised and disgusted by the lemming-like eagerness of the women, and the men as well, to divulge personal details of their lives that God knows were interesting only to them. The various revelations of what passed through their digestive tracts and how it reached its final destination would make a gastroenterologist blush.

The psychologist was young and eager but fell short of the mark on life experience or even group leadership experience and any deviation from the week's outline caused her great agitation.

What we were drinking was always referred to as The Product (reverential tone and genuflection), while I squirmed in my plastic chair and wondered how high the drug company shares were climbing.

Being pent up in that ship of fools was bad enough but when one fiftyish business executive lyrically discussed his bout of influenza and his consequent hunger and craving for the comfort of a soft-boiled egg, I was ready to bolt. Instead of just eating the darn egg and having some juice and a lie-down, this fellow had been trained so well by the Fatspeak program, he called the office and spoke to a *secretary,* who told him to drink hot tea. And he did. Like a good little boy.

Folks, I don't know what the answer is. I only know what it isn't. For me. For now. I thought a women's group experience (I had not expected the men) would help us to deal with anger, depression, and self-hatred. I thought we could transcend talk about junk food. I thought we would discuss sexuality and life changes and not just regurgitate what some smart ad executive wrote up in the manual.

I agree with something Barbara Edelstein, M.D., wrote many years ago in *The Woman Doctor's Diet for Women*. "My feeling is that the overweight female responds best to a one-to-one relationship where you can challenge her, refute her without embarrassing her, and compel her to come to grips with herself, her own tricks and evasions."

So what am I eating and what's really eating me? I am nibbling back to the basics. Low fat, low calorie diet, and moderate exercise, for which I will pay no one. Many women volunteered to talk to me about their dieting successes. I rejoice with them while mourning my own perceived failure. Perhaps I will find a therapist who does not take my problem lightly. As for my dollars perpetuating the bloated diet industry, well, I am just fed up.

Medical Readings

The History and Physical Examination

by John H. Dirckx, M.D.

General Appearance. The physical examination report usually begins with a description of the patient's general appearance.

The general features noted by the diagnostician in performing a physical examination include body build (muscular development, proportions, skeletal deformities), nutritional status, apparent age and general state of health, skin color (pallor, cyanosis, jaundice), alertness and responsiveness, mood, posture, gait, mobility, grooming and personal hygiene, quality and clarity of voice and speech, evidence of distress (dyspnea, signs of pain or anxiety), abnormal odors of breath or body, and any other readily observable abnormalities (facial scars, absence of a limb).

Some of these features are evident merely on inspection, some require more elaborate techniques, perhaps involving the collaboration of the patient, and some depend on inference. Although the physician's appraisal of a patient's general condition is often reduced to a formula in the physical examination report, it is safe to say that in most cases a number of unrecorded and perhaps not consciously noticed impressions and clues contribute to his overall diagnostic conclusions.

A comparison of the patient's stated age with his apparent age provides a broad general notion of his lifestyle, state of nutrition, and general medical condition. Obesity can be quantified to some extent by measurement of skin folds at selected standard sites with a caliper. Facial expression, speech, and manner offer clues to the patient's mental state as well as to the integrity of his central nervous system. Some of the physician's observations and conclusions about alertness, orientation, and emotional equilibrium will go into the record of the psychiatric (mental status) examination, if one is made.

The patient's body posture, stance, mobility, and gait are of particular interest during the orthopedic and neurologic examinations, but gross abnormalities such as hemiparesis, spinal rigidity, tremors, or a shuffling or staggering gait will be noted as part of the general appearance.

Laboratory Medicine: The Endocrine Glands

Endocrine glands are those that release their secretions, called hormones, directly into the circulation. Arriving at its target (or end) organ, a hormone exerts some stimulant (occasionally suppressant) action on a specific type of cell or tissue. The chief importance of diseases of the endocrine glands lies in the effect they can have on the level of hormones in the circulation.

Degenerative or destructive lesions of a gland may lead to a deficiency of its hormone, while functioning neoplasms of glandular tissue often produce excessive levels of hormone.

There are five anatomically discrete endocrine glands—the pituitary gland, the thyroid gland, the parathyroid glands, the adrenal glands, and the pineal gland.

Pituitary gland. The pituitary gland, also called the hypophysis, is situated beneath the brain in a bony receptacle on the floor of the skull called the sella turcica. It consists of two entirely distinct masses of tissue: the posterior lobe and the anterior lobe. The **posterior lobe** or neurohypophysis produces oxytocin which stimulates the contraction of the uterine muscle during labor, and vasopressin or antidiuretic hormone (ADH) which promotes reabsorption of water in the renal tubules.

The **anterior lobe** of the pituitary gland produces growth hormone and prolactin (a hormone involved in lactation), thyroid stimulating hormone (TSH), adreno-corticotropic hormone (ACTH), follicle-stimulating hormone (FSH), and luteinizing hormone, LH.

Thyroid gland. The thyroid gland is a flattened, shield-shaped structure incompletely divided into right and left lobes and situated in the front of the neck just above the breastbone. Thyroxine, the principal hormonal secretion of the gland, regulates tissue metabolism.

Thyroid tissue can be obtained for study by needle biopsy, but most specimens consist of whole glands or lobes removed for the treatment of thyroid hyperfunction or malignancy.

Deficiency of thyroid hormone (hypothyroidism) beginning before or shortly after birth causes cretinism. When thyroid deficiency begins later in life, the result is myxedema. In this condition the pulse and blood pressure are low, the skin coarse and dry, the hair thinned, the face and hands puffy, speech hoarse, slow, and slurred, mental functioning retarded, gonadal function impaired, and serum cholesterol elevated.

Hyperthyroidism (hyperactive thyroid), also known as Graves' disease, causes symptoms of weight loss, nervousness, and exophthalmos (bulging of the eyes). In hyperthyroidism the heart becomes dilated, flabby, and pale. In adulthood the commonest causes of myxedema are surgical removal of the thyroid gland and drug treatment of an overactive thyroid gland.

Parathyroid glands. Attached to the thyroid capsule but structurally distinct from the thyroid gland are the four parathyroid glands. The secretion of the parathyroid gland, parathormone, regulates calcium and phosphorus metabolism by increasing the reabsorption of calcium in the renal tubules, decreasing the reabsorption of phosphorus, and mobilizing calcium from bone.

Adrenal glands. The adrenal glands are paired, one being situated atop each kidney. The cortex contains cords of cells that produce cortisol for the regulation of carbohydrate and protein metabolism, aldosterone for the control of electrolyte (sodium and potassium) balance, and androgen, which affects the growth of body and facial hair. The adrenal medulla produces epinephrine (adrenalin).

Pineal gland. The pineal gland or epiphysis is a cone-shaped body less than 1 cm in greatest dimension, which is attached by a stalk to the roof of the third ventricle of the brain. Its principal secretion, the hormone melatonin, apparently plays a role in sexual maturation and in maintenance of diurnal bodily rhythms.

Pineal neoplasms occur typically before age 25 and are more frequent in males. The rare teratoma of the pineal may be associated with precocious sexual development.

Pharmacology: Endocrine Drugs

The endocrine system consists of many glands which secrete hormones into the bloodstream. Those of major importance in drug therapy include the thyroid gland which secretes thyroxine (T_4) and triiodothyronine (T_3); the pituitary gland which secretes growth hormone and vasopressin; and the adrenal gland whose cortex secretes aldosterone and corticosteroids. When these glands malfunction due to disease processes, they may release either a decreased or increased level of hormone. Drugs may then be given either as supplements to normalize hormone levels or to counteract increased hormone levels.

Thyroid gland drugs. Thyroid supplements are used to treat hypothyroidism. These drugs are obtained from natural sources such as desiccated (dried) ground animal thyroid glands or may be synthetically manufactured.

These thyroid supplements contain T_3 and T_4:
> desiccated thyroid
> liotrix (Euthroid, Thyrolar)
> thyroglobulin (Proloid)

The supplement liothyronine (Cytomel) contains only T_3. The supplement levothyroxine (Synthroid) contains only T_4.

Drugs used to treat hyperthyroidism act by inhibiting the production of T_3 and T_4 in the thyroid gland. Hyperthyroid drugs include:
> propylthiouracil
> methimazole (Tapazole)
> radioactive sodium iodide 131

Pituitary gland drugs. The pituitary gland secretes growth hormone. Decreased levels of this hormone inhibit skeletal growth in children. Drugs used as replacement therapy include:
> somatrem (Protropin)
> somatropin (Humatrope)

The pituitary gland also secretes vasopressin which

inhibits the excretion of water by the kidneys. Vasopressin is also known as ADH or antidiuretic hormone because of its action as described. A lack of ADH results in diabetes insipidus. Drugs used as replacement therapy include:

> desmopressin (DDAVP)
> lypressin (Diapid)
> vasopressin (Pitressin)

Adrenal gland drugs. The adrenal gland secretes many hormones, but one of particular interest which exhibits low levels due to the disease process of Addison disease is that of aldosterone. Drugs used as replacement therapy include:

> desoxycorticosterone (Percorten)
> fludrocortisone (Florinef)

The adrenal cortex also secretes hydrocortisone and cortisone, powerful anti-inflammatory hormones. These and other synthetic anti-inflammatory agents are known as corticosteroids. They are commonly prescribed to systemically inhibit inflammatory reactions throughout the body. These oral corticosteroid drugs include:

> betamethasone (Celestone)
> cortisone
> dexamethasone (Decadron)
> hydrocortisone (Cortef, Hydrocortone,
>   Solu-Cortef)
> methylprednisolone (Depo-Medrol, Medrol,
>   Solu-Medrol)
> paramethasone (Haldrone)
> prednisolone (Delta-Cortef)
> prednisone (Deltasone)
> triamcinolone (Aristocort, Kenacort, Kenalog)

Antidiabetic drugs. Diabetes mellitus results when the pancreas fails to produce any insulin (type I diabetes mellitus) or produces too little (type II diabetes mellitus). Type I diabetes mellitus is also known as insulin-dependent diabetes mellitus or juvenile-onset diabetes mellitus. Type II diabetes mellitus is also known as non-insulin-dependent diabetes mellitus or adult-onset diabetes mellitus. Type I must always be treated with subcutaneously injected insulin; type II may be treated with insulin or, more commonly, with diet and/or oral antidiabetic drugs.

Insulin is secreted by beta cells in the islets of Langerhans in the pancreas. This hormone plays an essential role in sugar metabolism. Insulin is derived from beef or pork pancreas or from human insulin (which overcomes the potential for allergic reactions). Human insulin is genetically produced using recombinant DNA techniques.

Regardless of the original source, all insulins are classified according to how quickly they act (which depends on the size of the insulin crystal) and how many hours their therapeutic action continues (which is lengthened by the addition of protamine).

Rapid-acting insulins include:

> regular (Regular Iletin, Humulin BR,
>   Humulin R, Novolin R, Velosulin)
> semilente (Semilente Iletin)

Intermediate-acting insulins include:

> NPH (NPH Iletin, Humulin N, Insulatard
>   NPH, Novolin N)
> lente (Lente Iletin, Humulin L, Novolin L)

Long-acting insulins include:

> protamine zinc (PZI)
> ultralente (Ultralente Iletin, Humulin U)

Mixtures of 70% NPH and 30% regular insulin are also available as:

> Humulin 70/30
> Mixtard 70/30
> Novolin 70/30

Note: The trade name for all human genetically produced insulins is Humulin.

Insulin is given subcutaneously once or twice a day at various sites on the arms, thighs, or abdomen. It can also be administered directly into the bloodstream by an implantable computerized insulin pump. Insulin dosages are always measured in units.

Oral antidiabetic agents. A patient with type II diabetes mellitus has a pancreas which is still producing limited amounts of insulin. With diet control and weight loss, this amount of insulin may be sufficient. If not, an oral antidiabetic agent may be ordered.

Contrary to popular opinion, oral antidiabetic agents are not insulin but act to stimulate the pancreas to produce more insulin. Oral antidiabetic agents are not effective for a patient with type I diabetes mellitus whose pancreas no longer produces any insulin.

Oral antidiabetic agents include:

> chlorpropamide (Diabinese)
> glipizide (Glucotrol)
> glyburide (Diaßeta, Micronase)

Laboratory Tests and Surgical Procedures

17-ketosteroids   Urinary breakdown products of adrenal cortical hormones, increased in certain disorders of the adrenal gland.

acetone, urinary   Acetone in urine can be measured with a dipstick. Small amounts are found in starvation and other abnormal metabolic states, larger amounts in uncontrolled diabetes mellitus.

blood sugar   The level of glucose in the blood.

Chemstrip bG   A dipstick used to measure blood glucose.

Clinistix   A dipstick used to measure urine glucose.

Dextrostix   A dipstick used to measure blood glucose.

fasting blood sugar (FBS)   Determination of serum glucose in a specimen drawn from a patient who has been fasting for several hours, usually overnight.

glucose tolerance curve   A curve plotted on graph paper from measurements of blood sugar made at various intervals after ingestion of a standardized carbohydrate meal. Distinctive abnormalities are seen in diabetes mellitus, hyperinsulinism, and malabsorption.

glucose tolerance test (GTT)   Same as *glucose tolerance curve*.

glucose, urinary   Usually detected with a dipstick, any amount of glucose in the urine is abnormal and ordinarily indicates an abnormally high blood sugar, as in diabetes mellitus.

glycosylated hemoglobin   A measurement of the amount of glucose bound to the hemoglobin of red blood cells, useful in monitoring the long-term control of diabetes mellitus.

GTT (glucose tolerance test).

ketones, serum   A group of waste products resulting from abnormal metabolism of fat in uncontrolled diabetes. Normally ketones cannot be detected in the serum. Elevation is associated with the condition of diabetic acidosis or ketoacidosis, also called diabetic coma when unconsciousness occurs. Ketones may be called ketone bodies, or the term *acetone* (the principal serum ketone) may be applied to ketones in general.

T3, T_3 (triiodothyronine)   Thyroid hormone.

T4, T_4 (thyroxine)   Thyroid hormone.

TFTs (thyroid function tests)   T3, T4, and TSH.

thyroidectomy   Surgical removal of the thyroid gland as a treatment for hyperthyroidism.

thyroid-stimulating hormone (TSH)   A hormone secreted by the anterior pituitary gland that stimulates the thyroid gland and promotes its normal function.

thyroxine   Principal hormone of the thyroid gland. Also called T_4.

Visidex II   A dipstick used to determine blood glucose.

Anatomy/Medical Terminology

Medical Terminology Matching Exercise

Complete the following matching exercise to test your knowledge of the word roots, anatomic structures, symptoms, and disease processes encountered in the medical specialty of endocrinology.

Instructions: Match the term in Column A with its definition in Column B.

Column A	Column B
A. thyroxine	____ oral antidiabetic drug
B. parathyroid gland	____ secreted by the adrenal cortex
C. Diabinese	
D. islets of Langerhans	____ female hormone
	____ insulin-dependent
E. Graves' disease	____ a thyroid hormone
F. estrogen	____ non-insulin-dependent
G. Humulin	____ male hormone
H. corticosteroids	____ enlarged thyroid
I. diabetes mellitus, type I	____ thyroid supplement
	____ regulates serum calcium levels
J. androgen	
K. goiter	____ hyperthyroidism
L. diabetes mellitus, type II	____ antidiabetic injection
	____ produce insulin
M. Synthroid	

Anatomy: The Endocrine Glands

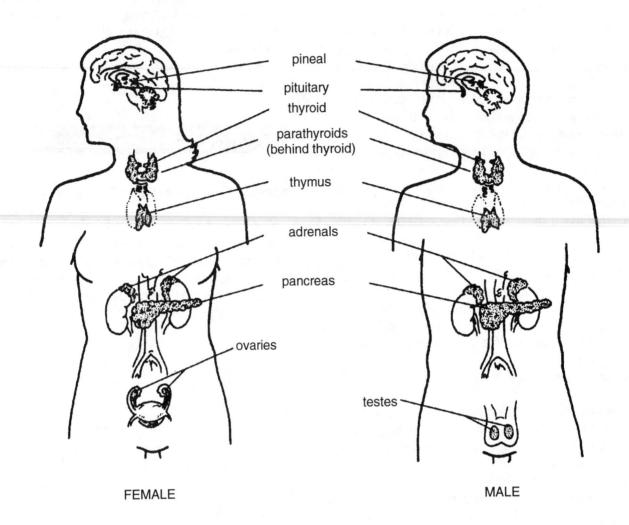

FEMALE   MALE

Abbreviations Exercise

Common abbreviations dictated in the body of a medical report may be transcribed as dictated. Uncommon abbreviations must be spelled out, with the abbreviation appearing in parentheses after the translation. All abbreviations (except laboratory test names) must be spelled out in the Diagnosis or Impression section of any report.

   Instructions: Define the following endocrine abbreviations. Then memorize both abbreviations and definitions to increase your speed and accuracy in transcribing dictation from endocrinology.

ADA   _____

AODM   _____

FBS   _____

GTT   _____

IDDM   _____

NIDDM   _____

OGTT   _____

TFT   _____

TSH   _____

Transcription Guidelines

Numbers

1. **Roman numerals.** Roman numerals are rarely used in technical medical reports. Some notable uses, however, are the following:

cancer stages	stages I through IV
cranial nerves	II through XII
EKG limb leads	I through III
factor	factor VIII (blood clotting)
type	diabetes mellitus, type II

2. **Arabic numerals.** Technical medical reports generally use arabic numerals rather than words to express numbers with greater precision and accuracy.

3. **Numbers and dates.** Arabic numerals are used to express dates, and a comma pair is used to set off a date in the month/day/year format (June 15, 1993) within a sentence. If the date is presented in the day/month/year format (15 June 1993), a comma pair is not needed. Although the date *May 3* is pronounced *May third*, it is not acceptable to type *May 3rd, 1993*.

She is scheduled for surgery on June 15, 1993, at Valley General Hospital.
She is scheduled for surgery on 15 June 1993.

4. **Numbers and age.** Arabic numerals are used for all ages. Hyphenate the age when it appears before the noun it modifies. Do not hyphenate an age that appears after the noun it modifies. Spell out terms which do not give a precise age.

The patient is a 36-year-old white male.
The patient is 36 years old.
She is in her early twenties.

Tip: When *years* is used instead of *year*, a hyphen is not used.

5. **Numbers and time.** Measures of time such as *years, months, weeks, days, hours, minutes,* and *seconds* take arabic numerals. Use a colon to express hours and minutes, but do not use a colon or *a.m.* and *p.m.* with military time.

The patient was admitted to the emergency department at 2:20 a.m.
The patient was admitted at 1420.
The needle was inserted at the 4 o'clock position.

6:15 a.m.	0615
6:15 p.m.	1815

6. Use only whole numbers when the time is followed by *o'clock.*

6 o'clock	a 2 o'clock incision

7. **Numbers and temperature.** After a patient's temperature, you may type either a degree sign or the word *degrees.* It is also acceptable to type only the numerical value. If the physician dictates *Fahrenheit* or *centigrade,* you may spell it out if you spell out the word *degrees.* If you use the degree sign, you must abbreviate *Fahrenheit* as *F* and *centigrade* as *C.* Do not place a space between the numeral, the degree sign, and the letter *F* or *C.*

Temperature 98.4.
Temperature 98.4°.
Temperature 98.4 degrees.
Temperature 98.4 degrees Fahrenheit.
Temperature 98.4°F.
Temperature 37.5 degrees centigrade.
Temperature 37.5°C.

Numbers Exercise

Instructions: Circle the correct term from the items in parentheses in the following sentences.

1. Patients in their early (40s, forties) should begin annual mammograms.

2. This (6 year old, 6-year-old) boy appears healthy but his sister who is (3 years old, 3-years-old) appears malnourished.

3. The patient spiked a temperature to 103 (degrees F, °Fahrenheit, °F) and was given ampicillin.

4. If you come in at 3:00 (p.m., o'clock), the doctor will see you.

5. Her next appointment is for May (10, 10th, tenth) at 10:15.

Proofreading Skills

Instructions: In the paragraphs below, circle the errors. Identify misspelled and missing medical and English words and punctuation errors. Write the correct words and punctuation in the numbered spaces opposite the text.

1	This 67 year old male was evaluated in the	1. 67-year-old female
2	emergency departmt at approximately 06:30	2. _____
3	hours for complains of repeeted episodes of	3. _____
4	vomiting, numberign at least 5 during the	4. _____
5	preceeding 8 or so hours.	5. _____
6		6. _____
7	She is a known diabetes and has taken	7. _____
8	fingerstick reedings of 423 and 241 at home.	8. _____
9	She is on multiple medication including	9. _____
10	Regular Insulin 10 units in the a.m., along	10. _____
11	with Ultralente 16 units at h.s. She also ad-	11. _____
12	mits to some chest pane, somehwat burning in	12. _____
13	nature, without radiation into her fase, neck,	13. _____
14	or arms. There is no history of diarhea. She	14. _____
15	has a previous history of coranary artery	15. _____
16	bypas sugrery some 4 years earlier.	16. _____
17		17. _____
18	PHISICAL ASSESMENT reveals her temp to	18. _____
19	be 98.2 pluse 60 respirations 20 and bloood	19. _____
20	pressure 102/50. Initialy her color was pale.	20. _____
21	Her mucus membranes did appear dry. Her	21. _____
22	hart rate was regular without murmurs. There	22. _____
23	was a well healed cikatrix to the anterior	23. _____
24	midsternial region. Lungs were clear to	24. _____
25	ausculation. The abdomin was soft with	25. _____
26	generalizd tenderness. No unusual pulsating	26. _____
27	masses. Lower extremties are free of any	27. _____
28	pretibial edema.	28. _____
29		29. _____
30	IMPRESSION:	30. _____
31	1. Diabetes melitus, out of control.	31. _____
32	2. Dehydration.	32. _____
33	3. Electrolyte balance.	33. _____

Terminology Challenge

Instructions: The following terms appear in the dictation on Tape 6A, Endocrinology. Before beginning the medical transcription practice for Lesson 12, become familiar with the terminology by looking up each term in a medical or English dictionary. Write a short definition of each word.

ACE inhibitors (angiotensin converting enzyme)
Addison's disease
adenoma
  follicular
  Hürthle cell
androgen level
bibasilar
cold nodule
congenital
Cortef
cortisone acetate
Cytomel
Diaßeta, DiaBeta
diabetes mellitus
  type I, type II
diaphoresis
discoid atelectasis
Dyazide
emesis
escutcheon
euthyroid
exophthalmos
extraocular movements
ferrous sulfate
fine-needle aspiration
Florinef Acetate
furosemide
goiter
  colloid
  nontoxic

Graves' disease
Humulin insulin
hyperkalemia
hyperthyroid
hypoglycemia
hypothyroidism
I.M., IM
Inderal
Kayexalate
lobectomy
metabolic acidosis
oral hypoglycemic agent
periareolar
pneumonitis
prerenal azotemia
PTU
Quinidex Extentabs
sodium bicarbonate
Solu-Cortef
surgical staples
Synthroid
tetracycline
thyroid function test
  T3
  T4
  TSH
thyroidectomy
Ultralente insulin
uptake scan
Vasotec

Sample Reports

Sample endocrinology reports appear on the following pages.

Transcription Practice

After completing all the readings and exercises in Lesson 12, transcribe Tape 6A, Endocrinology. Use both medical and English dictionaries and your Quick-Reference Word List as resource materials for finding words.

Proofread your transcribed documents carefully, listening to the dictation while you read your transcripts.

Transcribe (*NOT* retype) the same reports again without referring to your previous transcription attempt. Initially, you may need to transcribe some reports more than twice before you can produce an error-free document. Your ultimate goal is to produce an error-free document the first time.

BLOOPERS

This child will probably be shorter than he wants to be, but he should have picked different parents.

Physical examination revealed a garrulous, obese woman who was short of breath on motion but not on talking.

The patient had waffles for breakfast and anorexia for lunch.

At 2 a.m. the patient was found dead in bed after otherwise having had a good day.

THOMAS MORGAN   #090438   DATE OF OFFICE VISIT: 7/25/92

INITIAL HISTORY AND PHYSICAL EXAMINATION

This 36-year-old man was doing well until 3 years ago when he developed progressively severe fatigue. At that time he had been in a stressful job situation. However, these symptoms have persisted and gotten worse, although the stress has improved. There is no relation to meals or time of day, although he is somewhat more tired in the afternoons. He sleeps 7 to 8 hours during the week and 12 hours on weekends. Chem-2, CBC, Epstein-Barr studies, and thyroid function tests have been normal. He was tried on Thyrolar 1/2 grain because of low normal T4, but there was no benefit. He has received Parnate, Nardil, and other antidepressants, including vitamin B_{12} injections, without any benefit. He has a 3-year history of constant burning in the eyes. An ophthalmologist did not find anything wrong.

REVIEW OF SYSTEMS: He has periodic dizziness, particularly when standing up rapidly, occasional tinnitus, frequent constipation, and occasional diarrhea, nocturia x 2 or 3, cold extremities, and dry skin of relatively recent onset. He has some anxiety and insomnia and is depressed, apparently in relation to his condition.

FAMILY HISTORY: The father has heart disease. The brother has retinitis pigmentosa.

HABITS: He drinks coffee. His diet is balanced and low in sugar.

EXAM: Height 6'1", 190 pounds. Blood pressure 130/72, pulse is 68. HEENT, neck, heart, lungs, abdomen, pulses, extremities, gross neurologic, and skin are normal. Rectal not done.

ASSESSMENT:
1. Chronic fatigue.
2. Burning eyes.
3. Depression.
4. Signs of possible hypothyroidism.
5. Constipation and diarrhea.

PLAN: Will check basal temperatures and begin thyroid prescription if low. Gave therapeutic trial of 6 cc vitamin C, 4 cc calcium/magnesium, 1 cc of B_6, B_{12}, B_5, and B complex intravenously. Will repeat if helpful. Other recommendations as noted. Return in 4 weeks.

_____

JEANNE CRANE, M.D.

JC:hpi
d: 7/25/92
t: 7/26/92

CHART NOTE

EMILY JANE MORGAN   Age: 42   12/14/92

CHIEF COMPLAINT: Increasing fatigue, nocturia, and vaginal pruritus.

HISTORY OF PRESENT ILLNESS: Brief exam for this obese 42-year-old female patient with a 2-year history of mild hypertension and NIDDM, controlled by diet. Medications include Ortho-Novum 10/11. The patient was started on hydrochlorothiazide 50 mg 2 weeks ago because of elevated diastolic pressures.

Blood sugar by glucose meter is 417. Urine negative for ketones. Apical pulse of 90. Blood pressures are 144/94 and 140/98. Height 5'2", weight 186.

PHYSICAL EXAMINATION: Unremarkable.

RECOMMENDATIONS:
1. Instruction to patient to push fluids for the next several days.
2. Discontinue hydrochlorothiazide and birth control pills to end possible drug-induced hyperglycemia.
3. Start Micronase 2.5 mg q.o.d. and Capoten 25 mg b.i.d.
4. Set up an appointment on Friday for FBS.
5. Patient to see the nurse practitioner for fitting of a diaphragm and nutritional counseling on a 1200-calorie A.D.A. diet.

JC:hpi

Learning Objectives

Medical

- Describe the symptoms a physician looks for when performing a physical examination on an orthopedic patient.
- Describe the action of the following classes of orthopedic drugs: salicylates, NSAIDs, skeletal muscle relaxants.
- Given an orthopedic root word, symptom, or disease, match it to its correct medical definition.
- Given a cross-section illustration of the skeleton, memorize the names of the bones.
- Demonstrate knowledge of anatomical, medical, and adjectival terms by completing the exercises in this lesson.

Fundamentals

- Describe common orthopedic tests performed in a physical examination.
- Name three problems encountered in transcribing orthopedic dictation.
- Demonstrate the correct use of numbers in editing medical sentences.

Practice

- Accurately transcribe authentic physician dictation from the specialty of orthopedics.

A Closer Look

Transcribing Orthopedic Dictation

by Carolyn Cadigan, CMT

The transcription of orthopedic dictation is not unlike the transcription of other medical specialties—some love it, others don't. But once you have mastered the terminology of bones, muscles, tendons, ligaments, and surgical instruments (many of which sound as if they belong in carpentry), you may find that you have also developed a unique sense of humor. Orthopedic transcriptionists look forward to rainy days (arthritis complaints) and icy and snowy days (accidents, strained muscles). They count the number of injuries while watching sports events.

Colorful terminology. Orthopedic terminology is relatively constant: the names of the bones, muscles, tendons, and ligaments do not change, names of fractures and sprains remain basically the same, and orthopedic instrument names remain relatively constant. The most significant changes occur when new orthopedic appliances are developed, and when doctors themselves coin and create new terminology for specific purposes.

Orthopedic terminology tends to be descriptive. Should a patient present with a complaint of a painful knee, it is common to hear the physician dictate the following: *snap, crack, pop, clink, clunk, grind, tear, catch,* and *giving way.* And from the list of instruments used in orthopedic procedures, one would think the surgeon was building a house instead of repairing or replacing a joint: screws, washers, rods, plates, burs, drills, rasps, saws, chisels, tamps, clamps, and cement. On a follow-up postoperative office visit, it is not unusual for the physician to dictate that the patient is able to bend, flex, lift, A-B-duct (abduct), A-D-duct (adduct), and perform the normal activities of daily living.

Assessment and treatment. The orthopedist carries out a physical examination that may differ from the patient's expectations. The orthopedic physician does not usually listen to the patient's lungs or take the pulse, but may ask the patient to sit, stand, walk, squat, cross legs, and bend forward.

What can a physician determine from such tests? From bending forward, scoliosis; from a hairy patch on a child's spine, spina bifida or myelomeningocele; from heel and toe walking, Achilles tendon involvement; from holding the hands in an inverted prayer position, carpal tunnel syndrome.

Orthopedic tests. Some common orthopedic tests include the following.

anterior drawer test—With the patient supine (lying face up), the injured knee is bent to 90 degrees. The physician then grasps the upper end of the tibia and pulls it anteriorly. Excessive movement means the anterior cruciate ligament within the knee joint is damaged or torn.

Lachman test—Similar to the anterior drawer test but performed with the patient's knee flexed only to 15 or 20 degrees; also used to evaluate anterior cruciate ligament stability.

pivot-shift test—With the patient supine, the foot is held in the physician's hand. The physician then turns the foot inward while pushing on the outside of the knee with the opposite hand, at the same time flexing and extending the patient's leg. This test is also used to evaluate anterior cruciate ligament stability.

straight leg raising—With the patient supine, the leg is elevated with the knee straight to the point where pain is experienced in the back or leg itself, or dorsiflexion of the foot causes an increase in pain. This test is done to determine if nerve root irritation is present. Also known as Lasègue sign or test.

crossed (or contralateral) straight leg raising—With the patient supine, the unaffected leg is held straight and flexed at the hip. If sciatica is present, the patient will experience pain in the opposite, affected side.

McMurray's test or **sign**—The physician manipulates the patient's knee using circumduction motion. If clicking of the cartilage is present, the McMurray's test is positive.

To locate specific orthopedic tests in a medical dictionary, the transcriptionist should look under *test, sign, maneuver,* or under the name of the test itself listed alphabetically.

Occasionally the orthopedist will order x-rays of the involved site in an attempt to determine or verify the presence of a tear, rupture, fracture, dislocation, or foreign body. X-rays may include AP, PA, oblique, and lateral projections, as well as such exotic-sounding views as *sunrise, sunset, tunnel,* and *coned-down.*

Treatment modalities used in orthopedic cases vary widely but are generally conservative. Before recommending surgery, the orthopedist usually tries any one of a number of conservative treatments—splints, casts, supports, physical therapy, exercises, heat or ice applications, dressings (such as Unna's boot), braces (such as cowhorn, Milwaukee, DonJoy), and shoes (such as open toe, straight last, reverse last).

References. As with any other specialty, orthopedists have their own language—words and phrases and abbreviations which are specific to orthopedics. In addition to a number of helpful orthopedic references, I have come to rely heavily upon the patient's chart as well as the surgical and central supply departments of the hospital for information on orthopedic devices. The handwritten operating room record, which is prepared on every patient having surgery, lists all instruments used during the procedure, including the names of orthopedic pins, rods, prosthetic devices, and so on. Surgical components frequently arrive in the central supply and surgical departments direct from the manufacturer, with the name of the company and the product boldly printed on the outside of the box. In addition, the physical therapy/rehabilitation department of the hospital can provide you with the names of braces, supports, exercises, and other terms.

Remember to keep your own personal dictionary as you go along. You will find that in time you rely on it more than other reference books, if the entries you make are thoroughly checked for accuracy before you write them in.

The following terms are provided to help you start your own personal dictionary.

spline—a variety of flat nail that is placed across a fracture or bone osteotomy to hold it in place. It has been hammered flat while held in a vise.

rasp versus **raspatory**—There is really no difference between a rasp and a raspatory. One orthopedist commented that the word *raspatory* was simply a strange semantic perversion of the word *rasp* and should really not exist in the English language.

bone wax—a gel-like material that is exactly like wax that you would use in the kitchen. It has the ability to seal little pores in the bone that are exuding blood.

Although there are a variety of other thrombotic materials, such as thrombin and Avitene, none of these can plug pores with the waxy effect of bone wax.

Transcribing orthopedic dictation. Now, let's discuss specific tips on transcribing orthopedics, beginning first with the skeletal system, then the muscular system, followed by specific anatomic areas.

An illustration of the skeletal system (such as a plate of the human skeleton in a medical dictionary) would lead one to believe that skeletal terminology is rather straightforward; however, each bone has specific areas that are not usually found on skeletal charts. A single spinal vertebra, for example, has anatomic landmarks such as the spinous process, vertebral arch, transverse process, vertebral foramen, vertebral body, articular process, posterior tubercle, anterior tubercle, lamina, articular facet, and dens.

Most orthopedic patients complain not of broken bones but of aches and pains in the back, giving way of the knee or hip, peculiar snapping, clicking, or grating (crepitus) of a joint. It is not unusual for the orthopedic transcriptionist to transcribe a fractured bone report only occasionally.

Fracture types are fairly straightforward and can be found in medical dictionaries under the heading *fracture*. Some exceptions are hockey-stick fracture, dog leg fracture, stairstep fracture, and other coined terms.

A great many orthopedic terms are difficult to confirm in reference books. For example, when an orthopedist dictates on a fractured lateral malleolus, the transcriptionist may not have a clue as to what part of the body is involved since this structure is not listed under the heading *bone* in a medical dictionary. What the transcriptionist does find is that *malleolus* is listed under its own heading alphabetically, defined as a rounded prominence on either side of the ankle. (Do not confuse *malleolus,* the ankle bone, with *malleus,* one of the bones in the middle ear, also known as the *hammer.)*

The same problem occurs when *scapholunate* is dictated. This term is not listed under *bone,* and a further search reveals that, although both *scaphoid* and *lunate* are listed separately under *bone,* the transcriptionist is referred to the Latin forms of each word for a definition. A check under the heading *os* reveals *os scaphoideum* (scaphoid) is the most lateral carpal (wrist) bone and that *os lunatum* is the lunate bone. Therefore, a scapholunate dissociation is an abnormal separation between the scaphoid and lunate bones of the wrist.

Terminology involving the muscular system may present a challenge as well. When the phrase *vastus lateralis* is dictated, how does the transcriptionist know where to look?

It is important to know that medical dictionaries usually have both an English and a Latin listing for certain anatomic structures. For example, a specific muscle may be found under the listing *muscle* as well as under *musculus.* And in the case of *vastus lateralis,* which is obviously Latin, the transcriptionist would search under *musculus* (Latin) as opposed to *muscle* (English) to locate the definition.

For tendons, there are also two listings: *tendo* (Latin) and *tendon* (English). However, there are many more tendons in the body than are listed in the dictionaries. To find *extensor carpi radialis longus tendon* (not listed under *tendon),* the transcriptionist does a bit of detective work. The word *tendon* is the first clue. Although this phrase is not actually listed under *tendon,* the definition of a tendon is a cord which attaches a muscle to a bone. The transcriptionist would then know to look under the listing for muscle, or in this case *musculi,* because the phrase is in Latin.

Other important English-Latin listings include:

English	Latin
bone	os
condyle	condylus
nerve	nervus
ligament	ligamentum
articulation	articulatio
artery	arteria
vein	vena

Anatomic review. Beginning with the head and working downward, let's consider the various anatomic body parts and what orthopedic terminology the transcriptionist might encounter.

Orthopedic surgeons rarely perform surgery on the head. Patients with problems in this area will be referred to a neurosurgeon, dentist, otolaryngologist, or plastic surgeon. A solid basic background in facial structures and nerves in general will quite often suffice for the orthopedic transcriptionist.

Orthopedic terminology becomes more involved as the physician deals with the nerves, tendons, muscles, and small bony structures within a small area, such as the hand. Treatment of the hand is where most transcriptionists encounter terms such as *fisticuffs* and *anatomical snuffbox* for the first time. The former can be found in a standard English dictionary and the latter in *Dorland's* under *box.* For procedures involving the upper extremities, my favorite reference is Blauvelt's *A Manual of Orthopaedic Terminology,* which includes such terms as Bristow-May procedure, Girdlestone procedure, and Maquet procedure.

Transcribing dictation on the spine can be difficult and therefore time-consuming, if one does not know the terminology. The first step is to become familiar with the basic make-up of the spinal column: the cervical spine (C1 through C7), the thoracic spine (T1 through T12), the lumbar spine (L1 through L5), and the sacral spine (S1 through S5). It is common to hear reference made to the L6 vertebra, which is identified as either lumbarization of S1 or the sacralization of L5. Additionally, some physicians dictate *D-spine* for *dorsal spine.*

There are different ways to transcribe vertebrae and their identifying numbers. Many references join the vertebra and number without a hyphen (for example, T12) and use a hyphen for vertebral interspaces (L5-S1). However, in the hospital where I work, the transcriptionists have been instructed to use hyphens between the vertebra and the number, e.g., L-4; and to use hyphens and slashes for vertebral interspaces, e.g., L-5/S-1.

Some related spine terminology includes phrases such as *herniated nucleus pulposus, dural sac, facet, foramen and foramina, disk space, pedicle, ligamentum flavum, spinous process, transverse processes,* and *annulus fibrosus* (*not* fibrosis).

Orthopedic surgery on the spine may involve the correction of scoliosis. Instruments may include Luque or Harrington rods, C-washers, screws, clamps, and so on. The spellings for some of these instruments may be difficult to locate, but many of them are listed in reference books specializing in orthopedic terminology.

In hip surgery, the transcriptionist may encounter terms such as *femoral prosthesis, acetabular component, Knowles pinning,* and *figure 4 position.* An orthopedic reference book such as Blauvelt's will help the transcriptionist identify Knowles as the brand name of a type of pin used in setting hip fractures. The definition of *figure 4 position* is more difficult to locate. Imagine yourself lying on your left side. Now bring your right ankle up until it is resting on your left knee. This is the figure 4 position.

Another interesting term is *triple diapering,* which is used in the treatment of congenitally dislocated hips of newborn infants if the defect is detected at a very early age. The application of three layers of diapers holds the infant's legs in external rotation to properly seat the femoral heads back into the acetabular cups.

The language of knee surgery can be most descriptive. On examining the knee joint during arthroscopy, the physician may describe *parrot-beak tear, buckethandle tear, crabmeat-like appearance, horseshoe appearance, choppy sea sign, spongy appearance,* and *medial shelf* or *lateral shelf. Along with this descriptive terminology, the physician will also use anatomical and medical words such as meniscus, chondromalacia, Gerdy tubercle,* and the *master knot of Henry.*

Some of the above terms are difficult to locate. *Gerdy tubercle* can be found under *Gerdy* but not under *tubercle.* The *master knot of Henry* is not listed under *master knot* but is listed as the *ligament of Henry* in one reference. In this instance, the support of another transcriptionist or the physician is of the greatest help in providing verification.

Orthopedic abbreviations. When it comes to orthopedic abbreviations, one can quickly get lost within the first sentence without a good reference book and a personal list of abbreviations.

For example, ''The patient presented with a chief complaint of MTA and ITT.'' Here the transcriptionist is given no clues. Since it is unlikely the patient is complaining about the Mass Transit Authority or IT&T Financial Services, the transcriptionist must consult a reference book of abbreviations.

Unfortunately, MTA is hard to find, and ITT is usually defined as insulin tolerance test. The transcriptionist would know that an orthopedist would not likely be seeing a patient with a chief complaint involving an insulin tolerance test, so this definition can be quickly ruled out. The transcriptionist must either consult another trancriptionist, check the patient's chart if possible, or ask the physician.

Once the transcriptionist discovers that MTA and ITT stand for *metatarsus adductus* and *internal tibial torsion,* respectively, the next step is to insert these definitions into a personal dictionary so that they will be readily available the next time.

Another interesting abbreviation includes *DB bar* or *Denny Browne bar* for *Denis Browne bar.* The transcriptionist will find a *Denis Browne splint* listed in orthopedic references but not in medical dictionaries.

Another example: ''The patient was scheduled for AAA (or 3-A or triple A) procedure.'' Many reference sources define the abbreviation AAA as *abdominal aortic aneurysm.* This definition would not be appropriate for a scheduled orthopedic surgery. By asking another transcriptionist or the physician, or by consulting the patient's chart, the transcriptionist will see that the patient is scheduled for a diagnostic **arthroscopy,** operative arthroscopy, and possible operative **arthrotomy**.

Spelling. Certain orthopedic words present spelling controversies for medical transcriptionists. Some of these include bur/burr, disc/disk, and orthopedic/ orthopaedic.

bur—In medical usage this spelling is preferred in both English and medical dictionaries when referring to the small rotary instrument used in orthopedic surgery or dentistry.

disk—In medical usage this spelling is preferred by medical dictionaries when referring to the intervertebral disk of the spinal column. Some surgeons may prefer the alternative spelling *(disc)* and the transcriptionist may use that spelling instead.

orthopedics—Medical dictionaries show *orthopedics* as preferred spelling over *orthopaedics,* although if you work for an orthopedic hospital or for an orthopedic surgeon, you may be asked to use the *ae* form. (The American Academy of Orthopaedic Surgeons prefers the *ae* spelling.)

Main entries, subentries, and sound-alikes. To assist the new orthopedic transcriptionist, a list of alternative locations where a particular word or phrase may be found in medical dictionaries is provided below. For instance, if the physician dictates *Charcot-Marie-Tooth syndrome,* the transcriptionist can find this entity under *syndrome* or *disease* or *sign.*

If a physician dictates:	Also look under:
device	apparatus
	bandage
	component
	prosthesis
	splint
procedure	amputation
	approach
	flap
	graft
	maneuver
	operation
	technique
reflex	phenomenon
	sign
	test
syndrome	disease
	sign

Sound-alike words can create real problems for both novice and experienced medical transcriptionists. Errors in medical meaning can result unless the transcriptionist is aware of potentially confusing sound-alikes and can discriminate between them to select the correct term.

Listed below are some common sound-alike words encountered in orthopedic transcription.

epineural—designates an area beside the neural arch structure on a vertebral body
epineurial—pertains to the connective tissue (epineurium) that covers a nerve

perineural—designates the general area surrounding a nerve
perineurial—pertains to the connective tissue (perineurium) which covers individual bundles of fibers within a nerve

Hohmann retractor—used in hip surgery and other large bone areas
Hoen retractor—used for small bone areas, such as in the hands; an old-style type of retractor that has been replaced by mini-Bennett and other newer retractors.

Kirschner wire (K wire), suture, traction
Kuntscher nail, pin, reamer, rod

Arthropor cup prosthesis
Autophor ceramic hip prosthesis

Blount retractor
blunt retractor

Cofield shoulder prosthesis
Sofield osteotomy

A final word. If you cannot interpret an orthopedic term in the dictation, and have carefully researched it in all the available resources, leave a blank temporarily and continue with the transcription. Chances are that the physician will dictate the word again later, and it will be clearer, and then you can fill in the blank. Or if it is an abbreviation that you cannot translate, the physician may translate it the next time or give more clues to its meaning.

The History and Physical Examination

by John H. Dirckx, M.D.

Examination of Back and Extremities. A full orthopedic examination requires considerable cooperation from the patient in assuming various positions and performing various movements. In performing the orthopedic examination, the physician looks for any developmental or traumatic deformities not previously noted and any evidence of generalized conditions such as muscle wasting or weakness, stiffness, or tremors. The terms *varus* and *valgus* refer to abnormal deviations in joints of the extremities. In a varus deformity, the bone distal to the affected joint is deviated inward; hence genu varum means bowleg. Valgus is outward deviation of the distal bone; hence genu valgum means knock-knee.

The physician puts joints through passive range of motion and has the patient put them through active range of motion, with or without resistance by the examiner. Muscles are assessed for development, bilateral symmetry, strength, tone, and spasm or tenderness. Bones are assessed for deformity, masses, or tenderness. A joint is not simply the place where two bones are hooked together but a complex structure with highly specialized tissues, subject to many injuries and diseases. The physician examines joints for swelling, stiffness, thickening of synovial membranes, fluid, tenderness, and instability. The range of movement in a joint can be quantified with a goniometer, a simple device consisting of two arms jointed at their ends, with a scale that reads in degrees of rotation.

In examining an injured extremity the physician notes any swelling, deformity, cutaneous trauma, ecchymosis, or hematoma formation. The age of subcutaneous hemorrhage is judged by its color. Muscular and skeletal structures are palpated for tenderness, spasm, deformity, or discontinuity, and active and passive ranges of motion are checked. Joints are palpated for crepitus or effusion and tested by manipulation for ligamentous laxity. The circulation and sensation of the part are also carefully evaluated.

The back is examined first with the subject standing and facing away from the examiner. Any spinal curvature or developmental deformities are noted, as well as any surgical scars. The heights of the iliac crests are compared as a rough test of leg length equality. The spinous processes of the vertebrae, the sacroiliac joints, and the sciatic notches are assessed by palpation for tenderness, the muscles for tenderness and spasm. The examiner notes the range of spinal movements as the subject bends forward, backward, and to the sides. The subject then lies down on his back on the examining table and the physician tests for disorders of the sacroiliac and hip joints and for sciatic nerve irritation by manipulation of the lower extremities.

Pharmacology: Orthopedic Drugs

Drugs prescribed to treat various orthopedic conditions, such as arthritis (rheumatoid and osteoarthritis), bursitis, tendinitis, gout, and muscle spasms, include aspirin, nonsteroidal anti-inflammatory drugs (NSAIDs), gold salts, and skeletal muscle relaxants, among others.

Drugs used to treat arthritis inhibit the production of prostaglandins. These drugs include salicylic acid compounds such as aspirin, NSAIDs, gold salts, and corticosteroids.

Salicylic acid compounds. The oldest drug used to treat arthritis is aspirin. Aspirin is also known as acetylsalicylic acid, abbreviated ASA. It has anti-inflammatory, analgesic, and antipyretic actions which make it useful in treating many diverse medical conditions. Drugs which contain aspirin or related compounds and are used to treat arthritis include:

Anacin
Arthropan
A.S.A. Enseals
Ascriptin A/D
Bayer Aspirin
Bufferin
Cama
diflunisal (Dolobid)
Easprin
Ecotrin

Because salicylic acid compounds such as aspirin are irritating to the stomach and long-term therapy with such drugs has been shown to induce ulcers, some manufacturers have taken precautions to reduce this irritation. Ecotrin is manufactured as an enteric-coated tablet which will not dissolve in stomach acid; it dissolves only when it comes into contact with the higher pH environment of the duodenum.

Ascriptin A/D, Bufferin, and Cama contain magnesium and aluminum in the tablet to act as an antacid.

Although acetaminophen (Tylenol) is an analgesic and antipyretic like aspirin, it is seldom prescribed for rheumatoid arthritis because it is not an anti-inflammatory; it lacks the ability to inhibit the production of prostaglandins.

Nonsteroidal anti-inflammatory drugs. NSAIDs have analgesic effects and also inhibit the production of prostaglandins, but they have less of a tendency than aspirin to cause gastrointestinal side effects such as ulcers. They are similar enough to aspirin structurally that patients allergic to aspirin cannot be given NSAIDs. Nonsteroidal anti-inflammatory drugs include:

> diclofenac (Voltaren)
> fenoprofen (Nalfon)
> flurbiprofen (Ansaid)
> ibuprofen (Motrin, Rufen) prescription
>   (Advil, Medipren, Nuprin) over-the-counter
> indomethacin (Indocin)
> ketoprofen (Orudis)
> ketorolac (Toradol)
> meclofenamate (Meclomen)
> naproxen (Anaprox, Naprosyn)
> piroxicam (Feldene)
> sulindac (Clinoril)
> tolmetin (Tolectin)

Note: The ending *-profen* is common to some generic nonsteroidal anti-inflammatory drugs.

Corticosteroids used to treat the inflammation associated with arthritis, bursitis, and tendinitis, are given orally. Some can be injected directly into the joint (intra-articular administration). Corticosteroids include:

> betamethasone (Celestone)
> cortisone (Cortone)
> dexamethasone (Decadron)
> hydrocortisone (Cortef, Hydrocortone, Solu-Cortef)
> methylprednisolone (Depo-Medrol, Medrol, Solu-Medrol)
> prednisolone (Delta-Cortef)
> prednisone (Deltasone)
> triamcinolone (Aristocort, Aristospan, Kenacort)

Skeletal muscle relaxants. Acute musculoskeletal conditions such as strains, sprains, and "pulled muscles" can be treated with analgesics and anti-inflammatory drugs; but the physician may prescribe a skeletal muscle relaxant in addition to rest and physical therapy. Skeletal muscle relaxants most specifically relieve muscle spasm and stiffness. In addition, some have a sedative quality. These drugs include:

> carisoprodol (Soma)
> chlorzoxazone (Parafon Forte DSC)
> cyclobenzaprine (Flexeril)
> diazepam (Valium)
> metaxalone (Skelaxin)
> methocarbamol (Robaxin)
> orphenadrine (Flexon, Norflex)

Combination drugs include:

> Norgesic (orphenadrine and aspirin)
> Robaxisal (methocarbamol and aspirin)
> Soma Compound (carisoprodol and aspirin)

Anatomy/Medical Terminology

Medical Terminology Matching Exercise

Instructions: Match each item in Column A with its definition in Column B.

Column A

A. osteoarthritis
B. arthro-
C. kypho-
D. tendon
E. lordo-
F. osteosarcoma
G. lumbo-
H. strain
I. osteo-
J. scolio-
K. osteomyelitis
L. ligament
M. peroneo-
N. osteoporosis
O. costo-
P. subluxation
Q. malleolo-

Column B

____ lateral curvature of spine
____ dorsal curvature of thoracic spine
____ connects bone to bone
____ ankle bone
____ overstretching of muscle
____ fibula
____ joint
____ anterior curvature of lumbar spine
____ decreased bone density
____ bacterial infection of bone
____ degeneration of joint and cartilage
____ bone
____ incomplete dislocation
____ lower back
____ connects bone to muscle
____ rib
____ malignant bone tumor

Anatomy: The Human Skeleton

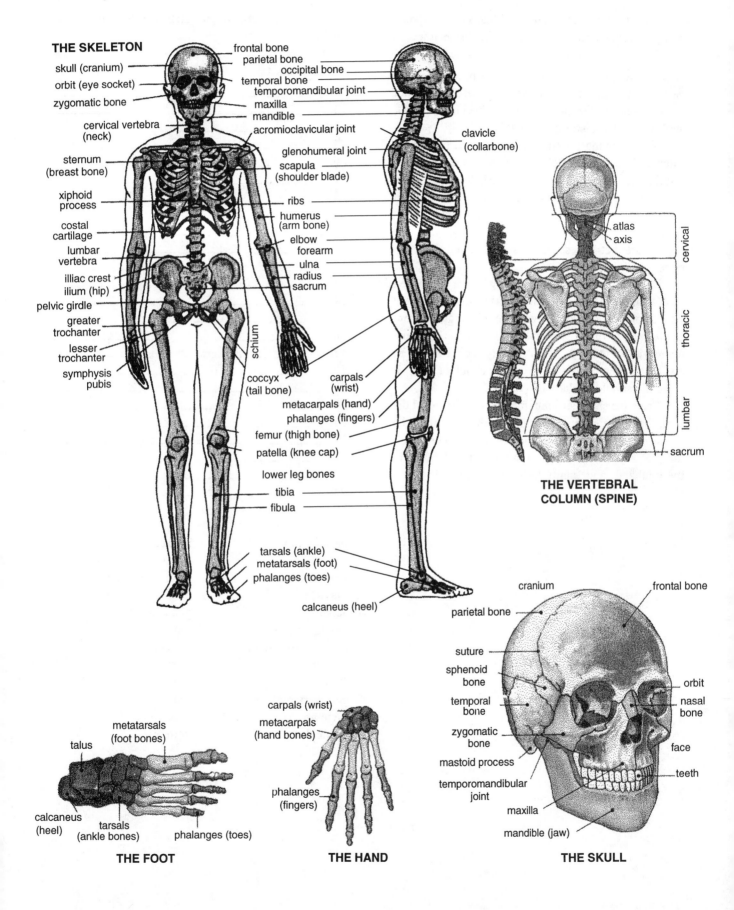

THE SKELETON

- skull (cranium)
- orbit (eye socket)
- zygomatic bone
- cervical vertebra (neck)
- sternum (breast bone)
- xiphoid process
- costal cartilage
- lumbar vertebra
- illiac crest
- ilium (hip)
- pelvic girdle
- greater trochanter
- lesser trochanter
- symphysis pubis

- frontal bone
- parietal bone
- occipital bone
- temporal bone
- temporomandibular joint
- maxilla
- mandible
- acromioclavicular joint
- glenohumeral joint
- scapula (shoulder blade)
- ribs
- humerus (arm bone)
- elbow
- forearm
- ulna
- radius
- sacrum

- ischium

- clavicle (collarbone)

- coccyx (tail bone)
- carpals (wrist)
- metacarpals (hand)
- phalanges (fingers)
- femur (thigh bone)
- patella (knee cap)
- lower leg bones
- tibia
- fibula
- tarsals (ankle)
- metatarsals (foot)
- phalanges (toes)
- calcaneus (heel)

THE VERTEBRAL COLUMN (SPINE)

- atlas
- axis
- cervical
- thoracic
- lumbar
- sacrum

THE FOOT

- metatarsals (foot bones)
- talus
- calcaneus (heel)
- tarsals (ankle bones)
- phalanges (toes)

THE HAND

- carpals (wrist)
- metacarpals (hand bones)
- phalanges (fingers)

THE SKULL

- cranium
- frontal bone
- parietal bone
- suture
- sphenoid bone
- temporal bone
- zygomatic bone
- mastoid process
- temporomandibular joint
- maxilla
- mandible (jaw)
- orbit
- nasal bone
- face
- teeth

Fill-in Exercise: The Bones

Instructions: The numbered blanks correspond to the numbers in the narrative paragraphs. Fill in the blanks with the correct entry from the word list below.

Beginning with the toes or (1), one proceeds along the foot, encountering the bones of the midfoot (2) and bones of the ankle (3), to the heel bone or (4), and then to the ankle bone or (5).

Next, moving proximally, the (6) and (7) are located in the lower leg, followed by the kneecap or (8), and then the (9) in the upper leg. The ball of the femur, also known as the (10), fits snugly in the (11) or socket in the pelvic bone. The lower part of the pelvic bone, including the seat bones, is called the (12), while the upper part that flares widely and is called the "hip bone" is the (13).

Moving up the spinal column, which is composed of (14) and (15), one encounters the ribs. There are 12 pair of ribs, of which 7 pair are joined at the front of the body to the breast bone or (16). Superior to the manubrium and the first ribs is the (17) or collarbone. As the clavicle continues across the shoulder joint, it joins the shoulder blade or (18).

From the shoulder joint, moving distally down the arm, the bones encountered include the (19), then the elbow or (20), then the two bones of the lower arm— the (21) and 22), to the (23) in the wrist, the (24) in the midhand, and finally to the fingers or (25).

1. <u>phalanges</u>
2. _____
3. _____
4. _____
5. _____
6. _____
7. _____
8. _____
9. _____
10. _____
11. _____
12. _____
13. _____
14. _____
15. _____
16. _____
17. _____
18. _____
19. _____
20. _____
21. _____
22. _____
23. _____
24. _____
25. _____

acetabulum	metacarpals
calcaneus	metatarsals
carpals	olecronon process
clavicle	patella
femur	phalanges (2)
fibula	radius
greater trochanter	scapula
humerus	sternum
ilium	tarsals
intervertebral disks	tibia
ischium	ulna
malleolus	vertebrae

Adjective Exercise

Adjectives are formed from nouns by adding adjectival suffixes such as *-ac, -al, -ar, -ary, -eal, -ed, -ent, -iac, -ial, -ic, -ical, -lar, -oid, -ous, -tic,* and *-tous.* In addition, some adjectives have a different form entirely from the noun, which may be either Latin or Greek in origin.

Test your knowledge of adjectives by writing the adjectival form of the following orthopedic words. Consult a medical dictionary to select the correct adjectival ending.

1. muscle _____
2. bone _____
3. spine _____
4. vertebra _____
5. cartilage _____
6. rib _____
7. pelvis _____
8. humerus _____
9. radius _____
10. ulna _____
11. clavicle _____
12. femur _____
13. tibia _____
14. fibula _____
15. patella _____
16. malleolus _____
17. phalanx _____
18. ligament _____
19. tendon _____
20. arthritis _____

Lay and Medical Terms

ankle bone	malleolus
collar bone	clavicle
breast bone	sternum
elbow	olecranon process
kneecap	patella
shoulder blade	scapula
hip bones	iliac crests
tail bone	coccyx
seat bones	ischium
shin bone	tibia
slipped disk	herniated nucleus pulposus

Root Word and Suffix Matching Exercise

Instructions: Combine the following root words with suffixes to form words that match the definitions below. Fill in the blanks with the medical words that you construct.

Root Word	Suffix
kypho-	-osis
lordo-	-itis
osteo-	-desis
myelo-	-oma
scolio-	-algia
arthro-	
myo-	

A. pain in a muscle

_____

B. condition of humpback curvature of the spine

_____

C. condition of swayback curvature of the spine

_____

D. inflammation of the bone marrow
(Tip: Use 2 root words and 1 suffix.)

_____

E. condition of sideways curvature of the spine

_____

F. inflammation of the joints

_____

G. surgical fusion of a joint

_____

H. tumor of the muscle

_____

Transcription Guidelines

1. **Metric numbers.** It is customary to abbreviate metric measurements in medical reports. Abbreviations for metric measurements contain no periods and have the same form for both singular and plural.

cm	centimeter, centimeters
g	gram, grams
mL	milliliter, milliliters

   Note: The new SI abbreviations for gram and milliliters (*g* and *mL*, respectively) replace the older abbreviations *gm* and *ml*.

2. Metric numbers less than one should be preceded with a zero and a decimal point for clarity, even if the zero is not dictated.

   0.5 mm in diameter

3. In a series of metric measurements, the units of measure that accompany the numerals should be listed in a consistent fashion.

   If dictated: 3.3 cm x 1 x 4
   Transcribe: 3.3 cm x 1 cm x 4 cm   OR
   3.3 x 1 x 4 cm

4. Do not use an abbreviation with a metric measurement if no specific numeral is dictated.

   The scar was several centimeters in length.

5. **Numbers and English units of measure.** Standard English units of measure are usually spelled out.

   inch   foot   pound

6. **Numbers and plurals.** It is not necessary to add an apostrophe when pluralizing a number, although it is acceptable to do so.

   100s or 100's   4 x 4s or 4 x 4's

7. **Numbers and suture sizes.** Suture sizes may or may not be dictated with a number sign (#). As a general rule, transcribe as dictated. When the suture size is a single whole number, the number sign can be added for clarity. In the following examples, the numbers are dictated as "two oh" or "two zero," and "number one." Be consistent in styling in a report.

   00 or 2-0 or #2-0 Dexon suture
   #1 Tevdek suture

8. **Numbers and blood pressure.** The blood pressure reading contains two numbers separated by a slash or virgule (/). The dictator says "over" to indicate the slash. The abbreviation for the unit of measure used with blood pressure is *mmHg* (millimeters of mercury). *Hg* is the chemical symbol for mercury. There is no space between *mm* and *Hg*.

   If dictated: Blood pressure 120 over 80 millimeters of mercury.
   Transcribe: Blood pressure 120/80 mmHg.

9. **Numbers and verb forms.** Use a singular form of a verb with units of measure.

   Approximately 50 cc of fluid was aspirated from the peritoneal cavity.

10. **Numbers and hyphens.** The use of hyphens with metric measurement abbreviations is optional.

    5 cm laceration   OR   5-cm laceration

11. **Numbers and "x."** The symbol "x" may be used to represent the dictated words "times" or "by." It is written as a lowercase letter with spaces on either side.

    If dictated: Bleeding times 3 days
    Transcribe: Bleeding x 3 days

    If dictated: The ulcer is 2 by 4 cm in size.
    Transcribe: The ulcer is 2 x 4 cm in size.

12. **Numbers and lists.** The dictator may number the diagnoses in a long list to be presented vertically. Sometimes a dictator will give the first several numbers and then say "number next" rather than trying to remember the next number. The transcriptionist may elect to enumerate a long list of diagnoses, even if numbers are not dictated. If, however, there is only one diagnosis dictated, it should not be numbered.

Exercise on Numbers and Measurements

Instructions: In the sentences below, find and correct the errors involving numbers and units of measure.

1. LABORATORY DATA showed a total bilirubin of .5 mg.

2. There is another mole several mm away from the malignancy that we will need to check periodically.

3. She is 5.5 feet tall and weighs 160.5 pounds.

4. A 2 cms nodule is noted in the left lower lung.

5. I closed the wound with 1 Dexon.

6. The patient's blood pressure is 160 over 82 millimeters of mercury.

7. The decubitus ulcer on her buttocks is 5 by 7 cms in size.

Transcription Tips

1. There are several sound-alike terms in the musculoskeletal system. Memorize their meanings so that you can select the appropriate term for a correct transcript.

   peroneal (pertaining to the fibula)
   perineal (pertaining to the area between the genitalia and rectum)
   peritoneal (cavity located within the abdomen)

   humeral (pertaining to the humerus, an arm bone)
   humoral (pertaining to immunity from antibodies in the blood)

   humerus (the arm bone)
   humorous (funny)

   ilium (the hip bone)
   ileum (part of the small intestine)

   malleolus (ankle bone)
   malleus (bone of middle ear)

2. Orthopedic physicians commonly dictate "a-b-duction" and "a-d-duction." These are not slang terms. The physician is simply spelling the first two letters of the term and then pronouncing the rest as a word. This is done to avoid error because it is often very difficult to differentiate between these two terms when spoken.

3. Several nouns pertaining to the musculoskeletal system change their spelling when forming derivatives.

   femur becomes *femora* or *femurs* (noun) and *femoral* (adjective)

   foramen becomes *foramina* (noun) and *foraminal* (adjective)
   tendon becomes *tendinitis* (noun)

4. Paget's disease of the bone is different from Paget's disease of the nipple of the breast, although both are spelled the same.

5. The following words have more than one acceptable alternative spelling.

Preferred	Acceptable alternative
orthopedics	orthopaedics
orthopedist	orthopaedist
disk	disc

   Note: *Orthopaedic* is from the Greek. Unless specified by the dictating physician, omit the *a* in the diphthong *ae*. Exceptions: The official name of the American Academy of Orthopaedic Surgeons, some orthopedic groups and hospitals.

6. Memorize the spellings of these difficult orthopedic words:

   psoas muscle (silent *p*)   bony (*not* boney)

7. Drug spelling tips: The names of several gold salts drugs contain *au*, the chemical symbol for gold: **au**ranofin, Rid**au**ra, **au**rothioglucose. *Flexeril* is often misspelled as *Flexoril* because of association with the flexor muscle.

8. Transcribe these slang terms correctly when encountered in dictation.

Slang	Translation
K wire	Kirschner wire
tib-fib	tibia-fibula (noun) or tibial-fibular (adjective)

Terminology Challenge

Instructions: The following terms appear in the dictation on Tape 6B. Before beginning the medical transcription practice for Lesson 13, become familiar with the terminology below by looking up each word in a medical or English dictionary. Write out a short definition of each term.

abduction pillow
acetabular
adduction
affected
aforementioned
AML hip prosthesis
analgesics
anterior cruciate ligament
anti-inflammatory
arthroplasty
arthroscopy
avascular necrosis
axial weight loading
bone cement
bone densitometry studies
calcitonin
commensurate
compression fracture
· correlate
crutch ambulation
debridement
disk (disc) space
electromyogram (EMG)
endpoint
epidural
extension
external rotation
femoral condyle
flexion
ganglion
ganglionectomy
genu valgum
hemarthrosis
implant stimulator
inhibition
internal rotation

Jewett hyperextension
brace
kyphosis
L1
L3
long leg immobilizer
lordosis
medial retinaculum
musculoskeletal deficit
osteochondral
osteochondroplasty
osteoporosis
patellar tilt
precipitated
Q angle
Rush rod
S1 (back)
Sjögren's disease
spine
  cervical (C)
  dorsal (D)
  lumbosacral (LS)
  lumbar (L)
  sacral (S)
  thoracic (T)
  thoracolumbar
steroid
T11
TENS unit
vitamin D complex
VMO (vastus medialis
  obliquus)
VMO advancement
VMO instability
weightbearing

Sample Reports

Sample orthopedic reports appear on the following pages, illustrating a variety of formats.

Transcription Practice

After completing all the readings and exercises in Lesson 13, transcribe Tape 6B, Orthopedics. Use both medical and English dictionaries and your Quick-Reference Word List as resource materials for finding words.

Proofread your transcribed documents carefully, listening to the dictation while you read your transcripts.

Transcribe (*NOT* retype) the same reports again without referring to your previous transcription attempt. Initially, you may need to transcribe some reports more than twice before you can produce an error-free document. Your ultimate goal is to produce an error-free document the first time.

WILMA WOODS

#081948

Admitted: 8/25/92

Discharged: 8/26/92

DISCHARGE SUMMARY

ADMITTING DIAGNOSIS: Tensor fasciae latae syndrome, left thigh.

DISCHARGE DIAGNOSIS: Same.

OPERATION PERFORMED: Excision, trochanteric bursa, and division, fascia lata, left thigh.

HISTORY: The patient has had difficulty since June or July and has had a variety of treatments, including physiotherapy and local injections, none of which produced any substantial or ongoing relief.

PHYSICAL EXAMINATION: There is restricted range of motion in the left hip.

LABORATORY WORK: The patient has a slightly elevated uric acid at 6.9, and a slightly elevated cholesterol, 212.

The pathology specimen was unreported at the time of discharge. Segments of the trochanteric bursa were sent to the laboratory for evaluation.

HOSPITAL COURSE: On the day of admission, the patient was admitted for a 23-hour-day case, and the hip was opened through a rather extensive lateral incision down to the greater trochanteric bursa. This was excised together with an oblique incision distally through the tensor fasciae latae, actually distally and proximally. The subcutaneous tissues other than the fascia were closed together with an intracuticular stitch in the skin. The patient had more pain than anticipated and was hospitalized.

CONDITION ON DISCHARGE: At the time of discharge, the patient was ambulatory on crutches. She did, however, have a low-grade temperature but had no clinical symptoms. The wound appeared entirely satisfactory.

POSTOPERATIVE PLAN: The patient should be on crutches, increasing her weightbearing gradually.

JACK OLDYCE, M.D.

JO:hpi
d: 8/25/92
t: 8/27/92

MICHAEL JORDAN

#052562

DATE OF OPERATION: 9/25/92

OPERATIVE REPORT

PREOPERATIVE DIAGNOSIS:
1. Left knee medial collateral ligament tear.
2. Anterior cruciate ligament tear.
3. Possible meniscus tear.

POSTOPERATIVE DIAGNOSIS: Same.

PROCEDURES:
1. Exam under anesthesia.
2. Diagnostic arthroscopy.
3. Debridement, anterior cruciate ligament stump.
4. Repair, lateral meniscus, arthroscopically.

ESTIMATED BLOOD LOSS: Minimal.

TOURNIQUET TIME: Two hours.

INDICATIONS: This is a 38-year-old white male who sustained an injury to his left knee
3 days prior to admission when he was jumping from a boat onto a dock and had an external
rotation injury with his foot planted. On clinical examination, he was noted to have increased
valgus stress with end point, slightly increased Lachman; however, the patient was quite
guarded on exam. In addition, he had a hemarthrosis. It was felt he would benefit from exam
under anesthesia and diagnostic arthroscopy and repair of structures as necessary.

PROCEDURE: The patient was taken to the operating room, placed in a supine position on the
operating room table, and turned in the left lateral decubitus where an epidural anesthetic was
placed. Once this had taken, the patient's left leg was examined under anesthesia and noted to
have an increased valgus laxity with end point, a positive Lachman test, and positive pivot-shift
test.

The patient's left lower extremity was then prepped and draped in the normal fashion,
exsanguinated, and the tourniquet applied to 350 mmHg. The knee was then insufflated with
fluid, a large trocar placed in the medial suprapatellar pouch, and two parapatellar portholes,
one lateral and one medial, just above joint line were made. The knee was thoroughly irrigated
with fluid using the arthroscopic sheath, and then using the 25° 0.5 mm arthroscope, visualization of the joint was begun. Beginning in the suprapatellar pouch, there was no significant
abnormality noted or loose bodies. The undersurface of the patella showed some mild wear
laterally. It was noted to ride in the femoral groove in a centrally directed fashion without
deviation. Exam of the medial joint revealed a medial plica which was not fibrous or inflamed.
Exam of the medial gutter revealed no loose bodies. Exam of the medial joint line revealed the

(Continued on page 2)

MICHAEL JORDAN

#052562

DATE OF OPERATION: 9/25/92

Page 2

OPERATIVE REPORT

meniscus to be intact, being probed in its entirety, and good femoral and tibial articular carti-lage noted. The meniscus was well visualized due to the medial collateral ligament injury. The deep collateral ligament was visualized and noted to be stretched but not completely torn. The posterior horn of the medial meniscus was examined through the notch using a 70° scope, and no evidence of meniscal synovial tear was noted.

Examination of the notch revealed the anterior cruciate ligament to be completely avulsed from its femoral attachment. The remaining tendon was debrided using the automated shaver. Atten-tion was then turned to the lateral joint line where the posterior horn of the lateral meniscus was torn in its periphery. The remainder of the meniscus was noted to be intact. The popliteus tendon was visualized and noted to be intact. The femoral and tibial articular cartilage was noted to be intact. Exam of the lateral gutter revealed no loose bodies or abnormalities.

Attention was then turned to the lateral meniscus where, using a meniscal shaver, the tear was debrided. Using the arthroscope, the posterior horn of the lateral meniscus was then sutured with two mattress-type sutures of nonabsorbable 2-0 material. This was accomplished, making a two-inch lateral incision in order to visualize the posterolateral joint, including the fascia lata distally. The sutures were then tied over the posterolateral capsule, and visualization with the arthroscope revealed the meniscus to be in excellent position and stable. Once this was accomplished, the wound was thoroughly irrigated. The subcutaneous tissue was closed using 3-0 Vicryl suture in an interrupted fashion and the skin with a 3-0 nylon running stitch. The knee was irrigated with copious fluid and closed using 4-0 nylon suture in an interrupted fashion. A sterile compressive dressing was applied. The patient was placed in TED hose and Watco brace, setting the brace between 40° and 60° of free motion. He was then taken to the recovery room in stable condition. The instrument, sponge, and needle counts were correct.

JACK OLDYCE, M.D.

JO:hpi
d: 9/25/92
t: 9/26/92

Lesson 14. Orthopedics

Learning Objectives

Medical

- Describe common orthopedic problems in pediatric and elderly patients.
- Discuss the purpose and technique involved in performing common orthopedic laboratory tests and surgical procedures.
- Define common orthopedic abbreviations.
- Given a cross-section illustration of the muscular system, memorize the names of the muscles.
- Given a category of orthopedic drugs, indicate which drugs belong to that category.
- Differentiate between various orthopedic sound-alike terms.

Fundamentals

- Discuss the cause and prevention of repetitive strain injury (RSI).
- Demonstrate the correct use of hyphens in punctuating medical sentences.
- Given a medical report with errors, identify and correct the errors.

Practice

- Accurately transcribe authentic physician dictation from the specialty of orthopedics.

A Closer Look

Promoting Wellness, Preventing Injury

by Elaine Aamodt

In recent years repetitive stress injury (RSI), also known as cumulative trauma disorder (CTD), has become one of the fastest growing occupational hazards in the U.S. Only 13 years ago, Department of Labor statistics showed RSI accounting for 20 percent of all occupational injuries, but since then that figure has increased to over half.

Such injuries have long been common among butchers, carpenters, and assembly line workers; however, with the advent of widespread computer use, RSI has now become the scourge of the white collar world as well. A job such as medical transcription, which was only recently performed on a typewriter, is now done on computer, and unlike the typewriter of old, the computer allows its user to sit at the keyboard for entire shifts, striking keys four or five times per second without even the occasional break to change paper and ribbon or to hit the carriage return. Such a work environment can easily lead to repetitive stress injuries, and those involved in the transcription field must become aware of the possible risks as well as ways to avoid those risks.

Repetitive stress injuries arise precisely as their name indicates, from repetitive stress, and any job in which continuous repetitive motion is required is a potential offender. Among keyboard users, one of the most common cumulative trauma disorders is carpal tunnel syndrome (CTS). In fact, it was estimated in 1990 that 15 percent of all workers in high-risk industries (such as medical transcription) would develop carpal tunnel syndrome.

Carpal tunnel syndrome develops when the median nerve leading to the hand becomes pinched by swollen tendons or tissue in the carpal tunnel—the narrow tunnel in the wrist formed by the carpal bones. The results are numbness, tingling, pain, or burning sensations in the fingers and hand.

CTS injuries vary both in severity and longevity. In some cases, symptoms subside with such self-help treatments as rubbing or shaking the hand, running warm or cold water over the hand, ice packing, elevation, or rest. Symptoms may return when the stressful motions of the job are resumed. In other cases, symptoms are more severe, often becoming especially painful at night, and can make even the simplest daily task, such as buttoning a shirt, strenuous if not impossible. If further damage is not prevented, pain can also travel to the shoulders, neck, and upper back.

Symptoms of carpal tunnel syndrome usually appear gradually and, in the early stages, are often hard to distinguish from arthritis. However, it is extremely important that anyone suspecting CTS development take preventive steps and see a doctor as soon as possible because symptoms that go ignored over time can lead to permanent disability.

Not only is this a frightening prospect from a health perspective, it is also a potential financial disaster. The American Academy of Orthopaedic Surgeons in 1990 estimated the cost of cumulative trauma disorder related injuries in medical bills and lost workdays at approximately $27 billion. Estimates indicate that direct cost to employers in worker compensation claims, increasing insurance premiums, and medical expenses would average $20,000 per injured worker in just one year, and some cases would exceed $200,000.

These are the simple, easy-to-measure costs. More difficult to quantify is the suffering of the victims. I recently spoke with a transcriptionist in Texas who was plagued with CTS for over a year before doctors were able to diagnose her condition. During that year, because her pain was not diagnosed as resulting from a work-related injury, she was ineligible for worker compensation. (She had been told that pain without an actual diagnosis of injury was not an acceptable reason for missing work.) Unable to continue in her job, she was forced to go on unemployment until a diagnosis was finally made several months later. Since that time, she has undergone surgery on both wrists, and while her condition has improved greatly, the damage done is permanent. Not only will she never be able to work at a keyboard again, she can no longer do simple household chores such as wash dishes or hang clothes in the closet without experiencing severe pain. No price tag can be put on that kind of suffering.

Because carpal tunnel syndrome can be so debilitating and costly, in both human and financial terms, it is something that cannot be ignored in any high-risk field. And while treatments do exist, their results are not always guaranteed. As with most injuries, an ounce of prevention is worth a pound of cure.

Most preventive measures are fairly simple, but they must begin with education (both of management and employees) to be effective. There has to be an atmosphere in the workplace of understanding and an acknowledgment of CTS as a legitimate health concern. Too often employers do not take complaints about pain seriously, and employees are afraid to discuss or even admit discomfort for fear of losing their job. This kind of production-first/workers-last environment is not only dehumanizing, it greatly increases the risk for work-related injuries.

Fostering a positive environment, on the other hand, can lead to improved morale and higher productivity in the long run. The crucial element of education will help transcriptionists to recognize the signs and dangers of wrist pain while still in the early, reversible stages. Understanding and compassion will keep lines of communication open and allow supervisors and transcriptionists to work together to find ways of resolving a problem before it becomes a disaster.

Preventing injury. A good first step is evaluation of the work environment. A transcription service owner recently hired a physical therapist to counsel her employees in the office. With a biofeedback machine, the therapist was able to demonstrate for the transcriptionists how tension is built or released depending on chair position, hand position, screen position, and so on. In this way the transcriptionists became aware of the possible flaws in their usual working positions and consequently learned how to minimize stressful positions and movements.

Often medical transcriptionists who have been working for years feel that they have no need to make any adjustments. To an extent that may be true; a transcriptionist who has been working for ten years or more and hasn't gotten CTS probably never will, according to the medical experts. However, all transcriptionists should be trained to minimize stress and to find the position with the lowest tension, reducing their risk for injury.

Sitting. The workplace must, of course, be completely adjustable. Chairs, for example, must be comfortable and fit their occupants. The jury is still out on what comprises the perfect chair; however, many ergonomists now say that a chair should be adaptable to the diversity of every human body type and seating preference that comes its way. The ergonomically correct chair, they say, should come with an operator's manual and have about 150 parts. Proper seating will not only help stave off CTS, it will also assist in prevention of lower back pain and other injuries.

Once seated, transcriptionists should have the computer screen at eye level so that they will not have to crane their necks this way or that. Wrists should be in a level position, and feet should be comfortably planted on an appropriate footrest. However, even this supposed cure-all position which was once touted as the only correct way to sit has its shortcomings.

According to Marvin Dainoff, Director of the Center for Ergonomic Research at Miami University in Ohio, "Static posture is the enemy." Quoted by Steve Lohr in an informative article in the *New York Times,* "Sit Down and Read This (No, Not in That Chair!)" (July 7, 1992), Dainoff explains that remaining perfectly still in any position for too long is not good for anyone. Small movements, called "micromovements" (wiggling and fidgeting), are important in that they help relieve stress on the back, shoulders, hands, and wrists. This will not only help avert CTS, but also will help reduce other injuries related to long periods of sitting.

In *Sitting on the Job* (Houghton Mifflin, 1989), author Scott Donkin also recognizes the problem: "People who sit a great deal tend to develop weak abdominal, buttock, and front and inner thigh muscles. Their neck, shoulder, and back muscles tend to be tense, and their spinal movements are usually restricted." Exercise and the freedom to move about and to take stretching breaks are crucial in combating repetitive stress injury.

Breaks. Not only are breaks a vital part of CTS avoidance, but the manner in which breaks are taken actually makes a difference as well. Statistically, it appears that people working in a mentally or emotionally stressful environment are more prone to developing CTS due to the general effects of stress on the body. Psychologically, and consequently physically, it is therefore crucial that supervisors and service owners not only allow, but actually encourage or mandate frequent breaks for employees. The feeling that breaks are encouraged helps employees feel that their well-being is a top priority (as well it should be) which improves morale and can actually contribute to the healing effect in and of itself.

The *Los Angeles Times* office, where nearly 40 percent of its editorial staff was suffering from CTS to varying degrees, has seen positive results from having messages programmed into the computer terminals that automatically remind employees to take a break every fifty minutes. The newspaper office also provides a break room where employees have access to exercise equipment and a refrigerator with ice packs to help them ease the pressure in their wrists.

Self-help. If symptoms of CTS do appear, there are some self-help efforts that can be very effective. However, if implemented incorrectly these same efforts can actually do more harm than good. For example, wearing a forearm splint works well for some, but if used improperly, this same splint can increase pressure on the wrist and increase damage. Similarly some researchers have asserted that a vitamin B_6 deficiency is a leading cause of CTS. However, trying to treat your CTS by taking B_6 supplements on your own can be extremely dangerous since high B_6 intake can lead to permanent nerve damage. Exercise is also important in combating CTS, but the wrong kinds of exercise will also lead to further damage. For reasons such as these, it is wise to consult a physician or physical therapist and to do plenty of research on your own while planning your attack on carpal tunnel syndrome.

If your office cannot afford state-of-the-art ergonomic chairs, fully adjustable work stations, and all the other available gadgetry, there are still many simple steps that can be implemented quickly and easily that will reduce the chance of injury in your workplace.

A medical transcription service owner suffering from CTS found that a good wrist pad running along the lower edge of the keyboard was enough to get her back on the job. Such a pad helps prevent the wrists from flexing or bending in unhealthy ways and generally costs only about $30.

It is also important to give your hands frequent breaks from the keyboard in order to stretch. If possible, consult a physical therapist or physician to find out about specific exercises you can do both at home and at the keyboard to keep carpal tunnel syndrome at bay. You may also find such exercises in the popular literature. Scott Donkin's highly recommended book *Sitting on the Job* (Houghton Mifflin, 1989) contains detailed diagrams of exercises for back, neck, shoulder, and hands, as well as diagrams and descriptions of healthful sleeping positions, sitting positions, and even breathing exercises for relaxation.

While there are many new and innovative ergonomic products on the market, we must realize that, while these products can be very helpful, a major component in fighting carpal tunnel syndrome is *attitude.*

Everyone involved must become educated about carpal tunnel syndrome and accept the fact that some fundamental changes will have to be made in the way we go about our work before this problem can be eliminated.

The Arms Race

by Bron Taylor

I had a chance encounter with a phlebotomist friend of mine the other day, and he started a line of thought I can't shake. He's working under difficult conditions—40 hours a week in a hospital, with no benefits, at a salary below that of most beginning transcriptionists. He does a job which the hospital cannot function safely without (without blood being drawn, few lab tests can be done and modern medicine can't be practiced). In the small lab he works in, there are many accidental needlestick injuries a year, and one of his co-workers has already converted to HIV-positive status. I asked him how he could stand it. "I need the job. After a year, I'll go some place better," he said. Then he told me that he had recently told his supervisor, "I will only work as fast as I can concentrate and do a safe job. If you want faster work than that, get somebody else." (They kept him.)

There are many parallels to transcription in his remark. Over the 20 years I've been transcribing (at a major university medical center, a large private hospital, a small private hospital, and as a proofreader/transcriptionist for two services), I've seen quotas rise inexorably. I think we're nearing or possibly at the point where we need to say, "Enough." We're not, of course, at the same level of risk as the phlebotomists, but there are two problems in this uncontrolled "arms race" we're now engaged in.

I remember when it was different. My best job was at the university, where I had the great good fortune to have Vera Pyle as my supervisor. This was in the years before DRGs and the increased pressure on hospitals to cut costs, and they were, as Vera calls them, truly "the Golden Years." We had in-service education lectures from every specialty. We were allowed to watch surgery from inside the operating room whenever we wanted. We were considered to be doing our job if to research a new term we got up and went to the bookstore or the library or on a search for the dictators themselves. The goal was to produce immaculate reports with no medical errors.

Well, isn't that the goal everywhere? Unfortunately, at many of the places I've worked in recent years, no. At one hospital, I saw "*methadone*-resistant Staph. aureus" come off the printer on a co-worker's report. I asked my supervisor if she would diplomatically explain that it would have to be changed, and was told that it was the doctor's responsibility to read the report before he signed it and to "get back to your terminal." I've also frequently heard remarks from fellow transcriptionists such as "They don't pay us enough to pay attention" (from salaried MTs) and (from production MTs) "I can't make any money if I have to proofread what I'm doing."

I may be a maverick, but I think at the point where we're going so fast that things like this get out into the world, we're going too fast. Perhaps I have an unorthodox view of our function. Certainly we are medical language specialists. Of course we are voice recognition experts. There is no question that the work we produce quickly allows for good patient care, is useful for research purposes, and aids in timely payment to physicians and hospitals, which helps keep the doors open to patients.

Nevertheless, I think the primary reason we go to continuing education lectures and learn as much as possible about medicine is that we really are part of the healthcare team. When not pressed to superhuman speed, we can function as the last healthcare workers in a position to catch a tired physician's inversions, slips, and errors from fatigue, and produce the record the dictator intended, if not exactly the one dictated. Medical records are special documents, protected by confidentiality, and used by a great many people. They must be accurate. If a tired or pressed transcriptionist transcribes a drug, for example, that rhymes with what was intended, a lot of damage might be done. We all know that sometimes the doctors sign without reading the record. Particularly in these days of computers, when the records look so beautiful, it's tempting for doctors to assume that what looks right is right.

There is another aspect to the question of the push for more and more speed. At another hospital where I worked, every two weeks we were given productivity slips, comparing our production to that of our fellow workers, to two decimal places. This was the only criterion by which our work was measured. No attention was paid to difficulty of dictation, environmental variables, or clerical duties. Soon several of us developed nightmares about these production comparisons. Others developed repetitive strain injuries. Interestingly, none of us reported these injuries, although they were clearly job-related, because in the current climate we were afraid of losing our jobs. That's the situation in many hospitals where my friends work.

In some transcription services, where one's ability to earn is directly correlated with one's speed, the problem is even worse. Naturally, the response is to go faster and faster, to compete, to stay within acceptable limits, which rise ever higher.

What's the problem with this? Who among us hasn't done work for an orthopedist, hand surgeon, or neurologist and heard that the patient works at a computer keyboard, without thinking "uh oh"?

I can't be the only transcriptionist who has seen a great rise in the number of cases of carpal tunnel syndrome, de Quervain's, or even outlet syndrome of the shoulders, from this daily mad pace at the keyboards. I can't be the only one reading of workers waking in the night from the pain. Recently I've read reports from hand surgeons suggesting that the worker slow down (and how does one explain this to one's supervisor?) or be retrained for a non-keyboard position.

What's going on here? Medically, we're being afflicted by an overuse syndrome, I think. Carpal tunnel syndrome is the most common. The problem is that in that small tunnel, formed by the transverse retinacular ligament and the carpal bones, run the median nerve and nine extrinsic flexor tendons. My favorite orthopedic book gives 24 possible causes for entrapment neuropathy (which carpal tunnel is); one of them is overuse syndrome and another is wrist fracture. I haven't heard of too many transcriptionists fracturing their wrists, but I have seen overuse syndrome.

Carpal tunnel syndrome can be diagnosed by electrodiagnostic tests, but outlet syndrome and de Quervain's are mostly diagnoses of exclusion, when the tests are negative and the pain remains. The orthopedic text author cheerfully goes on to say that most of these compression neuropathies cure themselves within six weeks, assuming no work is done at the keyboard, but what happens when the individual has to return to full-time high-speed work is not discussed.

Overuse syndrome seems to occur mostly in transcriptionists who have been working for many years, but need we lose their valuable experience? Certainly there are palliative measures, such as wrist rests, special keyboards, and ergonomic chairs, but they seem to be more discussed than employed. This can certainly change.

Possibly even more important than ergonomically poor equipment is job stress. I read an article recently in which the author cites a study in which 6 percent of workers at one group of keyboards were injured on the job, while 36 percent of similar workers were injured in a different department, with different management. The author felt that attitudes of supervisors to workers, pressure for speed, and fear of layoffs were factors in the injuries. He also states that some of these injuries can cause pain sufficient to end careers, which is very traumatic for someone who loves to transcribe.

Stress would be greatly reduced if transcriptionists slowed down to the point where they could use their brains as well as their fingers. I think we'd have a sense of having done the job better. I think without using our brains we have no right to call ourselves medical professionals. Why do we go to meetings to learn—if not to be helpful? Are we really medical professionals, or speed-typing machines? These days "faster is better" is becoming the ideal for transcriptionists, and, having seen the results as a proofreader, I know that's not right. I've seen some errors on reports from high-speed transcriptionists that would shock you, yet I know they'll argue they have the right to be paid for their exceptional speed, and of course they do.

Still . . . medical records are unique and we have a responsibility to produce them as accurately as possible. I feel that lately the only skill wanted from us is speed, not the ability gained from meetings and study and long experience to determine what the dictators really intended when they make unintentional errors. That used to be one of our skills too, possibly our chief skill, and I mourn its loss. When all that our supervisors want from us is speed, regardless of quality, we have reverted to being mere "girl typists," rather than medical professionals. (No offense to the many excellent male transcriptionists who have joined our ranks; this applies to them, too.)

When we are monitored like children, we've lost any control over our work, and there's a tacit sense that we're not responsible enough to do an honest day's work without the amount being closely checked and the quality ignored completely. This is precisely what causes the stress.

In no way am I suggesting that we go back to the plodding pace of old. All experienced transcriptionists are fast; we've learned how to use the reference books and get back to the keyboard quickly. We're aware of the pressures on hospitals and transcription services to produce more work, faster, and we're caught up in all of that. But what is the answer for medical transcriptionists, and when is The Arms Race going to end?

Proofreading Skills

Orthopedic Practice and Surgery

by Michael A. Ellis, M.D.

Modern orthopedics can be defined as the medical discipline that deals with problems of bones, joints, and muscles. The specialty of orthopedics originally evolved to help crippled children—to correct their deformities, to make them straight. The word *orthopedic* literally means "straight child"—from the Greek *ortho-* (straight) and *pais* (child).

One of the most interesting facets of orthopedics is that it is a medical discipline subject to great change—change for the better, which is why I find the practice of orthopedics exciting and enjoyable.

An orthopedic physician who sees ambulatory patients or outpatients in the office will recommend surgery only about one in twenty times. This average increases, of course, for the orthopedist whose caseload includes trauma victims. In a general orthopedic practice, approximately one-half of patients require emergency surgery for trauma, infections, or tumors. The rest are cases in which surgery is done electively, after nonsurgical approaches to the problem are unsuccessful.

Treatment of children. A general orthopedist, whose training is about 20 percent in pediatric orthopedics, frequently encounters children with orthopedic difficulties. The worst of these is noticeable right at birth and often includes such problems as clubfoot and congenital dislocation of the hip. In addition, birth trauma may result in orthopedic complications, particularly fractured clavicles.

Babies with fractures require little treatment. Their blood circulation is so efficient that one can almost see the healing process taking place. For instance, collar bone fractures occur frequently at birth but heal within four or five days, and without the use of an immobilizer. Unfortunately, our blood circulation gets steadily worse from the day of birth until we die, so that a fracture requiring only a few days to heal in a child may take six to eight weeks to heal in an adult.

Tradition once mandated that a child with clubfoot (a condition in which the foot is bent downward and inward) would receive no treatment until walking age. Frankly, the rationale for this was the blind hope that the foot would improve on its own. Even as recently as ten years ago, treatment of clubfoot was delayed until the child was a year old, requiring an average of four operations between ages one and 15 years. Usually these attempts were unsuccessful, leaving the patient with a fused foot that would not bend normally.

Today it is recognized that surgical intervention for clubfoot should be carried out at an early age. By the time the infant is three months old, the physician is able to assess whether cast technique or nonsurgical methods will be effective in the treatment of clubfoot. If nonsurgical treatment is unsuccessful by age three months, surgery is carried out. The procedure is not performed on the newborn because the stress of anesthesia and surgery is considered detrimental and is better tolerated when the infant is older.

The trend in orthopedic treatment includes not only earlier operations but also far more aggressive surgical techniques. For instance, clubfoot used to be treated with two separate operations—one to correct the downwardness and one to correct the inwardness, at ages one and two, respectively. And it would take one year beyond that before results were apparent. Today both procedures are performed during one operation, and the results are usually excellent. If good position is maintained after surgery with casting, the chances are 90 percent that the clubfoot will grow as a normal foot, albeit several sizes smaller than the opposite, unaffected foot. This smallness does not reflect failure of surgical treatment; it is rather that the same birth defect that caused the clubfoot produces other abnormalities in the same leg. Thus, a clubfoot that has been surgically corrected will look a bit different from a normal foot.

Children with a congenital discrepancy in leg length present an entirely different challenge to the orthopedic surgeon. In the past, the usual method of leg length equalization was time-consuming, debilitating, and required frequent hospitalization that often necessitated withdrawing the child from school for approximately two years. The surgery consisted of shortening the longer leg by cutting a segment out of it. Or, if the child was still growing, staples were placed across the epiphyseal growth plate to slow the growth of that leg until the legs equalized in length.

These procedures were arduous and fraught with complications, including interruption of the blood or nerve supply to the leg. The surgery was so debilitating that it was performed only when leg length discrepancy was severe enough that amputation was the only alternative. And today, when tallness is considered a positive rather than a negative social trait, physicians cannot convince a child or the child's parents to consider leg shortening surgery.

Presently the treatment of this condition is undergoing rapid evolution. A Russian physician by the name of Ilizarov (eh-liz'-a-rov) has developed a most innovative method of leg lengthening. It involves inserting metallic pins through the leg above and below the area to be lengthened, creating a surgical fracture, and then stretching the healing fracture apart. As the fracture heals, the soft new bone is literally stretched, and huge differences in leg length—up to several inches—can be corrected. There are none of the complications that were so prevalent with previous procedures.

The Ilizarov technique represents a genuine advancement in orthopedic practice. Orthopedic surgeons in the western hemisphere are now beginning to use Dr. Ilizarov's method, and I personally did my first Ilizarov procedure in September 1988.

Future pediatric orthopedic innovations will likely include in utero surgery to correct congenital malformations and deformities. Although we can't currently treat these conditions (today's instruments are too large to fit into the womb), this technology is up and coming and definitely on the horizon of orthopedic surgery. And further down the road is genetic manipulation that will totally prevent congenital abnormalities from developing at all.

The elderly orthopedic patient. The orthopedic physician sees many elderly patients who develop age-related injuries and conditions. Yet surprisingly, most of these people not only survive surgery but do very well. An elderly person in good general and mental health, with prospects for living five or more years, is a candidate to undergo even an arduous orthopedic procedure. The average age of elderly patients in my practice is 77, and there are many who are over 100 years of age!

About 12 years ago a 94-year-old lady who lives on a small farm came to see me, because she fell off her roof while she was trying to repair it to keep the rain off her and her 30 cats. She had broken her hip in the fall and required an artificial hip. She did very well after surgery, except that she complained of back pain and insisted that her back was broken. A back x-ray was taken, but her bones were so arthritic that it was impossible to detect a fracture. Our medical opinion was that her pain was due to severe arthritis, and I said to her, "Your're awfully old—94—your back ought to hurt! But there are no fractures on the x-ray, and your back pain is probably caused by arthritis." Her reply was, "Oh no, Dr. Sonny" (her name for me, since I was just 38 at the time), "I know my back

is broken." Three months later we took a followup x-ray, and there was the fracture!

At age 94, she went on to heal the back fracture as well as the artificial hip. She is now 106 years old and comes to see me occasionally, saying that she's still around and doing well, and reminds me, "I want you to know that I fixed that roof!"

The most prevalent surgical problem of the aged is that of stress fractures due to osteoporosis (thin and brittle bones). Older people, especially women, are not accustomed to falling; they do not employ their bodies in an agile way to prevent fractures when they fall. Complications and fractures resulting from falls are a staple of life for the aging person, especially the woman with osteoporosis.

A fallacy often repeated is that patients with osteoporotic fractures heal slowly. In actual fact, their fractures heal nearly as rapidly as those of a 30-year-old; the rate of healing for both is about the same. It is the *quality* of healing that is different. While the young patient heals with strong bone, the osteoporotic patient heals with bone of poor quality.

Osteoporosis is not necessarily limited to the elderly. Hyperthyroidism and other states that change the body's metabolic capacity may cause osteoporosis in a younger person as well.

There is now a very sophisticated medical test for osteoporosis called *bone densitometry,* and some osteoporosis centers charge upwards of $1,000 a visit for this service. In general, however, there is a tried-and-true test that doesn't require formal evaluation and is effective for the vast majority of older people, and that is, simply, an x-ray of whatever part of the body has pain.

Osteoporosis is demonstrated on x-ray by bone volume loss of 50 percent or more. By adding up the millimeters of thickness of the bone cortices (the outer bone coatings), the sum of the two cortices should at least be equal to the diameter of the intramedullary canal. If the sum of the two cortices is one-third or less the diameter of the intramedullary canal, severe osteoporosis is present. The experienced orthopedist will know at a glance if advanced osteoporosis is present on x-ray.

Osteoporosis cannot be reversed, even with today's state-of-the-art technology. The best we can do with current treatment is to arrest its progression. And despite all the talk about calcium supplementation, this will not reverse osteoporosis. Why aren't calcium supplements effective in reversing osteoporosis? Because bones are not made primarily of calcium. Bones are comprised of calcium hydroxyapatite, which is a mineral suspended in a living matrix of cells and other "bone glue" such as collagen fibers. Calcium supplementation does not affect the quality of these components.

What calcium supplements *can* do is arrest the progression of osteoporosis. The diet of most elderly people is deficient in calcium and protein in any case, and calcium supplements just add to the diet what should already be there. There is no question that an inadequate intake of protein and calcium will result in the production of poor quality osteoporotic bone. For a woman, the quality of bone at the time of menopause primarily determines whether or not she will become osteoporotic in later years.

If one added up all of the factors that deal with the strength of bone and the determination of osteoporosis—the amount of calcium in the body, protein in the diet, dietary substrates and bone-making materials, hormones that promote bone formation—and weighed them against exercise alone, the scale would tip more than 90 percent in favor of exercise. In my studied opinion, lack of exercise is the vastly underrated factor in osteoporosis.

If you inspect the lifestyle of the average woman with osteoporosis, you would discover that she walks less than one-half mile per day and does little lifting. Axial stress upon the bony skeleton—the loading of vertical weight—is very important in keeping bones strong. Bedridden people develop osteoporosis. Even a 15-year-old, who is metabolically superior and has a high calcium intake, will develop severe osteoporosis within a month if all physical activity sudden ceases (from paralysis, for example).

In addition to osteoporosis and fractures, elderly patients present with a wide variety of other orthopedic problems. Degenerative arthritis of the joints is a common presenting complaint of the elderly. In the mid-1950s, older people with hip fractures were simply put to bed—and nearly every person died within three months from pneumonia or other complications of forced bed rest, including the mental disorientation that older people experience when they are subjected to major stress.

Today, the ultimate orthopedic solution is to replace the joint, and joint replacement surgery has evolved to the point where hip, knee, elbow, and wrist joints can be replaced with quite satisfactory results. Even very elderly patients opt for joint replacement surgery when the prospect of regaining mobility and independence is offered. The death rate in orthopedic surgery of the elderly is surprisingly low—about 2 percent, which is actually comparable to the risk from a stroke or coronary. These statistics support the opinion that aggressive treatment for severe orthopedic problems is better than marginal treatment or no treatment.

Total hip replacement. When artificial hip surgery first came into vogue, there was only one brand of prosthesis—an artificial hip invented by Dr. Charnley of England and manufactured of stainless steel in Switzerland. Today there are many choices in hip prostheses, and the best ones are made of titanium rather than stainless steel. Titanium is durable, lighter, and its flexibility is more like that of real bone. (A metal apparatus that is rigid and cannot deflect will work its way loose or break the bone.)

Great controversy currently rages regarding the use of cemented hip prostheses versus press-fit prostheses. The press-fit prosthesis fits very snugly into the bone, within 1/1000 of an inch, and requires no cement. With the use of a porous-coated press-fit prosthesis with fine pores—on the order of 100 to 400 microns—the patient's own bone grows into the pores, resulting in true biologic binding that is not dependent upon cement. This is currently favored, and I believe it is a better process since a biologic bond does not have the inclination of cement to crack and ultimately fail.

Most prostheses are placed within the cavity of a bone, and the orthopedist must make the patient's bone fit the prosthesis. However, the technology for computerized bone cavity measurement is under development, and soon we will be able to fit the prosthesis to the bone—a prosthesis with a custom fit that will last the patient's lifetime.

Hemophilia. Why would a hemophiliac be under the care of an orthopedic surgeon? Blood contains enzymes that break down cartilage and impair the generation of lubricating material by the synovium. By the age of five, a hemophiliac child will have experienced thousands of bleeds into the joints, leading to destruction of the joints by the late teen years or early adulthood.

The high motion and weightbearing joints are the first to degenerate, beginning with the knees and usually followed by elbows, ankles, and hips. As the joints become deformed and contracted, the patient is left with only partial movement and characteristic body posture—walking on the toes with knees, elbows, and hips bent. In previous years, 20 percent of my hemophiliac patients required joint replacement surgery per annum.

During the past year the bottom has fallen out of elective surgery for joint replacements, and I have not operated on any hemophiliacs except in acute emergencies.

AIDS. AIDS has become a serious health risk for hemophiliacs. Current treatment for hemophilia consists of administration of clotting factors (factor VIII for classic hemophilia, factor IX for Christmas disease). The clotting factors are obtained through plasmapheresis—extracting plasma from large pools of donated whole blood, with hundreds of donors for each unit of clotting factor. By the age of five the hemophiliac child will likely become contaminated with the AIDS virus. In fact, every known hemophiliac in my private practice is seropositive for the AIDS virus.

There is an ethical problem related to surgically treating the hemophiliac patient: the orthopedic surgeon is at risk for contracting AIDS. Most orthopedic surgeons have had hemophiliac blood all over them during surgery, and surgeons frequently nick or cut themselves with contaminated scalpels. In 1988 over 15 percent of San Francisco's orthopedists tested positive for the AIDS virus.

Osteogenesis imperfecta. More rare than hemophilia, osteogenesis imperfecta is a genetically transmitted disease of collagenous tissue that leads to fractures and disfigurement early in life.

Patients with osteogenesis imperfecta are said to have "blue eyes and brittle bones." Collagen tissue in the eye is so deficient that light is able to penetrate the sclerae, revealing underlying blue veins, and thus the whites of the eyes appear blue. These patients have so many fractures that their bones often curve and shorten by the time they are young adults.

Treatment for osteogenesis imperfecta requires intramedullary rodding with multiple osteotomies—in lay terms a shish kebab operation. The curved bone is re-broken in multiple places, a rod is inserted down the middle, and the bones are allowed to heal in a straightened position.

Ollier's disease. Ollier's disease is a rare hereditary disorder in which there is defective conversion of cartilage within bones during childhood. Bones become weakened and are subject to frequent fracturing, and there may be visible lumps of cartilage that interfere with joint fusion. A child with this condition may have dozens of these lumpy tumors, and, unfortunately, surgical removal is not a practical consideration.

Sports medicine. Sports medicine is simply good medicine applied to people who play sports. That it has become a subspecialty is faulty, I believe, since there are no new or different treatments offered to the sports individual that are not offered to any other orthopedic patient.

When I was the team physician for the Baltimore Bullets, a professional basketball team, I used the same medical treatment for the professional athletes as I did for my nonathlete patients. The basic difference lay not in the treatment but rather in the patient. The athlete is usually in better overall physical condition, is more motivated in getting through treatment, and in setting post-treatment goals.

Podiatry. Podiatrists are trained in the mechanics of performing operative procedures on the foot, but they do not have any formal surgical training. I believe that podiatrists have a valid role as paramedical people with medical training in foot anatomy, and that they offer services that other medical disciplines do not provide adequately or optimally. For instance, when an older patient with diabetes develops corns or calluses that need treatment, the podiatrist is an appropriate care giver. However, I do not believe that podiatrists are fully capable of surgically treating diseases involving the foot. Surgery requires detailed technique based on an extensive background of medical knowledge, and no part of the body should be approached on a purely mechanical basis. I believe that the role of the podiatrist should be essentially nonsurgical.

Neurosurgery. In nonmetropolitan areas, spinal surgery frequently falls under the care of the orthopedist. Conversely, in larger hospitals and medical centers, neurosurgeons characteristically do all spinal surgery except for fusions and fracture repairs.

I personally do fracture repairs with rods and grafts, and do spinal fusions on those patients who have deteriorating disk disease. I leave the actual treatment of nerves and nerve roots to the neurosurgeons.

Pediatric orthopedics. Orthopedic surgeons who are interested in pediatric orthopedics take an extra year or two of specialized training. I believe that pediatric orthopedics is a valid subspecialty and warrants extra training. After all, doing major reconstructive surgery on a foot that is only two inches in length is a great deal different than operating on a foot that is ten inches long.

Orthopedics is an exciting medical and surgical specialty in an era of evolution. It is a discipline which offers much more today than it did 20 years ago, and 20 years from now will offer much more than it can today. For me, that is exciting to contemplate.

Laboratory Tests and Surgical Procedures

alkaline phosphatase   An enzyme whose level in the serum is often increased in bone disease and obstructive liver disease. Sometimes dictated "alk. phos."

ANA (antinuclear antibody)   An antibody detected by immunofluorescence in patients with rheumatoid arthritis, lupus erythematosus, and other autoimmune diseases.

arthroscopy   A surgical procedure which involves an incision into a joint and the insertion of an arthroscope to view the structures inside the joint.

Bessey-Lowry units   Units used to measure serum alkaline phosphatase.

bone scan   A nuclear imaging test which, following the intravenous administration of technetium, uses a scanning device to detect areas of abnormal uptake in the bones to identify fractures.

densitometry   Determination of variations in density (for example, bone density) by comparison with that of another material or with a certain standard. See *dual photon densitometry*.

dual photon densitometry   A quantitative assessment of a patient's bone density, and comparison with normal ranges for persons of the same age and sex.

EMG (electromyogram)   A test to determine the response pattern of muscles when stimulated by an electrical impulse from needle electrode inserted into the muscle.

erythrocyte sedimentation rate (ESR)   The rate at which red blood cells settle to the bottom of a specimen of whole blood that has been treated with anticoagulant. The rate is expressed in mm/h (millimeters per hour), as measured in a standard glass column. Elevation of the sedimentation rate occurs in various inflammatory and malignant diseases but is diagnostic of none. An acceptable brief form is *sed rate.*

ORIF (open reduction and internal fixation)   A surgical procedure to correct a fracture that requires alignment and fixation with a plate, pin, or screw.

RF (rheumatoid factor)   An antibody present in the serum of patients with rheumatoid arthritis and other autoimmune disorders.

sed rate   See *erythrocyte sedimentation rate.*

uric acid, serum   A breakdown product of purine metabolism, increased in gout and other disorders.

x-ray   The most common and least expensive diagnostic tool for assessing bone structure and integrity. Also called *radiograph* and *film*.

Anatomy/Medical Terminology

Orthopedic Questions

1. What is the difference between an orthopedist, osteopath, chiropractor, and rheumatologist?

2. The generic drug ibuprofen is very popular. Can you name its famous prescription trade name as well as two of its popular nonprescription, over-the-counter trade names?

Abbreviations Exercise

Common abbreviations may be transcribed as dictated in the body of a report. Uncommon abbreviations must be spelled out, with the abbreviation appearing in parentheses after the translation. All abbreviations (except laboratory test names) must be spelled out in the Diagnosis or Impression section of any report.

Instructions: Define the following orthopedic abbreviations. Then memorize both abbreviations and definitions to increase your speed and accuracy in transcribing dictation from orthopedics.

AAA _____

AK amputation _____

BK amputation _____

C1 to C7 _____

T1 to T12 _____

L1 to L5 _____

CTD _____

CTS _____

DTR _____

EMG _____

HNP _____

NSAID _____

ORIF _____

PIP _____

RF _____

RSI _____

TENS unit _____

VMO _____

Anatomy: The Muscular System

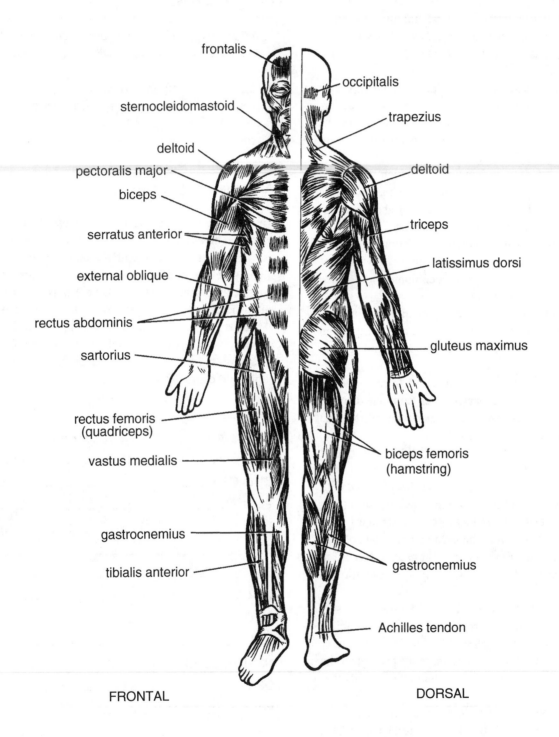

frontalis

occipitalis

sternocleidomastoid

trapezius

deltoid

pectoralis major

deltoid

biceps

triceps

serratus anterior

latissimus dorsi

external oblique

rectus abdominis

sartorius

gluteus maximus

rectus femoris
(quadriceps)

vastus medialis

biceps femoris
(hamstring)

gastrocnemius

tibialis anterior

gastrocnemius

Achilles tendon

FRONTAL

DORSAL

Drug Matching Exercise

Instructions: Match the drug category in Column A with the generic and trade name drugs in Column B. Note: Drug categories are used more than once.

Column A	*Column B*
A. corticosteroid	_____ Flexeril
	_____ ibuprofen
B. aspirin + antacid	_____ Bufferin
	_____ Meclomen
C. nonsteroidal anti-inflammatory	_____ Soma
	_____ Decadron
	_____ Voltaren
D. muscle relaxant	_____ Skelaxin
	_____ Clinoril
	_____ cortisone
	_____ Parafon Forte
	_____ Feldene
	_____ Cama
	_____ Robaxin
	_____ Orudis

Sound-alikes Exercise

Instructions: Circle the correct term from the sound-alikes in parentheses in the following sentences.

1. On the x-ray, the bony (apophysis, epiphysis) was closed in this 12-year-old precocious child.

2. The patient shattered the calcaneal (apophysis, epiphysis) when he jumped from the roof and landed on his feet.

3. The seventh (cervical, surgical) vertebra was fractured when the patient dived into the river and hit a submerged rock.

4. The humerus was fractured in its upper portion just at the (cervical, surgical) neck.

5. The child's right femoral (diaphysis, diastasis, diathesis) measured 13 cm, the left measured 11.5 cm.

6. On strength testing, the (flexor, flexure) muscle of the right arm was weaker than the left.

7. The patient had a (callous, callus) on his (heal, heel).

8. The thenar (eminence, imminence) was not visualized on the x-ray.

9. The ischium and (ileum, ilium) were shattered, the hip totally dislocated.

10. The remainder of the median nerve dissection was done under (loop, loupe) magnification.

11. The (metacarpal, metatarsal) bones of the patient's right hand were slightly calcified.

12. The left second (metacarpal, metatarsal) was fractured and the toe deviated to the right.

13. On x-ray, the line between the epiphysis and (metaphysis, metastasis) was not visible.

14. (Osteal, Ostial) density was thin and the bone porous in this postmenopausal woman.

15. (Axis, Obvious, Osseous) overgrowth of the (pen, pin) in the hip was noted.

16. The pain started in the buttocks and traveled along the peroneal nerve down into the patient's left (side, thigh).

17. The cowboy had a pronounced genu (valgum, varum) deformity.

18. The child was knock-kneed, genu (valgum, varum), and pigeon-toed, talipes (valgus, varus).

Word Search

Instructions: Locate and circle the orthopedic terms hidden in the puzzle horizontally, vertically, and diagonally, forward and backward. A numeral following a term in the word list indicates the number of times it can be found in the puzzle.

```
T  X  M  M  U  S  C  L  E  G  T  A  E
A  S  R  U  B  P  L  S  H  I  N  L  L
O  K  A  S  O  R  U  S  U  B  E  U  B
T  S  A  C  N  A  B  L  L  K  M  B  O
N  I  T  L  E  I  F  D  N  B  A  I  W
I  D  Q  E  R  N  O  J  A  A  G  F  R
O  S  T  E  O  P  O  R  O  S  I  S  A
J  H  N  S  G  M  T  V  A  N  L  U  L
S  B  I  R  Z  A  Y  F  E  M  U  R  L
U  C  O  N  D  Y  L  E  M  G  F  W  E
R  C  J  H  G  E  L  I  L  I  U  M  T
E  I  U  K  X  C  U  Y  T  I  B  I  A
M  N  B  I  S  D  N  I  A  R  T  S  P
U  G  O  U  S  I  S  Y  H  P  A  I  D
H  N  M  B  N  O  D  N  E  T  H  C  S
```

arm	femur	osteoporosis
bone (2)	fibula	osteomyelitis
bursa	flexion	patella
cartilage	hip	rib
cast (2)	humerus	ribs (2)
clubfoot	ilium	shin
condyle	joint (2)	sprain
diaphysis	leg	strain
disk (2)	ligament	tendon
elbow	lumbar	tibia
EMG	muscle (3)	ulna (3)

Hyphens

1. The trend in contemporary usage is to avoid the use of hyphens when they are not needed for clarity. Many coined words commonly used in medical reports do not appear in dictionaries, and it is up to the transcriptionist to decide whether to hyphenate them for clarity. For example, neither *weightbearing* nor *weight-bearing* (a term commonly used in orthopedic reports) appears in standard or medical dictionaries. The hyphenated word *follow-up* appears as a noun and adjective in *Webster's* and as two words without a hyphen as a verb. Some choose to omit the hyphen in *follow-up* by analogy to *workup*, a noun which does not have a hyphen.

   She is scheduled for follow-up in one week.
   Her follow-up appointment is in one week.
   She will follow up with the therapist in one week.

2. **Hyphens and numbers.** The use of hyphens with adjectives followed by metric measurement abbreviations is optional.

   2 cm laceration   OR   2-cm laceration

3. **Hyphens and adjectives.** Compound adjectives are hyphenated when the last letter of the first part is the same as the first letter of the second part.

   nonsteroidal anti-inflammatory drug

4. Traditionally, compound adjectives are hyphenated when they precede the noun and not hyphenated when they follow the noun.

   This 22-year-old patient was admitted yesterday.
   The patient was 22 years old.

   The patient is a well-developed, well-nourished 57-year-old white female appearing her stated age.

   The patient is well developed and well nourished.

5. Permanent compounds containing *self* retain the hyphen whether they precede or follow the noun they modify.

   a self-inflicted wound
   a wound that is self-inflicted
   self-conscious, self-restraint

6. Do not use a hyphen with compound adjectives formed with adverbs ending in -*ly* plus a participle or adjective.

   poorly developed and poorly nourished patient
   highly complex symptoms

7. **Hyphens and a complex modifying phrase.** In a complex modifying phrase that includes a prefix or suffix, hyphens are sometimes used to avoid ambiguity.

   non-insulin-dependent diabetes mellitus
   non-brain-injured patient

8. **Hyphens and ages.** Hyphenate ages when they appear before the noun they modify.

   The patient is a 36-year-old white male.

9. Do not hyphenate ages that appear after the noun they modify.

   The patient is 36 years old.

   Clue: When *years* is used instead of *year*, a hyphen is not used.

10. **Hyphens and prefixes.** When the prefix *post* (after, behind, posterior) is used as an adjective before a noun, it is connected to the root word without a hyphen.

    The postoperative assessment was negative.
    postacetabular, postsacral, posttraumatic

11. The word *post* in the phrase *status post* stands alone as a compound not connected to the noun it modifies.

    The patient is status post closed fracture of the left leg.

12. When two prefixes combine with the same root word, the first may be hyphenated. Alternatively, the root word may be repeated for clarity.

    The pre- and postoperative diagnoses were the same.
    The preoperative and postoperative diagnoses were the same.
    a 10- to 12-week history of symptoms

13. The use of hyphens with *mid* varies. The word *mid* may stand alone as an adjective or combine with a root word without a hyphen.

    mid and left forefoot
    midfoot, midline

14. **Hyphens and suffixes.** When *like* and *most* appear as suffixes, they are attached to the root word without a hyphen. If the root word ends with the same letter as the first letter of the suffix, hyphenate the word for clarity. If the root word has more than one syllable, hyphenation is optional.

    bandlike pain   yeastlike fungus
    shell-like growth   barrel-like chest

    seizure-like, seizurelike
    anterior-most, anteriormost

15. **Hyphens and single letters.** A hyphen is not needed to connect a single letter and noun combination, although it is acceptable to do so.

    J sign   C-section   T wave

16. A hyphen is used to join a single letter and an adjective or participle modifying a noun.

    Y-shaped incision

17. **Hyphens and clarity.** A hyphen is used to clarify medical meaning, when needed. In the following example, placing the hyphen between *large* and *bore* makes it clear that the physician is referring to the size of the bore, not the size of the needle.

    A large-bore needle was selected.

Hyphens Exercise

Instructions: Correct errors in the use of hyphens and numbers in the following sentences.

1. This 25 year old woman was admitted with a history of pain in the shoulder over the last 24 hour period.

2. This well developed and well nourished 13 month old boy was referred to the pediatric clinic for follow up.

3. The patient's pain medication was self administered as needed.

4. After the patient was prepped and draped, we entered the leg with a Y shaped incision.

5. She complains of a continual stabbing like pain over a three week period.

6. He is status post open reduction and internal fixation procedure with an additional post operative diagnosis of osteomyelitis.

7. The x ray demonstrates an intra articular fracture.

8. Her initial follow up appointment was canceled due to illness, so she has rescheduled and will follow up on June 15.

Proofreading Skills

Instructions: In the paragraphs below, circle the misspelled medical and English words and punctuation errors. Write the correct words and punctuation in the numbered spaces below the text.

1	The patient comes to clinc today becuase of
2	problems with recurent bursitus. What's
3	troubling him at this time is recurrent
4	tindonitis to the left arm. This has been
5	injected successfully with Cortisone on
6	multiple occasions as well as intermitent
7	problems of left hip pain which also seems to
8	be tendinitus/bursitus in nature.
9	
10	EXAM: The patietn has marked trigger point
11	on the lateral epicondyle. His hip is a sympto-
12	matic at this time, and exam is benine.
13	
14	After discussing the different posibilities, I
15	elected to try conservative theraphy. Tennis
16	elbow armband is placed to the right arm. He
17	is begun on anaprox DS on a trial basis. If
18	this gives adeqaute releif I would have him
19	use it on a p.r.n. basis. If he continus to have
20	signifcant pain would recomend retern to
21	clinic for trigger point injection.

1. _____
2. _____
3. _____
4. _____
5. _____
6. _____
7. _____
8. _____
9. _____
10. _____
11. _____
12. _____
13. _____
14. _____
15. _____
16. _____
17. _____
18. _____
19. _____
20. _____
21. _____

Terminology Challenge

Instructions: The following terms appear in the dictation on Tape 7A, Orthopedics. Before beginning the medical transcription practice for Lesson 14, look up each term in a medical or English dictionary and write out a short definition of each term.

18 gauge wire (18-gauge)
110 mm screw (110-mm)
150° four-hole plate
Acufex rasp
Acufex tibial guide
aluminum splint
anteromedially
apex
articular surface
basal neck
Betadine
bicortical screw
BK (below-knee)
  amputation
bur
bursitis
carpal tunnel syndrome
closed reduction
coagulase-negative
  staphylococcus
coagulated
copious
curet
decubitus position
Depo-Medrol
digital
Dupuytren's contracture
EMG (electromyogram)

erythema
Esmarch
exsanguinated
fascia lata
femur
Gore bit
Gore-Tex prosthesis
Gore-Tex tape
gouge (noun)
guide wires
hemostasis
Hemovac drain
intercondylar notch
intermuscular septum
internal fixation
interosseous membrane
intertrochanteric fracture
joint line
lateral epicondyle
lateral meniscus
long-standing
medial compartment
mediolateral
meniscectomy
mmHg
notchplasty
nubbin
osteomyelitis

outflow
palmar fascia
Penrose drain tourniquet
peroneal nerve
Phalen's test
piecemeal
PIP (proximal inter-
  phalangeal joint)
Polysporin
popliteal recess
posterior horn (of medial
  meniscus)
radialized
rasp
ray
reamed
Richards screw
Robert Jones dressing

Streptococcus viridans
subperiosteal
superomedial
synovium
tendinitis
tendinous
test
  anterior drawer
  Lachman
  pivot shift
tetanus
tibia
ticarcillin
Tinel's sign
vastus lateralis
well-leg holder
X-Acto knife

Transcription Practice

After completing all the readings and exercises in Lesson 14, transcribe Tape 7A, Orthopedics. Use both medical and English dictionaries and your Quick-Reference Word List as resource materials for finding words.

Proofread your transcribed documents carefully, listening to the dictation while you read your transcripts.

Transcribe (*NOT* retype) the same reports again without referring to your previous transcription attempt. Initially, you may need to transcribe some reports more than twice before you can produce an error-free document. Your ultimate goal is to produce an error-free document the first time.

BLOOPERS

Incorrect	Correct
Rectal exam showed hyperactive ankle jerks.	Peripheral exam showed hyperactive ankle jerks.
No evidence of fracture or osseous mythology.	No evidence of fracture or osseous pathology.
Treated with Parafon #4 tape.	Treated with Parafon Forte.
There is full range of emotion.	There is full range of motion.

Lesson 15. Obstetrics and Gynecology

Learning Objectives

Medical

- List common gynecologic symptoms and disease conditions mentioned in the Physical Examination section of an H&P.
- Describe the action of these drugs: uterine relaxants, uterine stimulants, oral contraceptives, and estrogen replacement therapy.
- Given a cross-section illustration of the female reproductive system, memorize the names of the anatomic features.
- Describe the process of fertilization and growth of the ovum.
- Given an Ob–Gyn root word, symptom, or disease, match it to its correct medical definition.
- Given a category of Ob–Gyn drugs, indicate which drugs belong to that category.

Fundamentals

- Describe the technological advances currently in use to increase productivity in medical transcription.
- Given a medical report with errors, identify and correct the errors.

Practice

- Accurately transcribe authentic physician dictation from the specialties of obstetrics and gynecology.

A Closer Look

The New Technology

by Judy Hinickle, CMT

In medical transcription, as in many aspects of the health information field, the trends in medical technology seriously impact those utilizing and managing that technology. We have high tech tools now to improve quality and measure quality, to increase production and measure production, to improve productivity and measure productivity, to improve access to dictated and transcribed reports, to measure the actual access or restriction of the reports, and even the means to measure the effect of applying improvement and measurement techniques.

But, without care, utilizing the technology available to us in medical transcription can bury, burn out, or belittle the most important element in the process—the medical transcriptionist.

An examination of the technologies and their advantages illustrates how they assist the medical language specialist in performing the unique task of interpreting what a medical dictator states and putting it into appropriate medical and English language. When utilized well, our new technologies can provide tools for improved quality and efficiency. And new technology can help to preserve the physical and mental health of the dwindling and perhaps endangered resource we know as a medical transcriptionist.

Among the new technologies available to us, we have ergonomic workstations, machine shorthand, voice recognition, digital dictation, and word processing advances.

Ergonomic workstations are of interest from two viewpoints: health and efficiency. Keyboards with a lighter touch and alternative arrangements of the keys can enable fewer and easier keystrokes. Others with unique designs (molding the shape of the keyboard, or changing its shape considerably) may provide relief from carpal tunnel syndrome and tendinitis. When combined with articulating keyboard arms, wrist rests, foot rests, adjustable chairs and desk heights, and lighting considerations, the enhanced comfort of the transcriptionist will certainly improve quality and efficiency. Fatigue and discomfort are, after all, major contributors to production lag and errors.

Machine shorthand has become available to the medical field through the use of computer-assisted technology. There are many graduates of court reporting schools desiring outlets other than legal for their keyboarding skills. If they are provided with appropriate, extensive medical transcription training, they may be excellent additions to the field.

It is wise to remember, however, that medical transcription cannot be accomplished any faster than the dictation can be heard, understood, and correctly reinterpreted into appropriate medical and English language. Claims that medical reporters will transcribe at fabulously multiplied rates over traditional keyboarding methods are exaggerated. Keyboarding skills are not the overriding measure of value, skill, and ultimate productivity. It is the medical language reinterpretation process which slows down all medical transcriptionists, even the most accomplished.

Voice recognition is viewed by many as a threat to the medical transcription industry; however, when viewed from the physical implications as above, we may find it an appropriate keyboarding alternative which will free up the time and energy needed for medical language specialists to apply their most valuable asset—the ability to interpret what dictators mean from what they say, and to type what is meant in appropriate medical and English language.

A transcriptionist does not merely recognize a voice but utilizes medical knowledge to discriminate meaning, and to clearly integrate that information with the dictator's style in order to reflect the actual patient care. Voice recognition will allow the transcriptionist to listen to dictation and edit the computer's reports without the physical stress presently associated with keyboarding. It will also allow easily standardized reports, requiring only a few words from the dictator and less medical language discrimination in keyboarding, to be done by clerical or secretarial workers rather than medical transcriptionists. This would be a boon in these times when skilled transcriptionists are a rarity.

We need to cooperate with this technology development to ascertain that it produces medically and grammatically sound reports. These reports need to accurately reflect patient care, and to do so without limiting the creativity and style of the dictator—medical art collaborating with medical science.

Digital dictation has enhanced the sound quality of most dictation, which is certainly an aid in sound discrimination and therefore quality. It has also enabled more demographic information to be easily available for inclusion in the document—a time-saver. Other important contributions affecting the transcription quality and productivity seem to be in the arena of management. Work type assignment can be done with more equality. Weight values can be applied to level of difficulty, where appropriate.

Turnaround times per work type can be achieved, assuring timely information on the patient record. Stat reports can be easily identified, accessed, and processed. Management reports can be generated to demonstrate turnaround time by work type and also by physician. Transcription time can be measured per transcriptionist and then compared to work type or dictator time to determine difficulty factors.

The more important influences here are those affecting quality. But productivity cannot be ignored, as transcriptionists are always working against the clock. Average improved productivity results from digital implementation have varied around the country, with reports of improvement ranging from 0 to 15%. Much depends on the antiquity of the preceding system, and the efficiency of management before the transition.

Word processing is certainly the field having the greatest impact on quality and productivity. Widespread use of PCs and electronic typewriters has greatly affected quality issues. Spellcheckers, English and medical, are available in many assortments and can often be appended, permitting more extensive medical dictionaries appropriate to the individual setting. Although this doesn't help if a wrong word in context has been chosen, it certainly catches typographical errors. Soon there will also be on-line medical dictionaries available, simplifying the process of word research and, more importantly, readily enabling an educational process.

Word wrap and justification have simplified mechanics, thus saving time. Formats can be standardized and selected with one keystroke, eliminating time-consuming report set-up time. The available editing techniques (copying, moving, inserting, deleting, word searching, global formatting, spellchecking, and abbreviating) have helped tremendously in achieving quality standards and greater efficiency.

More important than technology, however, is the need for ethical application of the knowledge gained from technological tools. Our focus should not be on the mechanical or physical aspects of people, but on the mind and spirit. The most significant contribution to quality and productivity in medical transcription will not be technological advances, but effective and continuing education.

Medical Readings

The History and Physical Examination

by John H. Dirckx, M.D.

Female Reproductive Tract. In women the examination of the external and internal genitourinary organs and the rectum and anus is normally performed with the patient in the lithotomy position. The patient lies on her back on a specially equipped examining table with her feet in stirrups, her thighs flexed sharply on her abdomen, and her knees spread wide apart. If she cannot assume the lithotomy position, the left lateral (Sims) position may be used instead.

The physician inspects the pubes and vulva for hair distribution, developmental anomalies, cutaneous lesions, swellings, and signs of inflammation. The urethral meatus and Bartholin's and Skene's glands are inspected and palpated. The physician tests for weakness of the pelvic floor by having the patient bear down while he observes for cystocele, rectocele, or uterine prolapse. He also notes any vaginal discharge and inspects the perineum and anus.

The physician then inserts a warmed and lubricated bivalve speculum into the vagina and by spreading its blades and adjusting its position obtains a view of the cervix, fornices, and vaginal walls. Specimens may be taken for cultures or cytologic study at this point. A gynecologist may use a colposcope, which provides bright light and strong magnification, to inspect the cervix.

After removing the speculum, the examiner inserts one or two fingers of his dominant hand, gloved and lubricated, into the vagina and places his other hand on the patient's abdomen (bimanual pelvic examination). He can thus assess the size, shape, and position of the uterus and detect any masses or tenderness in the pelvis. Normal ovaries and tubes can seldom be felt.

The physician concludes his examination of the female subject by performing a digital rectal examination. With the patient in the lithotomy position, the examiner inserts one finger in the vagina and another in the rectum at the same time (rectovaginal exam).

If the patient is pregnant the examiner performs certain additional diagnostic procedures. He attempts to determine the duration of the pregnancy by a consideration of uterine size. He assesses the size and shape of the pelvic outlet to judge whether the fetus will fit through it during labor. If the pregnancy is sufficiently advanced, he attempts to learn by palpation (Leopold's maneuvers) the position in which the fetus lies within the uterus. Finally, again if the pregnancy is sufficiently advanced, he listens for fetal heart tones by auscultation through the mother's abdomen. A special stethoscope (fetoscope) may be used for this purpose.

Laboratory Medicine: Diseases of the Female Reproductive System

Endometriosis is a condition in which functioning endometrium is located ectopically, most often on the pelvic peritoneum and in the ovaries. Adenomyosis refers to ectopic endometrium within the myometrium. The origin of this aberrant tissue is unknown. Menstrual changes occurring in it may cause severe pelvic pain. Microscopic examination shows a well-developed endometrial stroma and functioning glands. Hemorrhage and cyst formation are common. In the ovary, endometrial cysts contain brown fluid derived from degenerated blood (chocolate cysts).

Cysts and neoplasms of the ovary. Non-neoplastic cysts in the ovary may also arise from germinal follicles. **Follicular cysts** form from unruptured, atretic follicles. In the Stein-Leventhal syndrome (polycystic ovary syndrome), many such cysts occur in both ovaries, in association with hirsutism and failure to ovulate.

The **corpus luteum cyst** develops from a normal germinal follicle after expulsion of the ovum and formation of a corpus luteum. A serous fluid gradually replaces the blood normally found in a corpus luteum, and if the lesion remains for a long time without spontaneous rupture it may become quite large, its walls of luteinizing theca cells being replaced by fibrosis. **Theca-lutein cysts** are similar but are multiple lesions in both ovaries induced by excessive levels of chorionic gonadotropin formed in functioning tumors of the chorion (hydatidiform mole, choriocarcinoma).

Neoplasms of the ovary are of two types: teratomas, which take origin from germ cells, and tumors of nongerminal origin. A teratoma, developing from highly undifferentiated and pluripotential cells, may incorporate virtually any kind of tissue. Epithelium and other structures of ectodermal origin (hair, teeth, nerve cells) are usually present, and cartilage, bone, and glandular formations may also be found. In **cystic teratoma** (dermoid cyst), ectodermal elements preponderate, and the lesion consists largely or entirely of a multiloculated cyst lined by stratified squamous epithelium and filled with semisolid sebaceous debris.

The most important ovarian tumor arising from nongerminal tissue is cystadenocarcinoma, a bulky, nodular malignancy containing many cysts. Two forms are distinguished. In **serous cystadenocarcinoma,** thin-walled cysts are lined with cuboidal epithelium and filled with serous fluid. In **mucinous cystadenocarcinoma** the cysts contain mucoid material and are lined with mucin-secreting columnar cells. These tumors typically occur during or after middle age, and may arise either as malignant tumors or by malignant change in histologically benign serous or mucinous cystadenomas. They may become very large and typically invade contiguous structures and the pelvic wall besides metastasizing to distant sites.

Diseases of the uterus and tubes. The term **pelvic inflammatory disease** (PID) denotes a symptom complex of fever, pelvic pain, and evidence of inflammation in the uterine tubes (salpingitis), endometrium (endometritis), or both, along with focal pelvic peritonitis.

Salpingitis usually occurs by extension from the lower genital tract. The primary infection is either a sexually transmitted disease due to gonococcus or *Chlamydia* or a complication of childbirth, abortion, or instrumentation of the uterine cavity. Gonococcal salpingitis is manifested by hyperemia, edema, neutrophilic infiltrates and purulent exudate. The tube may become grossly dilated with pus (pyosalpinx), and infection may extend to the ovary (tubo-ovarian abscess), the pelvic peritoneum, and even the upper abdominal quadrants (Fitz-Hugh–Curtis syndrome or gonococcal perihepatitis).

Repeated infections lead to fibrotic thickening of the tube, with stenosis or occlusion of its lumen. Peritoneal scarring may lead to formation of fibrotic bands (banjo-string or violin-string adhesions). Salpingitis due to *Chlamydia trachomatis* is similar to gonococcal infection but elicits less inflammation and suppuration and is less likely to result in late complications.

Scarring of the uterine tube after chronic or recurrent salpingitis leads to infertility or sterility and predisposes to **tubal pregnancy.** Tubal pregnancy occurs when a fertilized ovum becomes implanted in the uterine tube because its expected migration to the endometrial cavity has been delayed. The trophoblast and chorionic villi invade the tubal wall, including the muscularis, and eventually cause hemorrhage, perforation, or both. Other possible sites of ectopic pregnancy are the ovary and the abdominopelvic cavity (with implantation on the peritoneum).

The myometrium is frequently the site of **fibromyomas** (fibroids), benign tumors containing both muscular and fibrous elements. Often several fibroids appear in the same uterus. The typical location is intramural (within the muscular wall), but subserosal and submucosal tumors also occur frequently. Enlargement of fibroids often takes place during pregnancy, and after menopause fibroids often calcify.

Endometrial adenocarcinoma, a disease primarily of the postmenopausal years, is more common in women with hypertension, diabetes mellitus, thyroid gland disorders, and carcinoma of the breast, and in those who have never been pregnant. The risk is also increased by prolonged administration of estrogen. The tumor occurs in both diffuse and localized forms, sometimes being limited to a single polyp, so that diagnostic curettage often proves curative. The tumor invades the myometrium, may spread to the tubes, ovaries, and vagina, and metastasizes to pelvic lymph nodes, lung, bone, and brain.

Sarcoma botryoides is a malignant tumor of mixed mesodermal origin arising in the cervix or vagina, less often in the bladder. The tumor occurs usually in children and appears as a grapelike cluster of rapidly growing tumor nodules. Hematogenous metastasis occurs early, particularly to the lung, and the prognosis is poor.

Diseases of the cervix. Benign lesions of the uterine cervix are common and their chief importance lies in the need to distinguish them from malignant neoplasms. **Cervical polyps** are single or multiple, sessile or pedunculated masses consisting of a fibromyxomatous stroma and covered by benign hyperplastic epithelium. This lesion is more common during pregnancy. A **nabothian cyst** is a small yellowish mass consisting of a dilated endocervical gland and appearing generally at the external cervical os. Condylomata acuminata, ulcers of herpes simplex, and syphilitic chancres may appear on the cervix.

Cervical erosion denotes a condition in which part of the normal squamous epithelium has been destroyed and replaced by columnar epithelium. This may be difficult to distinguish from **cervical eversion** (or ectropion), in which endocervical mucosa pouts out of the external cervical os.

Squamous metaplasia is a focal or diffuse replacement of mucus-secreting surface and glandular epithelium by squamous epithelium, which may grow into and completely line glands (epidermidization).

Squamous cell carcinoma of the uterine cervix is still an important cause of morbidity and mortality in women, despite the possibility of detecting dysplastic changes by means of the Papanicolaou smear years before invasive carcinoma develops. The risk of cervical carcinoma is increased by infection with herpes simplex or papova (wart) virus, by early age of first intercourse, and by repeated intercourse with an uncircumcised partner.

Cervical intraepithelial neoplasia (CIN) denotes dysplastic changes confined to the epithelial layer of the cervix. Foci of anaplastic cells with altered, erratic polarity and large, hyperchromatic, irregular nuclei may be found throughout the epithelium, but stromal invasion does not occur even though extension into endocervical glands is common. This lesion is most likely to occur at the squamocolumnar junction.

Cervical intraepithelial neoplasia is classified on the basis of depth as follows:

CIN I: Up to 1/2 of the epithelial thickness (mild dysplasia).

CIN II: From 1/2 to 3/4 of the epithelial thickness (moderate dysplasia).

CIN III: From 3/4 to full thickness (severe dysplasia; carcinoma in situ).

Typically a latent interval of years elapses between the development of CIN and evidence of invasion. Invasive squamous cell carcinoma may present as a flat, infiltrating lesion, as an ulcer, or as a nodular excrescence. Microscopic study shows proliferation of moderately well-differentiated, generally nonkeratinizing epithelium. The tumor spreads to the pelvic wall, vagina, bladder, rectum, and regional lymph nodes.

The FIGO (International Federation of Gynecologists and Obstetricians) staging of cervical carcinoma is as follows:

Stage 0:   Carcinoma in situ.

Stage I: Carcinoma invading basement membrane but confined to cervix.

Stage II: Carcinoma extending beyond cervix but not to pelvic wall or lower third of vagina.

Stage III: Invasion of pelvic wall and lower third of vagina, bladder, rectum, extrapelvic structures.

Disorders of pregnancy. Abnormalities of pregnancy develop often, many of them resulting in fetal loss. **Spontaneous abortion** is defined as an accidental termination of pregnancy before the time of fetal viability. Although it may be due to infection, trauma, hormonal disorders, or other causes, spontaneous abortion most often results from some inherent abnormality of the fertilized ovum (blighted ovum). An aborted fetus is usually expelled along with its membranes, but by exception it may remain within the uterine cavity indefinitely (missed abortion). A lithopedion is a retained dead fetus that has calcified.

Hydatidiform mole is an infrequent development from a fetus that has died before four weeks of gestation. The chorionic villi display an extreme stromal overdevelopment, while the fetus undergoes degeneration and necrosis. The hypertrophic villi form a friable mass consisting of a grapelike bunch of small transparent vesicles attached to the endometrium.

Malignant change in a hydatidiform mole (or, rarely, in the chorion of a normal pregnancy) generates a neoplasm called choriocarcinoma (chorioepithelioma). In this tumor, chorionic villi are absent, and masses of malignant chorionic epithelial cells invade locally and metastasize to lungs, brain, and liver.

Pharmacology: Obstetric and Gynecologic Drugs

Drugs that are used to treat women with obstetric and gynecologic problems include drugs for infertility and vaginal infections, drugs which stimulate or suppress labor contractions, drugs which correct menstrual disorders and endometriosis, estrogen replacement therapy, and birth control agents prophylactically prescribed.

Uterine relaxants. Premature delivery greatly increases morbidity and mortality in infants. Premature labor contractions may be inhibited by using uterine relaxing drugs which act on beta$_2$ receptors in the smooth muscle of the uterus to effect relaxation. These drugs decrease both the frequency and strength of contractions: ritodrine (Yutopar), terbutaline (Bricanyl).

Uterine stimulants. Women who are in labor and whose membranes have ruptured may be given the uterine stimulant oxytocin if their uterine contractions are too weak to effect delivery. Oxytocin is normally produced by the pituitary gland and directly stimulates the uterus by binding to special oxytocin receptors in the uterine muscle. Oxytocin increases both the frequency and strength of uterine contractions. When prolonged labor is due to cephalopelvic disproportion, oxytocin (Pitocin) is not indicated.

Postpartum bleeding is due to too great a degree of uterine relaxation which results in increased bleeding at the site of placental separation. Uterine stimulating drugs are also used to treat this condition. These drugs include:

> oxytocin (Pitocin)
> ergonovine (Ergotrate)
> methylergonovine (Methergine)

Drugs used to treat endometriosis. Endometriosis is caused by uterine tissue which implants within the pelvic cavity and on the ovaries and other organs. It continues to remain sensitive to hormonal influence, secreting blood when the uterus begins menstruation. Endometriosis causes pelvic pain, inflammation, and cyst formation. After using drugs to suppress the menstrual cycle for several months, endometrial implants may atrophy. Drugs used to treat endometriosis include:

> danazol (Danocrine)—oral administration
> nafarelin (Synarel)—nasal spray

Oral contraceptives. Birth control pills exert a hormonal influence to prevent pregnancy and are 95% effective if taken as directed. Most oral contraceptives contain a combination of estrogen and progesterone (or progestin) which is taken for 21 days. During the final seven days of the 28-day menstrual cycle, the patient may take no tablets, or seven sugar-filled tablets or sugar tablets with iron may be included in the pill case. Other oral contraceptives contain only progesterone.

The monophasic group of oral combination contraceptives provides the same fixed amounts of progesterone and estrogen in every tablet for each day of the 21-day segment. The amounts of progesterone and estrogen are designated by two numbers following the trade name drugs. Example: Norinyl 1+50 contains 1 mg of progesterone and 50 mcg of estrogen in every daily tablet. Because there have been increased side effects (particularly thrombophlebitis) associated with higher estrogen dosages, a physician may elect to prescribe Norinyl 1+35 which contains 1 mg of progesterone and 35 mcg of estrogen in every daily tablet.

> Demulen 1/50   Demulen 1/35
> Loestrin 1.5/30   Loestrin 1/20
> Norinyl 1+50   Norinyl 1+35
> Ortho-Novum 1/50 Ortho-Novum 1/35

The triphasic group of oral combination contraceptives provides a fixed amount of estrogen on each day of the 21 days; the amount of progesterone increases or varies through the cycle. This is designated, at least in the case of Ortho-Novum, by the numbers 7/7/7 which show that the first seven tablets contain 0.5 mg of progesterone and 35 mcg of estrogen, the second seven tablets contain 1 mg of progesterone and 35 mcg of estrogen, and the last seven tablets of the 21-day segment contain 0.5 mg of progesterone and 35 mcg of estrogen.

> Ortho-Novum 7/7/7
> Tri-Levlen
> Tri-Norinyl
> Triphasil

Estrogen replacement therapy. As women enter menopause, the ovaries secrete decreasing amounts of estrogen. This can produce symptoms of vaginal dryness, hot flashes (due to vasodilation), and fatigue. Estrogen replacement therapy corrects the deficiency of this hormone. Estrogen may be given orally, by injection, or applied as a transdermal patch. A topical cream may be used to treat vaginal symptoms only. Examples:

> conjugated estrogens (Premarin)
> estradiol (Estrace, Estraderm)
> quinestrol (Estrovis)

Drugs to treat vaginal infections. Vaginal infections and vaginitis are commonly caused by *Candida albicans* (a yeast), *Trichomonas vaginalis* (a flagellated parasite), and *Haemophilus vaginalis*, also known as *Gardnerella vaginalis* (a gram-negative rod).

Drugs used to treat candidal infections include:

> clotrimazole (Gyne-Lotrimin, Mycelex-G)
> miconazole (Monistat)
> nystatin (Mycostatin, Nilstat)

Drugs used to treat *Trichomonas vaginalis* infections include metronidazole (Flagyl) (given orally).

Anatomy/Medical Terminology

Obstetrics–Gynecology Questions

1. What is the difference between a primipara and primigravida?

2. What is the difference between colposcopy and culdoscopy?

Anatomy: The Female Reproductive System

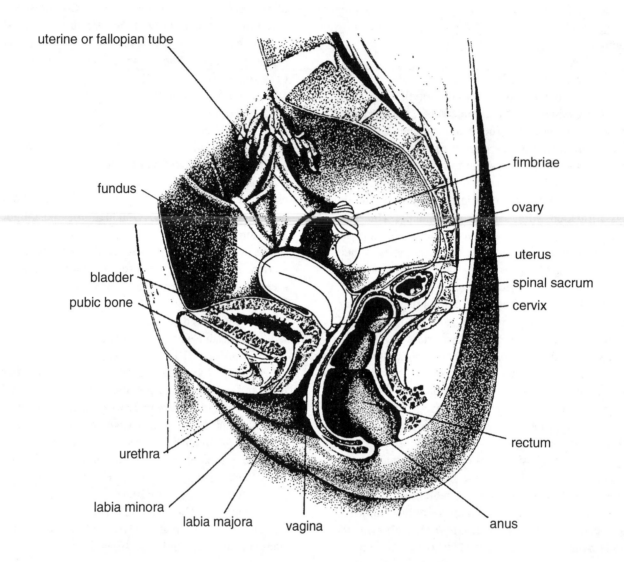

uterine or fallopian tube

fundus

bladder

pubic bone

urethra

labia minora

labia majora

vagina

fimbriae

ovary

uterus

spinal sacrum

cervix

rectum

anus

Adjective Exercise

Adjectives are formed from nouns by adding adjectival suffixes such as *-ac, -al, -ar, -ary, -eal, -ed, -ent, -iac, -ial, -ic, -ical, -ine, -lar, -oid, -ous, -tic,* and *-tous.* Medical transcriptionists must know which adjectival ending is the correct one for a particular word. In addition, some adjectives have a different form entirely from the noun, which may be either Latin or Greek in origin.

Test your knowledge of adjectives by writing the adjectival form of the following Ob-Gyn words. Consult a medical dictionary to select the correct adjectival ending as necessary.

1. ovary _____
2. uterus _____
3. tube _____
4. placenta _____
5. vagina _____
6. cervix _____
7. adnexa _____
8. embryo _____
9. fetus _____
10. gestation _____
11. labia _____
12. vulva _____

Fill-in Exercise: The Ovum

Instructions: The numbered blanks correspond to the numbers in the narrative paragraphs. Fill in the blanks with the correct entry from the word list below.

Each month, the ovary of a woman in her child-bearing years secretes an egg or (1). After (2) or the release of the egg, it is gathered in by the (3) or fingerlike projections on the end of the (4) tube, and passed to the uterus.

If fertilized, the egg implants in the inner lining of the uterus known as the (5). Estrogen and progesterone produced by the ovaries support the development of the fertilized egg. The (6) develops between the uterine wall and the developing (7), forming blood vessels that receive nutrients from the mother's circulation. Now, the placenta secretes the hormones estrogen and progesterone to support the pregnancy. If all goes well, a baby will be born after 40 weeks of (8).

The uterus is divided into three parts: the upper curved surface known as the (9), where the fallopian tubes enter; the body or (10); and the bottom neck or (11). This structure protrudes into the cavity known as the (12), which opens to the exterior of the woman's body.

1. ovum _____
2. _____
3. _____
4. _____
5. _____
6. _____
7. _____
8. _____
9. _____
10. _____
11. _____
12. _____

cervix	fundus
corpus	gestation
endometrium	ovulation
fallopian	ovum
fetus	placenta
fimbriae	vagina

Medical Terminology Matching Exercise

Complete the following matching exercise to test your knowledge of the word roots, anatomic structures, symptoms, and disease processes encountered in the medical specialties of obstetrics and gynecology.

Instructions: Match the term in Column A with its definition in Column B.

Column A

A. menopause
B. menarche
C. colpo-
D. episiotomy
E. gyneco-
F. primigravida
G. leiomyoma
H. hystero-
I. abruptio placentae
J. oophor-
K. ectopic pregnancy
L. salpingo-

Column B

_____ uterus

_____ incision made in perineum prior to delivery

_____ first pregnancy

_____ gradual end of menses

_____ fallopian tubes

_____ vagina

_____ ovary

_____ fibroid cyst of uterus

_____ female

_____ onset of menstruation

_____ implantation of fertilized egg in fallopian tube

_____ premature separation of placenta from uterine wall

Lay and Medical Terms

Lay Term	Medical Term
afterbirth	placenta
bag of waters	amniotic membranes and fluid
womb	uterus

Drug Matching Exercise

Instructions: Match the drug category in Column A with the drug names in Column B. Note: Drug categories are used more than once.

Column A	Column B
A. stimulates ovulation	____ Estrovis
	____ Demulen
B. prevents uterine contractions	____ Pergonal
	____ Ortho-Novum
	____ ritodrine
C. stimulates uterine contractions	____ Monistat
	____ Premarin
	____ oxytocin
D. oral contraceptive	____ Clomid
	____ Femstat
E. estrogen replacement therapy for menopause	____ Norinyl
	____ Gyne-Lotrimin
	____ Pitocin
F. treats vaginal yeast infections	____ Estraderm
	____ Mycelex-G
	____ Loestrin
	____ Bricanyl

Word Search

Instructions: Locate and circle the Ob–Gyn words and drugs hidden in the puzzle horizontally, vertically, and diagonally, forward and backward. A numeral following a term in the word list indicates the number of times it can be found in the puzzle.

```
M A E D T S I V O R T S E
V A G I S T A T H J N B S
B P G M P R E M A R I N T
L R G O F L A G Y L L I R
O E I L H J V B E A D C A
Z G H C G R C T R R T O D
A N I G A V S O L V A T E
N A D P E N I R D O T I R
A N I C O T Y X O O S P M
D C V P F G H L R L I I U
B Y O X L Y N I R O N L K
D A N A Z O L A R V O L Q
Z N E G O H T A T S M E F
```

AVC	Ogen
Bricanyl	oral
Clomid	Ovral
danazol (2)	oxytocin
Enovid	pill
Estraderm	Pitocin
Estrovis	Ponstel
Femstat	pregnancy
Flagyl	Premarin
HCG	RhoGAM
Lo-Ovral	ritodrine
Monistat	vagina
Norinyl	Vagistat

Proofreading Skills

Instructions: In the report below, circle the misspelled medical and English words and punctuation errors, and write the correct words and punctuation in the numbered spaces opposite the text.

1	FINAL DIGNOSIS:	1. DIAGNOSIS _____
2	1. Interuterine pregnancy, delivered.	2. _____
3	2. Periureteral tear.	3. _____
4		4. _____
5	HITSORY AND PHYSICAL: This is a 27	5. _____
6	year old secundagravida at term with blood	6. _____
7	type a positive who had a pregnancy com-	7. _____
8	plicated except for some first trimester	8. _____
9	bleeding. She was admitted after 5 hours of	9. _____
10	good labor and was bruoght to the delivry	10. _____
11	room, complete and pushing, with membraines	11. _____
12	still intact. Spontaneus rupture of membranes	12. _____
13	occurred only one minute pryor to delivery.	13. _____
14	The delivery was very rapid, though well con-	14. _____
15	trolled, and resulted in a superficil peri-	15. _____
16	urethral and labila tear which did not reqiure	16. _____
17	suturing. No episotomy required. The infant	17. _____
18	was suctioned well on the peritoneum. Blood	18. _____
19	loss was minimal, and both mother and infant	19. _____
20	were stabel following delivery.	20. _____
21		21. _____
22	HOSPTAL COURSE: Large urterine clots	22. _____
23	were expressed the first post partum day, and	23. _____
24	the initial post partum CBC reveeled a white	24. _____
25	count of 18.5 with 55 seggs, 17 bands, and	25. _____
26	23 lymphos.	26. _____
27		27. _____
28	The patient remained febrile with a temp of	28. _____
29	98.6 but had minimal uterin tenderness, and	29. _____
30	in light of the elevated white count, she was	30. _____
31	begun on ampicillian 500 mg q.i.d. for a 10	31. _____
32	day course. She was dischraged in stabel con-	32. _____
33	dition. Activity and diet as toleratd.	33. _____

Transcription Tips

1. Memorize these difficult-to-spell Ob–Gyn terms.

   cornua, cornual
   cul-de-sac
   endometriosis
   menarche
   menstruation (not *menestration*)

2. *Pap smear* is an acceptable brief form for *Papanicolaou smear.*

3. The term *adnexa* refers to the fallopian tubes and ovaries. The term is plural (adnexum is singular) and takes a plural verb.

   The adnexa were unremarkable.

4. The abbreviation *VBAC* (acronym for *vaginal birth after cesarean section*) is often pronounced "vee-back."

5. Both the Greek *hystero-* and Latin *metro-* mean *uterus.*

6. The slang term *primip* should be transcribed as *primipara*, and *multip* as *multipara.*

7. The terms *gravida* and *para* are used to describe a woman's reproductive history.

   The term **parous** describes a woman who has given birth either vaginally or by cesarean section after the 20th week of gestation; **parity** is the number of such deliveries.

   Gravida followed by a number refers to the number of pregnancies, including ectopics, hydatidiform moles, abortions, and normal pregnancies.

   Para followed by a number refers to the number of deliveries after the 20th week of gestation (live or stillbirth, single or multple, vaginal or cesarean) and does not correspond to the number of infants. A woman who has had only one pregnancy—even if she delivers twins or quintuplets—is still gravida 1, para 1. If she had an ectopic pregnancy and an abortion (less than 20 weeks' gestation) prior to a delivery, she will be gravida 3, para 1.

   Para may be expressed as a single number or may be a four-digit number, each digit representing a particular type of birth. The first number indicates term infants; the second, premature infants; the third, abortions or miscarriages; and the fourth, the number of living children. In the following examples, both sentences refer to the same patient.

   The patient is gravida 6, para 3. (Six pregnancies, 3 live births.)

   The patient is gravida 6, para 2-1-0-3. (Six pregnancies; 2 term infants, 1 premature, 0 miscarriages = 3 live births.)

   Another example: A woman who is para 0-3-0-2 could have had three separate pregnancies resulting in premature deliveries of which two children are now living, or she could have had triplets in one delivery with two living children, or even one premature and one twin premature delivery with two living children.

   Confused? Remember it this way. FPAL (Florida Power and Light): **F**ull-term deliveries, **P**remature (pre-term), **A**bortions, and **L**iving children.

   Another method of documenting the obstetrical history is an index called GPMAL. The letters refer to **G**ravida, **P**ara, **M**ultiple births, **A**bortions, and **L**ive births, and are replaced by numbers separated by hyphens to represent the specific information.

   Some physicians dictate para 3-2-0-1-2, which may be transcribed as gravida 3, para 2-0-1-2, or para 3, 2-0-1-2.

Terminology Challenge

Instructions: The following terms appear in the dictation on Tape 7B. Before beginning the medical transcription practice for Lesson 15, become familiar with the terminology below by looking up each word in a medical or English dictionary. Write out a short definition of each term.

abdominopelvic CT scan	hypertrophic
abstain	induration
adnexa	introitus
Advil	labium minus
ampicillin	large-cell carcinoma
Ancef	leukorrhea
anorexic	LMP (last menstrual
apex	period)
bimanual examination	mammogram
C-section	menarche
Candida	menometrorrhagia
cervicitis	Pap smear
Chlamydia enzyme test	para 3, 2-0-1-2
Colace	pelvic inflammatory
Compazine	disease (PID)
cryosurgery	pelvic relaxation
cystocele	postcoital
cystourethrocele	progesterone
D&C (dilatation and	rectocele
curettage)	rectovaginal septum
Darvocet-N 100	retroverted uterus
Demulen	Rh negative unsensitized
diplococci	Stadol
enterocele	STD (sexually transmitted
epithelial cells	disease) screen
extracellular	sulfa
exudate	TAH (total abdominal
fallopian tube	hysterectomy)
fibromyomata	Thayer-Martin test
finger cot	toluidine O
Flagyl	Trichomonas
flank pain	Tzanck smear
Fleet enema	urethrovesical angle
fundus of the uterus	uterine descensus
Gardnerella	vaginal vault
giant cell formation	vesicovaginal fistula
gonorrhea	Vicodin
gravida	zinc oxide ointment
herpes simplex	Zovirax

Sample Reports

Sample obstetric and gynecology reports appear on the following pages.

Transcription Practice

After completing all the readings and exercises in Lesson 15, transcribe Tape 7B, Obstetrics and Gynecology. Use both medical and English dictionaries and your Quick-Reference Word List as resource materials for finding words.

Proofread your transcribed documents carefully, listening to the dictation while you read your transcripts.

Transcribe (*NOT* retype) the same reports again without referring to your previous transcription attempt. Initially, you may need to transcribe some reports more than twice before you can produce an error-free document. Your ultimate goal is to produce an error-free document the first time.

CHART NOTE

SARAH TENCH   17 June 1992

SUBJECTIVE: Comes in today for annual exam. Menses are regular without intermenstrual bleeding. Her galactorrhea is unchanged. She continues to take bromocriptine 2.5 mg p.o. b.i.d. She takes chlorthalidone 50 mg daily and also daily potassium supplement. When seen a year ago she felt fatigued. Blood work at that time showed her to be hypokalemic. She resumed a potassium supplement at that time and felt much better. She has no headaches. She had some vaginal itching and discharge off and on during the summer but currently doesn't have any. She has never had a mammogram.

OBJECTIVE: Breasts without masses. There is bilateral galactorrhea. There was no axillary adenopathy. Abdomen soft and nontender. Pelvic: External genitalia are normal. Vagina rugous with a small amount of yellow discharge. Cervix clean. Uterus: Anterior, mobile, nontender, normal size, shape, and consistency. Adnexa clear, nontender. Rectovaginal exam confirms. Pap smear was obtained. Wet smear is unremarkable.

ASSESSMENT:
1. Long history of galactorrhea. Prolactins have been well controlled on Parlodel, as have her menses.
2. Has taken chlorthalidone daily for many years. This is for fluid retention.

PLAN:
1. Parlodel 2.5 mg p.o. b.i.d. is renewed for a year.
2. Chlorthalidone 50 mg daily and potassium supplement one daily is renewed.
3. Serum prolactin and serum potassium levels are obtained.

FB:hpi

MARIA GONZALEZ

#121359

DATE OF OPERATION: July 20, 1992

OPERATIVE REPORT

PREOPERATIVE DIAGNOSIS:
1. Intrauterine pregnancy, near term
2. Previous cesarean sections x 3
3. Diabetes mellitus controlled with 15 units of NPH Humulin insulin

POSTOPERATIVE DIAGNOSIS:
1. Intrauterine pregnancy, near term
2. Previous cesarean sections x 3
3. Diabetes mellitus controlled with 15 units of NPH Humulin insulin
4. Term birth living infant

Estimated blood loss: 500 cc

Anesthesia: Epidural

SURGERY PERFORMED:
1. Repeat low transverse cervical cesarean section
2. Bilateral tubal ligation, modified Pomeroy technique

PROCEDURE: The patient was taken to the operating room where she was given epidural anesthesia and properly prepped and draped. A midline incision was made through old scar and carried down to the fascia. Hemostasis was achieved by electrocautery. The fascia was entered by sharp dissection and extended superiorly and inferiorly. The peritoneum was entered with Metzenbaum scissors and extended superiorly and inferiorly. Lap pads were placed in both pelvic gutters, a right angle retractor in the upper abdomen, a bladder blade in the lower abdomen. The peritoneum was entered with Metzenbaum scissors and extended in a smile fashion, and the bladder was swept off the lower uterine segment.

A sharp scalpel was used to enter the uterus, and this incision was extended in a smile fashion with bandage scissors. Note: The placenta was under this lower uterine segment, and when inferiorly grasped, the vertex membranes ruptured spontaneously. The vertex was grasped, delivered with ease, and oral suction accomplished. The cord was clamped, cut, and tied, and the infant was handed to the doctor in attendance. Then we removed the placenta from the incision side superiorly to the anterior fundus. We wiped all membranes free with lap pad after the uterus was delivered outside of the abdominal cavity, and ring forceps were placed through the cervix to make sure it was open.

We then proceeded to close the uterine incision with #1 chromic suture in a running lock fashion, the second layer with #1 chromic suture in an inverting Lembert-type stitch. Good hemostasis was accomplished. We closed the peritoneum with #2-0 chromic suture in a running fashion.

(Continued on page 2)

MARIA GONZALEZ

#101359

DATE OF OPERATION: July 20, 1992

Page 2

We then inspected both tubes and ovaries which were normal. We grasped the tubes with Babcock clamps bilaterally, tied with one plain suture x 2 pulled bilaterally, excised the distal portions, and cauterized the proximal portions bilaterally. The uterus was then replaced to its pelvic position. All blood was wiped free with lap pads.

The cecum was grasped. The appendix had been removed previously. We palpated the gallbladder; no stones were felt. Both kidneys were palpated and within normal limits.

The patient tolerated the procedure well and left the operating room in good condition. Sponge count was correct.

FRANK BRIETZSCH, M.D.

FB:hpi
d: 7/20/92
t: 7/21/92

ANNIE OAKLEY

#092431

ADMITTED: 5 May 1992

HISTORY AND PHYSICAL EXAMINATION

CHIEF COMPLAINT: Uterine prolapse.

HISTORY OF PRESENT ILLNESS: This is a 64-year-old woman who is para 4, referred because of a large cystocele and uterine prolapse. The patient states that when she is on her feet, a bulge comes out of the vagina between her legs. She was found to have a large cystocele and a second-degree uterine prolapse, the cervix protruding through the os even with the patient lying down and when she strains. She does not have any significant problem with urinary tract control. She enters at this time for vaginal hysterectomy and A&P repair.

PAST HISTORY: Her general health has been reasonably good. She is taking Lanoxin 0.25 mg ½ tablet per day.

PHYSICAL EXAMINATION: Physical examination reveals a well-developed, well-nourished, slender white female at 131 pounds. Blood pressure was 130/70.
EARS: Negative.
EYES: Pupils small, react well to light. Sclerae clear.
MOUTH: I believe the patient has dentures. The throat is clear. The tonsils are absent.
NECK: Supple, no masses felt.
BREASTS: Quite good turgor for her age. No masses are felt.
LUNGS: Clear to P&A.
HEART: Regular rhythm, no murmurs.
ABDOMEN: Soft and nontender.
GYN EXAM: There is relaxation. When the patient strains, the bladder bulges down and out and the cervix comes out through the introitus.
RECTAL: Negative, no intrinsic masses. Moderate rectocele.
EXTREMITIES: No significant deformities are noted. No edema. Reflexes are physiologic.

IMPRESSION: Second-degree uterine prolapse, cystocle with some rectocele.

PLAN: Vaginal hysterectomy, anterior repair, and possibly posterior repair at the same time.

_____

FRANK BRIETZSCH, M.D.

FB:hpi

d&t: 5/5/92

Lesson 16. Obstetrics and Gynecology

Learning Objectives

Medical

- Describe common sexually transmitted diseases in women.
- Discuss the purpose and technique involved in performing common Ob–Gyn laboratory tests and surgical procedures.
- Define common Ob–Gyn abbreviations.
- Given an Ob-Gyn root word and suffix, combine them to match a given definition.
- Distinguish between Ob-Gyn sound-alike terms.

Fundamentals

- Demonstrate the correct use of apostrophes in editing medical sentences.

Practice

- Accurately transcribe authentic physician dictation from the specialties of obstetrics and gynecology.

A Closer Look

Kits and Caboodle

by Judith Marshall, MA, CMT

I had been sitting in the doctor's waiting room for over an hour. The phones rang incessantly with that electronic warbling toodle-toodle-toodle. A sound system jangled hard rock. Three secretaries at the carousel-like desk tried to chew gum and calm the patients at the same time. I was as unhappy as a squawling infant on a well-baby visit. Finally, one of Belkin's Bunnies, as I call them, screeched my name, "JU-DEE, JU-DEE, JU-DEE. The doctor is ready for you." They all think they are Cary Grant. Not a quiet "Mrs. Marshall" with a smile, but that odious nickname. "Oh, what's the use," I thought, "at least the waiting is over."

No, it wasn't. They got me with the old beauty shop trick. When the operator is running late, someone shampoos the patron who then waits some more, under a soggy, dripping towel. The doctor's office is worse. I was deposited in a cold, barren examining room, to sit shivering in a paper dress. I waited another twenty minutes, staring at the stirrups and contemplating the sort of weapon they would make. The doctor bounded in with a cheery, "How are we today?" "We are furious," I replied and told him why. He mumbled something about delays in surgery. "You're not a surgeon, Henry," I said. "All you've cut in fifteen years is roses from that garden of yours. But you are doing more overbooking than the airlines." A thorough annual physical examination was conducted in silence.

A few days later, one of Belkin's Bunnies stopped filing her nails long enough to send me a letter. The Pap test specimen did not have enough cells. It was just a technical problem with the slide, and would I just pop in soon and have the test redone?

No wonder do-it-yourself medicine is flourishing. The diagnostic home testing kits must have been invented by people who sat around in paper dresses freezing their tailfeathers. The manufacturers' incentive includes a market of over $300 million.

The educated consumer has come a long way from eating garlic and applying potato poultices (apologies to my grandmother), even if the chicken soup still works. Many people are fascinated by space travel, nuclear energy, and CAT scanners. I am more excited about Pampers, tampons, Velcro closures, and anything made with Gore-Tex. Women are always mopping something up. I adore those little twisty things that close bread wrappers and dog cookie bags. I went wild over the yellow stickies for scribbling (known by the pompous name of removable self-stick notes). Kiss your paper clips goodbye and join the twentieth century.

The frustration with traditional healthcare delivery systems and the ferocious cost in time and money led me to the shiny local drugstore, a wonderland of self-help tools. The first thing I bought was a pill splitter for six dollars. Why nick my precious pinkies, pulverize the pills, or have them shatter all over the floor? Then I bought a fancy blood pressure tester. It is lightweight, compact, and has batteries and a digital clock. I will take it to transcription and after the chief of orthopedics finishes his usual screaming, we can all take our pressure and monitor and adjust our medication, although some of my colleagues long to monitor and adjust the mouth of the chief of orthopedics. He has not been the same since his malpractice insurance increase.

There were two ovulation prediction tests on the shelf costing from $25 to $40 with an 85 to 99 percent accuracy. The happy consumer knows when magic time is approaching, not afterward. All right, this is not romance with roses and champagne, but for over four million couples with fertility problems, it is a shot at heaven. When a lot of us were trying to keep our spouses out of the 1961 military draft (Viet Nam was really heating up), all we had was a ridiculous chart and a roulette game with a thermometer I could never read anyway. The next thing I knew I was on a bus for visiting day at Fort Knox. I think a gypsy, wearing a kerchief and golden earrings, could have made a better set of predictions with a pack of cards.

The new thermometers are fabulous. One has the exact temperature visible in huge green digital numbers, instantaneously. This sure beats sitting on a squirming, screaming child whose forehead is hot, trying to keep a standard thermometer in place in any orifice handy. Ditto the crabby husband who can locate the break in eight thousand miles of pipe but can't find the underside of his tongue for a few minutes. In the future

I predict human beings will have a built-in pop-up thermometer, just like a turkey. (Where to implant it?) As soon as the body temperature reaches 100°F, bingo!

There are tests to determine pregnancy, quickly and effectively. There is a privacy and an immediacy to these top sellers, and a blessing for rabbits everywhere. Women don't need surprises or guesswork. They need fast, reliable, straightforward positives or negatives. The drug companies seem to have more faith in a woman's sense and ability to perform a test than the doctor who purses his lips and says, "Why not settle down and relax, Janie dear; it's probably just your nerves. If these so-called symptoms persist, call me in two weeks. You are just like your mother, so highstrung. Don't waste your money on a silly lab gimmick to use at home. It's much too complex for that pretty little mind of yours."

While there is nothing as effective as an actual blood-drawing kit, science is working on it. The Chemstrip bG and Tes-Tape help diabetics every day, and don't the dieters just whoop with joy when those Ketostix turn purple! Early colon cancer, our national obsession, now can be tested on the Hemoccult card and routinely mailed back to the doctor's office. This leads me to speculate on the ever-increasing amounts of what the Post Office is delivering in addition to the junk mail.

Alas, just when science discovers birth control pills and penicillin, "safe sex" remains elusive. AIDS, Chlamydia, and herpes fester in our highly mobile, less inhibited population. "What a wonderful anniversary, my darling. I love you madly, but before we get cozy by the fire, let's step into the bathroom so I can run a few tests."

I want to buy a program for my computer with questions and answers found on the routine history and physical. The system would utilize the information and apply the appropriate diagnosis, a magnificent Corpusearch to call my own, or we could name it "Narcissus." The machine would spit out an FDA-approved prescription, I could take the scrip to the pharmacist and fulfill my destiny. "Consumer, heal thyself." Think of it, a hypochondriac's paradise.

Where does all this leave the beleaguered physician, besides setting broken bones, applying leeches, and staying out of surgical malpractice cases? I asked Belkin what he thought. "Self-help methods are great, Mrs. M. I got rid of my medical transcriptionist. All I do now is dictate, plug the tape into a computer, and it prints out perfect dictation. Eliminates the middle person. You see, I bought this new kit. . . ."

Medical Readings

A Brief Look at STDs in Women

by John H. Dirckx, M.D.

A sexually transmitted disease (STD) is any infectious disease that is transmitted from one person to another through sexual contact. The only thing all STDs have in common is their mode of transmission. In other respects they vary widely among themselves.

Changes in national sexual mores have led to the emergence of sexually transmitted infections that were not previously known or recognized, such as chlamydia and AIDS, and to marked increases in the incidence of some formerly rare infections such as genital herpes and genital warts. Studies have revealed that the viruses that cause genital warts and genital herpes can induce cervical and other cancers.

All of the classically recognized STDs can be transmitted through vaginal intercourse. Most of them can also be transmitted through oral-genital contact and anal intercourse with resulting oropharyngeal, anorectal, or systemic infection. STDs affecting the skin (genital warts, pubic lice) or transmitted through the skin (syphilis, AIDS) can be acquired during intimate contact even though genital exposure is avoided or a condom is used.

The only absolute protection against acquiring an infection through sexual contact is lifelong celibacy or maintenance of a permanently and mutually monogamous sexual relationship. Some degree of protection against STDs is afforded by practicing "safe (or safer) sex"—which basically means using condoms and avoiding high-risk behaviors such as anal intercourse—and by limiting the number of sex partners.

The diagnosis and treatment of STDs are rendered more difficult by the reluctance of most people to discuss their sexual behavior with health professionals and by the refusal of many patients to believe that a sexual partner has become infected by some third person. Diagnosis often demands alertness and a high degree of suspicion on the part of the healthcare worker. History-taking must be searching but nonthreatening and nonjudgmental. Often the most suggestive point in the history is exposure to a new sexual partner within two months before the appearance of symptoms.

In treating any patient with an STD, the physician must reckon with two epidemiologic realities: the fact that at least one of the patient's sexual partners (and possibly all of them) is also infected, and the statistical probability that a person with one STD has other STDs. Failure to treat sexual partners prophylactically will lead to eventual reinfection of most patients. Moreover, unless both partners in a relationship are treated at the same time, they may keep reinfecting each other, a phenomenon known as "ping-ponging." STD screening tests are a standard part of prenatal care, as well.

Urethritis and pelvic inflammatory disease. Genital infections due to **chlamydia** are currently the most common of all bacterial STDs. Although, strictly speaking, chlamydia is the name of the causative organism, in clinical parlance genital infections due to this organism are often called simply "chlamydia." *Chlamydia trachomatis* is highly contagious: at least 50% of sexual partners of persons with chlamydia are also infected; 20% of men and 80% of women with the disease have no symptoms and do not know that they are infected (and infectious).

In women the most frequent form of chlamydial infection is mucopurulent cervicitis, which may cause slight bleeding or pain with intercourse but is often discovered only on routine pelvic examination. Chlamydia also causes acute urethral syndrome in women, in which symptoms of increased urinary frequency and urinary burning mimic cystitis, but urine cultures are sterile.

Because facilities for laboratory diagnosis of chlamydial infection are not altogether satisfactory, treatment must often be instituted on the basis of clinical suspicion. The organism cannot be grown on artificial media, and tissue culture is expensive and insensitive. In practice, a urethral or cervical smear is usually examined for chlamydial inclusion bodies (elementary bodies) within infected cells by a direct fluorescent antibody (FA) or enzyme-linked immunosorbent assay (ELISA) method. A genetic (DNA) probe procedure can also be used, and serologic tests are available.

As many as 20% of women with untreated chlamydia will eventually develop acute salpingitis, also called pelvic inflammatory disease (PID), due to spread of infection to one or both uterine tubes. PID is more likely to occur in a woman with an intrauterine device (IUD), and acute attacks are more common during menstruation. The symptoms of pelvic pain and fever are fairly nonspecific, but severe tenderness on manipulation of the cervix and on palpation of the uterine adnexa during pelvic examination are highly suggestive of the diagnosis. This is known as the chandelier sign; the term fancifully implies that the pain causes the patient to leap into the air and cling to the chandelier.

PID may progress to tubo-ovarian abscess or to perihepatitis (Fitz-Hugh and Curtis syndrome). A more common consequence of PID is scarring of the uterine tubes with resulting infertility or sterility and heightened risk of ectopic pregnancy.

Chlamydia responds to treatment with various antibiotics. Currently recommended drugs are doxycycline (Doryx, Vibramycin, Vibra-Tabs), tetracycline (Achromycin, Sumycin), or azithromycin (Zithromax), administered orally for 7-10 days. All of the patient's sexual partners must be treated prophylactically, regardless of symptoms or laboratory test results. Tubo-ovarian abscess and salpingitis that do not respond to antibiotics may require surgical treatment.

Gonorrhea is infection of the genital tract of either sex by *Neisseria gonorrhoeae*, a gram-negative diplococcus. This disease has been known for centuries and goes by the colloquial name of ''clap.'' Physicians often refer to the causative organism as the gonococcus, GC for short, and this abbreviation frequently stands for the disease itself in medical slang.

Like chlamydia, gonorrhea is an infection of the genital mucous membranes, causing urethritis in men but frequently asymptomatic in women; it too is capable of progressing to PID with its complications of tubo-ovarian abscess and Fitz-Hugh and Curtis syndrome and its aftermath of tubal scarring with resultant infertility or sterility and increased risk of tubal pregnancy. Also like chlamydia, gonorrhea can cause severe eye infection, resulting in blindness, in an infant born to an infected mother.

The diagnosis of gonorrhea can be made by examination of a gram-stained smear of urethral discharge for the typical intracellular diplococci or by culture of urethral, cervical, or other material on special media such as Thayer-Martin agar, which is designed to favor the growth of gonococci. The sensitivity of laboratory diagnosis, particularly in women, is enhanced by doing rectal as well as cervical cultures, because even without a history of anal intercourse, the organism often migrates to the rectum from a genital site of infection.

Increasing problems of resistance to penicillin have led to the abandonment of this drug in treatment of gonorrhea. Currently the drug of choice is ceftriaxone (Rocephin) in a single intramuscular injection of 250 mg. Other cephalosporins and some of the quinolones are also effective. All patients treated for gonorrhea are also treated prophylactically for chlamydia because of the high frequency with which these diseases occur together. In addition, all sexual contacts of patients with gonorrhea are treated prophylactically against both diseases, regardless of symptoms or results of tests.

Genital ulcers. Herpes simplex is a local infection of skin or mucous membranes caused by a virus. Type 1 herpes simplex virus (HSV-1) typically causes lesions of the lips and face (orofacial herpes, herpes labialis, cold sore, fever blister), while type 2 causes lesions of the genitals (**genital herpes**, herpes progenitalis). Although the types are distinguishable in the laboratory, there is no difference in their clinical effects, and a 10-20% overlap of their preferred infection sites occurs.

Transmission is by direct contact with an infected person. The incubation period may be as short as one week, but sometimes the virus remains dormant for months or years before causing symptoms. Apparently persons with latent infection (no active lesions) can spread the disease to others, at least in certain circumstances. Genital herpes is always spread through sexual contact.

Regardless of its location, herpes simplex appears as a small cluster of vesicles surrounded by a reddened zone of skin or mucous membrane. Itching or burning is often intense and may precede the appearance of lesions. Within a day or two the vesicles slough and become shallow, painful ulcers. A first attack of herpes simplex may be accompanied by swelling and inflammation of regional lymph nodes and fever. The lesions heal spontaneously after 1-2 weeks. However, the virus remains in the body for the life of the patient, lying dormant in spinal cord ganglia.

A recurrence of herpes simplex at the same site as the original eruption can be triggered at any time by various physical or emotional stresses, including fever, sunburn, menses, and fatigue. Recurrent herpes simplex is usually milder than the primary attack and of shorter duration, and fever and lymph gland involvement seldom occur. Recurrences may come at intervals of days, weeks, months, or years; many patients never experience any recurrences at all.

In women with genital herpes, severely painful vulvar lesions are the rule, but when the cervix is the site of the eruption it may go unnoticed. Anorectal lesions result from anal intercourse. Neonatal infection, acquired at birth by a child born to a mother with active genital herpes, often leads to disseminated disease with a high mortality rate.

Diagnosis of herpes simplex is usually obvious on direct examination. Confirmation may be obtained by means of a Tzanck smear, a stained preparation of material scraped or expressed from a lesion, which shows abnormal balloon cells with viral inclusion bodies. A Pap smear may also show these changes. These tests are relatively insensitive, however, and cannot distinguish between herpes and other viral eruptions (chickenpox, herpes zoster).

Treatment of genital herpes with acyclovir (Zovirax) shortens the period of clinical symptoms and of viral shedding, but does not eradicate the virus. Acyclovir is usually given orally, but it may also be applied in ointment form or administered parenterally. Long-term prophylaxis with oral acyclovir has been helpful for some patients with frequent recurrences.

Because genital herpes is a risk factor for cervical cancer, women with a history of this disease are advised to have regular Pap smears throughout life. A woman who goes into labor with active genital herpes is delivered by cesarean section to prevent transmission of infection to the newborn.

Genital warts. A wart is a benign skin tumor induced by infection with the human papillomavirus (HPV). Genital warts (venereal warts), occurring on the skin and mucous membranes of the genitals and anus, are spread almost exclusively through sexual contact. Perianal spread may result from anal intercourse but is often due to migration of virus from the patient's own genital lesions. Genital warts are highly contagious: 60 to 90% of sexual partners of persons with genital warts also have genital warts. They are the most common viral STD, and their incidence is increasing. Genital warts are more likely to develop during pregnancy and in persons with impaired immunity. In recent years the confirmation of a causal connection between genital warts and genital cancer has altered the way in which this disease is viewed and treated.

In men genital warts usually appear on the penis, occasionally within the urethra or about the anus. In women genital warts typically affect the labia and perianal skin but may involve the vaginal lining and cervix. The principal symptom of genital warts is their visible presence. Itching and vaginal discharge may occur, and warts sometimes ulcerate or become infected with skin bacteria.

HPV types 6 and 11 cause the classical genital wart known as condyloma acuminatum (plural, condylomata acuminata). This is a slender, often finger-shaped growth with a narrow attachment to the skin, a tapered tip, and a somewhat rough texture. HPV types 16 and 18 cause flat warts rather than classical condylomata acuminata. These viral types are associated with a high risk of dysplasia or cancer in affected genital skin or mucous membranes, particularly cervical intraepithelial neoplasia (CIN), which may progress to invasive carcinoma of the cervix.

Two-thirds of male partners of women with cervical dysplasia or cervical cancer have HPV-associated anogenital lesions. Partners of women with dysplasia or cancer of the cervix have a heightened risk of developing dysplasia or cancer of the penis. The second wife of a man whose first wife died of cervical cancer is at an increased risk of developing cervical cancer. Because of the contagiousness of HPV and the risk of malignant change, diagnostic procedures are now more elaborate and treatment more aggressive than they were just ten years ago.

Genital warts can usually be diagnosed by simple inspection, but many cases of latent infection are only recognized on Pap smear or cervical biopsy. A standard procedure for identifying genital warts and other lesions of the cervix is colposcopy, an inspection of the cervix with a low-power binocular microscope. In both sexes, visualization of small, flat, or atypical warts is enhanced by prior application of 5% acetic acid (white vinegar) for a few minutes to the area of skin or mucous membrane to be examined. Acetic acid causes blanching (acetowhitening) in typical HPV lesions. This procedure is not highly specific, but at least it helps the examiner to decide which lesions should be biopsied.

A wide variety of methods are used to treat genital warts, including surgical excision, electrodesiccation, cryosurgery, and laser ablation; application of liquid nitrogen, corrosive chemicals (trichloracetic acid, dichloracetic acid), or antimitotics (podophyllin, 5-FU); and intralesional injection of interferon. The choice of treatment depends on the site, character, and extent of involvement. Currently liquid nitrogen is favored for most lesions. Regardless of the method used, several treatments are usually needed to eliminate all warts, and rates of recurrence or treatment failure with all methods are substantial.

Vaginitis. Vaginitis is inflammation of the vagina (and usually also of the vulva) as manifested by vulvovaginal pain or itching and vaginal discharge that is abnormal in volume, consistency, color, or odor. Two forms of vaginitis are associated with sexual transmission of microorganisms.

Candida albicans, a yeastlike fungus, is present on the skin and in the digestive tract. Under certain circumstances candida can overgrow and invade epithelial surfaces, causing dermatitis, oropharyngeal infection (thrush), esophageal infection, or colitis.

Candidal vaginitis (vaginal candidosis or candidiasis) causes intense vulvar itching and a thick, white, curdy discharge. Like most other forms of candidal infection, candidal vaginitis is more likely to occur in diabetes, pregnancy, and immunodeficiency, and after antibiotic treatment. It is also more common in women taking oral contraceptives. While this condition is probably not usually acquired by sexual contact, the sexual partner of a woman with candidal vaginitis may have candidal dermatitis of the genitals, and may reinfect the woman after treatment.

Diagnosis is made by finding fungal elements on microscopic examination of vaginal secretions that have been treated with potassium hydroxide (KOH) to destroy human cellular material. Diagnosis may be confirmed by culture. Local treatment with various antifungal drugs in the form of cream or suppositories is promptly effective. Sexual partners may need treatment as well. Recurrences are common.

Although traditionally classed as a form of vaginitis, **bacterial vaginosis** or Gardnerella vaginitis causes little if any inflammation or itching. Usually the only symptom is a copious, gray, malodorous discharge. Like candidal vaginitis, this condition can arise with no prior sexual contact. However, it often appears shortly after intercourse with a new partner, and although men show no symptoms of infection, they can apparently harbor the pathogen and reinfect their partners.

Bacterial vaginosis is diagnosed by excluding other causes of abnormal vaginal discharge and by finding clue cells on microscopic examination of a wet preparation (wet prep) of vaginal secretions. Clue cells are vaginal epithelial cells studded with numerous Gardnerella organisms, which are coccobacilli (very short bacilli). Another typical finding is release of a fishy or amine odor when potassium hydroxide is added to secretions in preparation for examination for candida.

Treatment with oral or vaginal preparations of metronidazole (Flagyl, Protostat, MetroGel Vaginal) is promptly curative, but recurrences are common. Simultaneous treatment of male partners seems to improve outcome.

Laboratory Tests and Surgical Procedures

amniocentesis   A procedure to withdraw amniotic fluid through a needle from the uterus of a pregnant woman. The fetal cells and chemicals in the fluid are studied to identify fetal abnormalities.

amniotic fluid   The fluid medium surrounding a fetus. A sample withdrawn through a needle inserted into the pregnant uterus can be subjected to various chemical tests and to karyotyping of cells.

beta HCG   See *HCG* (human chorionic gonadotropin).

Candida albicans   A yeastlike fungus capable of causing superficial infection in the mouth (thrush) or vagina and on the skin. Also called *monilia*.

Chlamydia trachomatis   A gram-negative intracellular bacterium that causes sexually transmitted infections of the genital tract and other types of infection.

chocolate agar   A culture medium containing blood which, when autoclaved, turns chocolate brown. It is used to culture *Neisseria gonorrhoeae* and *Haemophilus influenzae.*

Coombs test, direct   A test to determine whether the patient's red blood cells have become coated with an antiglobulin. The test is positive in newborns with hemolytic disease due to Rh incompatibility and in others with acquired hemolytic disease.

Coombs test, indirect   A test to determine whether the patient's serum contains antiglobulin to red blood cells. This test is positive in the mother of an infant with hemolytic disease due to Rh incompatibility and in others with acquired hemolytic disease.

dark-field microscopy   A microscopic technique using special lighting that makes it easier to identify *Treponema pallidum*, the organism that causes syphilis.

estradiol   The principal estrogen (female hormone) secreted by the ovary. Measurement of its level in serum gives an estimate of ovarian function.

FSH (follicle-stimulating hormone)   A hormone secreted by the anterior pituitary gland that stimulates ovulation in women and spermatogenesis in men. Measurement of serum FSH is part of the evaluation of a patient for infertility or gonadal dysfunction.

FTA (fluorescent treponemal antibody) **test**   An indirect immunofluorescence test, highly specific for syphilis.

Gardnerella vaginalis   A gram-negative organism, formerly called *Haemophilus vaginalis,* which causes bacterial vaginosis.

HCG (human chorionic gonadotropin)   A hormone produced by the placenta and detected in various blood and urine tests for pregnancy. A more specific test detects only the beta subunit of this hormone, hence the term *beta HCG.*

Haemophilus vaginalis   Older name for *Gardnerella vaginalis.*

herpes simplex virus (HSV), **type 1**   The herpesvirus that causes cold sores, pharyngitis, conjunctivitis, and some skin infections; **type 2**   The herpesvirus that causes genital herpes.

hysterosalpingogram   A test to assess infertility in which radiopaque dye is injected into the uterus and fallopian tubes, and x-rays are taken to show if the tubes are patent (clear) or obstructed.

luteinizing hormone (LH)   A hormone produced by the anterior pituitary gland. In women it stimulates ovulation and formation of the corpus luteum, and in men it stimulates production of androgens in the testicle. Measurement of LH is part of the evaluation of a patient for infertility or gonadal dysfunction.

mammogram   An x-ray of the breasts. Used as a screening test in large numbers of women, particularly those over age 40, to detect breast carcinoma.

MMK (Marshall-Marchetti-Krantz)   An operation for urinary stress incontinence, performed retropubically.

Neisseria gonorrhoeae   The gram-negative diplococcus that causes gonorrhea.

Pap (Papanicolaou) **smear**   A smear of cells from the uterine cervix or other source, stained and examined for abnormal or malignant change.

RPR (rapid plasma reagin)   Test for antibody to *Treponema pallidum.* Used in the diagnosis of syphilis.

semen analysis   Examination of semen to determine the number, shape, and motility of spermatozoa as a part of an infertility evaluation.

spirochete   A spiral-shaped bacterium. The organisms that cause syphilis and Lyme disease are spirochetes.

STD screen   Sexually transmitted diseases screen.

STS (serologic test for syphilis)   A general term referring to any test used to identify syphilis by a serologic method.

Thayer-Martin agar   A culture medium containing denatured blood and antibiotics, intended to facilitate the growth of *Neisseria gonorrhoeae.*

TPI (*Treponema pallidum* immobilization)   A diagnostic test for syphilis.

Treponema pallidum   The spirochete that causes syphilis.

Trichomonas vaginalis   A protozoan parasite that causes vaginitis.

Tzanck smear   A stained smear of material from a cutaneous or mucosal lesion, intended to identify changes due to viral infection from herpes simplex or varicella.

VDRL (Venereal Disease Research Laboratory)   A serologic test for syphilis.

ultrasound   The use of sound waves to assess tumors of the ovaries or uterus as well as the fetus in pregnant woman.

Wasserman test   An older serum test for syphilis; now replaced by RPR and VDRL.

yeast   A one-celled fungus; often interchangeably used with *Candida albicans.*

Anatomy/Medical Terminology

Abbreviations Exercise

Common abbreviations may be transcribed as dictated in the body of a report. Uncommon abbreviations must be spelled out, with the abbreviation appearing in parentheses after the translation. All abbreviations (except laboratory test names) must be spelled out in the Diagnosis or Impression section of any report.

Instructions: Define the following Ob–Gyn abbreviations. Then memorize both abbreviations and definitions to increase your speed and accuracy in transcribing Ob–Gyn dictation.

CIN   _____

D&C   _____

EDC   _____

FSH   _____

GC   _____

HCG   _____

IUD   _____

LH   _____

LMP   _____

NSVD   _____

PID   _____

PMS   _____

STD   _____

TAH–BSO _____

TVH   _____

VBAC   _____

Root Word and Suffix Matching Exercise

Instructions: Combine the following root words with suffixes to form words that match the definitions below. Fill in the blanks with the medical words that you construct.

Root Word	Suffix
dys-	-itis
hystero-	-ology
gyneco-	-otomy
salpingo-	-oscopy
episio-	-ectomy
cervi-	-rrhea
meno-	
colpo-	

A. the study of the female reproductive tract

_____

B. surgical incision into the perineum prior to childbirth

_____

C. inflammation of the cervix

_____

D. surgical removal of the fallopian tube

_____

E. using a scope to visualize the vagina

_____

F. surgical removal of the uterus

_____

G. difficult or painful menstruation
(Tip: Use 2 root words and 1 suffix.)

_____

Word Search

Instructions: Locate and circle the Ob–Gyn terminology hidden in the puzzle horizontally, vertically, or diagonally, forward or backward. A numeral following a term indicates the number of times it can be found in the puzzle.

```
C O I T U S C U L D E S A C B E A
X U A D I V A R G I M I R P R M M
D M R B V T S A E R B S O P E B N
S U T E F E H Y R A V O B N A R I
N V F G T F A L L O P I A N S Y O
A O H S Y T A M T K Y R L D T O N
E V E B H B A P O J C T S Y C A O
R T A W O N F G X H N E D C G T I
A B O R T I O N E N A M O W C N T
S Q T J B D Y S M E N O R R H E A
E N I R E T U A I R G D A N D C U
C Z O B R A M W A X E N D A I A R
F I W E P M S V J M R E P S O L T
D U B O O I L A R A P V F J R P S
X U N G M U S C I R T E T S B O N
P E R D V E N I R E T U K L I M E
M A G S U D N U F U W O M B F J M
M D P G J S W D S L A C I V R E C
```

abort	endometriosis	ovary
abortion	fallopian	ovum
adnexa	fetus (2)	Pap
amnion	fibroid (2)	para
baby	FSH	placenta
breast (2)	fundus (2)	PMS
cervical	HCG	pregnancy
cesarean	IUD (2)	primigravida
coitus	labia	puberty
cul-de-sac	labor	sperm
curettage	LMP	testes
cyst	mammogram	toxemia
D and C	menarche	uterine (2)
dysmenorrhea	menopause	vulvar
EDC	menstruation	woman
egg	milk	womb
embryo	obstetrics	women

Sound-alikes Exercise

Instructions: Circle the correct term from the sound-alikes in parentheses in the following sentences.

1. Cesarean section was planned because the baby was in a (breach, breech) presentation.
2. The (cervical, surgical) neck of the uterus was reached, and the cervix (circumcised, circumscribed).
3. On (colposcopy, culdoscopy), the vulva and vagina were seen to be normal.
4. There was no free fluid or blood found in the cul-de-sac on (colposcopy, culdoscopy).
5. The patient had production of (claustrum, colostrum) immediately following delivery.
6. On examination of the breasts, there were no (discreet, discrete) nodules.
7. Examination of this 65-year-old woman reveals an absent uterus and an (atopic, atrophic, ectopic) vagina.
8. Following delivery of the 9-pound infant, the patient had a large (fissure, fistula) of the (perineal, peroneal, peritoneal) body.
9. The baby was delivered and laid momentarily on the mother's (perineum, peritoneum).
10. This grand multipara came in with complaints of "brown stuff" coming from her vagina. On examination, a rectovaginal (fissure, fistula) was found.
11. Following a Stamey urethral suspension, the patient developed a vesicovaginal (fissure, fistula).
12. The uterus was closed and placed back in the (perineum, peritoneum), and (perineal, peroneal, peritoneal) closure was accomplished with 0 Vicryl.
13. Exploration of the uterus with forceps resulted in no tissue, and (general, gentle) suction curettage was then done, yielding minimal tissue.
14. Examination of the urethra revealed a small growth, probably a urethral (furuncle, caruncle, carbuncle).
15. After the right fallopian tube was isolated, a small (knuckle, nuchal) was picked up between (loops, loupes) of suture, and excised.
16. The (lochial, local) discharge subsided after the first week postpartum.
17. The infant exhibited severe caput (molding, moulding) following a lengthy delivery.
18. Multiple uterine (myelomas, myomas) were noted upon examination of the uterine fundus.
19. The baby was delivered from the (vertex, vortex) position.

Transcription Guidelines

Apostrophes

1. Apostrophes are used to show possession.

   The laboratory tests were ordered by Dr. Jeppson's office.
   The patient was referred to Dr. Smith's office.

2. Apostrophes are used to show singular and plural possession or ownership, notably with units of time.

   She is to return to see me in one month's time.
   He has had a pain in the right groin of two months' duration.
   The uterus is the size of a 16-week pregnancy.
   The uterus is 16 weeks' size.

3. *It's* is a contraction for *it is*; use of the apostrophe indicates that a letter has been omitted. *Its* is the possessive form and does not use an apostrophe; the words *it is* cannot be substituted.

   It's (= it is) my opinion that she has an immune disorder.
   The fetus was noted to have its back to the camera on ultrasound. (Cannot substitute *it is*.)

4. Apostrophes are *not* needed when forming the plurals of abbreviations or numbers, except to avoid confusion when lowercase letters are made plural.

WBCs	EKGs	STDs	40s	CMTs
wbc's	rbc's	x's and y's		+'s

Apostrophe Exercise

Instructions: Insert apostrophes as appropriate in the following sentences.

1. Its too bad that the hospitals policy prohibits patients access to their own medical records.

2. Two sonograms were compatible with a fetus of 30 weeks gestation.

Continued ▶

3. On x-ray examination, the femur showed a fracture in its most distal portion of approximately two weeks duration.

4. Dr. Howards consultation was received two days before the patients surgery was scheduled.

5. Although its clear that the genus has been identified, the species has not.

Terminology Challenge

Instructions: The following terms appear in the dictation on Tape 8A. Before beginning the medical transcription practice for Lesson 16, become familiar with the terminology below by looking up each word in a medical or English dictionary and writing out a short definition of each term.

adenofibroma
amniotic fluid
anterior leaf of the
  broad ligament
Apgar score
axilla
bladder blade
blunt dissection
broad ligament
carcinoma in situ
cardinal ligament
caudad
cephalad, cephalic
cervical os
cervical stump
CIN-3 (cervical intra-
  epithelial neoplasia,
  grade 3)
condylomata acuminata
cystadenoma
deciduoid reaction
DeLee trap
dysplasia
exploratory laparotomy
exteriorized
fetal heart tones
fibrocystic disease, breasts
finger dissection
follicular cyst
forceps blade
frozen section diagnosis
fundal height
fundectomy
gestation
infundibulopelvic
  ligament

Kocher clamp
leiomyomata
linea alba
low cervical transverse
  C-section
mastitis
Mayo scissors
meconium
Mighty-Vac vacuum
  extractor
myoma
nonstress test (pregnancy)
O'Connor-O'Sullivan
  retractor
papilloma
pedicle
Pfannenstiel incision
placenta
Premarin
pretibial edema
Provera
reapproximated
rectus muscles
round ligament
salpingo-oophorectomy
secretory endometrium
subcutaneous mastectomy
suture
  chromic
  continuous
  figure-of-8
  imbricating
  interlocking
TA-55 articulator
tenaculum
toxemia
tubal pregnancy
uterine gutter
vaginal cuff
vector
vesicouterine reflection

Transcription Practice

After completing all the readings and exercises in Lesson 16, transcribe Tape 8A, Obstetrics and Gynecology. Use both medical and English dictionaries and your Quick-Reference Word List as resource materials for finding words. Proofread your transcribed documents carefully, listening to the dictation while you read your transcripts.

Transcribe (*NOT* retype) the same reports again without referring to your previous transcription attempt. Initially, you may need to transcribe some reports more than twice before you can produce an error-free document. Your ultimate goal is to produce an error-free document the first time.

BLOOPERS	
Incorrect	**Correct**
Periods of vaginal spotting with crabs.	Periods of vaginal spotting with cramps.
Genitalia showed evidence of exploration.	Genitalia showed evidence of excoriation.
Theological test for syphilis.	Serological test for syphilis.
Postpartum bladder acne.	Postpartum bladder atony.
Vaginal exam showed parasite left.	Vaginal exam showed parous outlet.
Diagnosis: Penile vaginitis.	Diagnosis: Senile vaginitis.
This Grandma Kipperus was given a sterno vaginal examination.	This grand multiparous was given a sterile vaginal examination.
Vaginal exam revealed a smug introitus.	Vaginal exam revealed a snug introitus.

Lesson 17. Otorhinolaryngology

Learning Objectives

Medical

- List common ENT (ear, nose, and throat) symptoms and disease conditions mentioned in the Review of Systems and Physical Examination sections of an H&P.
- Describe the action of these drugs: decongestants, antihistamines, antitussives, expectorants, and corticosteroids.
- Discuss the purpose and technique involved in performing common ENT laboratory tests and surgical procedures.
- Given a cross-section illustration of the ear, memorize the anatomic structures labeled.
- Define common ENT abbreviations.
- Given an ENT root word, symptom, or disease, match it to its correct medical definition.
- Given a category of ENT drugs, indicate which drugs belong to that category.

Fundamentals

- Discuss which type of working environment, compensation, and benefits package would be most attractive to you as a medical transcriptionist.
- Demonstrate the correct use of abbreviations, acronyms, and initialisms in editing medical sentences.
- Given a medical report with errors, identify and correct the errors.

Practice

- Accurately transcribe authentic physician dictation from the specialty of otorhinolaryngology.

A Closer Look

Who Nose?

Susan M. Turley, MA, CMT

If Bo knows football and baseball, then it might be correct to say that I now know noses. Recently I had the chance to see surgery from the other side—the patient's side.

After many years of extreme nasal stuffiness, I gathered my courage and decided to have a surgical correction or, as my mother-in-law so aptly put it, "go under the knife."

I mentioned my decision to my internist who specializes in natural medicine. With a shocked expression on his face, he described the surgery as "having a bulldozer up your nose." My feelings of courage began to evaporate. He insisted I cancel my upcoming appointment with the plastic surgeon. I solemnly considered that perhaps he was right, until, moving on to another of my medical problems, I asked him what he advised his patients to do for PMS. "Have a hysterectomy," he said with a perfectly straight face. "What?" I yelled. "You don't want me to have a simple nasal surgery but you recommend a hysterectomy for PMS!" He wasn't smiling. Obviously he had a hidden agenda. I kept my appointment with the plastic surgeon.

The plastic surgeon confirmed that my turbinates were grossly hypertrophied and were the cause of my inability to breathe. After we agreed that a turbinectomy would be beneficial, he then asked delicately if I had considered having any plastic surgery at the same time. Ever considered plastic surgery? Just since the day I was born! He gently asked what would I like to have done. "Hey," I said, "I have a list!" We started with number one on the list: a nose job. It was painful hearing him brutally describe the unacceptable aspects of my nose—bulbous tip, uneven width, drooping tip, drooping underside, excessive length—even though I had seen all these problems myself in the mirror.

258

Then there were finances to consider. My insurance would pay for the functional nasal surgery (turbinectomy and cartilage graft) but not for any cosmetic surgery. I would be responsible for the surgeon's fee, hospital's fee, and anesthesiologist's fee that pertained to the cosmetic part of the surgery. I was surprised to learn that the total cost of the cosmetic surgery could vary greatly (as much as $3000), depending on the hospital I selected. Naturally I chose the cheapest hospital where, my surgeon assured me, the care was excellent.

The surgeon's secretary informed me that his fee needed to be paid IN FULL ten days IN ADVANCE. That was a shock. I guess too many cosmetic surgery patients had stiffed him and walked away from their bills with their beautiful new noses in the air. At least that was what I liked to think. The alternative—that the bills were not paid because the patients were undergoing psychiatric treatment for a permanently botched-up nose—was too painful to contemplate.

On the morning of surgery, I found myself first paying the hospital's bill in full with my VISA card. I then undressed and was put in a recovery room bed where I could either watch TV or read. I chose to read; the nurse handed me a *Newsweek* in which the confidence-inspiring cover story was about doctors with AIDS. The anesthesiologist came in and started an I.V. in my right hand. He left before I could remind him that I was supposed to pay him in full before my surgery. I had no doubts, though, that he would return, and he did. With my right hand, I then laboriously wrote out a check to him for $700. Question: Did the first patient to undergo a rhinoplasty coin the phrase "paying through the nose"?

I reminded the anesthesiologist that the last time I had had general anesthesia (about eight years ago), I had been given Pentothal and asked to count backwards from 100. When I stopped counting I assumed I was asleep and so did the anesthesiologist who proceeded to intubate me. Not being fully asleep, however, I had to violently resist the urge to throw up. After surgery, two anesthesiologists came to my room and sheepishly asked me if I thought everything had gone well with my surgery. I told them what had happened and they apologized profusely, all the while throwing knowing looks at each other. This experience, I explained to the anesthesiologist, I had no wish to repeat. He assured me that that type of unfortunate accident was never supposed to happen. He hastily told me that he would be sure to give me an amnestic agent before the induction agent so that I would not remember anything.

After the anesthesiologist left, the plastic surgeon arrived to mark my nose and cheeks with a skin marking pen. I gave my checkbook (thank goodness, no one else needed to be paid) and glasses to the nurse, and was wheeled into the operating room.

The temperature in surgery was no warmer than 50 degrees, it seemed. Even the nurses were complaining of the cold. They gave me lots of warm blankets, though, and I was comfortable. Someone said, "How are you doing?" "Who, me?" I answered. Without my glasses I couldn't tell if the staff was talking to me or just chitchatting among themselves. "Me? I feel fine." That was all she wrote, as they say. I never felt drowsy; I never even knew when I fell asleep. That's what I call a smooth induction.

The next thing I knew I was in the recovery room. Disembodied voices kept calling my name and saying the surgery went fine. A nurse asked me how much pain I was having, and I said my nose felt like when I slammed my hand in the car door. She promptly provided a shot of Demerol and Compazine. (I had dry heaves for what seemed like hours.) I was very chilly, and the nurses wrapped warm blankets around me, even putting them on my head so that I could pretend I was hibernating in a warm cave.

When my husband and six-year-old son were allowed into the recovery room to see me, they maintained a respectful distance, not quite sure how to react to my extensively bruised face. From my eyebrows down to my cheekbones, the skin was pitch black, as if some prankster had poured indelible black ink all over my face. Later at home, my husband regained his sense of humor and cheerfully told well-wishers on the phone that I looked as if I had gone several rounds with Mike Tyson. Actually I thought I looked WORSE than that. But within five days, the bruising was barely noticeable.

The week following surgery had its own set of annoying problems. My glasses did not sit right over the nasal splint and, with my eyelids still swollen, it was nearly impossible to enjoy the new Tom Clancy book I had purchased especially for the occasion. My nose was filled with packing so that I mouth-breathed, snored, and coughed without getting much sleep for nearly a week. One small blessing was that the nasal packing now used is absorbable and does not need to be painfully pulled out of the nose.

As the swelling went down and the nasal splint came off, I began breathing more fully than I had in years, and I really liked my new nose. Would I do it again? Sure. By the way, where is that list?

Employment Enigmas

by Judy Hinickle, CMT

The possibilities of employment in the transcription field today have increased in scope and variety. Many people are faced with decisions or options not open to them even ten years ago.

Medical transcriptionists have always had opportunities to transcribe in hospital or clinic departments, services, and physician offices with traditional benefit structures. Many more now have taken the plunge into transcription supervision and management or teaching, or have become independent contractors, at-home employees, or self-employed service owners. Our respective employment opportunities include myriads of options such as flexible benefits vs. no benefits, job-sharing vs. part-time employment, incentive pay systems vs. hourly wages, and so on. Sifting through these options requires a conscious focus on the personal needs which drive us down the highway of employment.

Medical transcriptionists work to satisfy needs. Money is primary—usually to obtain family or personal needs (food, shelter, clothing, insurance, education, cars, retirement). Let's face it, would you be thinking of working as a medical transcriptionist if you won the lottery?

Secondary needs also play a part in employment motivation: a productive use of energy, a sense of accomplishment, fulfillment, achievement, power, or companionship and camaraderie. There are, of course, the needs met outside of work which will supersede employment motivations: family responsibilities and pleasures, mental and physical health, social needs. For example, the need to make more money may be set aside to work in a job which offers hours more conducive to spending time with spouse and children, as long as minimal monetary needs are met.

Each transcriptionist has an infrastructure of priorities at work. The energy a person is willing to apply to transcription, and the attitude surrounding it, are affected by the way in which the various needs are met. Some of these needs include the need for acceptance, the need to be praised, the need to be valued as a person, the need for a sense of security, the need to work hard and play hard, the need for a healthy environment and lifestyle. Certainly these emotional needs can be met outside a job. But because most of us need money, we work, thus requiring that our energy-absorbing job fulfill many of our emotional needs. A good employer recognizes these requirements.

The strengths a person calls upon within a job will be affected first by the fulfillment of the primary monetary need. For the most part transcriptionists are paid well throughout the country, whether they work for themselves or for someone else. There are variations as to how well, but the pay is good compared to other fields, given the level of formal education required. So the compensation for employees offers a variety of other options in the monetary fulfillment area.

Transcriptionists are paid in various employment settings by the hour, by production, by a combination of the two, or with the profits of self-employment. All sorts of personal needs are taken into consideration with each. Do you need the security of hourly wages or a salary? Or would you rather take risks that you will make more money when paid by production or through self-employment? Does a spotlight on production statistics cause you too much stress, or do you thrive on the challenge?

What about the other areas of compensation? Benefits are a major method of compensation, but perhaps we should consider whether an employer is the best choice for obtaining maximum benefits. Would you take a job because of the medical insurance, or the profit sharing, or the pension plan? Or would you rather make a better wage with a job having no benefits and make your own provisions for insurance, investment, and retirement?

We should analyze benefit opportunities in the light of today's society. Employment is in a fickle state these days. Employees job-hop and employers "re-organize" constantly. The days of working for one employer 25 years have passed for most employees. Our society is restless and mobile. Jobs may last less than five years. Careers may last only 10 or 20 years, then new paths are embarked upon. Are employees asking for long-term benefits from short-term employers? Do employees cling to making employers responsible for too much of their future financial security—possibly *expecting* that empowerment, yet *resenting* it at the same time?

Employers offer insurance and pension plans because they are needed in today's society. Is this the most efficient source for these benefits? It is of interest that employers target employee retention by using pension or profit-sharing plans which require a number of years for investiture. Is this building good employee relations, thereby saving the employer money? Or does it keep many people in jobs they don't like, just waiting for that benefit to mature? Could there be a resultant loss of revenue, with labor problems caused by unrest and dissatisfaction?

When looking at these wage and benefit issues, we need to consider trade-offs. If your choice of employment gives you none of the benefits which traditionally equate to 25 to 33% of your wages, are you then getting that in cash and applying it to those benefits? As an independent contractor with no benefits, are you making that additional 25 to 33% *after expenses* so that you can pay your taxes and also purchase the insurance and a pension plan independently? If self-employed, do your wages and profit *after expenses* equal or exceed an equivalent wage and benefit package in a traditional setting?

There are, of course, lifestyle and personal benefits to be considered in alternate employment settings, but we must be careful not to shortchange our financial future with short-sightedness now.

Once we get past wage and investment issues, personal ability and satisfaction become important. What kind of work hours does your lifestyle require? How much responsibility do you want to accept? Do you like to supervise? Teach? Do you like to ''plug in and tune out''? Would you rather not deal with people? Do you like taking risks? Do you think self-employment means there is no one to answer to? Do you want to work a certain number of hours per week and no more? All these questions are appropriate for various transcription opportunities.

Other issues surround our employment options:
- Self-employment and independent contracting tend to breed uneven cash flow and unreasonable hours, and can perpetuate poor future financial planning.
- Working at home takes great self-discipline and sometimes leads to a feeling of never getting away from work to relax.
- Employing others includes tremendous responsibility for their financial well-being, the quality of their work, the standards of their work environment, and making available enough steady work and benefits to keep them with you. Healthy cash flow is all-important to meet these responsibilities, and the paperwork can be overwhelming. Skills in marketing, accounting, and managing personnel are required. Clients may not have the bureaucratic drawbacks of an institutional employer, but their quality and timeliness expectations and their erratic quantity demands can be even more distressing.
- Working in a hospital or clinic setting can be anonymous, rigid, and sterile, with bureaucracy and remote supervision leaving you with no self-esteem or sense of accomplishment.
- Working in a transcription service can mean insecurity and a greater risk of layoffs.
- Working in a small office can be limiting and dictatorial.

Does this mean there are no good employment opportunities for medical transcriptionists? Of course not. There are excellent employment opportunities, but, as in most aspects of our lives, we have to take some bad with the good.
- Self-employment may offer a sense of achievement, freedom, flexibility, and more money if properly planned and executed. Long hours and uneven cash flow are accepted or compensated for in other ways.
- Working at home can be done profitably with application of self-discipline to hours worked and hours played.
- Employing others can create a sense of accomplishment, fulfilling a dream of doing something others cannot do, or cannot do as well. With proper planning and financial strategies, and many hours of hard work, cash flow and profit can come together. Marketing strategies can be utilized to equalize the work flow as much as possible. Clients can have clearly stated expectations met consistently.
- Working in a hospital or clinic can offer security of hours and benefits, and opportunities for career advancement. Sometimes it offers other perks such as convention and workshop attendance. With good supervision the employee is not anonymous, can find flexibility, and may find fertile ground for creativity in a financially sound environment.
- Working for a good transcription service can offer flexibility and excellent wages, generous benefits and profit sharing. Slow employment times may be compensated for during peak times. It may be especially profitable and fulfilling for part-time, high-energy professionals.
- Working in a small office can provide personal contact with appreciative dictators on a daily basis—a great source of self-esteem and security.

There are many things to consider in our employment decisions—certainly more than described here. Within each opportunity we need to balance the wage and benefit issues with the personal fulfillment and family issues, and the spirit of independence with the risks of less security. Being aware of our own personal needs and giving them priority levels, while keeping a watchful eye on the future, will help ensure fruitful decisions.

Medical Readings

The History and Physical Examination

by John H. Dirckx, M.D.

Review of Systems: Ears. The physician inquires about the duration, degree, and pitch range of hearing loss in one or both ears; ringing, popping, or other abnormal sounds heard by the patient; pain, pressure, itching, swelling, bleeding, or discharge; history of occupational, avocational, or military exposure to loud noises; history of injury to the ear, particularly perforation of the tympanic membrane; recent air travel or scuba diving; any previous operations on the ear; and use of a hearing aid. Pain felt in the ear can result from a wide range of nonotic diseases, including pharyngitis, laryngeal cancer, mumps, and brain tumor.

Vertigo and dysequilibrium, suggesting disease of the inner ear, are usually dealt with here also. The distinction between these two symptoms is sometimes difficult to make; lay persons refer to both as "dizziness." Vertigo is a constant or intermittent feeling that one is spinning ("like I just got off a merry-go-round"). In contrast, dysequilibrium means difficulty maintaining one's balance when standing or walking.

Review of Systems: Nose. The nasal history includes mention of any acute or chronic pain, swelling, obstruction, or discharge affecting the nose; sneezing, nosebleeds, or frequent colds; seasonal or occasional allergies; sinus infections; disturbance of the sense of smell; history of fracture or other injuries; submucous resection for deviated septum, removal of polyps, cautery for nosebleeds, or other surgical procedure; and regular or long-term use of decongestants or antihistamines for nasal symptoms, particularly inhalers, drops, or sprays.

Review of Systems: Throat. The throat includes not only the pharynx, the common channel shared by the respiratory and digestive tracts, but also the larynx. Important historical points include sore throat (the most common presenting symptom in many outpatient practices), postnasal drip, choking, and difficulty swallowing; atypical throat pain, which may be due to foreign body, abscess, tumor, or neurologic disease; hoarseness or other change in the voice; and history of tonsillectomy or other throat operation. Pain, swelling, or mass in the neck is included here for convenience.

Examination of the Head, Face, and Neck. The amount, distribution, texture, and color of scalp hair are observed, as well as the pattern of any hair loss. The scalp is inspected for scaling, dermatitis, signs of acute or past trauma, and other lesions. Any tremors or involuntary movements of the head are noted.

Facial configuration and symmetry can be distorted by various congenital syndromes. Paralysis due to peripheral neuropathy (Bell's palsy) or stroke can also cause facial asymmetry, as a result of impaired mobility of one part of the face. The examiner may instruct the patient to perform various movements such as wrinkling his forehead, showing his teeth, and pursing his lips to whistle, in order to test for facial muscle weakness or paralysis.

Pain in the lower jaw or difficulty in chewing or speaking will prompt an assessment of the mandible, the temporomandibular joints, and the muscles of mastication for mobility, spasm, swelling, crepitus, or tenderness.

Any swellings or masses are palpated for size, shape, consistency, mobility, pulsatility, and tenderness. Additionally, the entire neck is felt for enlarged lymph nodes, which may appear in any of several locations. Each anatomic group of nodes "drains" (receives lymphatic channels from) a specific region of the head, face, neck, or thorax.

The thyroid gland is felt and its size and consistency assessed. For this examination the physician may stand behind the patient and ask him to swallow in order to move the gland up and down under the palpating fingers. The larynx and the uppermost part of the trachea are also felt and any lesions or lateral deviation noted.

Examination of the Ears. For descriptive purposes the anatomist divides the human ear into three parts. The external ear consists of the pinna and the external auditory meatus or ear canal. The middle ear, or ear drum, is a hollow space within the temporal bone, lined with mucous membrane and communicating via the eustachian or auditory tube with the nasopharynx. The middle ear is separated from the external ear by the tympanic membrane, and it contains three small bones connected in sequence that transmit sound waves from the tympanic membrane to the cochlea. The inner ear consists of the cochlea, with receptors for the auditory division of the eighth cranial nerve; and the vestibular apparatus, with receptors for the vestibular division of the eighth cranial nerve, which is concerned with equilibrium.

Inspection of the ear canal and tympanic membrane is generally performed with an otoscope, a hand-held instrument with a light source, exchangeable cone-shaped specula of various sizes, and a magnifying lens. (A specialist may prefer to use a head mirror or head lamp and hand-held specula.) In order to get an adequate view of the tympanic membrane, the examiner must straighten the ear canal by pulling the pinna back and up with one hand while positioning the otoscope with the other. Because otoscopic examination can be performed with one eye only, there is no true depth perception. Accumulated wax (cerumen) or exudate, foreign material, swelling of the ear canal, and inability of the patient to tolerate the insertion of the speculum can all render otoscopic examination difficult or impossible.

Under ideal conditions the examiner inspects the ear canal for injection, edema, impacted cerumen, exudate, blood, and foreign material. The normal tympanic membrane appears gray or opalescent and nearly flat, but with recognizable landmarks. Behind it the manubrium (handle) of the malleus (hammer) can just be seen. Possible abnormalities are injection, bulging, retraction, or perforation of the tympanic membrane; discoloration by blood in the middle ear, which can result from basal skull fracture; a fluid level, bubbles, or both behind the tympanic membrane, indicating serous fluid in the middle ear; and tumors, such as cholesteatoma. Prior infections or perforations may have left scars on the tympanic membrane. A polyethylene tube placed in the tympanic membrane for chronic infection will be visible to the examiner.

Two tests of value in distinguishing types of hearing impairment are the Rinne and the Weber test, both requiring the use of a tuning fork.

In the Rinne test, the examiner notes whether the subject can hear the sound of the vibrating fork better (that is, longer, as it gradually ceases to vibrate) by air conduction or by bone conduction. Air conduction is tested by placing the prongs of the vibrating fork near the external auditory meatus. Bone conduction is tested by placing the shank of the vibrating fork against the mastoid process. With an intact acoustic nerve, a fork that can no longer be heard by bone conduction will still be audible by air conduction. When this is not the case, conductive hearing loss rather than neurosensory loss is likely.

In the Weber test the examiner touches the shank of the vibrating fork to the middle of the subject's forehead. If the sound of the fork seems louder in the ear whose hearing is impaired, the impairment is con-

ductive. If the sound of the fork seems fainter in the impaired ear, the impairment is neural.

Examination of the Nose. Examination of the nose begins with external inspection for developmental abnormalities, traumatic deformities, enlargement (rhinophyma), nodules, ulcers, and other cutaneous lesions. The interior of each nostril is then viewed with a beam of light from a head mirror or other source. When a head mirror is used, the nostril is gently dilated with a bivalve nasal speculum. Alternatively, a cone-shaped speculum larger than those used for ear examination can be attached to an otoscope. The interior of the nose is inspected for septal deviation or perforation; mucosal edema, injection, ulcers, erosions, or polyps; discharge, hemorrhage, foreign bodies, and tumors. The sense of smell can be tested if necessary by having the subject try to identify familiar substances such as coffee or cinnamon by smell alone.

Pharmacology: Ear, Nose, and Throat (ENT) Drugs

ENT drugs are prescribed for various conditions of the ears, nose, and throat ranging from swimmer's ear to nasal polyps to coughs and colds to seasonal or allergic rhinitis. ENT drugs comprise several distinct classes of drugs, including decongestants, antihistamines, antitussives, expectorants, corticosteroids, and antibiotics.

Decongestants. Decongestants act as vasoconstrictors which reduce blood flow to edematous tissues in the nose, sinuses, and pharynx; they achieve this vasoconstriction by stimulating alpha receptors in these tissues. Decongestants decrease the swelling of mucous membranes, alleviate nasal stuffiness, allow secretions to drain, and help to unclog the eustachian tubes. Decongestants are commonly prescribed for colds and allergies. They can be administered topically as nose drops or nasal sprays, or can be taken orally. Decongestants are often combined with antihistamines in cold remedies. Decongestant drugs include:

> oxymetazoline (Afrin, Duration)
> phenylephrine (Neo-Synephrine)
> pseudoephedrine (Afrinol, Sudafed)

Antihistamines. Antihistamines exert their therapeutic effect by blocking histamine (H_1) receptors in the nose, throat, and eyes. Histamine is released by the antibody-antigen complex that occurs during allergic reactions. Histamine causes vasodilation which allows blood vessels and tissues to become engorged, swollen, and red. Histamine also irritates these tissues directly, causing pain and itching. Antihistamines block the action of histamine at the H₁ receptors. This helps to dry up secretions, shrink edematous mucous membranes, and decrease itching and redness. A significant side effect of early antihistamines was drowsiness; however, newer antihistamines such as terfenadine (Seldane) and astemizole (Hismanal) have a different chemical structure that does not cross the blood-brain barrier to produce drowsiness. Antihistamine drugs include:

    astemizole (Hismanal)
    clemastine (Tavist)
    diphenhydramine (Benadryl)
    terfenadine (Seldane)

Antitussive drugs. Antitussives act to decrease coughing by suppressing the cough center in the brain. Their main purpose is to stop nonproductive dry coughs. They are not prescribed for productive coughs which are generating sputum.

    codeine
    dextromethorphan (Sucrets, Pertussin)
    hydrocodone (Hycodan)

Expectorants. Expectorants act to reduce the viscosity or thickness of sputum so that patients can more easily cough it up. Expectorants are prescribed only for productive coughs.

    guaifenesin (Robitussin)
    terpin hydrate

Corticosteroids. Corticosteroids have no antihistamine effect and are not prescribed for mild allergies. They have no effect on the common cold, but they are effective when administered intranasally to topically treat nasal polyps and nonallergic (vasomotor) rhinitis. Intranasal corticosteroids include:

    beclomethasone (Beconase, Vancenase)
    dexamethasone (Decadron Turbinaire)
    flunisolide (Nasalide)

Laboratory Tests and Surgical Procedures

ASO titer   A test to detect and measure antistreptolysin O in serum. This antibody is present during and shortly after streptococcal infections. The value is measured in Todd units.

audiogram   A test used to assess the completeness of the hearing response by having the patient indicate when sounds are audible in the upper, middle, and lower ranges of hearing.

beta strep (beta-hemolytic streptococcus)   Any strain of streptococcus that completely hemolyzes blood in a culture medium. The streptococci that cause streptococcal pharyngitis (strep throat) and rheumatic fever are of this type.

B strep   Slang term for beta-hemolytic streptococcus (beta strep).

Haemophilus influenzae (*H. influenzae*)   A gram-negative organism that causes respiratory and ear infections and is also an important cause of meningitis in children. Do not use *H. flu*, a slang term.

rhinoplasty   Surgical correction of nasal deformities for functional or cosmetic purposes.

Rinne test   Designed to test hearing by assessing the conduction of sound to the ear both through the skull bones and through the air. A vibrating tuning fork is placed behind the ear on the mastoid process to test bone conduction. A vibrating tuning fork is then placed near the external auditory canal, but not touching the ear, to test air conduction.

strep   An acceptable brief form for *streptococcus*. The term *strep throat* is commonly used.

streptococcus   Any of a group of gram-positive spherical bacteria usually found in chains. Streptococci are an important cause of soft-tissue infections, particularly abscesses with pus formation.

T&A (tonsillectomy and adenoidectomy)   Surgical removal of the palatine tonsils and adenoids in the throat due to chronic episodes of infection and hypertrophy.

tympanoplasty   Surgical repair of the eardrum and its connection to the bones of the inner ear.

Weber test   Designed to test hearing by comparing the conduction of sound to both ears through the skull bones. A vibrating tuning fork is placed in the center of the forehead.

Anatomy/Medical Terminology

Anatomy: The Ear

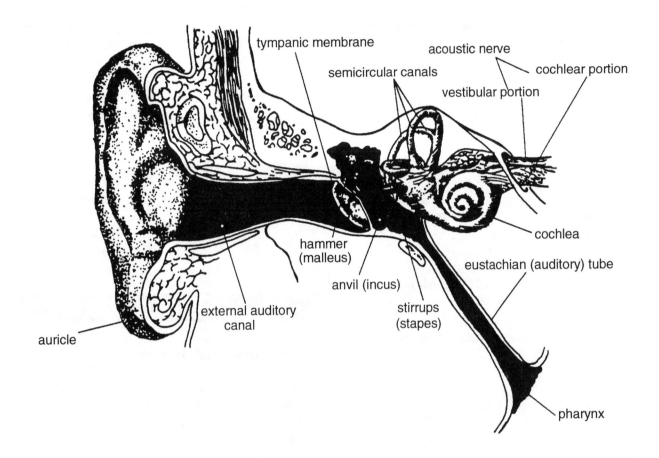

Abbreviations Exercise

Common abbreviations may be transcribed as dictated in the body of a report. Uncommon abbreviations must be spelled out, with the abbreviation appearing in parentheses after the translation. All abbreviations (except laboratory test names) must be spelled out in the Diagnosis or Impression section of any report.

Instructions: Define these common ENT abbreviations. Then memorize both abbreviations and definitions to increase your speed and accuracy in transcribing ENT dictation.

A.D.	_____
A.S.	_____
A.U.	_____
EAC	_____
ENT	_____
HEENT	_____
PE tube	_____
PND	_____
T&A	_____
TM	_____
TMJ	_____

Medical Terminology Matching Exercise

Complete the following matching exercise to test your knowledge of the word roots, anatomic structures, symptoms, and disease processes encountered in the medical specialty of otorhinolaryngology (ear, nose, and throat).

Instructions: Match the term in Column A with its definition or synonym in Column B.

Column A

Column B

A. tinnitus

_____ wax

B. pinna

_____ dizziness from sense of motion

C. myringo-

D. cochlea

_____ auricle or outer ear

E. cerumen

_____ hearing

F. oto-

_____ where sounds are translated into nerve impulses

G. epistaxis

_____ ringing in the ears

H. vertigo

_____ nosebleed

I. audio-

_____ eardrum

_____ ear

Lay and Medical Terms

Lay Term	*Medical Term*
ear wax	cerumen
eardrum	tympanic membrane
anvil, hammer, stirrup	malleus, incus, stapes

Drug Matching Exercise

Instructions: Match the drug category in Column A with the drugs in Column B. Note: Drug categories may be used more than once.

Column A   *Column B*

A. corticosteroid for intranasal use

_____ diphenhydramine

_____ Mycelex

_____ Seldane

B. decongestant

_____ Sudafed

_____ Beconase

C. antihistamine

_____ Nasalide

_____ Tavist

D. oral antifungal drug

_____ Afrin

_____ Benadryl

_____ Vancenase

_____ Mycostatin

_____ Dimetane

_____ Hismanal

Transcription Guidelines

Abbreviations and Symbols

Abbreviations, acronyms, and initialisms are frequently dictated in medical reports and are an integral part of the language of medicine. When abbreviations are dictated, students should consult reference books for their meanings and memorize them for future use.

A list of acceptable abbreviations is available in each facility where transcriptionists work. Many medical transcriptionists readily type abbreviations verbatim when dictated. Some transcriptionists prefer to translate almost all abbreviations and brief forms when dictated, believing that abbreviations obscure the clarity of the medical report and make it imprecise. Many facilities require the translation of abbreviations, especially when they appear in the Diagnosis or Impression section of a report.

In a few instances the translation of abbreviations may cause confusion rather than achieve clarity. For example, VDRL is readily recognized as a laboratory test for syphilis and it is not necessary or desirable to translate it, even in a Diagnosis or Impression.

With the following abbreviation guidelines in mind, students may opt to spell out abbreviations or type them as dictated when they are encountered in dictation.

1. Medical abbreviations are written in several ways. The three most common include all capital letters, a combination of capital and lowercase letters, and all lowercase letters with periods. Seldom are periods used with uppercase abbreviations. Periods are generally not used with combination uppercase and lowercase abbreviations, with the exception of Ph.D.

   p.o. b.i.d. (by mouth twice daily)
   q.h.s. (every night at bedtime)
   KCl (potassium chloride)
   PND (postnasal drainage)
   IV, IM; I.V., I.M. (intravenous, intramuscular)

2. The abbreviations for *intravenous* and *intramuscular* are written without periods (IV, IM) for simplicity by many transcriptionists, or with periods (I.V., I.M.) to avoid I.V. being misread as roman numeral four (IV). References are inconsistent, at times writing them with periods and at times without. Both forms are acceptable, but the transcriptionist should be consistent in usage within a report.

3. An acronym is a word formed from the first letters of other words. Acronyms are initially formed with capital letters, but after they gain acceptance as words, they are converted to lowercase letters and we then forget their origin as initialisms.

   AIDS (acquired immunodeficiency syndrome)
   CABG (''cabbage''—coronary artery bypass graft)
   ELISA (enzyme-linked immunosorbent assay)

   fabere test (flexion-abduction-external rotation-extension)
   laser (light amplification by stimulated emission of radiation)
   simkin analysis (simulation kinetics)

4. To make an abbreviation plural, simply add the letter *s* with no apostrophe if the abbreviation is in all capital letters. If the abbreviation ends in a period, either add *s* or an apostrophe and *s*.

   A series of CBCs (complete blood counts) was ordered.
   DTRs (deep tendon reflexes) were 3+ and equal bilaterally.

   IVs (or IV's) were ordered to run TKO (to keep open).
   Three M.D.'s were invited to speak.

5. When abbreviations are used with numbers for medication dosage times, use periods.

   | q.4h. | OR | q. 4 hr. (every 4 hours) |
   | q.12h. | OR | q. 12 hr. (every 12 hours) |

6. An abbreviation dictated at the beginning of a sentence or in the body of a report may be transcribed as dictated if its meaning is clearly understood—the names of lab tests, for example. If abbreviations are not dictated, the transcriptionist should not supply them, with the exception of metric units of measure which are routinely abbreviated.

   ST depression was noted on EKG.
   SGOT was elevated.
   CBC and electrolytes were within normal limits.

7. If the dictator abbreviates the title of a major heading within a report, the transcriptionist should translate the abbreviation.

   If dictated: HPI
   Transcribe: History of Present Illness

8. The first time an uncommon abbreviation or an abbreviation that has more than one meaning (such as PND) is used within a report, the transcriptionist should translate it for clarity and put the abbreviation within parentheses following the translation. The abbreviation may then be used in the report without translation, except in the final Diagnosis or Impression section.

   extracorporeal shock wave lithotripsy (ESWL)
   paroxysmal nocturnal dyspnea (PND)
   postnasal drainage (PND)
   total abdominal hysterectomy, bilateral salpingo-oophorectomy (TAH-BSO)

   If dictated:
   HIV-positive male with CA of the liver and PVH
   Transcribe:
   HIV-positive male with carcinoma of the liver and persistent viral hepatitis (PVH).

9. The symbol *x* represents the word *times* and also *by* in measurements.

   x = times: bleeding x 3 days
                oriented x 3

   x = by   a lesion measuring 3 x 5 cm

10. Abbreviating metric measurements is preferred in medical reports. Abbreviations for metric measurements contain no periods and have the same form for singular and plural usage.

    kg (kilogram)   mg (milligram)
    cc (cubic centimeter) mEq (milliequivalent)

11. Standard English units of measure (inch, foot, pound) are so short that they are usually spelled out, although *foot* and *pound* are correctly abbreviated *ft.* and *lb.*, respectively. The standard abbreviation for *inch* is *in.*, although it is recommended that it not be used in medical reports as it is too easily confused with the preposition *in*.

    Exception: It is common to use the abbreviation for pounds (lbs.) and single and double quotation marks for feet and inches in presenting weight and height figures in medical reports.

    Weight 120 lbs., height 5'2".

Abbreviations and Symbols Exercise

1. What is the difference between an abbreviation and an acronym? What is an initialism?

2. Why would you *not* translate such abbreviations as VDRL, SGOT, tPA, and DPT shot? (Before answering, find out what each abbreviation means.)

3. Abbreviations are rarely appropriate in which part of the report?

4. Translate the following abbreviations. Under what circumstances would you *not* translate the abbreviations? Under what circumstances would you always translate the abbreviations?

   ABG _____
   CHF _____
   COPD _____
   EKG _____
   MRI _____
   PID _____
   q.3h. _____
   t.i.d. _____

5. What are the abbreviations for the following?

   four times a day _____
   at hour of sleep _____
   urinary tract infection _____
   millimeters of mercury _____
   certified medical transcriptionist _____
   doctor of medicine _____

6. Correct abbreviation errors in the following sentences. Translate any abbreviations which you feel are inappropriate.

   A 0.5 cm. incision was made, but it proved too small, so a 1-in incision was made and the chest tube inserted. A total of 300 cc of fluid was obtained.

   Final Diagnosis: CHF with right pleural effusion, 300 cc of fluid removed.

   Disposition Patient placed on digitalis 0.25 mg. bid, hold IV D5W until the am.

Proofreading Skills

Instructions: Circle the errors in the report below. Identify misspelled and missing medical and English words and punctuation errors. Write the correct words and punctuation marks in the numbered spaces opposite the text.

#	Text	Answer #	Answer
1	This 17 year old female was seen in consul-	1.	17-year-old
2	atation with her mother regarding problems	2.	
3	referrable to her nose. The patient has had	3.	
4	progressive problems of congestoin and sniff-	4.	
5	ing with dificulty moving air through her nose	5.	
6	and sinsation of pressure. She is a ''mouth	6.	
7	brether'' and has a history of alergy to polens	7.	
8	and dust. Teh patient feels these problems are	8.	
9	becoming more severe. HER complaints are	9.	
10	fairly consistant.	10.	
11		11.	
12	EXAMNATION: She presents with a dema of	12.	
13	her nasal mucose, incraese in the size of the	13.	
14	turbenates, deviation of the nasal septum, and	14.	
15	a rather narrowed nasal airweigh.	15.	
16		16.	
17	DIGNOSIS:	17.	
18	1. Probable allergic rinitis with hypertrophy	18.	
19	of the turbinates.	19.	
20	2. Deviated nasal septa.	20.	
21	3. Narrow and adequate nasal airway.	21.	
22		22.	
23	COMMENTS:	23.	
24	1. I have discused with this patinent and with	24.	
25	her mother the sugrical approach to im-	25.	
26	proving her nasal airway with septoplasty,	26.	
27	possible submucus resection of deviated	27.	
28	portions of the septum, and possible reduc-	28.	
29	tion of the inferior turbenates. At the same	29.	
30	time, I would be performing a rinoplasty	30.	
31	procedure to smooth out the dorsal nose.	31.	
32	2. Becaus of the history of allergys to pollens	32.	
33	dust and environmental pollutants it is	33.	
34	quite possible the patient will continue to	34.	
35	have some snifing and consequently the	35.	
36	degree of improvemnt of her nasal airway	36.	
37	with surgery cannot be precisely determined.	37.	

Transcription Tips

1. Don't confuse the sound-alike prefixes *oro-* (mouth) and *auri-* (ear).

2. Both the Latin *auri-* (aural) and the Greek *oto-* (otic) mean *ear.*

3. Both the Latin *myringo-* and Greek *tympano-* mean *eardrum.*

4. Don't confuse *malleus* (bone of the middle ear) and *malleolus* (ankle bone).

5. The term *auricle* refers to the protruding flap of the external ear, also known as the *pinna.* However, *auricle* is also used as a synonym for the atrium of the heart.

6. When the term *mental* is used in ENT dictation, it refers to the mentum, or chin, *not* to thought processes.

7. When the term *alveolar* is used in ENT dictation, it refers to a ridge in the oral cavity, *not* to alveoli of the lungs.

8. Do not mistake *serous* (otitis media) for *serious*, especially in dictation of foreign dictators.

9. *Nares* is the plural form of the medical term for nostrils. *Naris* is the singular, not *nare* as is sometimes dictated.

Terminology Challenge

Instructions: The following terms appear in the dictation on Tape 8B, Otorhinolaryngology. Before beginning the medical transcription practice for Lesson 17, look up each term below in a medical or English dictionary and write out a short definition.

A.S.A.
adenoidectomy
adenoids
adenotome
Allis forceps
anterior pack
asymmetry
Betadine-impregnated
Blue Cross
bolus
Coumadin
counterpressure
dander
debridement
deviated nasal septum
electrocoagulation
epistaxis
external otitis media
exudate
flanged
fungus
Garamycin solution
genera
house dust mites
hydrogen peroxide
hypertrophied
immunotherapy
impedance
indirect visualization
injected (adjective)
iodoform gauze
irrigation
jugulodigastric areas
liquefaction
lymphoid hyperplasia
lymphoid plaques

malodor
mastoid
micro ear forceps
mold spores
myringotomy
nasal septoplasty
nasopharynx
operating microscope
otitis media
penicillin V potassium
pharynx
PND (postnasal
  drainage)
postauricular
posterior cervical
  nodes (neck)
pressure sponges
quadrilateral cartilage
rhinitis
rhinoplasty
S-shaped configuration
saline gargle
serous otitis media
silver nitrate
smell hallucination
Spectazole
strep screen
submucous resection
Teflon
tonsillar capsule
tonsillar fossa
tonsillar pillar
tonsillitis
tympanic membranes
ventilation tube

Sample Reports

Sample otorhinolaryngology reports appear on the following pages.

Transcription Practice

After completing all the readings and exercises in Lesson 17, transcribe Tape 8B, Otorhinolaryngology. Use both medical and English dictionaries and your Quick-Reference Word List as resource materials for finding words.

Proofread your transcribed documents carefully, listening to the dictation while you read your transcripts.

Transcribe (*NOT* retype) the same reports again without referring to your previous transcription attempt. Initially, you may need to transcribe some reports more than twice before you can produce an error-free document. Your ultimate goal is to produce an error-free document the first time.

BLOOPERS

Incorrect	Correct
History of enema associated with nosebleed.	History of anemia associated with nosebleed.
Six pricks on the chin.	Cicatrix on the chin.
Prognathism prevented proper masturbation.	Prognathism prevented proper mastication.
He has flapping of the left side of the face.	He has flattening of the left side of the face.
All fangs not inflamed.	Oropharynx not inflamed.

CHART NOTE

THOMAS MORGAN   Age 65   June 1, 1992

The patient comes in stating he has some irritation in his right ear. He does wear an ITE (in the ear) hearing aid on that side. He also has what he terms a smell hallucination in that there is kind of a musty smell in his nose when he inhales and exhales. He has been using some Ocean nasal spray from time to time.

PHYSICAL EXAM
EARS: Right ear: External canal is slightly irritated at the outer third, but the inner two-thirds is okay. Tympanic membrane is intact and not inflamed. Left ear is clear. There is no cerumen in either side.
NOSE: Airway is quite adequate. Septum slightly deviated to the right. No evidence of polyps or abnormal discharge.
THROAT: Normal mucous membrane, no evidence of inflammation.
NECK: No adenopathy.

IMPRESSION: Mild right external otitis.

DISPOSITION: Recommended 0.5% hydrocortisone cream in the outer ear and a couple drops of alcohol in the ear at night before he goes to bed to try to keep the canal dry. Nasal irrigation using a normal saline solution. He was asked to return if symptoms progress and we will go ahead and get a sinus view.

OF:hpi

January 21, 1992

Marisa Dulwicz, M.D.
2562 County Road
Dayton, OH 45429

Re: Constance Nipper

Dear Dr. Dulwicz:

This 21-year-old lady stated that she has been having some problems with a "swollen gland on the right side." She saw you about a week and a half ago, and you ruled out the presence of a stone within the saliva gland. She states the swelling "tends to go up and down."

Her general health is described as good, but she does have asthma. She is presently taking Motrin, Marax, and an inhaler.

Physical exam: Ears: Canals are clear, tympanic membranes normal. Nose: Airway adequate, no discharge. Throat: Normal mucous membrane, no postnasal drainage. Her right submandibular gland is slightly enlarged but soft and nontender.

Under the operating microscope, I was able to dilate Wharton's duct on the right, and after dilatation the gland resumed its normal size. There was no evidence of purulent discharge or calculi. Hopefully, this will do the trick.

I explained to her that we can only treat this either symptomatically or excise the gland, and I suggested that symptomatic treatment for awhile is indicated.

Thank you for the referral. If I can be of any further assistance, please let me know.

Best regards,

Otto Farengi, M.D.

OF:hpi

JEREMY RYAN

#090988

Date of Operation: 7/25/92

Preoperative Diagnosis: Chronic adenotonsillitis

Postoperative Diagnosis: Chronic adenotonsillitis

Operation: Adenotonsillectomy

Description of Procedure: The patient was brought to the operating room and general endotracheal anesthesia induced by Dr. Tang without difficulty. The patient was placed in the Rose position and the McIvor mouth gag was inserted in the routine fashion.

A red rubber catheter was passed transnasally and the adenoid bed was inspected with a mirror. Using the adenoid curets, the adenoid bed was then curetted to completed. Adenoid packs were placed and attention turned to the right tonsil.

The right tonsil was grasped with a tonsil tenaculum, and, using the electrocautery, a mucosal incision was created. Using scissors and a combination of sharp and blunt dissection, the tonsillar capsule was entered. The electrocautery was then used to free the mucosal and fibrotic attachments of the right tonsil. The right tonsil was then snared without difficulty and tonsil packs were placed. An identical procedure was carried out on the left side. The tonsillar beds were then dried up using the suction cautery.

The adenoid bed was then inspected and the suction cautery was used on the adenoid bed as well until cessation of any further bleeding.

The wounds were inspected. There was no further bleeding. The hypopharynx was carefully suctioned, the mouth gag was removed, and the procedure was deemed complete. The patient was transferred to the recovery room with all vital signs being stable.

_____

BRANDON KYLE, M.D.

BK:hpi

D: 7/25/92
T: 7/26/92

Lesson 18. Ophthalmology

Medical

- Describe common symptoms of ophthalmic disease as found in the Review of Systems and Physical Examination sections of an H&P.
- Describe common eye tests done in a physical examination.
- Describe the action of drugs used to treat eye inflammation and glaucoma.
- Discuss the purpose and technique involved in performing common ophthalmologic laboratory tests and surgical procedures.
- Given an ophthalmologic root word, symptom, or disease, match it to its correct medical definition.
- Define common ophthalmologic abbreviations.
- Given a cross-section illustration of the eye, memorize the anatomic structures labeled.
- Differentiate between ophthalmology sound-alike terms.

Fundamentals

- Discuss problems in terminology and style involved in ophthalmology transcription.
- Demonstrate the correct use of brief forms and the translation of slang terms in editing medical sentences.
- Given a medical report with errors, identify and correct the errors.

Practice

- Accurately transcribe authentic physician dictation from the specialty of ophthalmology.

A Closer Look

The Ophthalmology Medical Transcriptionist

by Mary Ann D'Onofrio, AMLS, ART, CMT

Physicians in private practice know the value of written communication and its place in the successful operation of their offices. For the general practitioner with only a small correspondence need, the office secretary/receptionist usually is quite capable of handling it. Medical correspondence for the specialist is quite another matter, however.

For the specialist, the dictated letter provides the documentation that often verifies or clarifies points discussed in person or via the phone with referring physicians. Documenting when and why a particular medical opinion was given is a legal record. It may verify for a community or governmental agency the need a patient has for services from that agency.

An accurately transcribed, attractive letter sent in a timely manner is a vital component of the physician's practice. The letter reflects the knowledge and judgment of the physician and, by inference, the quality of the staff. Having the right person available to carry out this task is the physician's prescription for success in maintaining communications with a vast array of people.

In the medical specialist's office practice, who is responsible for this very important correspondence? An ophthalmologist, for example, with a free-standing surgicenter as part of the practice, may employ up to a dozen people, including an office/business manager, billing clerk/bookkeeper, a reception staff, nurses and/or surgical assistants. None of these people generally have the time or training to handle the specialist's technical correspondence. These physicians need a professional familiar with the specialized material reflected in their medical correspondence. In short, they need a medical transcriptionist or a medical secretary with a strong background in medical transcription.

Medical specialists use technical language specific to their practice. For the ophthalmologist, this could include disease processes from anopsia to xerophthalmia, Adie-Holmes syndrome to Vogt-Koyanagi syndrome, Ault's line to von Graefe's sign. It might include a physical exam describing spots from Bitot's to Roth's, procedures from aqueous aspiration to Ziegler cautery, special medications from acetazolamide to Zolyse, or lenses from achromatic to X chrome. Technical language, indeed. The trained medical transcriptionist knows what it means and how to spell it.

Medical transcriptionists come with a variety of talents and experience. Knowing what is required in each job setting is the key to success. Which transcriptionist or medical secretary will get that job in the specialist's office? It all depends on what skills are required, and who is best equipped to do the job. The following scenario featuring two applicants illustrates these points.

An applicant currently taking a medical terminology course tries out for the job. She has been a secretary before and has good typing speed and produces letters that look good; however, her knowledge of medical terminology is still in its formative stages. She knows basic structures and diseases of the eye, but she lacks knowledge of a whole array of ophthalmic eponyms and pharmacologic terms. There are suture materials, types and manufacturers of intraocular lenses and instruments she has never heard of, and she lacks knowledge of the special language needed to describe refraction of the eye. She spends more time researching than transcribing. She is asked to reapply when her skills are improved, as the office cannot afford a full-time employee who produces so little.

Another applicant is interviewed and hired. She has been a medical transcriptionist in a small hospital and has transcribed many kinds of reports, including ophthalmology. Eponyms, surgical procedures, and ancillary terms, as well as a good grasp of pharmaceutical terms, are part of her background. When she took a general typing course, she received instruction in the art of correspondence and techniques for typing letters in a variety of styles. She has not used this skill in some time and has spent extra time at home brushing up on her little-used secretarial skills before applying for the job. She is soon producing excellent-looking and accurate correspondence for her ophthalmologist employer. She also suggests reference books for the office library which will assist in transcription.

Depending upon the practice and the office needs, a medical secretary or medical assistant with strong medical transcription skills may be the right choice for the office setting. If the practice is small she may have both front and back office duties. In a surgeon's office where I was employed, our staff of two handled reception, billing and bookkeeping, medical correspondence, and coding for insurance claims. At the same time we were also preparing examination trays, prepping patients, assisting with endoscopic procedures and preparing specimens for laboratory analysis. A medical transcriptionist may be taught the back office skills on the job if the office staff is small, yet the need for a variety of skills, including medical transcription, is vital to office function.

Not all specialists want or need in-office professionals to transcribe the physician's dictation. When the volume does not justify using an employee, the next logical choice is to have the dictation transcribed by an off-site transcription service which employs transcriptionists with a variety of skills, or the self-employed transcriptionist with skills in the area needed.

Whether working in the physician's office or in a private service office, this particular aspect of medical transcription is personally and financially rewarding. Preparing correspondence often involves all the skills of medical transcription found in hospital transcription: knowledge of laboratory values, pharmacology, operative terms, disease processes, radiologic noninvasive procedures, and more. Wages or fees should be comparable to those paid a hospital medical transcriptionist.

The special language skills, along with general secretarial letter preparation skills, are a winning combination for the medical transcriptionist or medical secretary to enhance the image of any medical specialist's office. These skills are the medical transcriptionist's prescription for success.

Abbreviations: O.D., O.S., O.U. (or o.d., o.s., o.u.)—simple, basic abbreviations for *oculus dexter* "right eye," *oculus sinister* "left eye," and *oculus uterque* "each eye." Curiously, not every major medical dictionary lists these abbreviations but they should be found in any good basic medical terminology or medical transcription program. The abbreviation for "millimeters of mercury," used by ophthalmologists to describe the intraocular pressure, is "mmHg."

Vision (distance and near). The basic description entails the patient's ability to read a Distance Vision Chart at 20 feet or 6 meters. (A Near Vision Chart is read at 14 inches or 35 cm to obtain the same results.) The person who can read the smallest line (J1:3 Point) on the Distance Vision Chart at 20 feet is said to have "twenty twenty" vision or 20/20. If a person with poor vision can read only the line at 20 feet that a person with perfect vision is able to read at 200 feet (J14:23 Point), the person with poor vision is said to have "twenty two hundred" vision or 20/200. The key to remember is that the first number will always be "20" followed by a second, usually the same or larger, number. Once it is clear what is meant by "twenty two hundred," there is no chance the transcriptionist will erroneously type "2200" or "22-100" when the physician dictates "The patient had vision in the right eye of 20/200."

Refraction. This refers to the sum total of "refractometry," or measuring the refractive error of the eye. It is the essential component needed prior to prescribing spectacles.

The refractive error in the right eye was a -0.50 +1.00 axis 113 with a reading add of 2.25 which gave a J1 reading.

The previous sentence describes the geometric calculations needed to establish the index of refraction for the manufacture of spectacles particular to the patient's needs. "Reading add" refers to the total dioptic power added to a distance prescription to supplement accommodation for reading.

NOTE: See the Sample Reports for examples of an ophthalmologic chart note and letter originally presented by Mary Ann D'Onofrio with this article.

Medical Readings

The History and Physical Examination

by John H. Dirckx, M.D.

Review of Systems: Eyes. A thorough review of ocular history elicits information about past or present symptoms such as blurring of vision, double vision, partial or complete loss of vision, difficulty of near adaptation, seeing spots or flashes, seeing haloes or rings around lights, undue visual impairment with reduced illumination, pain in, on, or behind the eyeball, redness, discharge, watering, abnormal sensitivity to light, swelling, drooping, itching, or crusting of lids,

as well as full details about the use of glasses or contact lenses and the date of the most recent eye exam.

Examination of the Eye. Normally the patient sits upright for the eye examination, if able to do so. The orbital margins are inspected for swelling or ecchymosis, and may be palpated for tenderness if any clue to recent trauma is noted. The lids are observed for evidence of deformity, swelling, discoloration, masses, crusting, or disorders of the lacrimal apparatus. Bulging or protrusion of one or both eyes (exophthalmos) can result from hyperthyroidism or orbital disease.

The anterior segment of the eye—the part in front of the lens—is easily studied with the help of a hand lamp. The physician looks for opacities in the cornea and anterior chamber, abnormalities of the iris, and irregularities in the shape of the pupil, incidentally observing whether the pupil constricts when light is shone directly into the eye. This procedure also serves as a test for photophobia.

A check of the accommodation reflex may also be made by asking the patient to look at a distant object and noting whether the pupils constrict. Astigmatism, a warping of the cornea out of its expected spherical form, can sometimes be detected by noting distortion in the reflection of some regularly shaped object on the cornea, but is usually determined by vision testing. The location of a lesion of the cornea or iris is indicated by the hour position to which it would be nearest if the eye were a clock dial (e.g., 5 o'clock).

Abnormalities of the white of the eye can be due to discoloration or disease of the sclera or of the overlying conjunctiva, usually the latter. Mild or early jaundice is typically more evident in the scleras than in the skin. Conjunctival swelling and discharge or lacrimation are noted, as well as the degree and distribution of any redness. Very thin scleras, such as occur in some connective tissue disorders, appear blue.

The visual field of an eye is that part of the space before it that it can see while held motionless. Abnormalities of visual field, which can be caused by retinal or neural disease or injury, represent partial loss of vision in the form of blind spots (scotomata) or narrowed range of vision. Visual fields can be roughly tested by the confrontation method. The subject is instructed to fix his gaze on the examiner's nose while first one eye and then the other is covered. The examiner moves his finger or a light from far to the side, or far above or below, into the subject's range of vision and the subject reports when he can see it. If the examiner fixes his gaze on the subject's nose (and if the examiner's own visual fields are normal), both should see the object at the same time. More elaborate equipment is needed for more precise mapping of visual fields.

The optic fundus is the portion of the interior of the eye that can be seen by an examiner looking through the pupil with an ophthalmoscope, a hand-held instrument with a light source and a set of magnifying lenses that can be quickly changed.

The principal features of the fundus are the retina, the optic disk or nerve head, and branches of the central retinal artery and vein. Retinal and optic nerve disease as well as the effects of systemic conditions such as diabetes, arteriosclerosis, and hypertension, are readily observed in the fundus.

Vision testing is usually performed with the familiar Snellen wall chart for far vision and a set of Jaeger test types for near vision. The subject reads the smallest letters he can see on the wall chart at a distance of 20 feet, and his performance is expressed as a fraction of normal. Thus 20/20 vision indicates normal far visual acuity, while 20/40 means that the subject can see no letters at 20 feet smaller than those that a normal person can see at 40 feet.

Firm palpation of the eyeball through the closed lids (moderately uncomfortable and slightly dangerous) can reveal undue hardness in glaucoma or softness in dehydration or diabetic acidosis. Alternatively, an instrument called a tonometer can be applied to the surface of the cornea, after local anesthetic drops have been instilled, to test its hardness. In some settings, tonometry is a routine part of the examination of persons over 40.

Pharmacology: Ophthalmic Drugs

Ophthalmic drugs may be applied topically to treat superficial infection or inflammation of the cornea and surrounding tissues, and to treat glaucoma; other ophthalmic drugs are taken systemically for severe infection or inflammation in the interior of the eye. All drugs intended for topical application in the eye are specially formulated in a base solution that is physiologically similar to fluids in the eye so as not to damage delicate eye tissues.

Corticosteroids. Corticosteroid drugs are used topically in the eye to treat the inflammation that results from trauma or contact with chemicals. These drugs include:

> dexamethasone (Decadron, Maxidex)
> prednisolone (Inflamase, Pred Forte)

Combination corticosteroids and antibiotic drugs include:

> Maxitrol (dexamethasone, neomycin, polymyxin B)
> NeoDecadron (dexamethasone, neomycin)
> Ophthocort (hydrocortisone, chloramphenicol, polymyxin B)

Drugs for glaucoma. Glaucoma is a disease whose presenting symptom is increased intraocular pressure. If untreated, it can lead to blindness. Drugs for glaucoma act either by decreasing the amount of aqueous humor circulating in the anterior and posterior chambers, or by constricting the pupil (miotic action) so as to open the angle of contact between the iris and the trabecular meshwork, allowing the aqueous humor to flow freely.

Direct-acting miotics cause pupillary constriction by stimulating the iris muscle around the pupil to contract. Miotic drugs used to treat glaucoma include:

> acetylcholine (Miochol)
> carbachol (Miostat)
> pilocarpine (Ocusert Pilo, Pilagan, Pilocar)

Other miotic drugs act by inhibiting cholinesterase, an enzyme which normally destroys acetylcholine. The increased levels of acetylcholine then result in miosis. Miotic drugs which act in this way include:

> demecarium (Humorsol)
> echothiophate iodide
> isoflurophate (Floropryl)
> physostigmine

Other topical drugs which do not constrict the pupil but increase the outflow of aqueous humor include:

> apraclonidine (Iopidine)
> epinephrine (Epifrin, Epitrate, Eppy/N)
> dipivefrin (Propine)

Another group of drugs used to treat glaucoma includes topical beta blockers. They act by blocking the production of aqueous humor to decrease intraocular pressure. They have no effect on pupil size and therefore do not cause the blurred vision or night blindness associated with other miotics which constrict and fix the pupil. Topical beta blocker drugs given for glaucoma include:

> betaxolol (Betoptic)
> levobunolol (Betagan)
> timolol (Timoptic)

Laboratory Tests and Surgical Procedures

keratoplasty   The surgical removal of cloudy cornea and replacement with a clear corneal transplant.

phacoemulsification   The use of ultrasonic waves in cataract surgery to break apart or emulsify the lens so that it can be removed.

scleral buckle   A surgical procedure used to treat retinal detachment. A silicone sponge, solid silicone band, or fascia lata is attached to the sclera and buried in it. The sclera then indents (or buckles) inwardly. Subretinal fluid can then be drained and the retina reattached.

Snellen chart   Used to test distance vision, this chart consists of lines of letters of various sizes. The patient stands 20 feet from the chart, and each eye is tested separately. If able to see only the top line (a very large letter *E*) clearly, the patient has 20/200 vision. Subsequent lines become progressively smaller in letter size. The 20/20 line contains letters that are clearly visible to patients of normal vision. A few additional lines identify those patients with better than average vision (20/15, etc.).

tonometry   Used to screen for glaucoma by detecting increased intraocular pressure, the tonometer is applied briefly to the cornea to take a reading. Types: applanation, Schiotz.

slit-lamp biomicroscopy   Using a strong light passing through a slit, this test permits a well-illuminated microscopic examination of the eyelids and anterior segment of the eye in a three-dimensional cross-section view.

slit-lamp examination   See *slit-lamp biomicroscopy.*

Anatomy/Medical Terminology

Lay and Medical Terms

Lay Terms	*Medical Terms*
crossed eyes	esotropia
wall-eyed	exotropia
double vision	diplopia
lazy eye	amblyopia
nearsightedness	myopia
farsightedness	hyperopia
white of eye	sclera

Medical Terminology Matching Exercise

Complete the following matching exercise to test your knowledge of the root words, anatomic structures, symptoms, and disease processes encountered in the medical specialty of ophthalmology.

Instructions: Match each term in Column A with its definition in Column B.

Column A	Column B
A. strabismus	_____ nearsightedness
B. oculo-	_____ clouding of the lens
C. cataract	_____ increased intraocular pressure
D. lacrimo-	
E. myopia	_____ deviation of one or both eyes
F. palpebro-	
G. glaucoma	_____ lens
H. presbyopia	_____ tears
I. phako	_____ decrease in visual acuity due to age
	_____ eye
	_____ eyelid

Abbreviations Exercise

Common abbreviations may be transcribed as dictated in the body of a report. Uncommon abbreviations must be spelled out, with the abbreviation appearing in parentheses after the translation. All abbreviations (except laboratory test names) must be spelled out in the Diagnosis or Impression section of any report.

Instructions: Define the following ophthalmology abbreviations. Then memorize both abbreviations and definitions to increase your speed and accuracy in transcribing dictation from ophthalmology.

EOM _____

EOMI _____

IOL _____

O.D., OD _____

O.S., OS _____

O.U., OU _____

PEARLA _____

PERRLA _____

Anatomy: The Eye

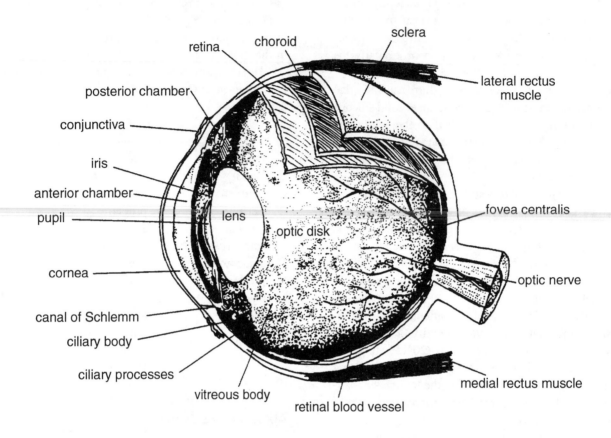

Sound-alikes Exercise

Instructions: Circle the correct term from the sound-alikes in parentheses in the following sentences.

1. Diagnosis: (Anisocoria, Anisophoria), left pupil being 1 mm, right being 1.5 mm.
2. On examination of the retina, the (aura, ora) was normal.
3. The patient had a (choreal, chorial, corneal) abrasion from the metal shaving that lodged in his eye.
4. Healon was (installed, instilled) into the eye, followed by a patch and shield.
5. (Intraocular, Intralocular) lens was (installed, instilled) after the native lens was removed.
6. The patient complained of unequal vision, with the plane of (cite, sight, site) in the left eye lower than the right, most likely due to (anisocoria, anisophoria).

Drug Matching Exercise

Instructions: Match the drug category in Column A with the trade name drugs in Column B. Note: Drug categories are used more than once.

Column A	*Column B*
A. glaucoma drug	____ Inflamase
	____ Betagan
B. corticosteroid	____ Herplex
	____ Miostat
C. antiviral drug	____ Pred Forte
	____ Amvisc
D. injected into anterior	____ Betoptic
chamber during surgery	____ Timoptic
	____ Viroptic
	____ Healon
	____ Maxidex

Transcription Guidelines

Brief Forms and Medical Slang

Brief forms are shortened forms of legitimate words that can be documented in a reputable dictionary. A slang term is either not listed in a dictionary or is designated as slang.

Medical slang should be avoided in medical documents for several reasons. The definition of a slang term may be obscure and might not clearly or accurately convey the intended meaning. Additionally, a slang term may be open to varied interpretations by different readers of the record, particularly obvious when a medical record is subpoenaed by legal process.

Slang terms used disparagingly to refer to patients should be avoided. Physicians do not intend for offensive or off-color remarks to be entered into the patient's medical record. If the transcriptionist is working for a medical facility or transcription company, and the policy for handling inflammatory remarks is known, the transcriptionist should adhere to that policy. If the policy is not known, the department supervisor should be consulted.

Brief forms can be easily confused with medical slang. A good rule to remember is, "When in doubt, write it out."

1. Brief Forms *(Acceptable)*

bands	band neutrophils
basos	basophils
eos	eosinophils
exam	examination
lab	laboratory
lymphs	lymphocytes
monos	monocytes
nitro	nitroglycerin
Pap smear	Papanicolaou smear
polys	polymorphonuclear leukocytes
prepped	prepared
pro time	prothrombin time
segs	segmented neutrophils

2. Medical Slang *(Not Acceptable)*

bili	bilirubin
CA	carcinoma
cath, cath'd	catheter, catheterized
coags	coagulation studies
crit	hematocrit
cysto	cystoscopy
diff	differential
fib	fibula
lytes	electrolytes
mets	metastases
peds	pediatrics
procto	proctoscopy
retic	reticulocyte
tib	tibia
tic	diverticulum
trach	tracheostomy

Brief Forms and Medical Slang Exercise

Instructions: Study the following examples of medical dictation. Decide which contain examples of brief forms that do not need to be changed and which contain medical slang that must be translated. Make the appropriate translation.

1. PLAN: An Rx was written for the above-mentioned medications.

2. LABORATORY DATA: Her crit was 35.

3. Rectal examination: On the right side of her anus, the patient has gangrenous internal and external hemorrhoids. A procto was done to help identify the pathology.

4. Her Pap smear showed carcinoma in situ.

5. The patient was cath'd and the urine specimen showed 1+ bacteria.

6. LABORATORY FINDINGS: The patient had a white count of 12,500 with a diff of 68 segs, 1 band, 13 lymphs, 17 monos, and 1 eo.

7. Her lab data will be forwarded to us, and we will have it in hand prior to her next scheduled follow-up exam.

Proofreading Skills

Instructions: Circle the errors in the report below. Identify misspelled and missing medical and English words and punctuation errors. Write the correct words and punctuation marks in the numbered spaces opposite the text.

1	SOAP NOTE	1. CHART NOTE
2		2.
3	S: This 36 year old man presents with the	3.
4	complant of teering and irritation of the	4.
5	left eye for about 48 hours. She has a	5.
6	thick mucus discharge which sticks the lids	6.
7	togehter overnight. Vision seems okay ex-	7.
8	cept for some bluring by mucous. She	8.
9	denies trauma or prior occular pathology.	9.
10	She denies any symptom of you or eye or	10.
11	alergy and does not wear contact lenses or	11.
12	glasses. She denies photofobia. She has not	12.
13	been around anyone with a pink eye.	13.
14		14.
15	O: The conjunctiva of the left eye is diffusely	15.
16	hypoemic and there is moderate cheimosis	16.
17	and lid edema. Traces of a mucopurulant	17.
18	dischrge are evident on the lid margins and	18.
19	lashes. EXam with pontocaine and	19.
20	Florescene reveal no corneal abrasion or	20.
21	ulcertion. No foreign bodies is noted on	21.
22	the palpable conjunctiva or on the globe.	22.
23	Pupil is round and reactive. The occular	23.
24	fundus is entirely normal. Slitlamp exam	24.
25	shows no pathology in the cornea anterior	25.
26	chamber or lens. Tenometry is defurred.	26.
27	Far point vision testing with the smelling	27.
28	chart is twenty twenty in each eye.	28.
29		29.
30	A: Acute bacterial conjunctivitus O.S.	30.
31		31.
32	P: 1. Sulamid opthalmic solution 2 drops O.S.	32.
33	q.i.d.	33.
34	2. Treat O.D. also at first sigh of	34.
35	symptoms their.	35.
36	3. Cold compreses O.S. ad lib. for	36.
37	comfort.	37.
38	4. Careful handwashig and avoiding close	38.
39	personal contact for 24 to 43 hours.	39.
40	5. Return p.r.n. as needed.	40.

Transcription Tips

1. Visual acuity at a distance is always dictated as two numbers separated by a slash, with the first number always being 20 (for the 20 feet between the vision chart and the patient). A dictated value which sounds like "twenty two hundred" is correctly transcribed as 20/200.

2. Memorize these difficult-to-spell ophthalmology terms.

accommodation	ophthalmology
fluorescein	pterygium (silent *p*)
funduscopy (not *-oscopy*)	ptosis (silent *p*)

3. When the dictator refers to both eyes, use the plural form of the anatomical structures.

   Scler*ae* and conjunctiv*ae* were normal.

4. The abbreviations PEARLA and PERRLA may be dictated as "pearl-la" rather than spelled out letter by letter.

5. Do not confuse the words *recession* and *resection*.

Terminology Challenge

Instructions: The following terms appear in the dictation on Tape 9A. Before beginning the medical transcription practice for Lesson 18, look up the words in a medical or English dictionary, and write out a short definition of each term.

Abraham contact lens
anterior chamber
antiviral therapy
arteriolar narrowing
artificial tears
bacteriostatic water
Beaver blade
bipolar cautery
BSS (balanced salt
  solution)
capsulotomy
cataract
  mature
  nuclear
  secondary
Cavitron AIS irrigating-
  aspirating needle
coapted
corneal epithelium
corneoscleral scissors
cortisone
cystitome

cytomegalovirus
dermatomyositis
ecchymosis
ectropion
episcleral
examination
  ophthalmoscopic
  slit-lamp
exotropia
extracapsular cataract
  extraction with lens
    implant
extraocular motility
forceps
  angulated
  McPherson
Fox shield
fundus of disk
funduscopy
ganciclovir
Garamycin
Healon
HIV antibody
IDDM
Inderal
intraocular pressure
IOL (intraocular lens)
Iolab intraocular lens
Kenalog
laser
  argon
  coherent YAG
  YAG
lens cortex
lid speculum
limbus
macular degeneration
macular edema
Marcaine
medial rectus recession
mJ (millijoules)
molluscum contagiosum
muscle
  inferior oblique
  inferior rectus
  orbicularis
  medial rectus
  superior rectus
Nizoral
OU, O.U.
pentamidine aerosol

peripheral iridectomy
peritomy
Persantine
photocoagulation
Pneumocystis carinii
posterior capsulotomy
position
  3 o'clock
  9 o'clock
  12 o'clock
prednisone
prism diopters
protocol
Proventil
pseudophakia
pupillary constriction
retinitis
retinopathy
retrobulbar block
rheumatoid arthritis
selenium
serum RPR
Sinskey hook
stereo acuity
strabismus
subconjunctivally
suture
  10-0
  nylon
  silk
  traction
temporally
test
  four-dot
  Snellen
Theo-Dur
Timoptic
Toxoplasma
Van Lint lid block
vision
  20/20
  20/30
  20/40
  20/50+
  20/200
visual acuity
Wydase
Xylocaine
Zantac
Zeiss operating
  microscope

Sample Reports

Sample ophthalmology reports appear on the following pages.

Transcription Practice

After completing all the readings and exercises in Lesson 18, transcribe Tape 9A, Ophthalmology. Use both medical and English dictionaries and your Quick-Reference Word List as resource materials for finding words.

Proofread your transcribed documents carefully, listening to the dictation while you read your transcripts.

Transcribe (*NOT* retype) the same reports again without referring to your previous transcription attempt. Initially, you may need to transcribe some reports more than twice before you can produce an error-free document. Your ultimate goal is to produce an error-free document the first time.

BLOOPERS

Incorrect	Correct
Papal edema	Papilledema
Frequent changing of menses without benefit	Frequent changing of lenses without benefit

CHART NOTE

CORA LORAINE POWELL   Age 62   October 25, 1992

In May the patient had a diagnosis of cataracts and elevated intraocular pressures which were 24 mmHg right eye, and 23 mmHg left eye. She has undergone bilateral cataract operations and she also has keratitis sicca with a Schirmer's test of 3 mm O.U. She had bilateral cataract surgery with a good visual result of 20/40 right eye, and 20/25 left eye.

The refractive error in the right eye was a -0.50 +1.00 axis 113 with a reading add of 2.25 which gave a J1 reading. Her intraocular pressures were controlled on Pilocar 4% and Betoptic eye drops. More recently she was switched to Phospholine Iodide 0.125% b.i.d. in the left eye. Her intraocular pressure on this examination was 15 mmHg right eye, and 20 mmHg left eye. Her optic discs showed a 0.3 cup of each disc and the peripheral retinas were within normal limits.

In addition, the patient has a small chalazion, right upper eyelid. It is recommended that she begin hot moist soaks t.i.d. to the right eyelid as well as Tobrex ointment to the right upper eyelid b.i.d.

DIAGNOSIS: 1. Pseudophakia, O.U.
2. Bilateral open angle glaucoma.
3. Keratitis sicca.
4. Chalazion, right upper eyelid.

It is recommended she return in three weeks for a follow-up evaluation. If the chalazion does not improve or increases in size, she may need incision and drainage in the office.

OUS:hpi

May 17, 1993

Basil Wolfine, M.D.
2020 Clearview Way, Suite 20
Sewell, NY 12840

Re: Sarah Anna Ratley

Dear Dr. Wolfine:

The patient was seen in February of this year and followed with a diagnosis of aphakia, left eye, and early nuclear cataract, right eye, as well as narrow angle glaucoma suspect in the right eye. She was placed on Pilocar 1% q.i.d., right eye. Gonioscopy showed a grade III angle superiorly using Scheie classification, with grade II pigmentation. Her intraocular pressures were slightly elevated and she was placed on Pilocar 1% b.i.d. In April she underwent YAG laser peripheral iridotomy, right eye, for narrow angle glaucoma, with subsequent widening of the peripheral iridotomy.

Her cataract progressed and her visual acuity more recently has been 20/50 in the right eye. She has always had visual acuity in the left eye of counting fingers on the basis of aphakia and a pupillary membrane with updrawn pupil. Her optic discs have had a cup:disc ratio of 0.34 in each eye and the peripheral retinas have been within normal limits.

Recently she complained of redness and discomfort in both eyes on the basis of a moderate degree of superficial punctate keratitis and was placed on Lacri-Lube ointment at frequent intervals. Her intraocular pressure was 28 mmHg in the right eye, and 20 mmHg in the left eye. Therefore, she was begun on Betoptic b.i.d. and Eppy at h.s. to the right eye. Because of her superficial punctate and some allergic conjunctivitis, she was switched to Celluvisc q. 2 hours and cold compresses, and was continued on her glaucoma drops.

IMPRESSION:
1. Cataract, right eye.
2. Status post YAG peripheral iridotomy, O.D., for narrow angle glaucoma.
3. Glaucoma suspect, O.U.
4. Aphakia with pupillary membrane and updrawn pupil, O.S.
5. Keratitis sicca with ocular surface disease.

Thank you for the consultation on this patient. If I can be of any further help, please do not hesitate to contact me.

Best regards,

O. U. Seymour, M.D.

OUS:hpi

SUSAN ELLEN POWELL

#121496

DATE OF OPERATION: June 21, 1992

OPERATIVE REPORT

PREOPERATIVE DIAGNOSIS: Cataract of right eye

SURGICAL PROCEDURE: Extracapsular cataract extraction with lens implant of right eye.

PROCEDURE: The patient was placed in the supine position on the operating room table after having received preoperative sedation and dilating drops to the right eye. An O'Brien akinesia of the right eye was done using 4 cc of a mixture containing two-thirds Marcaine 0.75% and one-third Xylocaine 2% plain with Wydase. A retrobulbar block was given through the lower lid temporally using 3 cc of the same. Light digital pressure was applied for a few minutes, and satisfactory anesthesia was achieved. The right eye and face were prepped with a 0.5% Betadine solution and draped in a sterile fashion.

A lid speculum was inserted into the right eye, and 4-0 silk traction sutures passed through the superior and inferior rectus muscles and the Zeiss operating microscope swung into position. A conjunctival peritomy was opened over the superior 140° at the limbus, and episcleral bleeders cauterized. A groove was made in the surgical limbus with a #64 Beaver blade and a 7-0 silk suture passed at 12 o'clock. The anterior chamber was entered at 11 o'clock with razor blade knife and an irrigating cystitome used to do a 360° anterior capsulotomy. Dissection was completed with corneoscleral scissors, and the lens nucleus was expressed. The 7-0 silk suture was tied and cut, and an additional 8-0 Vicryl was placed 3.5 mm on either side of the silk. The Cavitron AIS irrigating-aspirating needle was placed into the anterior chamber, and using BSS (balanced salt solution) for irrigation, the lens cortex was removed and the posterior capsule remained intact. The posterior capsule was polished, and the capsular bag filled with Amvisc. The 7-0 silk sutures were removed.

An Iolab intraocular lens model G157E power +24.0 diopters, control #011288G157E5092, was inspected under the microscope and appeared to be grossly free of defects. It was grasped with angulated McPherson forceps and placed into the capsular bag. The implant was rotated to the 3 to 9 o'clock position with a Sinskey hook. The Amvisc was replaced with the BSS and the pupil constricted with Miochol. The incision was closed securely with nine additional 10-0 nylon sutures. The conjunctiva was drawn over the suture line and coapted at 3 and 9 o'clock with bipolar cautery. Garamycin 20 mg and 20 mg of Kenalog were injected subconjunctivally below, and a patch and Fox shield put in place. Prior to the patch, a drop of Timoptic was placed on the cornea. The patient tolerated the procedure well and returned to the outpatient surgery area in good condition.

_____

O. U. SEYMOUR, M.D.

OUS:hpi
D&T: 6/21/92

Lesson 19. Neurology

Learning Objectives

Medical

- List common neurologic symptoms and findings mentioned in a complete neurologic examination.
- Describe the action of drugs used to treat seizure disorders and Parkinson's disease.
- Given a cross-section illustration of the brain, memorize the anatomic structures.
- Construct the adjectival form of common neurologic terms.
- Describe the anatomic parts of the brain and their functions.
- Define common neurologic abbreviations.
- Given a neurologic root word, symptom, or disease, match it to its correct definition.

Fundamentals

- Discuss the qualities of professionalism for a medical transcriptionist.
- Given a medical report with errors, identify and correct the errors.

Practice

- Accurately transcribe authentic physician dictation from the specialty of neurology.

A Closer Look

Professionalism and the Medical Transcriptionist

by Kathy Donneson, MPA

What is professionalism? What qualities distinguish a professional from a nonprofessional? Professionals may be judged by their attitudes and conduct as they relate to matters of work, interpersonal relationships, and ethics.

Medical transcriptionists work independently and produce a product (the transcribed medical document) which reflects their care, integrity, and skill.

1. Professional medical transcriptionists function with minimal supervision while producing maximum results in both quantity and quality. While the majority of working transcriptionists do have an immediate supervisor responsible for quality control, the attitude of each transcriptionist should be one of independence and responsibility for his or her own work. Professionals take pride in the accuracy and completeness of their own work and gain satisfaction from a job well done, both in quality and quantity.

2. Professional medical transcriptionists demonstrate responsibility in their day-to-day working judgments by combining past experience, the powers of deductive thinking, and a vast store of medical knowledge to produce an accurate medical record. Taking the time to consult up-to-date references or other healthcare professionals is the distinguishing feature between the professional and others who cannot be bothered to be medically accurate as they carelessly and thoughtlessly transcribe.

3. Professional medical transcriptionists demonstrate ethical values when dealing with confidential or personal information contained in the medical record. The professional resists gossiping about personal information contained in medical records and protects the right to privacy and confidentiality for each patient.

4. Professional medical transcriptionists demonstrate a disciplined work attitude with dedication to the needs of the patient before personal needs.

5. Professional medical transcriptionists display a commitment to continuing education by setting a high standard of performance and knowledge. The professional welcomes new knowledge and readily participates in educational efforts, not only for personal enrichment, but also for the collective benefit of the entire healthcare team.

6. Professional medical transcriptionists view co-workers as valuable members of the healthcare team, treating them with dignity and courtesy.

Through their conduct and attitude, professional medical transcriptionists can demonstrate to the public and other medical professionals that they are indeed disciplined, knowledgeable, and dedicated members of the healthcare team.

Medical Readings

Neurology and Neurosurgery

Part 1

by John H. Dirckx, M.D.

Neurology is the branch of medicine that is concerned with the diagnosis and treatment of diseases, developmental disorders, and injuries of the nervous system, particularly the central nervous system (brain and spinal cord). Neurosurgery is the branch of surgery that is concerned with the surgical treatment of these conditions. Most of the patients seen by a neurologist or neurosurgeon are referred by other physicians, usually family physicians, internists, or pediatricians.

Neurologists treat a broad range of disorders affecting the nervous system, including developmental anomalies, injuries, toxic conditions, infections, circulatory and degenerative diseases, chronic headaches, seizures, and benign and malignant tumors. Just as a general surgeon is a physician specially trained to treat various diseases and injuries by surgical (manual, mechanical, instrumental) means, a neurosurgeon is a neurologist trained to apply surgical methods to the treatment of neurologic disorders.

In assessing a patient with symptoms suggesting disease or injury of the central nervous system, the neurologist or neurosurgeon obtains a neurologic history, performs a neurologic examination, and may also order laboratory tests, x-rays, scans, an electroencephalogram, an electromyogram, or other special diagnostic procedures.

The **neurologic history**, obtained from the patient if possible, begins with detailed information about the patient's principal complaint or problem—its nature, duration, onset, and suspected cause; whether it is constant, variable, or intermittent; the effect of position, movement, rest, medicines, or other factors. Typical presenting symptoms of neurologic disease include numbness, shaking, weakness, or paralysis of an arm or leg; disturbances of balance or gait; passing out or having seizures; and recurring headaches. The neurologist also inquires about the patient's past medical history, including problems at birth and abnormalities of growth or development; seizures or fainting spells; mental troubles; previous illnesses of any kind; injuries; surgical operations; the use of medicines, alcohol, tobacco, or drugs of abuse; and occupational exposure to toxic substances. A family history of neurologic disease may also be significant.

The **neurologic examination** is a set of diagnostic procedures by which the neurologist assesses the structural and functional integrity of the various parts of the central nervous system. Many of these procedures require the cooperation of a conscious patient, but some do not. Only a few simple instruments are used, such as a penlight to check the pupillary reflexes, a rubber hammer to test deep tendon reflexes, and a pin to test skin sensitivity.

A neurologic examination is part of any complete physical examination, but as performed by a neurologist it is usually more elaborate and yields more precise information. An important element in neurologic diagnosis is localization; exactly where in the nervous system is the lesion (site of disease or injury)? The nervous system might be thought of as an enormously complex electronic device with millions of microscopic components and miles of "wire" (nerve fibers). Most of the important circuits have been mapped out. By applying a knowledge of neuroanatomy to the findings in the individual patient, the neurologist can often deduce with remarkable accuracy not only the nature of the problem but also its location in the system.

The main divisions of the nervous system are the brain and the spinal cord (which together make up the central nervous system) and the peripheral nerves, which carry sensory impulses from various parts of the body to the spinal cord, and motor impulses from the spinal cord to the muscles. The neurologic examination is planned to test the functions of the various components of the system in logical sequence.

The cerebrum, the largest and most highly developed part of the brain, is concerned with perception, memory, reasoning, and voluntary movement. An important part of the neurologic examination is the **mental status examination**, by which the neurologist assesses the patient's level of consciousness, intelligence, memory, orientation, judgment, and language skills. The neurologist does this principally by asking the patient questions and assigning mental tasks such as counting backwards. An estimate of the patient's mental competence is crucial to neurologic diagnosis, since many neurologic tests require the patient's understanding and cooperation. The full mental status examination also evaluates the patient's mood, thought content, attention span, and insight into the nature of the problem.

Twelve pairs of **cranial nerves** emerge from the brain and serve functions in the head and neck, including vision, the pupillary reflexes, and eye movements; hearing, taste, and smell; skin sensation, facial expression, and swallowing. The cranial nerves are often referred to by roman numerals I through XII rather than by name. The neurologist checks the cranial nerves by applying simple tests to assess the function of each. Often the first cranial nerve, the olfactory nerve, which is concerned with the sense of smell, is omitted from consideration.

The spinal cord is a complex bundle of hundreds of thousands of nerve fibers passing up and down, within the protection of the spinal column, between the brain and the body below the level of the neck. Thirty-one pairs of **spinal nerves** emerge from the spinal cord in serial fashion, one pair above each vertebra. After various branchings and joinings, these spinal nerves form the peripheral nerves, which carry sensory impulses from the skin surface, the muscles, and other body areas to the spinal cord, and motor impulses from the cord to the voluntary muscles of the trunk, arms, and legs. The neurologist assesses the integrity of the sensory nerves by checking the ability to feel light touch and pinprick (sometimes also heat, cold, vibration, and limb position) in various areas of the body. Impairment of a motor nerve is indicated by atrophy (wasting), weakness, or paralysis of muscles innervated (supplied) by that nerve.

A number of the tests performed as part of the neurologic examination assess several structures or functions at once. For example, the **Romberg test**, in which the patient is asked to stand erect with eyes closed, requires a normal sense of balance as well as intact nerves and muscles in the back and legs.

A **deep tendon reflex** is an involuntary contraction of a muscle when its tendon is suddenly stretched or tapped, as with a reflex hammer. Examination of various deep tendon reflexes in the arms and legs gives the neurologist information about both the sensory and motor nerves at the levels tested. In addition, hyperactive (abnormally vigorous) deep tendon reflexes may indicate disease or injury of upper motor neurons in the cerebral cortex. Such a lesion may also cause the appearance of various abnormal reflexes, such as the **Babinski (plantar) reflex**, in which the toes curve upward when the sole of the foot is stroked.

Tests of coordination (performance of complicated or delicate movements or rapidly alternating movements) evaluate the cerebellum, the part of the brain especially concerned with coordination, but also require intact muscles and nerves and a conscious and cooperative patient.

Numerous other tests not discussed here enable the neurologist to look for specific abnormalities or evaluate specific problems.

After completing the neurologic examination, the neurologist may order various special diagnostic procedures to provide further information. **Laboratory tests** of blood and urine may show evidence of infection, systemic disease, or chemical poisoning. **Lumbar puncture** (insertion of a needle into the subarachnoid space between two vertebrae in the lumbar region) permits measurement of the pressure of the cerebrospinal fluid (CSF), the serumlike fluid that surrounds the brain and spinal cord, and withdrawal of a sample of fluid for laboratory study.

X-ray examinations (including CT scans, angiography with introduction of dye into the circulation, and pneumoencephalography with replacement of CSF by air) and magnetic resonance imaging (MRI) can be performed to show injuries, hemorrhage, cysts, tumors, and other structural abnormalities of the central nervous system and surrounding tissues.

An **electroencephalogram** (EEG) provides a tracing of the electrical activity of the brain, as detected by electrodes placed at various points on the scalp. The EEG is particularly valuable in the diagnosis of seizure disorders. A complete electroencephalographic study includes tracings taken during hyperventilation, photic stimulation (exposure to flashing lights), and sleep.

Electromyography is a diagnostic procedure in

which a weak electric current is applied to a muscle and the result of the stimulus measured and recorded electronically. **Nerve conduction studies** measure the rate at which electrical impulses are transmitted by peripheral nerves.

The following survey of neurologic disorders is meant to provide a broad overview of the conditions seen and treated in a typical neurology or neurosurgery practice. It is by no means a comprehensive catalog of such conditions.

The brain and spinal cord are subject to numerous **developmental anomalies** and malformations, most of which are evident at birth. A particularly serious congenital disorder is **hydrocephalus**, in which the pressure of the cerebrospinal fluid is abnormally high because of some obstruction to its circulation. As a result the head enlarges abnormally, and compression of brain tissue results in severe neurologic damage and, usually, death without treatment. The treatment of hydrocephalus is the surgical placement of a shunt between the cranial cavity and some other part of the body, usually the peritoneal (abdominal) cavity, to maintain normal CSF pressure by allowing drainage of excess fluid.

The neurologist is frequently called upon to evaluate and treat patients suffering from **vascular disease** affecting the central nervous system. Enlargement or rupture of an **aneurysm** (an abnormal dilatation of an artery) or other blood vessel malformation present from birth can cause circulatory compromise of the brain. Various forms of **arteriosclerosis** (hardening of the arteries), including those associated with aging, high blood pressure, and high blood cholesterol, can cause focal or diffuse narrowing of arteries supplying the brain or spinal cord. The neurologic consequences of this narrowing depend on its location and degree and also on the patient's general condition.

There may be gradual decline in mental function (**senile dementia**); intermittent spells of weakness, numbness, or dizziness lasting less than 24 hours (**transient ischemic attacks**, TIAs); or **stroke** (also called cerebrovascular accident, CVA), a sudden onset of severe neurologic deficit (loss of consciousness, paralysis) due to compromise of the cerebral circulation resulting from thrombosis (clotting) or hemorrhage (leakage of blood from a diseased vessel).

Frequent manifestations of a stroke are **hemiplegia** (paralysis of the arm and leg on one side of the body, resulting from disturbance in the cerebral cortex on the opposite side) or **hemiparesis** (weakness of one arm and leg without complete paralysis) and **aphasia** (inability to speak, due to damage to Broca's motor speech area, which is in the left cerebral cortex in most persons). A stroke may be rapidly fatal, but many patients survive, some with severe neurologic impairment and others with little or none.

The signs and symptoms of cerebrovascular disease are highly variable, but by considering them in the light of neuroanatomy, the neurologist can generally determine the location and extent of the lesion. CT scans and other diagnostic studies are used to confirm the diagnosis. Once cerebrovascular disease causes a stroke or other symptoms, it may be too late for medical intervention to reverse the damage. The role of the neurologist in such cases is to ascertain the type and degree of nervous system involvement, to prevent progression of the disease (such as by controlling high blood pressure and prescribing medicines that reduce the risk of blood clotting), and to supervise a program of rehabilitation to restore mental and physical functioning to as near normal as possible. Certain cerebral vascular disorders (aneurysms, localized blood vessel narrowing, or acute hemorrhage) may be amenable to neurosurgical treatment.

Head and neck injuries are among the commonest causes of severe disability and death in accidents occurring on the highway, in the workplace, and at home. The neurologic consequences of such injuries depend on the location and extent of damage to the central nervous system. A severe fracture of the skull or spine may cause little or no impairment of nervous system function, and on the other hand a blow to the head can cause a fatal intracranial hemorrhage with little or no external evidence of injury.

Cerebral concussion is a very brief loss of consciousness due to head injury. Although occasionally followed by transitory neurologic symptoms, concussion has no long-term consequences. In contrast, when there is **laceration** of brain tissue or **hemorrhage** into the brain or between the brain and the skull, severe, irreversible, and perhaps rapidly fatal disturbances of brain function can result.

Injury to the spinal cord frequently accompanies neck injury, especially when a fracture is present. **Transection** (severing) of part or all of the spinal cord causes instant and permanent paralysis, loss of feeling, or both in parts of the body supplied by nerves emerging from the spinal cord below the level of injury whose connections with the brain have been lost. The treatment of head and neck injuries may include surgical repair or stabilization of a fracture of the skull or spine when there is pressure on or potential damage to underlying nerve tissue, evacuation of intracranial hemorrhage, and rehabilitation to preserve or restore function.

Disk disease is an important neurosurgical disorder. A disk is a cushion of fibrocartilage between two adjacent vertebral bodies. If the central jellylike core (nucleus pulposus) of a disk herniates (bulges out of place), it may compress adjacent nerve roots emerging from the spinal cord and cause **radiculopathy**—pain, numbness, muscle weakness, or all of these in areas supplied by the nerve roots affected.

Most disk problems involve lumbar vertebral disks and cause low back pain and leg symptoms. An injury (often occupational) may be the event that precipitates herniation of a nucleus pulposus, but usually rupture of a disk implies some previous degeneration. Diagnosis is confirmed by CT scan, magnetic resonance imaging, or myelography (x-rays taken after injection of dye into the subarachnoid space at the level of suspected herniation). Mild disk problems may resolve with rest, but surgical treatment (laminectomy with decompression of nerve roots and excision of disk fragments) is often necessary.

Varying degrees of **impairment of consciousness** accompany a broad range of neurologic disorders, and may also be a manifestation of systemic, metabolic, or toxic conditions. Stupor or coma can be caused by cerebral vascular disease and head injuries, as already discussed, as well as by local or diffuse central nervous system disease (encephalitis, meningitis, Alzheimer's disease), diabetic acidosis, liver or kidney failure, circulatory collapse (shock), high fever, alcoholic intoxication, drug abuse or overdose, chemical poisoning, and other conditions. In assessing a comatose patient the neurologist must rely on any available history and diagnostic clues obtained by examination and testing performed without any help from the patient. Prompt, accurate diagnosis of coma may be lifesaving. (See Part 2 in Lesson 20.)

Pharmacology: Neurology Drugs

Various disease conditions of the central nervous system benefit from pharmacologic therapy. These include epilepsy, Parkinson's disease, and insomnia.

There is no one drug which has therapeutic effects against all types of seizures. Some drugs which are effective for controlling one type of seizure may actually provoke another type of seizure.

Barbiturates are a class of sedative drugs, some of which possess an anticonvulsant action. Barbiturates

used to treat seizures include:

    phenobarbital (Luminal)
    phenytoin (Dilantin)
    ethosuximide (Zarontin)
    carbamazepine (Tegretol)

Phenytoin (Dilantin) is the drug of choice for treating adults with tonic-clonic seizures, while phenobarbital (Luminal) is the drug of choice for treating children.

Valproic acid (Depakene, Depakote) is used to treat absence seizures, although ethosuximide (Zarontin) is the drug of choice.

Drugs to treat Parkinson's disease. Drug therapy for Parkinson's disease is divided into two main categories: drugs which increase or enhance the action of dopamine in the brain, and drugs which inhibit the action of acetylcholine. All these drugs act to restore the natural balance between dopamine and acetylcholine.

Drugs which increase the amount of dopamine, enhance its action in the brain, or directly stimulate dopamine receptors include:

    amantadine (Symmetrel)
    bromocriptine (Parlodel)
    carbidopa (Lodosyn)
    levodopa (L-dopa, Larodopa)

Drugs which inhibit the action of acetylcholine in the brain include:

    benztropine mesylate (Cogentin)
    biperiden (Akineton)
    ethopropazine (Parsidol)
    procyclidine (Kemadrin)
    trihexyphenidyl (Artane)

Combination drugs for Parkinson's disease include:

    Sinemet-10/100 (mg of carbidopa/
      mg of levodopa)
    Sinemet-25/100
    Sinemet-25/250

None of the drugs prescribed for Parkinson's disease can cure it. In fact, over time tolerance can develop to their therapeutic effects. Larger drug doses are then required to maintain control of parkinsonian symptoms; however, these also produce more side effects. When doses can no longer be increased or when side effects become intolerable, the physician will gradually withdraw all medication, placing the patient on a "drug holiday" for a few days. When drug therapy is again initiated, the patient will respond to lower doses of antiparkinsonian drugs.

Drugs for insomnia. Nonbarbiturate hypnotics depress central nervous system functions and promote sedation and sleep. They include chloral hydrate (Noctec), estazolam (ProSom), and flurazepam (Dalmane).

Anatomy/Medical Terminology

Anatomy: The Brain

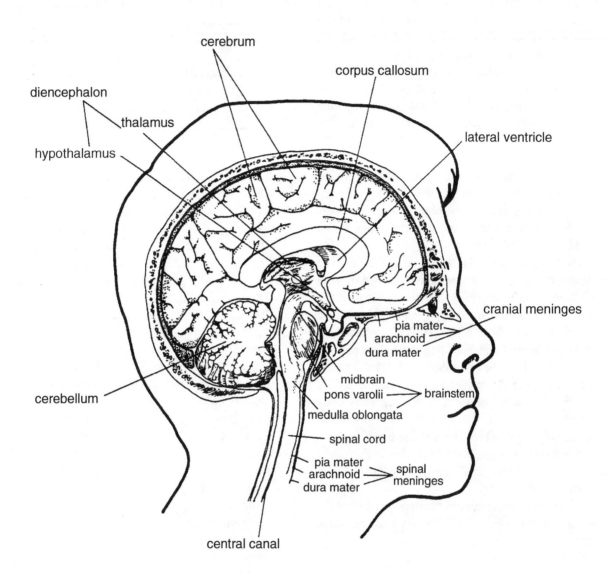

cerebrum

corpus callosum

diencephalon

thalamus

lateral ventricle

hypothalamus

cranial meninges

pia mater
arachnoid
dura mater

cerebellum

midbrain
pons varolii — brainstem
medulla oblongata

spinal cord

pia mater
arachnoid — spinal
dura mater   meninges

central canal

Adjective Exercise

Adjectives are formed from nouns by adding adjectival suffixes such as *-ac, -al, -ar, -ary, -eal, -ed, -ent, -iac, -ial, -ic, -ical, -lar, -oid, -ous, -tic,* and *-tous.* In addition, some adjectives have a different form entirely from the noun, which may be either Latin or Greek in origin.

Test your knowledge of adjectives by writing the adjectival form of the following neurology words. Consult a medical dictionary as necessary.

1. nerve _____
2. spine _____
3. cranium _____
4. cerebrum _____
5. cerebellum _____
6. meninges _____
7. paraplegia _____
8. hydrocephalus _____
9. epilepsy _____
10. ventricle _____
11. arachnoid _____

Fill-in Exercise: Central Nervous System

Instructions: The numbered blanks correspond to the numbers in parentheses in the narrative paragraphs. Fill in the blanks with the correct entry from the word list below.

The (1), or CNS, is the largest division of the nervous system and consists of twelve pairs of (2) nerves and 31 pairs of spinal nerves. The spinal (3), into which the spinal nerves enter, is protected by the spinal column, consisting of seven (4) vertebrae, twelve (5) vertebrae, five (6) vertebrae, and five (7) vertebrae. The end of the spinal cord is called the (8) because the ending group of nerves resembles the hair of a horse's tail.

There are three protective layers of membranes that surround the spinal cord and brain. The outermost layer, which is the thickest, is called the (9); the middle layer is the arachnoid membrane; and the innermost layer, which is thin and contains many blood vessels, is called the (10).

The brain itself is divided into several parts. The largest division is the (11) which is further divided into lobes: the (12) lobe in the forehead region, whose functions include memory and perception; the (13) lobe under the temporal bone of the skull, whose functions include hearing and understanding speech; the parietal lobe; and the (14) lobe at the base of the skull, whose functions include vision. Other parts of the brain include the thalamus; the (15), which regulates body temperature; the (16), which contains centers which automatically regulate breathing and heart rate; the (17), which connects the cerebrum to the cerebellum, and the (18), which is concerned with coordination of voluntary movements.

In the center and between the various lobes of the cerebrum are the (19), cavities filled with cerebrospinal fluid.

1. ____central nervous system____
2. _____
3. _____
4. _____
5. _____
6. _____
7. _____
8. _____
9. _____
10. _____
11. _____
12. _____
13. _____
14. _____
15. _____
16. _____
17. _____
18. _____
19. _____

cauda equina	lumbar
central nervous system	medulla oblongata
cerebellum	occipital
cerebrum	pia mater
cervical	pons
cranial	sacral
cord	temporal
dura mater	thoracic
frontal	ventricles
hypothalamus	

Abbreviations Exercise

Common abbreviations may be transcribed as dictated in the body of a report. Uncommon abbreviations must be spelled out, with the abbreviation appearing in parentheses after the translation. All abbreviations (except laboratory test names) must be spelled out in the Diagnosis or Impression section of any report.

Instructions: Define the following neurology abbreviations. Then memorize both abbreviations and definitions to increase your speed and accuracy in transcribing dictation from neurology.

CNS _____   LP   _____

CSF _____   MS   _____

CVA _____   RIND _____

EEG _____   TIA _____

Medical Terminology Matching Exercise

Instructions: Match the term in Column A with its definition in Column B.

Column A   *Column B*

A. concussion   _____ fissures in surface of brain

B. encephalo-   _____ painful sensation

C. sulci   _____ brain

D. dura mater   _____ nerve

E. neuro-   _____ paralysis of lower body

F. paresthesia   _____ malignant brain tumor

G. radiculo-   _____ brief loss of consciousness
                         after head injury

H. paraplegia
                   _____ largest division of the brain
I. multiple
   sclerosis   _____ numbness, tingling

J. -algia   _____ caused by demyelination
                         of nerves
K. syncope
                   _____ shows neurofibrillary tangles
L. Alzheimer's   of brain on autopsy
   disease
                   _____ spinal nerve root
M. cerebrum
                   _____ outermost meningeal layer
N. astrocytoma
                   _____ fainting

Drug Word Search

Instructions: Locate and circle the neurology terms hidden in the puzzle horizontally, vertically, and diagonally, forward and backward. A numeral following a term in the word list indicates the number of times the word can be found in the puzzle.

```
R  E  S  T  O  R  I  L  C  N  P  L  S
E  N  A  T  R  A  F  D  J  Y  R  A  Y
X  A  L  Y  J  J  O  O  A  T  O  R  M
D  M  G  H  S  R  T  P  R  O  S  O  M
E  L  U  I  A  P  O  A  V  L  O  Q  E
P  A  R  L  O  D  E  L  V  C  M  Z  T
A  D  D  N  O  I  C  L  A  H  A  N  R
K  I  X  V  U  L  L  M  I  R  S  I  E
E  P  E  R  M  A  X  O  O  P  I  L  L
N  L  N  D  E  N  H  N  T  Q  E  A  O
E  E  G  B  S  T  T  C  E  Y  I  T  R
E  J  O  N  L  I  N  S  O  M  N  I  A
G  H  C  E  N  N  O  C  T  E  C  R  L
```

Artane   levodopa
CNS   Noctec
Cognex   Nytol (2)
Dalmane   oral (2)
Depakene   Parlodel
Dilantin   Permax
Doral   pill
drug   ProSom (2)
EEG (2)   Restoril
epilepsy   Ritalin
Halcion   Soma
insomnia   Symmetrel
L-dopa   Zarontin

Lay and Medical Terms

Lay Term   *Medical Term*

fit, convulsion   epileptic seizure

stroke   cerebrovascular accident (CVA)

water on the brain hydrocephalus

Transcription Guidelines

Pronouns: Which, Who, That

1. The pronoun **which** used as a relative pronoun (a noun substitute used to introduce clauses) refers to animals and things. *Which* is often used in non-restrictive clauses, which are set off by commas and are not necessary to the meaning of the sentence:

   The medicine that he took, which he left at home in Virginia, was Dyazide.

2. The pronoun **who** (or whom) refers to people and sometimes animals.

3. The pronoun **that** can refer to any of the above. *That* is used almost exclusively to introduce restrictive clauses (clauses that are necessary for the understanding of the sentence and not set off by commas):

   The medicine that he took is unknown to me.

4. A good test of some restrictive clauses is to leave out the relative pronoun, and if the sentence still makes sense, it is an essential clause (example A). In example B, however, the relative clause is restrictive, but *that* cannot be omitted.

   A. The medicine that he took is unknown to me.
      The medicine he took is unknown to me.
   B. The chamber that receives oxygenated blood from the lungs is the left atrium.

5. *Who* and *whom* can be used in restrictive or non-restrictive clauses. *Which* and *that* can sometimes be interchanged, but *which* cannot be used to refer to persons.

Transcription Tips

1. An alternate acceptable spelling of *disk* is *disc.*
2. The word *diskectomy* is spelled only with a *k.*
3. Don't confuse *CNS* (central nervous system) with *C&S* (culture and sensitivity).

Proofreading Skills

Instructions: In the following partial report, identify the errors and write the correct medical and English words in the numbered blanks below the text.

```
 1  This is a 44-year-old married blackmail cold
 2  minor. He has been 6¢ April 7, when he
 3  enveloped a blue-light illness. Over the fol-
 4  lowing sick, weak period he had several recur-
 5  rents of abominable stress with apple soda
 6  Disney and nausea but no Emerson's. Coffin
 7  spells occurring mostly in mourning were
 8  predictive of prurient material. He also
 9  complained of knights, wets, and a casual
10  rigger. No, he mopped as is.
11
12  Passed history insignificant in that about two
13  years ago he spent two days in the icy ewe with
14  8-reel flutter. He is presently on pneumatic
15  rations. He was First Scene by me today and
16  omitted Perrier because of an apple soda
17  synchrony followed by this Orient nation.
18
19  Review of Symptoms: Denies headaches,
20  vertical, or prior apple soda sympathy. No food
21  and tolerance, weightless weakness, or mustard
22  skeletal complaints. No inner mitten clot
23  dictation.
```

1. _____ black male coal _____
2. _____
3. _____
4. _____
5. _____
6. _____
7. _____
8. _____
9. _____
10. _____
11. _____
12. _____
13. _____
14. _____
15. _____
16. _____
17. _____
18. _____
19. _____
20. _____
21. _____
22. _____
23. _____

Terminology Challenge

Instructions: The following terms appear in the dictation on Tape 9B. Before beginning the medical transcription practice for Lesson 19, look up the terms in a medical or English dictionary, and write out a short definition of each term.

abducens muscle
albeit
Alzheimer's disease
anticonvulsant
articulate
ataxia
basilar skull fracture
C5-6
cervical myelogram
circumlocutory
coherent
contrast media
cortical sensation
cranial nerves II
  through XII
cryptococcal antigen
CSF (cerebrospinal
  fluid)
CT scan
CVA (cerebrovascular
  accident)
déjà vu
dementia
Dilantin
diplopia
EEG (electroencephalo-
  gram)
extradural defect
foramen
frontal lobe (of brain)
gait
glioma
hemiparesis
insight and judgment
intractable
intrinsic brain stem lesion
jamais vu
lethargy
lightheadedness
lumbar puncture

meningitis
mental status
monotone
motor examination
MRI (magnetic resonance
  imaging)
myasthenia gravis
myelography
nerve root
neuroradiologist
NP leads
nuchal rigidity
PA and lateral chest x-ray
painful stimuli
postprandial blood sugar
reflexes
  deep tendon
  plantar
seizure
  generalized
  grand mal
sensory examination
sign
  Brudzinski's
  Kernig's
sleep-deprived EEG
SMAC
stereognosis
tandem walking
tangential
Tegretol
test
  finger-to-nose
  heel-to-shin
  Prostigmin
  psychometric
  Romberg's
  Tensilon
urine catecholamines
vertigo

Sample Reports

Sample neurology reports appear on the following pages.

Transcription Practice

After completing all the readings and exercises in Lesson 19, transcribe Tape 9B, Neurology. Use both medical and English dictionaries and your Quick-Reference Word List as resource materials for finding words. Proofread your transcribed documents carefully, listening to the dictation while you read your transcripts.

Transcribe (*NOT* retype) the same reports again without referring to your previous transcription attempt. Initially, you may need to transcribe some reports more than twice before you can produce an error-free document. Your ultimate goal is to produce an error-free document the first time.

CHART NOTE

AGNES SHAKLEE   Age 74   June 20, 1992

This very pleasant 74-year-old woman has rather advanced parkinsonism present for many years. It is affecting her daily living to a great degree. She has difficulty dressing, has frequent falls, occasionally related to freezing or to festination, but also occurring without any apparent cause. She has marked hesitancy on changing direction and unsteadiness with fatigue. She has a minor problem with sialorrhea, eating, and swallowing. She is able to maintain her personal hygiene without any difficulty. She has had some symptoms of depression along with her Parkinson's disease.

On neurologic exam she did have mild to moderate impairment in cognition and short-term memory, although she is oriented x 3. She has a mild tremor, worse in the left arm than the right. She has rigidity in the upper left extremity. She has marked poverty of movement with long delays in initiating movement and frequent freezing. She has a moderately flexed posture and cannot straighten to command. She has postural instability. Her speech is mildly dysarthric. She has a paucity of spontaneous facial expression. Her gait is characterized by shuffling strides with festination in propulsion. She does not need assistance with gait. She can arise from a chair with difficulty only after multiple attempts. She has micrographia. Deep tendon reflexes are symmetrical, and toes are downgoing. Cranial nerves are unremarkable.

She has been on Sinemet 25/100 t.i.d. for the last six years or so. She will be going on vacation soon and I would not attempt to add a second antiparkinsonian medication. However, I have asked her to increase her Sinemet dose to q.i.d. We will see how she does with Sinemet and plan to add bromocriptine 1 mg per day when she returns.

AF:hpi

NAME: MARIAN BARTLEY   **DATE:** 03/25/92

PREOPERATIVE DIAGNOSIS: Herniated nucleus pulposus, L5-S1.

POSTOPERATIVE DIAGNOSIS: Herniated nucleus pulposus, L5-S1.

OPERATION PERFORMED: Microdiskectomy of L5-S1.

PROCEDURE: After a satisfactory level of general endotracheal anesthesia was obtained, the patient was rolled prone on the Relton-Hall frame, and her back was prepared and draped in a routine manner. A midline skin incision was made about 2 inches long, a little longer than usual because of her obesity. The subcutaneous tissues were dissected out to the fascia. A deep retractor was necessary simply to retract the fat down to the fascia. An incision was made along the fascia. A towel clip was placed on the L5 spinous process confirmed by x-ray. The Grossman retractor was utilized to retract the paraspinous muscles on the left side. A microscope was draped out and brought into place.

The ligamentum flavum was excised. The medial aspect of the pedicle was exposed. A laminectomy was continued inferiorly because it was recognized preoperatively that the extrusion of disk material extended inferiorly into the spinal canal. The S1 nerve root was clearly identified and gently retracted medially. It was found to be under a great deal of tension. The annulus was tented up, an incision was made into the annulus, and a large amount of disk material that was herniated centrally was removed. The annulus was incised inferiorly enough to expose some inferior extrusion of disk. When all the centrally herniated disk material was removed, the canal was probed with a Murphy ball. The more caudal portion of the sacral canal was explored. There appeared to be a fragment of disk scarred up, or at least adherent to the dura ventrally. This was teased free with a blunt hook, and a massive fragment of herniated disk material was serially gently freed up with a blunt hook and gently pulled with a micro pituitary rongeur which seemed to free this massive fragment of disk material in its entirety. The spinal canal was probed with a Murphy ball, and no further free material could be identified. The wound was vigorously irrigated.

Dissection had been somewhat slow and tedious to assure freeing up the caudally herniated disk extrusion. Consquently the blood loss was 500 cc. Hemostasis, however, was satisfactorily achieved with gentle tamponade with Gelfoam and cottonoids. One epidural vein laterally in the canal did require electrocautery. There were excellent dural pulsations at the completion of the case. There seemed to be adequate epidural fat to cover the exposed nerve root, so no free fat graft was taken. Because of the blood loss during the case and the patient's obesity and anticipated oozing, it was elected to place a deep medium Hemovac drain that was brought out through the fascia and through a separate stab wound in the skin.

The midline fascial closure was made with 0 Vicryl, subcutaneous tissue with 2-0 Vicryl, and skin closure was made with a running subcuticular undyed 3-0 Dexon. Steri-Strips were applied. A sterile dressing was placed, and the patient was returned to the recovery room in satisfactory condition.

_____

ABSALOM FUSE, M.D.

AF:hpi
d&t: 3/25/92

Lesson 20. Neurology

Learning Objectives

Medical

- Describe common neurologic diseases and symptoms.
- Discuss the purpose and technique involved in performing common neurologic laboratory tests and surgical procedures.
- Given a category of neurologic drugs, indicate which drugs belong to that category.
- Given a neurologic root word and suffix, construct a term to match a given definition.
- Given a cross-section illustration of the spinal cord and nerves, memorize the anatomic structures.
- Differentiate between neurologic sound-alike terms.

Fundamentals

- Discuss the challenges and rewards of working as a medical transcriptionist in a foreign country.
- Demonstrate mastery of all areas of punctuation and editing by correcting and editing medical sentences.

Practice

- Accurately transcribe authentic physician dictation from the specialty of neurology.

A Closer Look

Transcribing Lines in the Sand

by Elizabeth D'Onofrio

Saudi Arabia. A land of sheiks and camels, of shifting sands, rugged mountains, and tropical beaches. Whisper the word "Arabia" and hear the lilting voice of Scheherazade in the cool of twilight. A world away in every respect. And endlessly exotic to our imaginations, awed from our early years by magic tales spun in dreamy Arabian nights. But Arabia in the light of day? Behold, a land of modern hospitals, striding in step with the rest of the world into the twenty-first century. Yet, the mystique remains as a sultry wink, promising adventure to those who dare.

Dee Sparkes, CMT, is one who dared. Coming upon a crossroad in her life and looking for a radical change from Seattle, she decided to ply her medical transcription skills in Saudi Arabia. Her relatives and friends thought it was a crazy idea. But dreams appear foolish to those who dare not dream.

Far from foolish, working in Saudi Arabia was for Sparkes a "wonderful experience" about which she says, "Even now I would go back." She saw it as a unique opportunity to encounter a culture she would not otherwise have experienced, a sentiment shared by every woman I interviewed. The other leading attraction was the monetary bonanza reaped from living on a tax-free salary with inordinately few expenses to pay. With the addition of generous vacation time, even the Navy would have a hard time competing with these medical transcriptionists' opportunities to "see the world."

As in the Navy, the work comes first. Work weeks generally contain forty-five hours spread over five and a half days; the weekend, in the Islamic culture, is on Thursday and Friday. Labor hours can expand to overtime in the case of overflow work since there are no temporary service agencies to handle a glut.

The work environment presents numerous challenges not encountered in the average American hospital. Though English is the official language, many variations abound in Saudi hospitals. Not all native speakers of English speak the same variety; the dialect of American English differs from British, Canadian, Australian, and New Zealander. Even the speech of the Northern Irish is different from that heard in the south of Ireland. Added to these different species of English are the accents of people for whom English is a second, third, or fourth language.

In the early 1980s, Saudi hospitals had American administrators and Western doctors, often trained in Great Britain, who followed a standard dictation style. Since mid-decade, however, when the oil situation changed and the Saudis' revenue dwindled, more Arab and third-world physicians have been hired. Mary Kay Loper of Panama City, Florida, counted doctors hailing from as many as thirty-two different nations at the Saudi hospital where she was assigned. Few of these doctors have Western training; those who do are usually trained in Germany. Thus, the dictation may travel through a mental maze of three or four languages before arriving in English.

Not surprisingly, the dictation in "English" is not always recognizable to American ears, and sometimes is mind-boggling without the chart on hand. One doctor reported her patient received "Bomg acetaminophen;" the transcriptionist was left to decipher the meaning as "80 mg acetaminophen." Another doctor insisted he "eksuh-MINED" his patient thoroughly. Of course, there are many doctors in the United States who speak English as a second language and have quirky pronunciations. A doctor of my acquaintance has been heard to examine a patient's "tee-roid" (thyroid) and report on how it "devva-LOPED."

In Saudi Arabia the turnover rate among physicians is currently rather high, and medical transcriptionists are not able to transcribe the same doctors long enough to master their idiosyncrasies. Raydene Boulton, CMT, of Tucson, returned from the King Faisal Specialist Hospital in Riyadh, found that the Arab doctors speak English only when necessary (almost only when dictating). Consequently, their mercilessly thick accents have few opportunities to get thinned.

The style of dictation may be far from orthodox, as well. One doctor had a "telegram" style; his habit was to say "stop" at the end of his sentences instead of "period." The poor transcriptionist had to listen to the tape five times before making sense of it. Dee Sparkes encountered a doctor at the King Fahd Armed Forces Hospital, in Jiddah, who did not like to dictate at all, possibly because his command of English was not fluent. She would take down the report in shorthand. Invariably, however, he would stop at certain words, unable to name them off the top of his head. He would recognize what he meant to say if she could name it for him. So the guessing would begin. They would go through "charades, pantomimes, and drawings" to get the dictation on paper.

Besides dealing with doctors, the transcription department itself is not immune to difficulties. Hospitals in Saudi Arabia are generally turnkey operations, i.e., the hospital is built and furnished by one company, which then turns the keys over to the managing company. The needs of management are not necessarily foreseen by the building company. This is apparent in the area of reference books. Good reference materials are not as near as the local bookstore; many transcription departments lack a decent medical library. The general rule to follow for having adequate reference books is BYOB (bring your own books).

For the supervisor, the staff members can be another challenge. Dee Sparkes supervised British, Irish, and Filipino women. Their previous training was more secretarial than transcription; their experience centered mostly on "ward notes" with few H&Ps or surgical reports. Consequently, they had to be retrained according to American standards. Lacking any formal, pre-packaged training programs, she had to make up reference reports herself, a labor-intensive task.

Dee Sparkes also found it necessary to train her staff to pay stricter attention to documentation. Since malpractice suits are not as prolific elsewhere as in the United States, scrupulous documentation had not been stressed in their earlier training.

Generally the Arabic language does not pose an obstacle to the medical transcriptionists working in Saudi Arabia. Having no direct contact with the patients, learning or not learning Arabic is not an issue. Most shopkeepers speak some English.

Problems can arise, however, when the Saudis take speaking and writing Arabic for granted, as at the military hospital where Jeanne Tucker, RRA, of Maitland, Florida, headed the medical record department in the 1980s. Her staff received sixty-three beautiful, brand new IBM Selectric typewriters—with Arabic characters and which operated right to left. There was a three-month delay for a ship to bring replacements with Western characters. On another occasion, dictating equipment requiring AC power was stocked by her hospital, which operated on DC power.

Repairs also present a problem. At a different hospital, a new loop Dictaphone system sat in a sandy warehouse. There were no Dictaphone technicians in the kingdom to service it, and the hospital had to wait six months for parts.

Despite problems and setbacks, the work itself offers a unique opportunity to learn medical terminology not commonly heard in the United States. Saudis are known to marry first cousins, resulting in unusual birth anomalies in their offspring. Diseases indigenous to the Arabian peninsula expose the medical transcriptionist to additional specialized terminology.

Of the many medical transcriptionists who obtain employment in Saudi Arabia, the lure is often the tax-free income, augmented by the virtual lack of expenses. Apart from food and clothing, all else is provided by the employer. Housing is rent-free and furnished, including linen, table settings, and cookware. The mode of housing varies from hotels or dormitories to apartments or villas. A two-bedroom apartment is the norm, shared with a roommate, although some accommodations are single or triple occupancy. Added perks include a washer and dryer and no utility bills.

Despite the difficulties or because of them, the Saudi experience has changed the lives of the women who have gone there. ''Careerwise, it made me appreciate what we have in the U.S.,'' says Dee Sparkes, also quick to add that the experience enriched her ''more as a person.'' These medical transcriptionists dared to take adventure by the hand and have returned home the better for it. We say thank you for daring; your experiences have enriched us now, too.

Medical Readings

Neurology and Neurosurgery

Part 2

by John H. Dirckx, M.D.

Infections of the brain (encephalitis) or its covering membranes (meningitis) can be life-threatening. Infecting organisms may be carried through the blood stream from elsewhere in the body or may invade the cranial cavity after head injury or from infected teeth, ears, or sinuses. **Encephalitis**, usually viral in origin, causes drowsiness, seizures, and other evidences of

neurologic impairment. Treatment is largely supportive and recovery is often complete. **Meningitis** may be viral, bacterial, or fungal. The usual symptoms of meningitis are severe headache, high fever, stiff neck, and drowsiness or stupor. Viral (aseptic) meningitis is typically benign, but bacterial meningitis due to pneumococcus, meningococcus, gonococcus, staphylococcus, or *Haemophilus influenzae* may be rapidly fatal or may lead to permanent neurologic impairment. Lumbar puncture with chemical and microbiologic examination of CSF is particularly helpful in diagnosis. Prolonged treatment with intravenous antibiotics is usually necessary.

Brain abscess is a localized accumulation of pus within the brain. The symptoms are those of an intracranial space-occupying lesion (tumor), often with fever and other evidence of infection. Prolonged antibiotic treatment may be curative, but surgical drainage of the abscess is sometimes necessary.

Tumors affecting the central nervous system may arise from nerve tissue or supporting structures, chiefly the meninges, or may metastasize (spread) to the brain from malignant tumors elsewhere in the body. Although many primary brain tumors are histologically benign, any of them can cause severe impairment or death by enlarging and compressing brain tissue. Increased intracranial pressure is a common early finding with most types of tumor. The symptoms, which may be subtle, include headache, nausea, seizures, personality change, and decline of mental function. The alert neurologist will carefully investigate these symptoms or any others suggesting the presence of a tumor within the skull. CT scans and MRI are invaluable in determining the size and location of a tumor. The treatment is usually surgical removal, but this may be difficult or impossible without damage to surrounding brain tissue. Treatment of malignant tumors of the brain or spinal cord may also include radiation and chemotherapy.

Chronic, recurrent, or severe **headaches** are a common reason for neurologic consultation. Although most headaches are due to stress, fatigue, or depression, a severe headache can be a symptom of an intracranial tumor, infection, or vascular accident, as well as of fever, metabolic disorders, and toxic conditions. **Migraine** headache is a recurrent and often disabling severe type of headache that affects as many as 15% of young women. It occurs with less frequency in men and older persons. The ultimate cause is unknown, but the mechanism of the headache is inappropriate flow of blood through intracranial vessels. The pain is typically throbbing and located in one temple. It may last many hours and be accompanied by dizziness, nausea, and blurring of vision. In many patients a warning (aura) occurs before the onset of headache, usually in the form of visual disturbances such as flashing lights or blind spots. Migraine headaches are often triggered by stress, fatigue, skipping meals, alcohol, or certain foods. The role of the neurologist in treating migraine is to rule out other causes of recurrent headache, advise the patient about triggering factors to be avoided, provide medicine to be taken at the first indication of headache in an effort to abort the attack, and often prescribe long-term prophylactic medicine to be taken regularly to prevent or mitigate headaches.

Epilepsy is a disorder of the central nervous system characterized by recurring seizures. A seizure is a temporary disturbance of brain function causing transitory impairment or loss of consciousness, local or generalized muscle twitches, jerks, or spasms, or some combination of these. Seizures are classified as either partial, due to a local disturbance of brain function, or generalized, in which the whole cerebrum is affected by an abnormal discharge of nerve impulses. A person experiencing a **partial seizure** may have numbness or twitching in one part of the body, sweating, flushing or hallucinations, with or without some transitory blunting of consciousness. A **generalized seizure** may consist of an abrupt and very brief impairment of consciousness or alertness (absence, petit mal), or complete loss of consciousness with falling and muscle rigidity followed by generalized muscular convulsions (grand mal). Other types of seizure are also recognized.

Seizures can result from any severe disease affecting the brain (CVA, tumors, infections), from head injury, or from fever, chemical poisoning, or various metabolic disorders (low blood sugar, kidney failure). However, in many persons with recurrent seizures no cause can be found, and a diagnosis of idiopathic or constitutional epilepsy is made. In this condition, the seizures usually begin before age 20. In evaluating a patient with seizures, the neurologist first tries to determine whether any treatable cause is present. Encephalography (EEG) is helpful in confirming the presence of epilepsy and in classifying the seizure disorder.

The treatment of idiopathic epilepsy consists of long-term administration of anticonvulsant medicine to prevent seizures. A number of chemically different anticonvulsants are available. The choice of drug depends on the type of epilepsy being treated, and the dose is titrated (adjusted) according to the patient's response and often also with the help of laboratory tests to determine the level of the drug in the patient's blood.

Dementia (organic brain syndrome) refers to significant impairment of mental function, particularly alertness, orientation, memory, and reasoning ability, caused by organic (physical) disease or injury rather than by mental illness (psychosis). Dementia may be due to intracranial tumors or infections, cerebral vascular disease, excessive or inappropriate drug use, and various metabolic and nutritional disorders. About two-thirds of elderly persons with dementia suffer from **Alzheimer's disease,** a progressive deterioration of mental function due to specific degenerative changes in brain cells. The cause is unknown but the condition seems to run in families.

Neurologists are often called upon to collaborate with psychiatrists, internists, and family physicians in evaluating patients with dementia. X-rays and laboratory tests may be needed to rule out treatable causes. For progressive and irreversible dementia the neurologist may prescribe medicines to control anxiety, depression, or other symptoms, and may work with caregivers, whether family members or professionals, to ensure the patient's comfort and safety and to maintain good nutrition and general health. Specific drug treatment of Alzheimer's disease has shown some promise, and research is underway to define the cause and find ways of arresting the disease.

Another important class of problem dealt with by neurologists includes various **disorders of movement**— conditions causing uncontrollable shaking, twitching, or writhing movements, sometimes accompanied by muscle rigidity, incoordination, or dementia. Tremors may occur in a variety of neurologic diseases, most of them of unknown cause.

Parkinsonism is a particularly common form of movement disorder that occurs typically after age 45 and is due to a specific biochemical imbalance in parts of the brain concerned with muscle control and coordination. A person with parkinsonism typically has shaking of one or both hands at rest, rigidity of muscles in the face, trunk, and extremities, and difficulty standing and walking. Treatment with drugs that partly correct the underlying biochemical imbalance may control symptoms but does not affect the progression of the disease.

Huntington's chorea is a familial disorder of unknown cause, characterized by chorea (twitching, jerking movements) and dementia. **Gilles de la Tourette's syndrome**, which typically first appears in childhood, causes motor tics (muscle twitches), most often affecting the facial muscles, and phonic tics (grunting, barking, or other vocal sounds). The treatment of these and most other conditions causing tremors or abnormal movements is purely symptomatic and supportive.

Multiple sclerosis is a chronic neurologic disease of highly variable symptoms, which frequently begins in early adulthood and is of unknown cause. Patches of degenerative and inflammatory changes at various sites in the brain and spinal cord, which can be demonstrated with MRI, are responsible for symptoms. Scattered muscle weakness, tingling or numbness, and visual disturbances occur in varying degrees of severity. Spontaneous remissions (periods of improvement) are common but usually temporary. In **amyotrophic lateral sclerosis**, motor cells of the spinal cord undergo degeneration for unknown reasons, with resultant weakness and wasting of muscles. As with other progressive degenerative diseases, treatment is largely symptomatic.

Myasthenia gravis is a disorder resulting from blockage of transmission of impulses from nerves to voluntary muscles. It is probably an autoimmune disorder in which antibodies are formed to the patient's own nerve receptors. Symptoms are muscle weakness, particularly affecting the eyelids and the muscles of chewing and swallowing. Weakness increases with use of the affected muscles and improves dramatically after an injection of edrophonium or neostigmine, which enhance receptivity of muscles to nerve impulses. Long-term treatment with similar medicines usually controls symptoms.

Although most of the conditions for which a neurologist is consulted affect the central nervous system, injuries and diseases of peripheral nerves constitute an important part of neurologic practice. **Neuropathy** is any disease of one or more peripheral nerves, with resultant loss of sensation, causalgia (burning pain), paresthesias (tingling or other abnormal sensations), and muscle weakness, paralysis, or wasting, in varying proportions. Electromyography and nerve conduction studies are important adjuncts in the diagnosis of peripheral neuropathies. **Mononeuropathy,** affecting a single peripheral nerve, is usually due to injury, local disease, or entrapment of the nerve at a pressure point by surrounding tissues. **Bell's palsy** is a mononeuritis affecting the facial nerve (the seventh cranial nerve) on one side. The cause is unknown. Symptoms range from mild weakness of muscles on one side of the face to complete paralysis, with inability to blink, smile, whistle, or wrinkle the forehead. Most cases resolve without lasting consequences, but some drooping or flattening of the affected side of the face may remain permanently.

Neuralgia is local pain due to abnormal stimulation of a sensory nerve by injury, local disease, exposure to cold, or, in many cases, by unknown factors. Most cases of neuralgia involve the head and face. Trigeminal neuralgia, affecting the trigeminal nerve (fifth cranial nerve), causes sudden attacks of severe, stabbing pain in the face; and glossopharyngeal neuralgia, affecting the ninth cranial nerve, causes similar pain in the throat. When medical treatment fails, these problems can sometimes be helped by neurosurgery.

Carpal tunnel syndrome, resulting from compression of the median nerve on the palmar side of the wrist, causes pain and tingling in and around the thumb, sometimes with numbness and eventual muscle wasting. This may result from injury or repetitive strain at the wrist, but the disorder is also commoner in patients with rheumatoid arthritis, thyroid disease, and diabetes. A number of nerve entrapment syndromes at other sites are recognized. Treatment is by surgical release of the trapped nerve, when a trial of rest and splinting fails to alleviate symptoms.

Polyneuropathy, affecting more than one nerve, is usually due to a generalized neurologic or systemic condition, such as diabetes mellitus, alcoholism with severe nutritional deficiency, and poisoning with industrial chemicals or certain drugs. **Guillain-Barré syndrome** is an acute polyneuropathy that often but not always follows a viral respiratory infection. The chief symptom is muscle weakness, but causalgia and numbness may also occur. Symptoms may be severe and even life-threatening, but most patients make a complete recovery. The neurologist's contribution to the care of Guillain-Barré syndrome is to make an accurate diagnosis by neurologic examination, lumbar puncture, and laboratory studies and to direct supportive and rehabilitative care until symptoms resolve.

Neurologists and neurosurgeons are consulted by other specialists for help in the diagnosis of a broad range of other injuries and diseases, including psychiatric disorders; problems with vision, hearing, and balance; chronic pain syndromes; and other conditions causing symptoms referable to the nervous system. Although many of the conditions for which neurologists and neurosurgeons are consulted are chronic, progressive, and incurable, practitioners of these specialties often achieve spectacular success in treating life-threatening diseases such as meningitis, brain abscess, and intracranial tumors and aneurysms, and in controlling such potentially disabling disorders as migraine headaches, epilepsy, and parkinsonism.

Laboratory Tests and Surgical Procedures

carotid arteriogram   An iodinated contrast dye is injected into an artery to demonstrate patency or occlusion of the carotid arteries on x-ray exam.

CSF (cerebrospinal fluid)   The fluid medium of the central nervous system (brain and spinal cord), which can be sampled by lumbar puncture (spinal tap) for chemical testing, cell counts, and culture.

EEG (electroencephalogram)   A recording of the electrical impulses of the brain which are able to be detected on the scalp by electrodes placed there. At least 21 electrodes are placed on the scalp using the International 10-20 System. An EEG is used to diagnose and classify seizure activity and may be done with the patient awake or asleep.

LP (lumbar puncture)   The use of a needle inserted between the third and fourth lumbar vertebrae to remove cerebrospinal fluid for analysis. Also called *spinal tap.*

opening pressure   A measurement of the initial pressure of the cerebrospinal fluid. Made during a lumbar puncture, using a manometer.

spinal tap   See *lumbar puncture.*

Anatomy/Medical Terminology

Drug Matching Exercise

Instructions: Match the drug category in Column A with the drug name in Column B. Note: Drug categories are used more than once.

Column A	*Column B*
A. drug for seizures	____ Sinemet
	____ Zarontin
B. drug for Parkinson's disease	____ Artane
	____ ProSom
	____ Tegretol
C. drug for insomnia	____ Cogentin
	____ Permax
	____ Dilantin
	____ levodopa
	____ Dalmane
	____ Parlodel
	____ Depakene
	____ phenytoin
	____ Symmetrel

Root Word and Suffix Matching Exercise

Combine the following root words with suffixes to form words that match the definitions below. Fill in the blanks with the medical words you construct.

Root Word	*Suffix*
meningo-	-gram
encephalo-	-oma
myelo-	-plegia
neuro-	-itis
quadri-	-opathy
para-	

A. paralysis affecting both legs

_____

B. inflammation of the brain

_____

C. disease condition of the nerves

_____

D. inflammation of a nerve

_____

E. paralysis affecting all four extremities

_____

F. inflammation of the membranes surrounding the brain

_____

G. tumor arising from the meninges

_____

H. record of a study of the spinal column using contrast medium

_____

I. disease condition of the brain

_____

Anatomy: The Spinal Cord and Nerves (Posterior View)

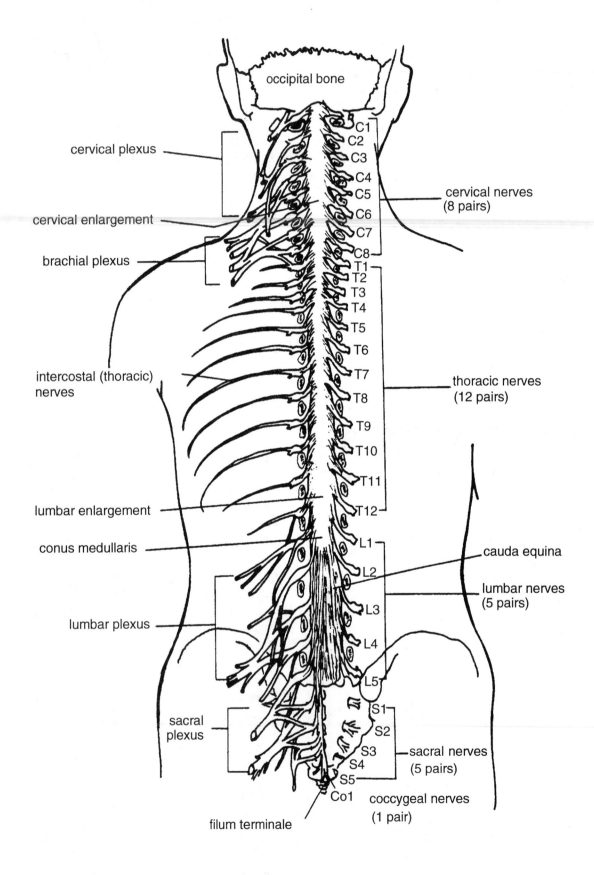

occipital bone

cervical plexus

cervical enlargement

brachial plexus

intercostal (thoracic)
nerves

lumbar enlargement

conus medullaris

lumbar plexus

sacral
plexus

filum terminale

C1
C2
C3
C4
C5
C6
C7
C8

cervical nerves
(8 pairs)

T1
T2
T3
T4
T5
T6
T7
T8
T9
T10
T11
T12

thoracic nerves
(12 pairs)

L1
L2
L3
L4
L5

cauda equina

lumbar nerves
(5 pairs)

S1
S2
S3
S4
S5
Co1

sacral nerves
(5 pairs)

coccygeal nerves
(1 pair)

Sound-alikes Exercise

Instructions: Circle the correct term from the sound-alikes in parentheses in the following sentences.

1. Following the stroke, the patient had (dysphagia, dysphasia, dysplasia), so we had to administer medicines by the intravenous route.

2. Due to the patient's (dysphagia, dysphasia, dysplasia), we were unable to get a complete history, but his neighbor said he was found on the floor in a pool of urine, (conscience, conscious) but confused.

3. (Accept, Except) for a slight weakness in the left arm, the patient had no residual symptoms of stroke.

4. This patient with Huntington's disease has continuous (corneal, choreal, chorial) movements.

5. There was blood mixed with cerebrospinal fluid coming from the basilar (cistern, system).

6. The patient's headaches were preceded by an (aura, ora) consisting of wavy, colored lines.

7. The patient was observed to have a (concussion, convulsion) by the paramedics who inserted a mouth gag to keep him from biting his tongue.

8. The parents were warned of the signs and symptoms of (concussion, convulsion) following a head injury and told if the patient became excessively sleepy to return.

9. The patient was not (conscience, conscious) when the EMTs arrived.

10. A seizure (diaphysis, diastasis, diathesis) of uncertain origin was diagnosed.

11. The ventricular (cistern, system) is well demonstrated on the MRI scan, and there appear to be no impingements or hemorrhages.

12. The (facial, fascial, faucial) sheath was picked up and the nerve examined.

13. This post-stroke patient has an ataxic (gait, gate).

14. With high fever, elevated white count, and (knuckle, nuchal) rigidity, meningitis is almost a certainty in this young male.

15. The patient was unresponsive to (noxious, nocuous) stimuli.

16. The neural (sheet, sheath) was inflamed and compressed.

17. On MRI scan of the brain, a (cellar, sellar) tumor was suspected.

18. A (fecal, thecal) injection of morphine failed to relieve the patient's intense pain.

19. A (facial, fascial, faucial) (tic, tick) involving almost continuous winking of the left eye was seen.

Word Search

Instructions: Locate and circle the neurology terms hidden in the puzzle horizontally, vertically, and diagonally, forward, and backward. A numeral in parentheses after a word indicates the number of times it can be found in the puzzle.

```
E S Y N C O P E T S X N C V A B O
J K P D O H N O R U E N R G L A I
M U O U M U R B E R E C A A L G I
A L N R A S A B V Y I J N N U N A
R L S A T W M E N G A I I G K A M
G L Z R O S O Q E R P I A L S O D
O Z O H S U C L U S Z C L I Y T E
L K P M E N P A R K I N S O N S T
E E R U Z I E S O G I Y F N C A F
Y L T Q R L M V N A L T I A O F A
M A I D E E G E R A J I F C P N O
Y R A X J Y M B R E D A O O E M A
A U R A G M J A X O N G L M L R T
Q D A E H E P I L E P S Y A A R T
```

Alzheimer	epilepsy	Parkinson
aura (2)	gait	pia
axon	ganglion	pons
brain	glioma	quadriplegic
cerebrum	gyrus	seizure
coma (2)	head	skull (2)
comatose	myelin	spinal
cranial	myelogram	stroke (2)
CVA	nerve (2)	sulcus
dura	neuron (2)	syncope (2)
EEG	paralysis	TIA (2)

Terminology Challenge

Instructions: The following terms appear in the dictation on Tape 10A. Before beginning the medical transcription practice for Lesson 20, look up the following words and phrases in a medical or English dictionary, and write out a short definition of each term.

10-channel EEG
affect (psychiatry)
alpha activity on EEG
annulotomy
annulus
aphasia
aseptically
attenuation
Babinski reflex
bursts (dysrhythmic)
cognition
cycles per second (6 to 7)
diminution
disk bulge
dura
dysrhythmic bursts
elicits
emesis
epileptic seizure
etiology
fontanelle
glioblastoma multiforme
Hastings frame
hemilaminectomy
hyaline membrane disease
hydrocephalus

hyperventilation
intraventricular
   hemorrhage
L3-4 interspace
L4-5 interspace
L5 disk
L5-S1 interspace
lamina
muscle
   sternomastoid
   trapezius
myoclonic-type
   movements
nerve root
neuropathy
palate
parkinsonian
peripheral neuropathy
phenobarbital
PIE (pulmonary inter-
   stitial emphysema)
position
   kneeling
   lateral decubitus
   prone
position sense

posthemorrhagic
posthyperventilation
   period
postural hypotension
radiation necrosis
radiation therapy
Reglan
retinopathy

rongeur
   downbiting
   pituitary
   straight
   upbiting
stance
stocking-glove
   distribution
vertebral body
VP shunt
   (ventriculoperitoneal)

Transcription Practice

After completing all the readings and exercises in Lesson 20, transcribe Tape 10A, Neurology. Use both medical and English dictionaries and your Quick-Reference Word List as resource materials for finding words. Proofread your transcribed documents carefully, listening to the dictation while you read your transcripts.

Transcribe (*NOT* retype) the same reports again without referring to your previous transcription attempt. Initially, you may need to transcribe some reports more than twice before you can produce an error-free document. Your ultimate goal is to produce an error-free document the first time.

BLOOPERS

Incorrect	**Correct**
Urologic exam disclosed orientation x 3.	Neurologic exam disclosed orientation x 3.
Apparently in pain by way of his surroundings.	Apparently in pain but aware of his surroundings.

Learning Objectives

Medical

- List the items tested in a mental status examination.
- Describe the action of categories of drugs used to treat neurosis, psychosis, and depression.
- Given a psychiatric symptom or disease, match it to its correct medical definition.
- Construct the adjectival form of common psychiatric terms.
- Define common psychiatric abbreviations.

Fundamentals

- Discuss the terminology problems encountered in psychiatric transcription.
- Distinguish between use of the psychiatric term *affect* and the general terms *effect/affect*.
- Given a medical report with errors, identify and correct the errors.

Practice

- Accurately transcribe authentic physician dictation from the specialty of psychiatry.

A Closer Look

Curve Balls

by Mary Ann and Elizabeth D'Onofrio

For the medical transcriptionist, the differences between general medical and psychiatric reports are more than mind over body. Psychiatry presents unique challenges requiring formats and knowledge not demanded by the other specialties. It is true that each specialty has its own unique tests, but psychiatry, and especially psychology, demands that the results be displayed in specific format. In addition, the content of many psychiatric reports is dotted with people and place names common to American culture, past and present.

General medical transcriptionists are ever so familiar with the ubiquitous laboratory data section of the discharge summary wherein multiple tests with their results are described by the physician dictator. These results, at least, can be transcribed in a narrative format. However, the transcriptionist who transcribes psychological evaluations must, for the most part, detail the results of the client/patient's tests in tabular form. Since each of these tests has its own unique set of parameters, varying at times in wording from psychologist to psychologist, the process of setting up the test results is tedious and laborious. A time-saving device for transcriptionists using word processors is the use of templates for this repetitive display of test data.

The unique demands of psychiatric transcription encompass challenges beyond those of format. The challenge goes so far as to leave the vocabulary of medicine altogether and enter the world of popular culture.

This is especially true in the area of chemical dependency. All medical transcriptionists are challenged to spell medications accurately, the psychiatric transcriptionist included. Transcriptionists in the field of cardiology are expected to know the correct spellings

Psychiatric Drugs: Street Names

These street drugs are drawn from *Psychiatric Words and Phrases* by Mary Ann and Elizabeth D'Onofrio (Health Professions Institute, 1990). The medical or chemical name is listed first, followed by street names.

amobarbital
  blue angels
  blue devils
  bluebirds
  blues
  Christmas trees
  double crosses
  double trouble
  greenies
  lilly
  rainbows
  tooies
amphetamine (AMT)
  A's
  bennies
  black beauties
  bumblebees
  cartwheels
  copilots
  crossroads
  double crosses
  footballs
  greenies
  hearts
  jelly beans
  peaches
  pep pills
  speed
  sugar daddys
  uppers
  whites
amyl nitrite
  amys
  pears
  poppers
  snappers
barbiturate
  barbs
  candy
  dolls
  downers
  fender bender
  goofball
  goofers
  peanuts
  sleeping pill
  yellow jacket
  yellows
butyl nitrite
  bolt
  bullet
  climax
  locker room
  rush

cannabis
  Acapulco gold
  Afghanistan black
  bhang
  dagga
  dope
  ganja
  grass
  hash
  hash oil
  hay
  joint
  kif
  Latin lettuce
  Lebanese red
  maconha
  marijuana
  Mary Jane
  Panama red
  pot
  reefer
  rope
  Salmon River Quiver
  sinsemilla
  Skunk Number 1
  smoke
  super grass
  tea
  Thai sticks
  THC
  tops
  Turkish green
  weed
cocaine
  bernies
  big C
  blow
  boy
  coke
  crack
  flake
  freebase rocks
  happy dust
  lady
  nose candy
  rock
  snow
  snowbirds
  white
cough preparations
   with codeine
  blue velvet
  Robby
  schoolboy

dextroamphetamine
  brownies
  Christmas trees
  dexies
  hearts
  wakeups
heroin
  big H
  black tar
  brown sugar
  gag
  girl
  H
  hard stuff
  horse
  junk
  mud
  skag
  smack
lysergic acid diethylamide
  acid
  blue heaven
  green dragon
  heavenly blue
  LSD
  microdot (blue or purple)
  orange sunshine
  pink wedges
  red dragon
  sandos
  strawberry hill
  sugar cubes
  white lightning
  window panes
marijuana
  Colombian
  Hawaiian
  homegrown
  Mexican
  sinsemillan
  Thai
mescaline
  barf tea
  big chief
  buttons
  cactus
  mesc
methamphetamine
  crank
  crystal
  crystal meth
  ice
  meth
  speed

methaqualone
  ludes
  sopors
morning glory seeds
  flower power
  heavenly blue
  pearly gates
morphine
  dope
  M
  Miss Emma
  morpho
  white stuff
nitrous oxide
  laughing gas
  nitrous
  whippets
opium
  Dover's powder
  licorice
  PG
pentobarbital
  nebbies
  yellow bullets
  yellow dolls
phencyclidine
  angel dust
  angel hair
  dust
  fairy dust
  hog
  killer weed
  loveboat
  lovely
  PCP
  peace pills
  zombie dust
phenobarbital
  phennies
  pheno
  purple hearts
psilocin or psilocybin
  business man's acid
  magic
  magic mushrooms
  mushroom
secobarbital
  Christmas trees
  double trouble
  pink lady; pinks
  rainbows
  red devils; reds
  seccy
  tooies

of such drugs as mexiletine and Streptase. Psychiatric transcriptionists, in turn, must know how to spell desipramine and Prozac; however, they may also be expected to spell "whippets," "tooies," or "sinsemilla." It is common for psychiatrists and psychologists to include in their dictations vernacular renderings of the illicit drugs used by certain patients. Because of regional variations and the continual coining of new slang terms on the streets, a complete universal list is impossible. (See the brief list on the following page.)

The impact of popular culture is also markedly apparent when one transcribes reports about adolescent patients. The environment in which patients live has direct influence on their personal development. And for the adolescent patient of today, the influences come predominantly from music, television, and video games. Transcriptionists working on reports in adolescent psychiatry, without children or grandchildren around to keep them "hip," would do well to have a television guide and the phone number of a local record store on hand.

In general medicine, the transcriptionist must know that when internists dictate "I and E okay," they mean "inspiration and expiration, satisfactory," not "INE-OK." The psychiatric transcriptionist, however, may encounter a physician dictating that the patient's favorite rock group is "In Excess," which is correctly spelled "INXS." The correct spelling of a rock group's name may seem frivolous, but there is a great difference between "The patient claims to listen to simple minds, and in excess, every day," and "The patient claims to listen to Simple Minds and INXS every day." Rock groups are notorious for inventing unique spellings for their names but even common names can require "expert" verification for accuracy. Paula is a common name, but when slurred by the dictator the question of gender needs to be clarified. Such was the case when the music therapist spoke of singer Paula Abdul.

Video games, too, find their way into psychiatric transcription. Only the pop-culturally aware transcriptionist will know to supply the almost silent initial "n" in "Nintendo." Even older toys like "fooseball" can present a spelling challenge. The psychiatric transcriptionist may do well to keep the phone number of a local toy store on file, too.

Child psychology provides another challenge. One projective attitude test, the so-called "magician question," requires a child to imagine himself as a magician capable of turning family members into animals; the animals he designates reveal a lot about how he perceives his family. Exposed to the multimedia environ-

ment of today, children are very sophisticated in their knowledge of unusual animals. Suddenly the medical transcriptionist becomes a zoological transcriptionist. Exotic names we encountered in dictation recently included cockatiel, peccary, and lemur. A quality thesaurus on the bookshelf provides accurate spellings.

Maps are also an excellent resource to have on hand—old as well as current. Invariably, patients were born in cities other than the city of treatment. A map or place name atlas will give the transcriptionist, in general medicine or psychiatry, accurate spellings. Psychiatric transcriptionists may find that maps of Viet Nam and Southeast Asia are especially helpful when veterans name the places where they have served.

Accurate medical reports are not only the goal of the medical transcriptionist, they are key to success in the field. The correct spellings of medications, operations, and instruments, to name a few, are of paramount importance to the verity of the legal document that is the medical report. In psychiatry and psychology, however, the pool of terminology floods over the borders of the merely medical and encompasses words and experiences from all walks of life. The challenge to the psychiatric transcriptionist is to maintain the field's high standards of accuracy in form and content by hitting the "curve balls" as well as the straight pitches.

The History and Physical Examination

by John H. Dirckx, M.D.

Review of Systems: Psychiatric. This part of the Review of Systems is often omitted from a general history and physical examination. The psychiatric history is even more intimate and sensitive, if possible, than the sexual history. A person with severe psychiatric impairment makes a most unreliable historian. For example, there is usually not much point in asking someone if he has experienced hallucinations or delusions, for these terms are used only by persons who are convinced of the unreality of the experiences. A person with even mild neurotic problems frequently resists talking about them. Hence part or all of the psychiatric history may have to be obtained from the patient's family or friends or from medical records.

At times it is hard to distinguish between psychiatric history-taking and psychiatric examination, since both make use of the same basic tool—interviewing the patient. When the patient's chief complaint is not psychiatric, inquiries about past or present mental illness or emotional disturbance are more clearly historical in intent. The interviewer asks about any prior diagnosis of mental, emotional, or nervous illness (anxiety, depression, schizophrenia, manic-depressive psychosis or bipolar disorder, alcoholism, drug addiction), and treatments used, including counseling, group therapy, drug therapy, hospitalization, and electroshock. A general notion of the subject's mental and emotional health history can be obtained by inquiring about family and marital harmony, school performance, job stability and satisfaction, social contacts, sleep pattern, drug and alcohol use, and general sense of well-being, self-esteem, and purpose in life.

The Formal Mental Status Examination. In recording the subject's general appearance at the beginning of the physical examination report, the physician usually comments briefly on his mental condition. If the patient displays psychiatric symptoms, the medical examination includes a more formal investigation of his mental status.

A thorough assessment of a patient's psychiatric condition can take weeks or months, and in a sense is never complete. The mental status examination performed in conjunction with a physical examination is a brief survey of selected aspects of the patient's mental health that can be evaluated without prolonged and intensive interviewing.

Most of the data for this kind of examination are gathered during history-taking. In addition to the basic historical interview, the examiner asks the subject questions specifically designed to test his mental status. The examiner records his findings and conclusions according to a fairly standard format. A psychiatrist or other physician with psychiatric leanings may use highly specialized, not to say extravagant, terminology. The following is a typical format for recording the results of the mental status examination.

Appearance: The examiner records any peculiarities of dress or personal grooming.

Sensorium: This refers to the subject's receptiveness and responsiveness to external stimuli. The physician judges his alertness, attention span, and ability to receive and process visual, auditory, and tactile stimuli.

Activity and behavior: Gait, posture, and general level of motor activity are assessed, and any bizarre or compulsive actions, mannerisms, or catatonic posturings are noted.

Mood: The subject's emotional state and his response to being interviewed are observed and recorded.

Thought content: The physician looks for evidence of unconventional thoughts, fantasies, phobias, hallucinations, delusions, obsessive ideas, or poverty of imagination.

Intellectual function: The physician tests the speed, coherence, and relevance of the subject's abstract reasoning by asking him to do simple mental arithmetic and to interpret proverbs such as ''Birds of a feather flock together.''

Orientation: The examiner ascertains the subject's awareness of time (time of day, day of week, date, season, year), place (state, city, exact present location), and person (who he is, identity of family or friends).

Memory: The subject's recall of recent and remote events is tested through questioning. The examiner also assesses his fund of information by asking about matters of general knowledge. (Who is President of the United States?)

Judgment: This term refers to the subject's competence or reliability in analyzing facts or situations and deriving conclusions and plans of action from them. (What would you do if you ran out of gas on the interstate?)

Insight: In psychiatry, insight means a patient's awareness that he is ill and his recognition of the nature and implications of his illness.

Orientation, memory, and judgment are often called the organic triad, because they are commonly affected in organic dementia. In addition to relatively unstructured interviewing, the subject may be given various formal, standardized tests of intelligence and personality.

Pharmacology: Psychiatric Drugs

Drugs for neurosis. The symptoms of neurosis include anxiety, anxiousness, and tension—all at a more intense level than normal—and a feeling of apprehension with vague, unsubstantiated fears. The neurotic patient, however, never experiences any loss of touch with reality.

The treatment of neurosis involves the use of **antianxiety drugs,** also known as anxiolytic agents or minor tranquilizers. The term **minor tranquilizer** is somewhat of a misnomer in that it carries the connotation that this class of drugs is somehow less effective in treating symptoms than the major tranquilizers (used to treat psychosis) or that the minor tranquilizers are only major tranquilizers given at a lower dose. In fact, minor tranquilizers are completely unrelated chemically to major tranquilizers. They are extremely effective drugs of great importance with specific therapeutic action in treating neurosis.

Benzodiazepines. The benzodiazepines are by far the most commonly prescribed drugs for the treatment of anxiety and neurosis. Examples:

> alprazolam (Xanax)
> chlordiazepoxide (Librium)
> clorazepate (Tranxene)
> diazepam (Valium)

Drugs used to treat psychosis. The symptoms of psychosis include a loss of touch with reality with resulting illusions, delusions, and hallucinations. Psychotic symptomatology may, in part, be based on an overactivity of the neurotransmitter dopamine in the brain either from overproduction of dopamine or from hypersensitivity of dopamine receptors.

The treatment of psychosis involves the use of **antipsychotic drugs**, which are also known as **major tranquilizers** or neuroleptics. These drugs block dopamine receptors in many areas of the brain including the limbic system which controls emotions. Antipsychotic drugs decrease hostility, agitation, and paranoia without causing confusion or sedation. None of the antipsychotic drugs are addictive; they are not schedule drugs.

Phenothiazine drugs for psychosis include:

> chlorpromazine (Thorazine)
> fluphenazine (Prolixin)
> thioridazine (Mellaril)
> trifluoperazine (Stelazine)
> haloperidol (Haldol)
> thiothixene (Navane)

Drugs used to treat affective disorders. The term *affect* refers to an emotional feeling or mood expressed by a patient's outward appearance. Affective disorders center on two major emotions: **depression** and mania. The depressed patient experiences insomnia, crying, lack of pleasure in any activity, loss of appetite, suicidal feelings, and feelings of helplessness, hopelessness, and worthlessness. Depression results from decreased levels of the neurotransmitters norepinephrine and serotonin in the brain. The treatment for depression involves the use of **antidepressant drugs.**

Antidepressants, or **mood-elevating drugs,** not only alleviate the symptoms of depression, they also increase mental alertness, normalize sleep patterns, help restore appetite, and decrease suicidal ideation. There are three main categories of antidepressant drugs: MAO inhibitors, tricyclic antidepressants, and tetracyclic antidepressants.

MAO inhibitors for depression. This older group of antidepressants prevents the enzyme monoamine oxidase (MAO) from breaking down the neurotransmitter norepinephrine in the brain. MAO inhibitor drugs are used infrequently due to the possibility of severe side effects. MAO inhibitors used to treat depression include:

> isocarboxazid (Marplan)
> phenelzine (Nardil)
> tranylcypromine (Parnate)

Tricyclic antidepressant drugs. The tricyclic antidepressants prolong the action of norepinephrine in the brain and correct its low levels which cause depression. The tricyclics are so named because of the triple-ring configuration of their chemical structure. The tricyclic antidepressants include:

> amitriptyline (Elavil, Endep)
> amoxapine (Asendin)
> desipramine (Norpramin)
> doxepin (Adapin, Sinequan)
> protriptyline (Vivactil)
> trimipramine (Surmontil)

Tetracyclic antidepressant drugs. Although different slightly in chemical structure, tetracyclic antidepressants have the same therapeutic effect as the tricyclic antidepressants. An example is maprotiline (Ludiomil).

Other antidepressant drugs which act to inhibit the uptake of serotonin in the brain so as to correct its low levels include trazodone (Desyrel).

The second emotion of affective disorders is that of **mania,** which is associated with increased levels of norepinephrine in the brain. The drug lithium (Eskalith, Lithobid, Lithotabs) is used exclusively to treat the symptoms of manic-depressive illness.

Case History

An alcoholic patient was admitted with delirium tremens. His doctor prescribed paraldehyde. . . . The nurse mixed the paraldehyde with orange juice in a plastic cup with a plastic spoon, not realizing that paraldehyde dissolves many plastics. As the patient was about to drink his medicine, he noticed that the cup and spoon were melting. He threw the cup down and shouted, ''I'm not taking that stuff. You're trying to kill me.''

—Michael R. Cohen, ''Medication Errors,''
Nursing 79 (October 1979, p. 56)

Anatomy/Medical Terminology

Medical Terminology Matching Exercise

Instructions: Match the term in Column A with its definition in Column B.

Column A

A. psychiatrist
B. manic-depressive
C. bulimia
D. obsession
E. psychologist
F. compulsion
G. affect
H. psychosis
I. neurosis
J. phobia

Column B

____ fear of particular objects or circumstances
____ cycles of binge eating and vomiting
____ inner feelings as expressed by facial features and voice
____ M.D. with further training in mental disorders
____ feelings of anxiety and fear
____ persistent idea that invades thought processes
____ loss of touch with reality
____ uncontrollable, repetitious act
____ also known as bipolar disease because of mood swings between two opposite poles
____ has master's degree or Ph.D. in psychology

Adjective Exercise

Adjectives are formed from nouns by adding adjectival suffixes such as *-ac, -al, -ar, -ary, -eal, -ed, -ent, -iac, -ial, -ic, -ical, -ive, -lar, -oid, -ous, -tic,* and *-tous.* Some adjectives have a different form from the noun, which may be either Latin or Greek in origin.

Instructions: Write the adjectival form of the following psychiatric words.

1. neurosis _____
2. psychosis _____
3. psychiatry _____
4. mania _____
5. compulsion _____
6. apathy _____
7. claustrophobia _____
8. paranoia _____
9. hypochondriasis _____
10. bulimia _____
11. autism _____
12. phobia _____

Abbreviations Exercise

Instructions: Define the following psychiatric abbreviations. Then memorize both abbreviations and definitions to increase your speed and accuracy in transcribing dictation from psychiatry.

ADD _____
CNS _____
IQ _____
MAO inhibitor _____
MMPI _____
SAD _____
WAIS _____
WISC _____

Drug Word Search

Instructions: Locate and circle the psychiatric terms hidden in the puzzle horizontally, vertically, and diagonally, forward and backward. A numeral following a word indicates the number of times it is found in the puzzle.

```
W  L  L  I  P  S  Y  C  H  O  S  I  S
M  C  S  D  R  U  G  I  X  L  O  E  R
C  A  D  R  O  M  V  A  L  I  U  M  E
S  Z  P  A  L  V  N  L  A  R  O  H  Z
R  O  M  I  I  A  E  V  D  A  A  N  I
T  R  A  N  X  E  N  E  R  L  I  O  L
E  P  O  A  I  A  S  E  D  L  K  F  I
N  V  F  M  N  Y  P  O  L  E  F  A  U
A  A  E  R  R  T  L  K  I  M  Y  R  Q
V  L  V  E  N  I  Z  A  R  O  H  T  N
A  I  L  I  T  H  I  U  M  D  C  E  A
N  U  J  D  T  B  L  I  V  A  L  E  R
E  M  J  K  N  A  U  Q  E  N  I  S  T
```

Ativan	MAO	psychosis
Desyrel	Mellaril	Sinequan
drug	Navane	Thorazine
Elavil	oral	tranquilizers
Etrafon	Paxipam	Tranxene
Haldol	pill	Valium (2)
lithium	Prolixin	Xanax
mania	Prozac	

Transcription Guidelines

Affect, Effect

1. The word *affect* is most often used as a verb and, as such, is pronounced as though it begins with a short *ah* sound. The accent is on the second syllable (ah fekt'). *Affect* means to change or to influence.

   The combination of narcotics affected (influenced) the patient's sensorium.

   The use of some drugs affects (changes) the effectiveness of others.

2. The verb *affect* is often accompanied by helping verbs, i.e., *was, is, shall, will, has, have*. The verb endings *-ed* and *-ing* may also be added.

   It is uncertain how the news of his terminal state will affect (influence) the patient.

3. The word *effect* is most often used as a noun. When used as a noun, it is preceded by the words *an, the, this, these,* as well as other adjectives such as *positive, good, poor.*

   It is uncertain what effect (outcome) the news of his terminal illness will have on the patient.

4. The noun *effect* is often the object of a verb. In one example below, it is not only the object of the verb *produced* but is preceded by *an adverse,* i.e., an article and an adjective. It means the outcome, result, product, sequel, or end of an action.

   The combination of drugs produced an adverse effect.
   The surgical procedure produced a good cosmetic effect.

5. Often, *effect* is used in the context of a drug's action or with names.

digitalis effect	Doppler effect
placebo effect	Tyndall effect

6. When used as a verb, *effect* is pronounced by some doctors as though it begins with a long *e* sound so that we will spell it correctly. As a verb, *effect* means to accomplish, to cause, to create, to do, or to execute in such a manner as to bring about a desired result.

   This therapy should effect a cure.
   Closure was effected (brought about) by interrupted sutures.
   This regimen effected (brought about) a reversal of the patient's symptoms.

7. In summary, *affect* is most often used as a verb; therefore, it will have verb endings (*-ed, -ing*), will be used with helping verbs (*has, is, was*), and will mean to change or influence.

   Effect is most often used as a noun and means the result or outcome of some action. It may be preceded by articles (*an, the*) and other adjectives (*this, these, good, placebo, ill, side, negative*).

8. In psychiatry, the word *affect* is commonly used as a noun, meaning an outward appearance of an inner emotion.

   The patient demonstrated a flat affect.

   Example A:
   This patient's affect has affected her ability to effect a normal relationship with others and work effectively, but has had no effect on her ability to care for herself.

   Explanation:
   This patient's *emotional state* has *changed* her ability to *achieve* or *accomplish* a normal relationship with others and work *with good results,* but has had no *result* on her ability to care for herself.

   Example B:
   The effects of transcribing difficult reports affect our affect to such an extent that we cannot effect transcription effectively.

   Explanation:
   The *results* of transcribing difficult reports *influence* our *emotional state* to such an extent that we cannot *accomplish* transcription *with good results.*

Proofreading Skills

Instructions: Circle the spelling errors in the sentences from psychiatric dictation below. Write the correct spelling in the numbered spaces opposite the text.

1 It was not unusul to expect that this	1. _unusual_
2 scizophrenic patient, given her diagnosis,	2. _____
3 would exhibit bazaar behavior.	3. _____
4	4. _____
5 The patient exhibitted the classic signs of	5. _____
6 depression: feelings of hoplessness,	6. _____
7 helplessness, and worthlessness. He also com-	7. _____
8 plains of iritability and easy fatigueability.	8. _____
9	9. _____
10 During the hospitalization, the patient's effect	10. _____
11 became more appropriate, although he still	11. _____
12 had some lose associations noted on mental	12. _____
13 status examination shortly preceeding	13. _____
14 discharge.	14. _____
15	15. _____
16 She has been on her perscription antianxiety	16. _____
17 medication, Zantac, since her last visit and	17. _____
18 reports that her symptoms have grately	18. _____
19 improved.	19. _____
20	20. _____
21 The patient was neetly groomed but exhibitted	21. _____
22 a blank, empty stair and masklike feces.	22. _____
23	23. _____
24 Today, for the first time, th patient	24. _____
25 demonstrated some insite by admiting that his	25. _____
26 beleifs may be dellusional in nature, although	26. _____
27 his overall judgment remains questionable.	27. _____
28	28. _____
29 DIAGNOSIS: Access I: Paronoia, chronic,	29. _____
30 severe, manifested by persistant fixed	30. _____
31 dellusions.	31. _____
32	32. _____
33 This intervenous drug abuser has a passed	33. _____
34 psychiatric history of illusions of grandeur,	34. _____
35 the history of which is well-detailed from past	35. _____
36 admissions.	36. _____
37	37. _____
38 He seems cooperative but with a degree of	38. _____
39 suspisiousness which appears to underly all his	39. _____
40 behavior.	40. _____
41	41. _____
42 HABITS: Denies the use of elicit drugs but	42. _____
43 does admit to smoking four packs of cigar-	43. _____
44 retes daily.	44. _____

Transcription Tips

1. Do not confuse the abbreviation *SAD* (seasonal affective disorder) with the emotion of *sadness*.

2. Do not confuse *allusion* (an indirect reference to something) and *illusion* (an unreal or misleading image or perception).

   The patient made frequent allusions to childhood molestation by her father.
   He made allusion to a history of some kind of tropical disease.

   The patient was suffering from the illusion that there were insects crawling over him.
   The patient suffered from illusions of being weightless and transparent.

3. The antidepressant drug Asendin allows patients to ascend from the depths of depression; however, note that the spelling of Asendin does not include the *c* in *ascend*.

4. There are many words in this medical specialty that begin with a silent *p*: psychiatry, psychiatrist, psychology, psychologist, psychoanalysis, psychogenic, psychomotor, psychoneurosis.

5. Notice the difference in pronunciation between the following pairs:

   psy **chi'** a try, psy'chi **at'**ric
   psy **chol'**o gy, psy cho **log'**i cal

6. Spell out the slang word *psych* as either *psychiatric* (adjective) or *psychiatry* (noun) in reports. Select the meaning that is appropriate for the context of the report.

7. A common expression in psychiatry is "oriented in 3 spheres," meaning the patient is oriented to time, person, and place. It is the same as "oriented x 3" (pronounced "oriented times 3").

8. The chief complaint in a psychiatric history is often quoted in the first person.

   CHIEF COMPLAINT:
   "I'm here because I can't stop crying."

Terminology Challenge

Instructions: The following terms appear in the dictation on Tape 10B. Look up each word or phrase in a medical or English dictionary, and write out a short definition of each term.

adjunct	Navane
adjustment disorder	neuroleptic medication
Axis I, II, III, IV, V	neuropraxic
bipolar affective	obtunded
disorder	PTCA (percutaneous
blunt trauma	transluminal coronary
clavicle	angiography
compliant	post-angioplasty
disoriented	psychogenic amnesia
flight of ideas	psychosocial
hallucinating	semi-comatose
hypoperfusion	stressors
ICU	subdural hematoma
illicit	suicidal ideation
incoordination	tibial plateau
intellectual functioning	tricyclic antidepressant
lithium	valproate
loose associations	valproic acid
manic phase	venous thrombosis

Sample Reports

Sample psychiatry reports appear on the following pages.

Transcription Practice

After completing all the readings and exercises in Lesson 21, transcribe Tape 10B, Psychiatry. Use both medical and English dictionaries and your Quick-Reference Word List as resource materials for finding words. Proofread your transcribed documents carefully, listening to the dictation while you read your transcripts.

Transcribe (*NOT* retype) the same reports again without referring to your previous transcription attempt.

NAME: HILDA SCHOPENHAUER   #010347

DATE OF ADMISSION: May 1, 1992

DATE OF DISCHARGE: May 14, 1992

CHIEF COMPLAINT: The patient was transferred from the emergency department where she was treated after deliberate suicide attempt on multiple medications.

HISTORY OF PRESENT PSYCHIATRIC ILLNESS: This is the first acute psychiatric hospitalization for this 45-year-old divorced white female, who was admitted to the locked unit on an involuntary commitment status for treatment of depression. The patient attempted suicide by taking an overdose of Asendin, lithium, Xanax, Elavil, and Trilafon. The patient was admitted with the following diagnoses: (1) Major depression with possible psychotic features. (2) Paranoid personality features. (3) Rule out subclinical dementia.

HOSPITAL COURSE: The patient was initially admitted to the locked psychiatric unit on May 1 and was started on Trilafon 8 mg p.o. at bedtime, Elavil 2 mg p.o. at bedtime, and Ativan 1 mg p.o. h.s. p.r.n. insomnia. The patient received regular individual psychotherapy and various group psychotherapies that were available on the unit. After several days of stabilization in the locked psychiatric unit, she was transferred to the acute adult psychiatric unit where the psychiatric treatment continued. The patient was seen in consultation by her family physician, Dr. Jeckel, and Dr. Hyde, a neurologist, as described above. Since the patient continued to complain of sleep difficulties, the dose of Elavil was increased to 75 mg which she tolerated without any side effects. The patient was started on Zoloft on May 9, which she tolerated without side effects during her hospital stay. The dosage of Elavil was further increased to 100 mg p.o. at bedtime on May 10. The patient remained quite depressed, tearful, anxious, and insecure during her hospitalization, especially during the first five days. The patient was allowed to hold individual therapy sessions with her outpatient psychotherapist during the last 2 to 3 days of her hospitalization. Since the patient remained quite anxious, she was started on Librium 5 mg p.o. daily a.m. on May 11. The patient was cooperative and compliant with all therapeutic assignments and expectations. She actively participated in individual and group therapy sessions and was able to bring up conflictual issues such as anger, dependency, and poor self-esteem and was able to begin to deal with these issues effectively. The patient successfully completed the treatment program and was discharged on May 14.

Evaluation prior to discharge revealed that the patient did not have any acute suicidal ideation, intent, or plan. Her mood at the time of discharge was significantly less depressed, with appropriate affect. She denied any feelings of hopelessness or helplessness. The patient was

(Continued on page 2)

DISCHARGE SUMMARY   Page 1 of 2

NAME: HILDA SCHOPENHAUER   #010347   Page 2 of 2

discharged with prescriptions for Eskalith CR 450 mg p.o. daily, dispense 20; Ogen 1.25 mg p.o. at bedtime, dispense 20; Synthroid 0.1 mg p.o. daily, dispense 20; Trilafon 4 mg p.o. at bedtime, dispense 20; Elavil 100 mg p.o. at bedtime, dispense 20; Zoloft 50 mg p.o. daily, dispense 20; Librium 5 mg p.o. a.m., dispense 20; and Bentyl 20 mg p.o. a.m., dispense 20, without refill. The patient had an appointment at the clinic the following day for outpatient follow-up. She was also strongly advised to obtain medical follow-up by her family medical doctor after discharge.

DISCHARGE DIAGNOSES:
1. Major depression, severe, single episode.
2. Mixed personality disorder with schizoid, hostile-dependent, and passive-aggressive features.

SF:hpi   DISCHARGE SUMMARY   SIDNEY FROID, M.D.
D: 5/15/92
T: 5/16/92

June 25, 1992

Department of Social Services
Disability Evaluation Division
1992 Golden Gate Blvd., Suite 9
San Francisco, CA 94132

                    Re: Rathany Yi   #123-45-6789

Dear Staff:

Thank you for referring to me the case of Ms. Yi for psychiatric evaluation.

The patient was examined in psychiatric consultation on June 22, with the aid of an interpreter. No physical examination was given. No psychological testing was given. All past medical records provided were noted and reviewed.

HISTORY OF PRESENT ILLNESS: Ms. Yi is a 44-year-old Cambodian refugee. She lives in an apartment with her husband and three children. She describes feeling sick all the time, too weak and tired, dizzy and depressed, to do anything except "rest." Currently she is taking a combination of five different medications under the care of two different physicians. She takes Theo-Dur for relief of asthma-like symptoms, analgesics, decongestants, and two different forms of tricyclic antidepressants. She feels that the medications are helping her. She is not receiving any formal psychiatric treatment with or without medication.

MENTAL EXAMINATION: The patient is a clean, neatly dressed, well groomed, western-style female. She understands English and responds to questions before they are translated. There is no evidence of any ambulatory difficulties or speech impediments. There is no evidence of history of alcoholism or illicit drug use. She is oriented to time, place, persons, and events. There is no evidence of any delusions or hallucinations at the present time and no history of such in the past. There is no evidence of any paranoia such as feelings of being persecuted or plotted against. Thought content is generally well organized, coherent, and relevant without flight of ideas or loose associations.

Depression is manifested by occasional crying periods usually occurring every other day. There is fitful sleep. There are occasional nightmares. There is no suicidal ideation or history of any suicidal attempts. Energy level is described as poor with description of fatigue with minimal exertion.

Memory for recent and remote events she feels is impaired. She cannot recall her social security number. She can recall her address and phone number. She can do simple arithmetic such as addition and subtraction between the sums of 1 and 10. General information and knowledge appear to be average.

Re: Rathany Yi   #123-45-6789   Page 2   June 25, 1992

It is my medical opinion that at Ms. Yi's current level of daily functioning she has minimal difficulty in relating to others. In appearance, she seems to have the ability to care for her personal needs. How much her interests, habits, and daily activities are constricted as a result of mental impairments is difficult to assess because it is my medical opinion that this represents a factitious disorder.

DIAGNOSIS:

AXIS I: Factitious disorder, not otherwise specified.
            Rule out post-traumatic stress disorder.
AXIS II: Diagnosis deferred.
AXIS III: No known documented physical illness.
AXIS IV: Degree of psychosocial stressors cannot be evaluated.
AXIS V: Highest level of adaptive functioning cannot be evaluated because of the factitious disorder.

It is my medical opinion that Ms. Yi's impairments regarding her ability to carry out work-related activities cannot be assessed because of the factitious disorder.

Very truly yours,

SIDNEY FROID, M.D.

SF:hpi

Lesson 22. Pathology

Learning Objectives

Medical

- List the parts of an autopsy report.
- List the parts of a pathology report.
- Describe the steps in performing an autopsy.
- Given a pathology term, match it to its correct medical definition.

Fundamentals

- Discuss how to prepare for a job interview.
- Write a letter of application and your resumé.

Practice

- Accurately transcribe authentic physician dictation from the specialty of pathology.

A Closer Look

Getting a Job

by Ellen Drake, CMT

Plan ahead. If you're like most students, you've been thinking about the job you want since your first days as a student, how much you're going to make, and how you're going to spend all that money. You probably have also been planning ahead and preparing your resumé, practicing for interviews, and learning all that you can so that you can make the best impression possible on a potential employer and live up to that impression.

Maybe you're not that well prepared, but it is foolish to wait until you have a certificate or diploma in hand to think about applying for a job. If you want to work as a medical transcriptionist in a local clinic, physician office, or hospital, you should be participating in the local professional association activities and getting to know MTs and supervisors.

If your school does not plan field trips to various hospitals and clinics, you may try to call transcription supervisors and ask if they have time to show you around their department. If working for a doctor's office appeals to you, talk to a few physician office transcriptionists and ask them for advice. Follow up with a handwritten, personal thank you note (not a preprinted card).

You may hear conflicting stories and sometimes negative comments about job openings, but don't be discouraged. The need for medical transcriptionists is well documented throughout the country. Even the want ads in the newspapers don't tell the whole story because many job openings are only periodically advertised or not advertised at all. The employers who need qualified transcriptionists often choose not to advertise because of the large number of unqualified applicants who respond or the fact that they pay a lot for the ads with no results.

322

Be aware that opportunities for transcription jobs are numerous and varied. Besides hospitals and doctors' offices, those needing qualified MTs include clinics, HMOs, free-standing surgical and radiology centers. laboratories, medical transcription services, nursing homes and visiting nurse associations, physical therapy centers, psychologists, podiatrists, chiropractors, and insurance companies. Even some dentists and veterinarians are now hiring transcriptionists.

One of the statements students often encounter is "I hire only experienced transcriptionists." This can be very discouraging. If every employer hires only experienced workers, how does one get experience? If your school offers work experience through internships, externships, or practicums as part of the medical transcription program, these usually improve your employability (and should be listed on your resumé under the heading "Experience").

If a school-sponsored work experience is not provided, you may want to create your own trainee position by agreeing to work in an office for two to four weeks at no charge, giving a potential employer a no-risk opportunity to see that your skills are sufficient for the job. Yes, you need to pay bills and eat, but sometimes it's necessary to look at the long-term benefits of just a short time more of sacrifice.

There are many sources of information to help you in preparing a resumé, writing an application letter, and putting your best foot forward in an interview. Your school may have classes to help you. The counseling office or learning/tutoring center at your school may be able to help. The library has numerous references, and even some student dictionaries give advice in the appendix on preparing resumés.

Application letters. Application letters are written to accompany resumés, indicate the job you want, highlight your strengths, and state your availability for an interview. They should be only a page long, no more. If you are sending your resumé to the Human Resources Department (formerly Personnel) of a large clinic or hospital, you may want to send a copy to the transcription supervisor, or at the very least, telephone to say that you have sent your resumé to the Human Resources Department. Be sure to proofread your letter and resumé carefully. In the area of transcription, quality is all-important, and many supervisors would look no further than the first error before discarding your application.

Resumés. The purpose of your resumé is to persuade an employer to interview you. It must look professional and present your qualifications in the best possible manner. It should be specific for the position for which you are applying. A resumé should be limited to one page if possible and should contain the following categories of information:

1. Personal data: Name, address, telephone number. Age and marital status are not included.

2. Educational background: Include name of schools, degrees, areas of special training, academic awards. You might also mention the medical specialties covered in your training program and that the dictation you transcribed was actual physician dictation (not reports read by actors or other readers).

3. Work experience: If work experience is unrelated to the position applied for, explain how the experience you've gained in the jobs you've held can be applied to the position you are seeking. Include any internship or practicum experience, and give dates.

4. References: Just list names and addresses; don't include actual letters at this point. Take the letters of recommendation to your interview. Be sure that you have contacted each of your references to be sure it is okay for you to list them. You do not want to list anyone who may give you a noncommittal or even negative recommendation.

5. Professional affiliations: Be sure to include professional association membership on the national, state/regional, and local level, any offices held, awards, and published works.

Portfolio. Some students create a portfolio to carry to an interview. A portfolio might include letters of reference and samples of your work. Be sure your work samples are of the highest quality and there is no patient/facility/physician identifiable information on any reports. It may also include copies of your certificate or diploma and awards, certificates of attendance at professional meetings, a more extensive description of the transcription you've done, and copies of any evaluations your instructor or work experience supervisors may have given.

Sample Resumé

Susan Bright
210 State Street
Orlando, FL 32820
(407) 555-9999

Education   Florida Community College, graduated 1993. Certificate in Medical Transcription. Other electives include Coding 1 and 2, Medical Law, and computer courses in word processing, dBase, spreadsheets, and desktop publishing.

Experience   Student Assistant to Dean of Vocational Education. Florida Community College, August 1992 to August 1993. Answered phone, typed correspondence, did general filing.

Medical Transcription Intern. E. W. Jones, M.D., Orlando. August 1993. Transcribed dictated reports and correspondence, scheduled surgery, coded and filed insurance reports for prominent orthopedist.

Medical Transcription Intern. Community Hospital, Health Information Management. July 1993. Transcribed dictated histories and physicals, clinical summaries, and operative reports from all specialties and staff physicians. Used WordPerfect 6.0 and became familiar with digital dictation and management system.

References   Jane Emeritus, CMT, Medical Transcription Program Director, Florida Community College, Sanford, FL 32771. Phone (407) 333-2456.

E. W. Jones, M.D., 2013 Main St., Orlando, FL 32820. Phone (407) 222-2456.

Joan Flagg, RRA, HIM Director, Community Hospital, Sanford, FL 32771. Phone (407) 444-2456.

Professional Affiliation Honors and Awards   *Student Member,* American Association for Medical Transcription, Florida Association for Medical Transcription, Central Florida AAMT Chapter, and Business/Vocational Students of America. *Awards:* Medical Transcription Scholarship from Central Florida AAMT Chapter, Florida Vocational Honor Student Society award, and Outstanding Vocational Student award from Florida Community College. *Publications:* "Origins of Cancer—Genetic or Virus," *The Communicator,* February 1993.

Sample Application Letter

September 13, 1993

Sandra Comp, CMT, CMA-A
Transcription Supervisor
Sunshine Medical Clinic
32 South First Street
Orlando, FL 32801

Dear Ms. Comp:

I saw your advertisement in the *Florida Sentinel* for a Medical Transcriptionist I, and I hope that you will consider me for the position.

You may recall that I met you when our class toured the medical clinic last April. I was very impressed with your facilities, equipment, and the efficiency with which your employees worked. I decided then that Sunshine Medical Clinic would be a great place to work.

You no doubt are already aware of the quality of the transcription program at Florida Community College. You will see from my resumé that I was one of the top students in the program. My typing speed is 95 words per minute copy typing, 80 words per minute on dictation. My grade point average is 3.90.

I am available for an interview at your convenience and look forward to speaking with you.

Sincerely yours,

Susan Bright
210 State Street
Orlando, FL 32820
(407) 555-9999

Medical Readings

Introduction to Pathology

Pathology is the branch of medicine that studies the structural and functional changes produced in the living body by injury or disease. Pathology is divided into several subspecialties, and the branch of pathology which involves the majority of medical transcriptionists is **cellular pathology.**

Cellular pathology is the study of organic tissue, and the cellular pathologist is a physician who specializes in the study of organic tissue. Using naked-eye (gross) observations and observations with a microscope, the pathologist can determine if structural or functional changes have occurred within cells, indicating a disease process.

An autopsy is the examination of a body after death (postmortem examination). An autopsy consists of detailed visual observations of external body tissues and internal organs, and microscopic analyses of the internal organs and structures following tissue dissection.

When a surgical specimen or a body is received by the pathologist, the gross examination is done first. Gross specimens are described by size, color, texture, and appearance. After a gross examination has been performed, the pathologist takes small samples of representative tissue (referred to as sections) and makes slides from the tissue for microscopic analysis. These slides are usually ready for viewing the following day. By examining these tissue sections through the microscope, the pathologist can perform a detailed cell structure analysis to determine the presence or absence of abnormalities.

In addition to analyzing gross and microscopic specimens, the pathologist is frequently called on to perform a *frozen section.* The pathologist receives a tissue specimen that requires an immediate microscopic diagnosis. The pathologist quick-freezes the specimen, cuts it, stains it, analyzes it under a microscope, and renders a *frozen section* diagnosis. Because a specimen processed in this manner is not satisfactory for detailed cell analysis, *permanent* sections are taken as well for routine microscopic examination.

The autopsy report. A gross autopsy report will typically include an external examination, an internal examination, a summary of findings, and one or more provisional diagnoses. Some pathologists also include a clinical history.

The external examination includes a systematic description of the decedent by body system, noting the presence or absence of clothing; the condition of eyes, teeth, skin, and appendages; the degree of decompositional change; the presence or absence of scars, wounds, or obvious trauma; and palpation of the usual anatomic landmarks.

The internal examination includes a detailed gross examination of all body cavities. The body is usually opened through a Y-shaped incision (literally in the shape of a Y), and the findings are described categorically by body system. These findings include a description of the endocrine, respiratory, cardiovascular, gastrointestinal, urogenital, and central nervous systems in their unaltered state; and a description of specific organs that have been removed for measurement and closer examination, including the lungs, heart, liver, spleen, pancreas, kidneys, and brain.

The results of available laboratory tests (for example, screening tests for drugs and alcohol) are often reported at the conclusion of the autopsy report, as are the provisional (tentative) and/or clinical diagnosis and cause of death, if determined. Additionally, tissue specimens taken for microscopic examination may be listed.

The microscopic autopsy is similar to the microscopic description of a surgical specimen. Using a microscope, the pathologist examines representative tissue specimens taken during the gross autopsy examination. A final pathologic diagnosis is then rendered.

Not included in student practice transcripts but encountered on the job is identifying patient information. Each report will have a preprinted or designated area for the patient's name, hospital number, pathology number, attending physician, and often the date of birth and/or age. Autopsy reports will also include the date and time (or estimated time) of death, as well as the date and time the autopsy was performed. The pathologist's name is typed at the bottom of each report, with a space above the name for the pathologist's signature.

The pathology report. The pathology report usually consists of three parts: the gross description, the microscopic description, and the diagnosis.

In most settings, the pathologist dictates several cases consisting of only gross specimens. The gross descriptions are transcribed and the pathologist reviews them for accuracy. When the microscopic descriptions have been dictated, the transcriptionist carefully matches each document with the appropriate patient and specimen, transcribing each microscopic description on the page of the corresponding gross description.

The tissue diagnosis should be dictated at the same time as the microscopic description. Some specimens (teeth, for example) do not require a microscopic diagnosis, and the dictation will consist only of a gross description and diagnosis.

Although some pathologists prefer to dictate their findings after the examination has taken place, many dictate as they perform the exam. A microphone, rigged to a headset or suspended from the ceiling, is remotely attached to dictation equipment, and a foot pedal controls the forward and reverse motion of the tape. This arrangement leaves the dictator's hands free to perform the exam while simultaneously operating the dictation equipment.

Laboratory Medicine: Anatomic and Clinical Pathology

by John H. Dirckx, M.D.

Pathology is a diagnostic science. Although a pathologist's findings and conclusions may strongly influence the course of treatment chosen for a patient, pathologists do not prescribe medicine or perform surgery. Their chief concern is to supply diagnostic information to the treating physician. Moreover, they make no attempt to assess symptoms such as pain, itching, or nausea, but rather confine their attention to those features of disease that can be objectively observed and perhaps even measured.

This emphasis by the pathologist on objective interpretation is reflected in a dual signification for many everyday diagnostic terms. For example, the clinician diagnoses pneumonitis (inflammation of the lung) on the basis of clinical symptoms—fever, chills, cough productive of purulent sputum, and chest pain—and of physical findings such as characteristic sounds heard through a stethoscope. Pathologists diagnose pneumonitis only when they have seen gross and microscopic evidence of inflammation in lung tissue—something no one is likely to do as long as the patient is alive.

History of pathology. The historical roots of pathology lie in the dim past when man first speculated about the causes of disease. Primitive peoples with little insight into the workings of nature are apt to attribute disease to evil spirits, divine vengeance, or witchcraft. Our remote ancestors entertained such beliefs, and members of some undeveloped cultures entertain them today.

The Greek physician Hippocrates (460-377 BC) is honored as the father of medicine because he argued that disease is a purely natural phenomenon, subject to rational explanation and amenable to rational treatment. The doctrines of Hippocrates, as modified and augmented by Galen (AD 129-199), dominated Western medical thought until the beginning of the modern scientific era.

According to Hippocratic medicine, health depends on a proper balance of four bodily "humors" (blood, phlegm, yellow bile, and black bile), and disease results when there is an excess of one or more of these with respect to the others. This abortive attempt to formulate reasons for the changes that take place when a person gets sick became the basis for a system of therapeutics that relied heavily on phlebotomy (bloodletting) and the administration of violent emetics and cathartics to rid the body of excessive or "peccant" humors.

Developments in anatomy, chemistry, and particularly microscopy during the eighteenth century led to a revolution in pathologic thinking. The old Hippocratic-Galenic theories were rejected in favor of a rigorously scientific pathology based on correlation of symptoms and physical findings with gross and microscopic changes detected on postmortem exam. The pioneer of this new anatomic pathology was an Italian physician and anatomist, Giovanni Battista Morgagni (1682-1771), whose epoch-making work, *The Seats and Causes of Disease,* was published in 1761. The German pathologist Rudolf Virchow (1821-1902) carried the science further by explaining disease in terms of changes in the behavior and interrelations of cells. His *Cellular Pathology* was published in 1858.

It was also during the nineteenth century that the French chemist Louis Pasteur (1822-1895) and the German physician Robert Koch (1843-1910) demonstrated conclusively that some diseases are caused by microorganisms that multiply in the body, produce toxic wastes capable of interfering with normal functions, and induce similar disease on being transmitted to healthy persons.

One of Virchow's most memorable contributions to modern pathologic thinking was his statement, "Disease is life under altered conditions." Although even today we find it hard not to think of a disease as a "thing" that someone "has," disease is merely an abstraction—a state, quality, or condition somehow different from that indefinable state, quality, or condition we call "health." The major premise of pathology is that specific causes of disease are consistently associated with specific changes in bodily structure and function. Often a further premise is that the specimen of blood, urine, or tissue submitted to pathologic study is representative of what remains in the patient's body.

Changes in form and structure are the province of the anatomic pathologist, while changes in function or activity, as observed or measured through laboratory study of blood, urine, and other body fluids, are the province of the clinical pathologist. The distinction is far from absolute, for each branch of pathology constantly makes use of the data and conclusions of the other. In each branch, a thorough familiarity with what is normal—that is, an appreciation of the full range of variations in form or function that are compatible with health—must precede any attempt to identify abnormality.

The diagnostic process. In performing a gross examination of a tissue specimen, the anatomic pathologist looks for departures from expected color, size, shape, surface texture, internal consistency, and homogeneity, as well as for any tumors, cysts, hemorrhage, exudate, tissue death, scarring, or abnormal deposition of materials such as fat or calcium. In examining microscopic sections of tissue he observes the type, size, shape, number, and distribution of cells present, the configuration and staining properties of their nuclei, cytoplasmic granules, vacuoles, or deposits, the type and distribution of intercellular material such as connective-tissue fibers, extravasated blood, fibrinous or other exudates, and any variations from expected tissue architecture.

Arriving at a pathologic diagnosis is not simply a question of recognizing certain patterns that are characteristic of certain diseases. This visual recognition is only the starting point for an analysis of all available data leading to a diagnostic formulation that includes, when possible, the cause of the disorder in this particular patient, its chronology and degree or extent, and its relation to other abnormal conditions, past and present. In examining tissue from a living patient, the pathologist regards the specimen not as a static product of past events but rather as a momentary glimpse of a dynamic process that is still going on.

The diagnosis may be purely local, referring only to the specimen submitted—for example, a basal cell carcinoma of the cheek, completely excised and contained in its entirety in the surgical specimen submitted. On the other hand, assessment of a small piece of tissue may enable the pathologist to diagnose a widespread or systemic condition. For example, certain findings in a lymph node may indicate a malignant process affecting the entire lymphatic system, and certain

changes in the kidney may point to a diagnosis of diabetes. More than once, an astute pathologist has diagnosed measles before the rash appeared by finding Warthin-Finkeldey giant cells in an appendectomy specimen.

General pathology is concerned with the investigation and description of classes or patterns of abnormal changes in tissues, regardless of the specific organ or region in which the tissue is located.

The scope and divisions of pathology. First, pathology is one of the principal basic sciences, along with anatomy, biochemistry, physiology, and pharmacology, learned during the preclinical years of medical school. Physicians' approach to the evaluation, diagnosis, and treatment of a patient is conditioned more or less strongly by their fund of knowledge regarding the effects wrought by specific diseases on the structure and function of specific organs and tissues.

Second, in their efforts to learn the nature, cause, and extent of disease in a particular patient, and also to assess the effects of treatment, physicians may subject various tissues, fluids, or other materials removed from the patient's body to pathologic examination. Tests of blood and urine are part of any thorough diagnostic evaluation. Organs and tissues removed during surgical procedures are routinely submitted to a pathologist for gross and microscopic study. The information obtained from this study helps to confirm the preoperative diagnosis and, in cases of malignancy, to determine the extent of disease and the adequacy of surgical removal.

A third application of pathology to practical medicine occurs when an autopsy is performed to discover the cause of the patient's death and to correlate the medical history with postmortem findings. Besides providing data for official certification of the cause of death, autopsy findings may have great legal importance—for example, in a case of suspected homicide. In addition, information about the cause of death and the precise nature of the patient's disease contributes to the unending learning process of the treating physician and of other health professionals who attend the autopsy as an educational experience.

Under ordinary circumstances, autopsies and pathologic examinations of tissue specimens are performed by pathologists—physicians with postdoctoral training and certification by the American Board of Pathology. The pathologist's examination of specimens is not limited to naked-eye inspection but also includes microscopic examination and perhaps chemical or other testing. For this reason, pathology is a laboratory-based specialty, and the majority of pathologists perform at least a part of their professional activities in hospitals.

The practice of pathology is divided into three principal branches. **Anatomic pathology** is concerned with the gross and microscopic changes brought about in living human tissues by disease. **Clinical pathology** refers to the laboratory examination of bodily fluids and waste products such as blood, spinal fluid, urine, and feces. **Forensic pathology** involves the application of knowledge comprised by the other two branches to certain issues in both civil and criminal law. The practice of forensic pathology is largely confined to official settings. The standard pathology residency lasts four years, the training time being variously divided between anatomic and clinical pathology. Pathologists who serve as medical examiners, coroners, or forensic consultants usually have additional training in forensic pathology.

Much of the day-by-day work in clinical pathology is done by medical technologists. These are specially trained nonphysicians who, under the supervision of a pathologist, perform routine laboratory examinations of blood, urine, and other fluids, and prepare tissue specimens for microscopic examination by a pathologist.

Certain terms related to anatomic pathology deserve clarification here. **Histology** is a division of anatomy concerned with the microscopic study of tissues. **Microscopic anatomy** applies the materials and methods of histology to specific organs and bodily structures. **Cytology** is the study of cells. **Histopathology** refers to the study of microscopic changes in tissue induced by disease or injury. **Histochemistry** is a specialized field in which chemical properties and reactions of tissues are observed microscopically. **Electron microscopy** is the study of specimens with an electron microscope, which uses a stream of electrons instead of a beam of visible light and allows much greater magnification than the light microscope used for routine laboratory work.

In practice, the term **histology** is often applied to the whole range of laboratory techniques used in preparing slides of tissue specimens for microscopic study by a pathologist. **Cytology** is often used in the narrow sense of a study of cells that have been detached from a surface for microscopic study, as in a Pap smear.

The pathologist's report of an autopsy or of examination of a tissue specimen is customarily dictated for subsequent transcription. This is in keeping with the usual practice of preserving permanent medical records in typewritten form. Typed records are more legible and more suitable for photocopying and microfilming than handwritten records and generally take up less space. In reporting the findings, a pathologist ordinarily describes not only the abnormal features of the specimen but also identifying anatomic characteristics, gross and microscopic. This practice not only serves to document the thoroughness of his assessment, but also is necessary for a complete diagnostic appraisal of the specimen.

Suppose, for example, that a surgeon submits a specimen for pathologic study which he believes to be a mesenteric lymph node but which is in fact just a mass of fat and connective tissue. If the pathologist merely states that the specimen contains no malignant cells or other signs of abnormality, without making it clear that it is not a lymph node, his report could seriously mislead the surgeon in his further management of the case.

Having described his gross and microscopic findings, the pathologist usually records a diagnosis or diagnostic impression, summarizing and coordinating those findings in the light of his specialized knowledge and experience. The diagnoses listed at the end of an autopsy report may number ten, twenty, or more. The diagnoses may be accompanied by code numbers referring to some standard system of disease nomenclature. In a case of malignancy, the pathologist's diagnosis will often include an estimate of the extent of the malignant process according to a standard grading or staging system.

The Autopsy. The autopsy, necropsy, or postmortem examination (sometimes called simply a "post") is the pathologic examination par excellence. During an autopsy, every part of the body can be opened and exhaustively studied, and any organ or tissue can be removed as necessary for processing and microscopic evaluation. Fluids and other materials are readily collected for culturing, chemical testing, and other clinical pathologic studies.

In nearly every case, the chief reason for doing an autopsy is to determine as precisely as possible the cause of death. It may already be known with a fair degree of certainty on clinical grounds that death was due, for example, to myocardial infarction or to irreversible brain damage sustained in an automobile accident. But an autopsy provides objective anatomic evidence to confirm the clinical diagnosis and to show the exact pathophysiologic mechanism of death.

Sometimes two life-threatening conditions are both present at the time of death—for example, severe pneumonitis and meningitis, both due to pneumococcus. The autopsy may supply information as to which condition actually proved lethal. Occasionally the autopsy discloses an unsuspected cause of death—for example, fatal hemorrhage from a peptic ulcer in a patient under treatment for acute myocardial infarction.

An exhaustive search for the cause of death may seem like misplaced effort, since no amount of information generated by an autopsy can bring the patient back to life. But the attempt to secure full, detailed, accurate information about the cause of death is not a mere academic exercise. In every jurisdiction in the United States, a death certificate listing the cause of death must be signed by a physician and filed with the authorities before a dead body may be embalmed and buried or cremated. Although by no means all deaths are investigated by autopsy, certification of the cause of death is more likely to be accurate and complete in those that are. The validity of public health statistics compiled from data entered on death certificates depends on the caution, diligence, and thoroughness with which the certifying physicians investigated the cause of death.

In certain cases (homicide, suicide, fatal accident, death due to poison or drug overdose, and others), the law requires that an autopsy be performed by or under the auspices of a coroner or medical examiner. In addition, an autopsy may be ordered by legal authorities when a person dies during the first 24 hours after hospital admission or after surgery, or when a person with no known health problems dies suddenly. Data supplied by a medicolegal autopsy may become evidence in a criminal prosecution, a wrongful death suit, or both. Statistics on accidental death gleaned from coroners' reports have been used to support legislation concerning, for example, automobile seat belts, motorcycle helmets, drunk driving, and legal drinking age.

In a teaching hospital (one whose mission includes the training of residents, medical students, nurses, and other health professionals), the autopsy serves as a unique learning experience. Physicians at all levels of training can profit by attending autopsies. Organs and tissues removed at autopsy may be preserved and reviewed days later at a pathology conference. Microscope slides made from these tissues may be used as teaching aids for years. For the physician or physicians who were responsible for the treatment of the patient, the autopsy provides invaluable, if not always comforting, feedback on the thoroughness and accuracy of diagnostic evaluation and the appropriateness of treatment. When death occurs in the postoperative period, an autopsy may show that it resulted from surgical complications or errors of technique. Recently implanted grafts, heart valve replacements, pacemakers, and other materials or devices must be examined for signs of rejection or malfunction. When death follows the use of any experimental treatment, an autopsy is of crucial importance.

Except in those cases where an autopsy is mandated by law and performed by a coroner or medical examiner, written permission must be obtained from the next of kin before an autopsy can begin. The law makes special provision for autopsy permission when the deceased had no known family.

Generally it is the responsibility of the attending physician to solicit and obtain autopsy permission. However, the pathologist must assure himself that a permission has been duly signed and witnessed before performing any examination of the body; otherwise he could be subject to legal reprisals for unauthorized mutilation of the dead. The permission form may restrict the pathologist to certain procedures only. For example, permission to open the skull may be withheld. Because microscopic examination of autopsy specimens is an integral part of the examination, the form must specify that the pathologist may remove and retain such tissues and body parts as he deems necessary.

Autopsies are performed in a hospital department set aside for this purpose. The autopsy room or morgue is usually located on a ground floor adjacent to a loading area for the convenience of undertakers, and it is equipped with refrigerated lockers for the storage of bodies pending autopsy or removal. Strong illumination and adequate ventilation are essential. The autopsy is performed on a specially designed operating table provided with running water and suction equipment. Attached to the table or immediately available in the room is a cutting board for the gross examination of organs as they are removed from the body. A scale is provided for weighing organs, and graduated containers for determining the volume of fluids. The instruments used are similar to surgical instruments—scalpels, scissors, forceps, clamps, and, for cutting bone, electric saws, chisels, and hammers. In addition, a knife with a very long flat blade is used to cut sections of uniform thickness from large organs such as the spleen and kidney. Specimen containers prefilled with fixative are on hand for immediate preservation of tissues removed.

The subject of an autopsy may be called the body, the cadaver, the deceased or decedent, the patient, the remains, or the subject. The person performing the autopsy is called the prosector, the dissector, the operator, the autopsy surgeon, or simply the pathologist. He is usually assisted by a morgue attendant or diener (German *Diener* 'servant'), who looks after the autopsy facility and its equipment, moves bodies to and from the autopsy table, and helps with the actual autopsy procedure as needed.

The autopsy room is usually equipped with a pedal-activated dictating machine so that the pathologist can dictate his findings while performing the autopsy. An autopsy report or protocol so dictated will naturally follow the sequence of examination procedures as they are actually done. This sequence varies from one prosector to another and may be modified in individual cases for various reasons. In virtually all cases, however, the autopsy follows the same basic plan.

After confirming the identity of the body by means of a wrist tag, a toe tag, or both, and satisfying himself that a valid consent for the performance of the autopsy has been given in writing, the pathologist weighs the body, if equipment is available for that purpose, and determines its length from crown to heel. The entire body surface is inspected and palpated, and note is made of the color and consistency of the skin, the color and distribution of head and body hair, any deformities, swellings, or injuries (open wounds, discolorations, needle punctures), surgical or traumatic scars, and any other departure from normal and expected appearances. The presence of endotracheal tubes, intravenous lines, and catheters is noted.

Rigor mortis refers to the stiffening of the muscles that comes on within a few hours after death and passes off after another few hours. **Livor mortis** (postmortem lividity, hypostasis) is a purplish discoloration of the skin due to engorgement of capillaries that occurs shortly after death. Lividity affects whatever parts of the body are lowermost, but does not appear in areas of the skin that have been in firm contact with a supporting surface.

The eyes and the cavities of the mouth, nose, and ears are inspected for evidence of disease, injury, or foreign material. If the eyes have been removed to provide corneal transplants, this fact is noted. The external genitalia are inspected for developmental abnormalities and signs of disease or injury. The body is turned over for inspection of the back and anus.

The thoracic and abdominal cavities are now opened. The prosector makes a Y-shaped incision through the skin and subcutaneous fat of the anterior body surface, the extremities of the Y being at the two shoulders and the pubic region. Some operators make the upper limbs of the Y above the breasts and nearly parallel to the clavicles; others cut below the breasts. Over the thorax the scalpel cuts all the way through skin and fat to the underlying breastbone and ribs.

Below the level of the breastbone the operator inserts two fingers into the peritoneal cavity and lifts skin, fat, and peritoneum away from the abdominal organs so that they will not be injured as he carries the incision down to the pubes (veering around the umbilicus).

The skin is retracted from the line of the incision on each side and dissected free of the underlying tissues until wide flaps have been reflected. The thickness of the subcutaneous fat is noted and recorded. The breasts and axillary structures are examined from within and specimens are cut from any abnormal or suspicious areas. The ribs and clavicles are then cut through near their attachments to the breastbone, and the front of the bony thorax is removed in one piece.

The thoracic and abdominal organs are first inspected in their natural positions and then removed for further study. The membranous surfaces of the thoracic and abdominal cavities—pleura, pericardium, peritoneum, diaphragm, omentum—are examined for abnormalities of color or texture, adhesions, or tumors. Any blood or fluid in a body cavity is noted and if possible measured. Each organ is severed from its attachments, weighed, and opened. As the heart is removed, ligatures are placed around the stumps of the great vessels to facilitate embalming of the body by the undertaker. The intestine is removed in its entirety from just below the stomach to just above the rectum. Both solid and hollow organs are opened for inspection of internal detail. Selected features—for example, the thickness of the walls of the cardiac chambers—are measured.

Representative pieces of tissue from each organ are immediately placed in fixative. Entire organs may be preserved in large jars or buckets of fixative if they are needed for a pathology conference or ''organ recital'' to be held later. Blood may be withdrawn directly from the chambers of the heart for testing. Specimens may be taken for culture or other laboratory procedures, and the contents of the digestive tract may be submitted for chemical analysis. Before incising a solid organ to take material from inside for a culture, the prosector sears the surface with a hot spatula to destroy any microorganisms there, which might contaminate the culture. Any solid material removed from the body and not needed for subsequent study is placed in a large plastic bag, which is sealed at the conclusion of the autopsy and placed inside the body before it is closed.

If an examination of the brain (''head post'') is to be performed, the operator makes an incision across the top of the head from ear to ear, turns flaps of scalp forward and backward, and removes the top of the skull like a cap by cutting around it with an electric saw and detaching the cap with a chisel. The brain and its membranes are observed, and any swelling, deformity, tumor, or hemorrhage is noted. The brain is cut free of its attachments and placed intact in fixative. Usually it is allowed to harden in fixative for several days before being cut for gross and microscopic study. If necessary, the spinal cord or specimens of bone can be removed by further manipulation of the saw and chisel. At the conclusion of the autopsy, the attendant sews the incisions shut with heavy thread or cord in a continuous or "baseball" stitch and washes the body.

Occasionally an autopsy is performed on a body that has already been embalmed. In this case, the pathologist's examination will disclose evidence of the embalmer's activities. Embalming consists of two basic procedures: replacement of the blood in the circulatory system with a preservative fluid that incidentally imparts to the skin a cosmetically acceptable hue, and introduction of a similar fluid into the thoracic and abdominal cavities through one or more punctures made with a hollow instrument. Before instilling cavitary fluid, the embalmer removes as much as possible of the contents of the digestive tract by suction through the instrument. After the instrument is withdrawn, the skin puncture site is closed with a plastic plug to prevent leakage.

Anatomy/Medical Terminology

Medical Terminology Matching Exercise

Complete the following matching exercise to test your knowledge of the terms and procedures in the medical specialty of pathology.

Instructions: Match the term in Column A with its definition in Column B.

Column A	Column B
A. patent	____ mass of cells misplaced during embryonic development
B. toe tag	____ material spread thinly over microscopic slide
C. punch biopsy	____ thickened
D. formaldehyde	____ malignancy still within original area of growth, not metastasized
E. smear	____ commonly used tissue fixative
F. curettage	____ scraping with a sharp instrument to obtain cells for examination
G. diener	____ used to identify patient's body
H. in situ	____ the cause of a disease
I. amorphous	____ container for holding tissue specimens
J. etiology	____ open, unobstructed
K. friable	____ allows pathologist to make diagnosis while the patient is still in operating room
L. inspissated	____ without shape
M. rest	____ another name for an autopsy
N. post	____ morgue attendant
O. cassette	____ uses cylindrical instrument to obtain plug of tissue for examination
P. frozen section	____ crumbly

Transcription Tips

1. Do not confuse C&S (culture and sensitivity) with CNS (central nervous system).

2. Tissue specimens are often labeled as Block #1, Block #2, and so on. Do not confuse this with the term *en bloc* (in a lump; as a whole).

3. Avoid using slang terms in pathology reports.

Slang	*Translate to read*
tabby	TAB or therapeutic abortion
CA	carcinoma
mets	metastases

4. These brief forms are acceptable as dictated and need not be translated:

bands	band neutrophils
basos	basophils
blasts	very immature leucocytes
eos	eosinophils
lymphs	lymphocytes
monos	monocytes
polys	polymorphonuclear leukocytes
segs	segmented neutrophils
stabs	another name for bands; from the German word *Stab* (band)

5. All of the following terms are synonymous and interchangeable:

   neutrophils
   polymorphonuclear leukocytes
   PMNs
   polys
   segs
   segmented neutrophils

6. Do not confuse *rigor mortis* and *livor mortis*. Both are Latin terms, with *mortis* meaning *of death*. *Rigor mortis* refers to the stiffening of muscles that comes on a few hours after death. *Livor mortis* refers to the purplish discoloration of areas of the body closest to the ground.

Terminology Challenge

Instructions: The following terms appear in the dictation on Tape 11A. Before beginning the medical transcription practice for Lesson 22, look up the following words and phrases in a medical or English dictionary and write a short definition of each term.

accumulation	interventricular septum
adrenal gland	kidney architecture
aerated	leptomeninges
antecubital fossae	lobular parenchyma
aspiration trocar	medulla, medullae
atypical biliary ductules	medullary zone
autolytic	mesenteric soft tissue
autopsy	mesocolonic fat
calices	muscularis propria
calvarium	orbital aspect
cerebellum	pachymeninges
cerebral hemispheres	paravertebral
cerebrum	parenchyma
columns of Bertin	parietal pericardium
concretions	pelves
configuration	pelvic brim
coronal sections	pericardial sac
cortex, cortices	perisplenic
description	pleural
gross	portal triads
microscopic	postmortem
disseminated intravas- cular coagulation	psoas ("so'us")
	pulmonary edema
dura	refractile material
embolus	scaphoid
endocardium	splenic flexure
ependymal lining	striated
epicardium	subarachnoid space
fascicles (muscle)	subendocardial
fibrillar	symphysis pubis
foci	tension pneumothorax
free foamy fluid	thrombus
frothy	toxicology
Glisson's capsule	trocar plug
gyrus, gyri	umbilicus
hemoperitoneum	valve cusps
hemothorax	Virchow-Robin spaces
hilar aspect	viscid
incision	visceral pericardium
thoracoabdominal	vitreous
Y-shaped	valve leaflet

Sample Reports

Sample pathology reports appear on the following pages.

Transcription Practice

After completing all the readings and exercises in Lesson 22, transcribe Tape 11A, Pathology. Use both medical and English dictionaries and your Quick-Reference Word List as resource materials for finding words. Proofread your transcribed documents carefully, listening to the dictation while you read your transcripts.

Transcribe (*NOT* retype) the same reports again without referring to your previous transcription attempt. Initially, you may need to transcribe some reports more than twice before you can produce an error-free document. Your ultimate goal is to produce an error-free document the first time.

OMAR KATT

#122442

PATHOLOGY REPORT

CLINICAL HISTORY: Thrombocytopenia.

MATERIAL SUBMITTED: Spleen.

GROSS DESCRIPTION: The specimen is labeled "spleen." Received in formalin is an 80 g spleen measuring 10.0 x 7.0 x 2.5 cm. The external capsule appears discretely lobulated and wrinkled purple-gray without evidence of lacerations or discolorations. A small amount of attached fatty tissue is present throughout the hilum. Upon sectioning, the parenchyma appears glistening dark red, with pinpoint bulging follicles, and unremarkable trabecular architecture. No areas suggestive of infarction or hemorrhage are grossly noted. Representative sections are submitted in four cassettes (A-D).

MICROSCOPIC EXAMINATION: Sections from the spleen reveal somewhat attenuated white pulp regions with only a rare small germinal center found. The sinuses are slightly congested with slight infiltration by neutrophils. Occasional plasma cells are also found. Small collections of two and three foamy histiocytes are found in some areas. A rare megakaryocyte is also present. There is no evidence of capsular fibrosis, granuloma formation, or malignancy in the tissue submitted.

DIAGNOSES:

> SPLEEN: Benign splenic tissue demonstrating mild sinus congestion together with small aggregates of foamy histiocytes.
>
> No evidence of malignancy.

JORGE CASTRIOTI, M.D.

JC:hpi
d&t: 11/06/92

NAME: PIETRE BONAFACIO   #060109   EXPIRED: 11/23/92

AUTOPSY, GROSS DESCRIPTION

EXTERNAL EXAMINATION:
The body is that of an adult white male. The body has been embalmed. The head is
normocephalic. There is gray hair distributed over the scalp. The ears are without lesion. The
nose is without lesion. The eyes have been capped. The mouth has been sealed. At the right
base of the neck there is a sutured embalming wound. The chest is symmetric and stable. The
abdomen is rounded. There is an old healed surgical wound between the umbilicus and the
pubis in the midline. The scar expands to as wide as 8 cm and is associated with a ventral
hernia that measures approximately 15 cm x 12 cm x 8 cm. The upper extremities are without
lesion. There is a yellow metal ring present on the fourth finger of the left hand. The lower
extremities are well formed. The back is without lesion. The external genitalia are adult male.
The penis is uncircumcised. The testicles are descended into the scrotum and are without
masses. Along the left hip there is a 25 cm in length recently healed surgical wound.

INTERNAL EXAMINATION:
The body is opened by the usual Y-shaped incision, revealing approximately 5 cm of
subcutaneous fat present at the level of the umbilicus. The ventral hernia sac is filled with
yellow, clear, low-viscosity fluid. The walls of the hernia sac are shiny and trabeculated. The
pleural spaces are without abnormal accumulations of fluid. Fibrous adhesions are not present.
The peritoneal cavity is smooth and glistening. There are no abnormal accumulations of fluid.
No significant fibrous adhesions are observed.

RESPIRATORY SYSTEM: The larynx is palpated in situ and is without lesion. The trachea is
patent and without lesion. The major bronchi are well formed. The right and left lungs are
heavy. The visceral pleura is smooth and glistening. Bilaterally the posterior aspects of both
lungs are congested. At the lateral base of the right lower lobe there is a 3 cm in diameter
white metastatic tumor mass. In the right upper lobe and in the left upper and lower lobes,
there are numerous small metastatic white tumors, none exceeding 0.5 cm in diameter. The
carinal lymph nodes are enlarged to approximately 3 cm in diameter and filled with gray
tumor. The parenchyma of the lung reveals severe panlobular and centrilobular emphysema
with extensive anthracotic pigmentation.

CARDIOVASCULAR SYSTEM: The pericardium is lightly adhesed to the surface of the heart.
The pericardial space is obliterated by fibrinous adhesions. These are easily broken. The heart
appears slightly enlarged with dominance of the left ventricle. The myocardium is red and
meaty. No evidence of scarring or past infarction is observed. The right atrium is well formed.
The tricuspid valve is well formed and without lesion. The sinus and conus of the right ventricle are well formed. The right ventricular free wall measures up to 0.7 cm in thickness. The
pulmonary valve is well formed. The pulmonary arteries fail to reveal blood clots. There are
four pulmonary veins which return to the left atrium. The mitral valve is well formed. The left
ventricle is well formed. The left ventricular free wall measures up to 2.1 cm in thickness. The
aortic valve is without lesion. The coronary arteries are distributed over the heart in the usual
fashion, and there is no significant atherosclerosis observed. The aorta runs the usual course
and reveals only mild atherosclerosis. The great veins are without blood clot or other

abnormality. The lymph nodes, right and left of the aorta, from the pelvic floor to the diaphragm are markedly enlarged, up to 5 cm in diameter, white, and filled with tumor.

GASTROINTESTINAL SYSTEM: The esophagus runs the usual course and is without lesion. The stomach is well formed. The small intestine and large intestine are well formed. The appendix is present and without lesion.

LIVER: The liver is of the expected size, shape, and position. Glisson's capsule is smooth and glistening. The hepatic parenchyma is slightly buttery in character but shows no evidence of metastatic tumor and no evidence of cirrhosis. The gallbladder is present in the usual position and contains approximately 70 ml of greenish-black viscid bile. No stones are observed. The extrahepatic biliary ducts are of the expected caliber and run the usual course.

SPLEEN: The spleen is enlarged and weighs approximately 400 g. The splenic capsule is intact. The splenic parenchyma is red, meaty, and uniform. No metastatic tumor masses are observed.

PANCREAS: The pancreas is of the expected size, shape, and position and is without specific gross abnormality.

ADRENAL GLANDS: The adrenal glands are of the expected size, shape, and position. Both the cortices and medullae are well formed.

THYROID GLAND: The thyroid gland is palpated in situ and is without lesion.

UROGENITAL SYSTEM: The kidneys are of the expected size, shape, and position. The capsules are smooth and glistening and strip with ease. The renal parenchyma is well formed. The cortex is greater than 0.5 cm in thickness. The pelves and calices and pyramids are all well formed. The ureters run the usual course and are of the usual caliber. The bladder is contracted and trabeculated. The prostate appears to be about 20 g in weight and is gray and uniform.

CENTRAL NERVOUS SYSTEM: The central nervous system is not examined in this dissection.

PROVISIONAL ANATOMIC DIAGNOSIS:
1. Bilateral bronchopneumonia.
2. Malignant tumor of unknown primary, with metastases to:
   a. Periaortic lymph nodes.
   b. Left and right lungs.
   c. Carinal lymph nodes.
3. Past history of bladder carcinoma.
4. Myocardial hypertrophy with left ventricular thickening.
5. Splenic hypertrophy.

MS:hpi   MATTHEW SCANDERBERG, M.D.
d:11/25/92
t:11/26/92

PATHOLOGY REPORT

HEART: Sections of the heart show a thin epicardium. There is marked hypertrophy of the myocardial fibers. Nuclei are quite large and irregular in size and shape. Many hyperchromatic nuclei are seen. Focal areas show moderate disarray of the myocardial fibers. Multiple focal areas of fibrosis are present, particularly in the subendocardial areas. Inflammatory cells are not seen. Some of the myocardial fibers show only a thin shell with a pale, vacuolated, somewhat finely granular cytoplasm. These changes appear to be more marked in the inter-ventricular septal area.

LUNGS: Multiple sections of lung show large distended alveolar spaces filled in some areas with a fibrinous exudate and numbers of neutrophils. The alveolar walls are thickened and edematous. The vessels are congested, and moderate numbers of neutrophils are in the alveolar wall. Other areas show the lumens to be filled with an abundance of protein-rich fluid with little inflammatory reaction. Some areas show marked congestion of the vessels with hemorrhage into the alveoli. Cross-section of a small artery shows the lumen to be filled with a thrombus. Some of the bronchi are quite dilated. They have thin walls and are lined by a low columnar epithelium. They are filled with an abundance of purulent material. Focal areas of fibrosis of the lung are also noted.

SPLEEN: The spleen has a thin fibrous capsule. Malpighian bodies are indistinct. The sinusoids are moderately widened.

LIVER: Sections of the liver show a thin fibrous capsule. Portal spaces are fairly small in size. Multiple small fatty vacuoles are noted in the cytoplasm of the hepatocytes, particularly in the peripheral zones. There is mild widening of the sinusoids in the central zones as well as of the central vein. A few scattered neutrophils are in the sinusoids in the liver.

PANCREAS: The pancreas shows a normal lobular pattern. The acini are not remarkable. The interlobular fibrofatty tissue shows no noteworthy change.

KIDNEYS: The kidneys have a thin capsule. The cortices show glomeruli of normal appearance. The tubules are not remarkable. The interstitial tissue shows no noteworthy change. The pelves are not remarkable.

ADRENAL: The adrenal has a cortex of moderate thickness. The cells are not remarkable. The medulla shows no noteworthy change.

DIAGNOSES:
1. Hypertrophic cardiomyopathy.
2. Edema and congestion of lungs.
3. Hypostatic bronchopneumonia, bilateral.
4. Small infarct of lung.
5. Congestion of spleen.
6. Fatty change of liver.
7. Surgical absence of gallbladder.
8. Surgical absence of uterus.

Medical

- Describe the procedures used in the pathology lab to examine gross specimens, frozen specimens, and specimens prepared for microscopic examination.

Fundamentals

- Discuss the ethical dilemmas that may face medical transcriptionists in their work.
- Demonstrate correct grammar usage in subject-verb agreement.

Practice

- Accurately transcribe authentic physician dictation from the specialty of pathology.

Transcriptionists Are People, Too

by Kathy Rambo, CMT

Medical transcription is my profession. It's what I do seven, eight, sometimes eleven or twelve hours a day. Having one's ears bombarded that long every day by one account of sickness after another isn't good for one's psyche unless there are also leisure-time activities to offset the strain of listening to so many different doctors with so many different accents and so many different speaking peculiarities.

One of my hobbies is writing. There are also days when I consider myself a feminist: Women Hold Up Half the Sky, and all that. Thus, when the assignment for a writing class I was taking was to go somewhere in Southern California I hadn't been before and write about it, I immediately thought of the Women's Building in Los Angeles. I'd wanted to go there for a long time but was shy enough to need an excuse. The class assignment was that excuse. Before I was able to get to L.A., however, something intervened. My trip was much shorter, though it was to a place I'd never been before.

One of my transcription clients was the pathologist of a small nearby hospital. I was in the lab to pick up the day's work when the pathologist came out of his office. "Hi, got a few minutes?" he asked. I nodded. "I'm just starting on the specimens from today's tabbies. Want to watch?" (TAB is an acronym for therapeutic abortion. No one could tell me why it had been corrupted to "tabby." The medical world is not the most reverent of places. Too much sickness and death can desensitize a person.) I shrugged and followed the pathologist back into his cigar smoke-filled office.

I believe a woman's body is her own and should be free from regulation by any government, but I'm still more unsure than most of my feminist and liberal friends whether the body within the woman's body is also hers to do with as she would. Then there was the strictly physiological fact that watching specimens of any kind be cut up might make my stomach react, but my curiosity had to be satisfied.

Several containers the size and shape of large cottage cheese cartons sat on the black-tiled counter. Next to them was what looked like a small footstool (it turned out to be the dissecting bench) covered with paper towels, on top of which lay several scalpels, a pair of throwaway plastic gloves, and a metric ruler. The pathologist clipped a small mike to his tie, donned the gloves, switched on his dictating equipment, and opened the nearest container. The smell of formalin mixed with the stale cigar smoke. My stomach jumped in acknowledgment, but I knew I would stay.

"Well, this is what all that messing around comes to," he said, as he lifted the fetus from its cottage cheese carton and laid it on the table. I had seen pictures of babies in the womb before. I had seen premature babies in the hospital nursery. This specimen was similar to both, yet not quite the same as either. It was grayish-pink and mottled, and when the doctor pulled its legs or touched its head, it squeaked like a rubber toy.

He turned to me, one hand squeaking its head, and smiled. "Pink scalpel or blue?" I giggled, a high nervous sound, then asked if he could really tell what the fetus's sex was. "Of course," he said, taking it by its head and stretching its legs out. "See?" It squeaked again. I saw. "World's got too many women in it, anyway," he said, using the metric ruler to measure its length. He told me its crown-to-rump and crown-to-heel measurements, but I didn't remember them: My eyes were closed, and I was struggling to control the heat in my face.

"Now comes the fun part," the pathologist said, and I opened my eyes in time to watch the scalpel (not pink or blue, only shiny stainless steel) slit its way into the top of the rubber head and slide, squeaking, down and back, to the neck. I was determined to stay. He put a thumb on either side of the knife's path and opened it slightly. I could tell he was enjoying the moment of suspense, but I would stay. He pulled the sides apart slightly and looked at me. "Sex should be something done in a dark closet," he said. I turned toward the door.

"Leave it open, will you?" he called after me. "It's getting a little stuffy in here." He was chuckling as I walked away. I was thinking I should have gone to the Women's Building as I had originally intended.

Well, I thought as I pushed open the double doors and walked outside, at least I have something to write about. And maybe I can find a nice quiet ophthalmologist to replace this account.

I took a deep breath. The air smelled of a stage II alert.

Medical Readings

Laboratory Medicine: The Gross Examination of Tissue

by John H. Dirckx, M.D.

The purpose of this section is to present an overview of what anatomic pathologists do and how and why they do it. The materials examined by an anatomic pathologist fall into two major classes: specimens taken from living patients, and autopsy specimens. At autopsy it is feasible to remove vital organs such as the heart and the liver in their entirety and subject them to thorough, destructive dissection. Specimens from living patients are necessarily limited in type and volume. Such specimens are either tissues or organs removed during surgical operations or samples of material (biopsy specimens) removed from the living body for the purpose of examination.

Whereas the pathologist himself obtains and selects autopsy material for examination, specimens from the living patient are generally obtained by other physicians and submitted for study to the pathologist. Virtually all tissue specimens, regardless of how and by whom they are obtained, are subjected to certain routine procedures. As soon as possible after being removed from the body, the specimen is placed in a glass, plastic, fiberglass, or aluminum bottle, jar, or bucket containing a fluid called a **fixative.** The fixative has several purposes: to arrest the process of decomposition that begins almost at once in devitalized tissue, to kill bacteria and fungi in or on the specimen, and to begin hardening the tissue to facilitate preparation for microscopic study.

The most commonly used fixative is a 10% aqueous solution of formalin. Because formalin is made by bubbling formaldehyde gas through water, it is often called simply "formaldehyde." Formalin is inexpensive and highly suitable for most purposes. However, several other fixatives are available and may be preferred for special applications. The following list includes most of the fixatives in general use as well as certain chemicals that are included in the formulas of several fixatives.

absolute alcohol	Gendre's solution
acetic acid	glacial acetic acid
acetone	glutaraldehyde
Altmann's solution	Helly's Zenker-
Bouin's solution	formalin solution
buffered formalin	Jores's solution
Carnoy's solution	Kaiserling's solution
Carson's solution	Maximow's solution
chlorpalladium	Millonig's phosphate-
chromic acid	buffered formalin
Delafield's solution	Müller's solution
Flemming's solution	neutral (buffered)
formaldehyde	formalin
formalin	osmic acid
formalin-alcohol	osmium tetroxide
formalin-ammonium	picric acid
bromide	potassium bichromate
formol-Müller's	(or dichromate)
solution	Tellyesniczky's solution
FU-48 Zenker's	Zenker's solution
solution	

In performing an autopsy, the pathologist removes organs one by one and subjects them to an immediate gross examination, opening them with a knife and inspecting their internal features. In this way he can observe any abnormalities of size, shape, color, or consistency and any nodules, injury, hemorrhage, degeneration, scarring, or other significant local changes. In addition, he can select those portions of the organ most likely to be useful for microscopic study.

The pathologist's initial examination of a surgical or biopsy specimen is usually performed after the specimen has been placed in fixative. Although the fixative alters the color and consistency of the tissue to some extent, gross pathologic features can still generally be recognized. Occasionally specimens are brought directly from the operating room to the pathologist without being placed in preservative or fixative.

The pathologist performs his examination at a cutting board, which protects the top of the workbench from knife cuts and from the chemical action of fixatives. He handles the specimens with rubber gloves or with forceps, soaking up excess fluid with paper towels or other absorbent materials. He uses scalpels, razor blades, and scissors to open specimens for

further examination and to trim them to the proper size for processing. One dimension, at least, of the trimmed specimen must be no more than 3-4 mm to allow penetration of processing chemicals. The trimmed pieces of tissue are placed in small flat round or oblong cassettes of perforated metal or plastic with lids of the same material, in which they will remain during the first stages of processing.

The pathologist dictates his findings during or immediately after the gross inspection and cutting of surgical specimens. This dictation typically follows a set pattern:

Identification of the specimen. The dictation always begins with basic identifying data: the patient's name as shown on the label of the container and on the laboratory requisition accompanying the specimen, and a general indication of what material has been submitted. At every step in the handling of a specimen, care is taken to ensure that it is correctly identified. The container in which it is placed by the pathologist, surgeon, or operating room technician is labeled with the patient's name, the nature of the specimen, and often the date, the name of the person obtaining the specimen, and other information. Alternatively, a serial number or accession number may be assigned to the specimen container and the pertinent data kept in a register. If only one specimen is taken during an operation, as in an appendectomy, it may be unnecessary to identify it other than by the patient's name. When anatomically indistinguishable specimens are submitted, such as abdominal lymph nodes taken from several areas and possibly containing metastatic malignancy, they must be kept carefully separated and distinguished as to their origins.

In removing a specimen, the surgeon may cut it to a certain shape to indicate its origin or its orientation in the patient's body. Orientation may also be indicated by placement of a suture (surgical stitch) at a certain place in the specimen, such as at the uppermost point of a tumor excised from the skin. In cutting autopsy specimens from paired organs such as the lungs and the kidneys, the pathologist may indicate by the shape of the specimen which side it came from—for example, triangular for left, square for right.

After identifying the specimen, the pathologist may include clinical information (patient's medical history) in his dictation if this is available to him; often it is entered on the requisition.

Dimensions. The size of each specimen as submitted is usually determined and recorded in three planes in metric units (cm or mm). Solid organs or tumors may be weighed, if practicable, and the weight recorded in grams (g). The volume of any contained fluid (as in a cystic cavity) may be measured or (more often) estimated, and recorded in milliliters (ml) or cubic centimeters (cc).

Gross description. The pathologist then describes the physical features of the specimen, with particular attention to any abnormalities such as swelling, hemorrhage, scarring, or tumor. The description typically includes mention of the color, texture, and consistency of both the exterior and the cut surfaces of the specimen. Any well-defined abnormality (nodule, cyst, ulcer, perforation, scar, pigmentation) is measured as precisely as possible. Not only the exact size and location of any tumor, but also its relation to the margins of the surgical specimen, must be carefully determined to document the adequacy of removal.

Microscopic examination of certain kinds of surgical specimen is routinely omitted unless the pathologist's gross examination shows abnormalities needing further study. Surgically removed tissues that are not usually sectioned for microscopic study include hernia sacs, blood clots, varicose veins, healthy bone (e.g., a section of rib removed for access to thoracic organs), and teeth. If microscopic examination will not be done, the pathologist dictates a diagnostic impression at the conclusion of his report on gross findings.

Because the tissue specimens taken by the pathologist in the autopsy room are generally too large to be handed over directly to a histology technician for preparation of microscope slides, these specimens are subjected to further examination and selective cutting in the pathology laboratory, just as with surgical specimens. Ordinarily, however, the pathologist does not dictate a report after this second inspection and cutting of autopsy specimens, since gross findings are included in the report of the autopsy.

The histopathology laboratory and the microscopic examination of tissue. The preparation of microscope slides from a gross tissue specimen is a complex and exacting process consisting of many steps, some of which are performed by automatic machinery.

The process actually begins when the specimen is placed in fixative. The fixative arrests decomposition and hardens tissue. Before the tissue can be cut into transparent sections, it is necessary to make it still harder by replacing its water content with a rigid material such as paraffin or cellulose. (Bone, however, is too hard for sectioning. A specimen containing bone must be decalcified with either dilute acid, an ion exchange resin, or a chelating agent, or by electrolysis,

before it can be processed. The same is true of teeth and soft-tissue specimens such as sclerotic arteries and scar tissue containing calcium.)

When the paraffin method is used, the tissue specimen is first dehydrated by immersion in a graded series of solutions of an organic solvent such as acetone, Cellosolve, ethyl alcohol, or isopropyl alcohol, which replaces the water. The dehydrated tissue is then immersed in a clearing agent such as xylene (xylol), benzene, cedarwood oil, or chloroform, which replaces the dehydrating agent and renders the tissue transparent. Certain agents (dioxane, tetrahydrofuran) can serve as both dehydrating and clearing agents. After clearing, the tissue is transferred to a bath of melted paraffin, which replaces the clearing agent and infiltrates the tissue spaces. When this infiltration is complete, a technician removes the specimen from the paraffin bath with warmed forceps and embeds it in a cube-shaped mold containing fresh melted paraffin.

When the mold has cooled, the result is a block of paraffin inside which the tissue is embedded with all its water replaced, and its empty spaces filled, by paraffin. This paraffin block is then trimmed to appropriate dimensions and cut on a microtome, a precision instrument on the order of an electric meat slicer, which makes transparent slices that are only about 5 microns (0.005 mm) thick. For technical reasons, sections are usually made by cutting across the broadest flat surface of the tissue specimen, unless the pathologist has given special instructions for an edge cut or cross section. Usually only one or two sections from each paraffin block are chosen to be made into slides. Sometimes serial sections (for example, every tenth or twentieth slice) are taken so as to provide the pathologist with a three-dimensional concept of a tissue or lesion.

Immediately after cutting, the paraffin sections are floated on a bath of warm water, which helps to smooth out wrinkles and curled edges. Each section is affixed to a separate microscope slide (a thin strip of clear glass about 1″ x 3″) by means of a film of albumin solution or other suitable adhesive. The slides are identified with labels bearing names or numbers matching those of the containers in which the gross specimens were submitted.

Substances other than paraffin are sometimes used to infiltrate and embed tissue for sectioning. With Carbowax, which is water-soluble, the dehydration and clearing steps can be omitted. However, obtaining satisfactory sections with Carbowax demands a high degree of technical skill. Celloidin is a suspension of a cellulose derivative in a volatile solvent. Because infiltration and embedding with celloidin do not require heat, there is less distortion of tissue than with the paraffin and Carbowax methods. However, celloidin takes much more time; as much as a month may elapse between fixation and sectioning. Commercially available embedding media besides Carbowax include Epon, Paraplast, and Parlodion.

Microscopic examination of the slide at this stage would yield little information, because all of the tissue spaces are filled with the infiltrating medium. This must be removed and replaced with water or some other suitable fluid by a reversal of the procedures used in making the block. Once the infiltrating agent has been removed and the tissue section rehydrated, the slide is immersed in one or more coloring solutions called stains. These impart a more or less intense coloration to the tissues, which greatly facilitates microscopic examination.

Seldom is only a single color applied. Different stains have affinities for different components of tissue, depending on their chemical properties. Hence it is usual to apply at least two contrasting colors. The use of standard combinations of stains enables the pathologist to recognize normal and abnormal microscopic features of tissue consistently and confidently.

In practice, staining usually involves a number of steps besides immersion of the prepared slide in a coloring agent. First a **mordant** may be applied to render the tissue chemically more receptive to staining. Many fixatives have mordant properties. After the first stain has been applied, the slide is immersed in or washed with a **decolorizer,** which removes stain from all parts of the tissue to which it has not become chemically bound. The slide is then treated with a **counterstain** of a contrasting color, which is taken up by tissues decolorized in the preceding step. A **polychrome** stain is a mixture of two or more coloring agents in one solution. With a polychrome stain, differential staining of tissue components takes place even though the tissue is exposed to all of the coloring agents simultaneously. A **metachromatic** stain is one that changes color on becoming chemically bound to certain tissues.

By far the most commonly used combination of stains for routine histopathology work is hematoxylin and eosin (H&E). Hematoxylin is a deep blue stain which imparts various shades of blue and purple to cell nuclei and other tissue components of slightly acidic nature. Eosin stains most of the other components pink to red. Many special stains and techniques are available to bring out certain features (nerve tissue, reticular fibers, lipid material, pathogenic microorganisms) that are not shown by routine stains. In submitting a tissue block to the histology technician, the pathologist may write instructions regarding the use of special stains. Some staining operations can be done by automatic machinery but often part or all of the staining process is performed manually. Slides are placed vertically in tall narrow glass containers called Coplin jars, which are filled with stain or other solutions.

After staining and drying, the tissue section on the slide is ordinarily protected with a cover slip, a very thin sheet of glass about 7/8″ square. A film of balsam or other mounting medium is first placed over the tissue section, and the cover slip is gently dropped into place. The balsam eventually hardens around the edges, but under the cover slip it remains fluid indefinitely, preserving the section in a clear, homogeneous, refractile medium. Mounting media in common use are Apathy's medium, (Canada) balsam, Clarite, and Permount.

In most laboratories, slides are available for the pathologist's examination 24 to 72 hours after the tissue is removed from the body. Processing is speeded and simplified by the use of automated machinery that dehydrates, clears, and infiltrates tissue during the night. The preceding day's specimens are then embedded, sectioned, and stained on the following morning.

The pathologist examines or "reads" slides with a light microscope, using various magnifications as needed. The standard magnifications are scanning power (X35-50), low power (X100), and high power (X450-500). The greater the magnification, the more the detail that can be distinguished, but the smaller the zone of tissue that can be viewed without moving the slide. After reviewing the slides, the pathologist dictates his microscopic findings and then states one or more diagnoses or diagnostic impressions.

Since gross and microscopic reports are dictated on different days, they are seldom transcribed at the same session. Ordinarily the gross report is transcribed on the top half of a standard surgical pathology form. This transcription is made available to the pathologist when he examines the slides of the tissue. His dictation of microscopic findings and diagnosis is then transcribed on the bottom half of the form, and the form is returned to him for review and signature.

Anatomy/Medical Terminology

Word Search

Instructions: Locate and circle the pathology terms hidden in the puzzle horizontally, vertically, and diagonally, forward and backward. A numeral following a term in the word list indicates the number of times it can be found in the puzzle.

```
W  S  R  E  B  I  L  A  C  C  Y  S  T  D  W  B  O
S  M  R  T  U  M  O  R  H  E  L  U  S  P  A  C  K
H  E  A  R  T  S  D  I  E  N  E  R  Y  A  Y  I  P
W  A  C  C  K  R  S  E  M  X  J  X  C  T  M  P  G
A  R  S  T  A  I  N  I  A  G  K  C  O  L  B  O  T
S  Z  L  C  I  V  Q  M  T  D  G  L  A  N  D  C  E
H  F  S  I  K  O  I  J  O  U  O  G  F  D  O  S  D
I  I  O  B  V  N  N  T  X  G  M  R  B  I  A  O  A
N  S  S  R  A  E  M  S  Y  S  P  O  T  U  A  R  W
G  I  L  T  M  N  R  G  L  D  D  S  R  L  N  C  D
S  S  I  U  O  A  O  R  I  Y  O  S  L  F  E  I  S
C  O  D  C  E  L  L  I  N  E  M  B  A  L  M  M  Y
N  N  E  N  O  B  O  I  S  O  J  S  M  R  I  O  Z
W  G  J  T  O  L  C  G  N  I  I  Z  E  O  C  R  O
C  A  S  S  E  T  T  E  Y  C  C  S  D  V  E  G  H
B  I  O  P  S  Y  G  N  O  P  S  N  E  I  P  U  C
H  D  N  I  G  R  A  M  J  P  U  P  I  L  S  E  A
```

autopsy	diagnosis	livor
biopsy	diener	margin
block	DOA	mass
body (2)	edema	microscopic
bone	embalm	morgue
caliber	examination	pupils
capsule	fluid	scar (2)
cassette	formalin	sections
cavity	gland	slide
cell	gross	smear (2)
CIN	heart	specimen
CIS	hematoxylin	spongy
clot	histology (2)	stain
cyst (2)	incision	tissue
cytology	lesion	tumor (2)
dead	liver	washings

Transcription Guidelines

Subject-Verb Agreement Exercise

Review the guidelines on correct subject-verb agreement in Lesson 10, page 167, and complete the following exercise.

Instructions: Circle either the singular or plural form of the verb or pronoun in the pairs in parentheses to demonstrate correct subject-verb agreement.

1. The endocervical canals are patent, and each (connect, connects) with (its, their) respective (uterus, uteruses). (Note: The patient was didelphic.)
2. Examination of sections of both right and left lung (show, shows) severe vascular congestion but (is, are) otherwise unremarkable.
3. Sections of the remaining breast tissue (show, shows) atrophy without evidence of additional tumor.
4. Acute blood clot and old organized and degenerate blood clot (is, are) observed.
5. The wound was explored for foreign bodies, none of which (was, were) found.
6. The compression of the renal pelvis and deviation of the left upper ureter (is, are) essentially the same as seen on the intravenous pyelogram.
7. The nodules in the left lower lobe (has, have) not changed in size.
8. Approximately 10 cc of straw-colored fluid (was, were) obtained and sent for appropriate microbiologic studies.
9. We have no way of telling what the exact relationship of this mass to the subclavian vein and subclavian artery (is, are).
10. The sulci in the region of the temporo-occipital area on the right side (is, are) slightly effaced.
11. There (is, are) minimal degenerative change in the articular facets.
12. No definite adenopathy or masses (is, are) seen in the chest or around the chest wall or axilla.
13. Multinucleate giant cells and nuclear changes consistent with herpes or other viral infection (is, are) encountered.
14. Focal areas of necrosis with some slight pseudo-palisading (is, are) present.
15. Blocks #11 through #14 (is, are) periaortic node.

Terminology Challenge

Instructions: The following terminology appears in the dictated reports on Tape 11B. Before beginning the medical transcription practice for Lesson 23, look up each word or phrase in a medical or English dictionary, and write out a short definition of each term.

adjacent
aggregates
apocrine
bisected
bosselated
cancerization
carcinoma
  bronchogenic
  duct cell
  large-cell
  oat cell
  small-cell
  undifferentiated
cell
  infiltrating
  inflammatory
  plasma
chromatin
clefting
cone biopsy
curettings
cytologic features
cytoplasm
diffuse
ectasis
embedded
endocervical
endometrial
eosinophilic
excisional biopsy
fibrocartilage
follicular
formalin
frozen section
germinal center
H&E stain

hyperchromatic
infiltrate
keratinization
lumen
meniscus
metaplasia
mitotic rate
mucous cyst
nonkeratinizing
nuclear-cytoplasmic
  ratio
nucleolus
nucleus
opacified
opaque
ovoid
Pap smear
papillary
parafollicular
pleomorphic
polymorphonuclear
  leukocytes
proliferation
squamous epithelium
stratified
subepithelial
subjacent
synovitis
synovium
tissue
  fibrofatty
  fibrous
  grumous
tonsillar crypt
transepithelial migration

Transcription Practice

After completing all the readings and exercises in Lesson 23, transcribe Tape 11B, Pathology. Use both medical and English dictionaries and your Quick-Reference Word List as resource materials for finding words. Proofread your transcribed documents carefully, listening to the dictation while you read your transcripts.

Transcribe (*NOT* retype) the same reports again without referring to your previous transcription attempt. Initially, you may need to transcribe some reports more than twice before you can produce an error-free document. Your ultimate goal is to produce an error-free document the first time.

Lesson 24. Radiology

Learning Objectives

Medical

- Given a radiology term, match it to its correct medical meaning.
- Define common radiologic abbreviations.
- Discuss the purpose and technique involved in performing common radiologic procedures.

Fundamentals

- Describe some of the challenges and rewards of working as a radiology transcriptionist.

Practice

- Accurately transcribe authentic physician dictation from the specialty of radiology.

A Closer Look

The Radiology Transcriptionist

by Kathy Rambo, CMT

I was typing in the hospital radiology department, my earphones hooked up to the transcribing unit, when a transcriptionist from the medical records department spoke to me. "Kathy, how can you stand to transcribe x-rays all day? How boring it must be!" She was on her way home after spending her day transcribing histories and physicals, consultation and operation reports, and discharge summaries. She thrived on the diversity and had told me more than once that she would probably die of boredom if she "had to transcribe the same thing over and over."

That was about 15 years ago, and I still specialize in radiology. And I still don't find it boring. To the contrary, because of the many advances in computer and medical technology, radiology transcription has become one of the most exciting areas in which to work. The chorus of "It's boring" is no longer sung. Many transcriptionists are humming a new tune.

Over twenty years ago, I moved to California from Ohio with three years of a college English major and four years as a newspaper ombudsman under my belt and no plans for the future. I landed my first job in the medical field as an orderly and darkroom technician for a local community hospital's x-ray department. The hospital was small, with only 67 patient beds. The radiology department had one room where the x-rays were taken, a darkroom for developing them, and an office where they were read by a radiologist. The office also did duty as the reception area, the chief tech's office, and the transcription area.

Because of the size of the department, from the beginning I was exposed to more than the specialized x-ray terminology. I was present when the radiologists explained their findings to a patient's attending physician and when the reports were dictated. I heard the technologists discuss positions and views among themselves and with the radiologists. I listened in when the interning students from the community college radiology technology program were taught about both the technical and medical aspects of the various x-ray exams. I learned a great deal about the importance of positioning and the reasons for an adequate preparation for certain tests.

I had been on the job for about six months when the radiology transcriptionist quit and I was asked if I would be interested in learning her job. From then on, my experience is not too different from that of most medical transcriptionists before the advent of the American Association for Medical Transcription (AAMT) and college courses in the field. I received on-the-job training, learning new terminology as I went on to other radiology departments and as the field of radiology itself advanced and expanded.

One of the biggest advantages to radiology transcription is how easy it is to find information. Unlike the generalist, whose office is located in the medical records department, the radiology medical transcription specialist often works in the radiology department. This affords quick access to the physician who dictates the reports (and, in many cases, performs the exams), the technologist who either performs the exams alone or assists the radiologist, and other x-ray reports on the patient.

Many radiologists are eager to help the transcriptionist with further explanation of the terms or exams, and many techs will take the time to review what positions a patient was placed in or what views were taken. The availability of the reports for previous exams on a patient has many times helped me to decipher something in the dictation.

It is true there are days when a radiology transcriptionist hears no more exciting dictation than normal chest x-rays and a few decidedly uninteresting broken bones (just as there are days when the generalist transcribes nothing but normal H&Ps and a few decidedly uninteresting metatarsal resections). But the ever-advancing field of radiology, with all of its new technologies, has become one of the most exciting specialties a medical transcriptionist can choose.

An overview of radiology. It all began in 1895, when German physicist William Conrad Roentgen discovered a strange form of electromagnetic radiation which was similar to visible light but had a shorter wavelength. Roentgen discovered these mysterious rays could penetrate soft tissue but would be absorbed by bone. The first "roentgenogram" was of his wife's hand. It wasn't long before x-rays were being used to diagnose fractures.

By the time I became a radiology transcriptionist in 1970, hospital x-ray departments were routinely offering bone and soft tissue examinations; fluoroscopy procedures (direct x-ray examination of deep structures such as the stomach and intestine using a fluorescent screen); and tomography (examination of thin layers of body tissue at varying depths—body section radiography, planography, laminography).

Fluorescent screens soon went the way of all obsolete technology, and now image intensifiers combine with spot and overhead films to produce such examinations as upper gastrointestinal and barium enema series.

A radiologist dictating a tomographic report may use the term "plane," referring to a selected level of the body. In other instances, the dictator may refer to a "plain" film, an x-ray unaided by the use of a contrast medium or special procedure. (The latter is frequently heard in examinations such as an intravenous pyelogram, or IVP, when the doctor describes the appearance of the abdomen in the preliminary or scout film—the "plain" film taken before contrast medium is injected.)

But what used to be known as the x-ray department has changed a lot over the years. With so many new techniques and procedures now available, many hospitals and radiology offices have opted to change the title to Diagnostic Imaging.

Besides the standard x-ray examinations, today's field of radiology offers procedures which sound as though they came straight from a Ray Bradbury novel:

nuclear medicine
ultrasonography
computerized axial tomography (CAT or CT)
magnetic resonance imaging (MRI)
balloon angioplasty
positron emission tomography (PET)
digital subtraction angiography (DSA)

A basic knowledge of these procedures makes the job of transcribing the reports much more interesting. More importantly, it also arms the radiology transcriptionist with an extra tool in the constant monitoring which must be done to ensure an accurate medical record.

Nuclear medicine was the first subspecialty I learned as a fledgling transcriptionist. With the use of radioactive isotopes either injected or ingested, the technologist scans the vessels or organs of interest. The uptake of radioactivity is then counted and interpreted as an image by a computer.

As I moved from hospital to hospital and grew in my knowledge of radiology transcription, the list of subspecialties also grew, and the next special procedure I learned was ultrasonography (echography, sonography, ultrasound).

Medical ultrasound is a direct result of the use of sonar during World War II. With the use of transducers of varying size, sound waves inaudible even to the superhuman ear of the medical transcriptionist pass into the patient and are bounced back to the transducer, then recorded as computer images. Ultrasound exams may utilize many different methods: gray-scale ultrasound, real-time imaging, Doppler ultrasound, and A-mode, B-mode, M-mode.

Recent years have seen even more science fiction brought to science fact in **diagnostic imaging.** Depending on the size of the facility where they work, radiology medical transcriptionists may encounter any or all of several other Bradburyesque modalities.

Computed tomography (CT) is probably the only imaging procedure to generate so many cartoons because of its other acronym—the CAT scan. CAT stands for either computerized axial tomography or computer-assisted tomography. The CT is also variously referred to as reconstructive tomography, computed transmission tomography, and computerized transverse axial tomography (CTAT). CT scans convert x-ray pictures into video images using a spinning x-ray tube and computer graphics.

Magnetic resonance imaging (MRI) uses magnetism instead of radiation. Misaligning and realigning the atoms in the body, an MRI scan can produce extremely fine detail in places that CT cannot. MRI is less often referred to as nuclear magnetic resonance (NMR).

Two of the newest imaging procedures are the **positron emission tomography** (PET) and the **single photon computed emission tomography** (SPECT). As with the other modalities, PET and SPECT use computers to aid imaging and diagnosis. These two procedures could be classed under the nuclear medicine subspecialty, since both employ radioactive isotopes. SPECT depicts blood flow; PET does that as well, and also measures metabolism.

All of the aforementioned modalities fall under the general description of special imaging procedures. New diagnostic and therapeutic procedures have also been developed in recent years, most notably in the area of **interventional radiology.** These procedures are interventional because of the introduction of catheters into various vessels.

The ability to intervene via catheter has led to **digital subtraction angiography** (DSA), also known as **digital vascular imaging** (DVI). Iodinated contrast material is injected via venous catheter, and a computer subtracts out all the tissues until only the vessels visualized by contrast material are left. Any vessels blocked by occlusion or stenosis are then readily apparent.

With the knowledge gleaned from the DSA, a radiologist can insert an even smaller balloon-tipped catheter. The balloon is inflated, and the occlusion or stenosis is reduced by compression into the vessel wall.

The catheterization technique can also be used to stop GI bleeding by infusing medication, to minimize bleeding during surgery by blocking a vessel, to remove kidney stones, or to circumvent renal and biliary stenosis and allow for drainage from the urinary system.

A radiology transcriptionist may not be exposed to all of the subspecialties in the field. But confronting one of these subspecialties and all of its accompanying strange, new terminology can be exciting—IF the medical transcriptionist knows how to find the definitions and correct spelling of that terminology.

Resources. One of the best sources for a deeper understanding of any diagnostic imaging examination and its attendant terminology is the technologist who performs or assists the radiologist in performing the various studies. A good technologist who has the time is usually willing to explain the details of a study or define any difficult technical terms. Many times there are technical books in the chief technologist's office that a transcriptionist can peruse for further information.

If the department is busy, you may not have much chance to ask a radiologist for more than the explanation of a word or two, but most radiologists are eager to help the radiology transcriptionist when time permits.

Other good sources of information include sales representatives for products and equipment, magazines and newsletters of the various radiology subspecialties and professional associations, hospital video libraries, and the catalogs of pharmaceutical and medical equipment companies.

The most often used source of knowledge, however, is the personal reference library. The radiology specialist is always on the lookout for new books, word lists, and other materials. Unfortunately, radiology is a transcription specialty that used to have few reference books available. Perhaps this is because the field advances so rapidly. In the past, what most radiology transcriptionists had access to was what, for the most part, they dug out.

My personal reference library consists of three sections: the basics, which I think any medical transcriptionist should have; a second classification of materials which each medical transcriptionist chooses to add to the basics; and those materials which deal exclusively with radiology.

The third segment of my reference library consists of those materials which relate to radiology. In addition to these books, my radiology reference material includes copies of all the ''normal'' reports used by all the radiologists for whom I've ever transcribed (A ''normal'' is a report for any exam which failed to show any abnormalities on the radiologist's reading. Each radiologist usually has an individual normal for each exam done in the department.); lists of isotopes which I obtained from a radiopharmaceutical company; and lists of patient positions, film views, and body planes gleaned from the offices of several chief x-ray techs for whom I've worked.

Over the years, each medical transcriptionist builds up a personal medical reference library from newly published texts and by adding to the terminology notebook begun by each of us in our first days on our first transcription job. We hound the book sales representatives who visit the hospitals, we attend association conventions and seminars, and we network with our peers to ensure that our knowledge of our specialty is kept up-to-date. We do all of this because we find our work exciting and we see ourselves as professionals.

Transcription practices. There is another aspect of the radiology specialty which is unlike most other areas of medical transcription, and which can separate the truly professional medical transcriptionist from one who looks on the radiology specialty as merely a boring job.

Radiology dictation is usually accompanied by an examination request form. This requisition slip contains patient information (age, medical record and/or hospital number, attending physician), and the radiology examination ordered. Many times, it will also list the patient's admitting diagnosis and the reason for the requested exam. This is information which a professional radiology transcriptionist reviews and keeps in mind while transcribing the report.

A busy radiologist can easily dictate ''greater trochanter'' when the exam is of a shoulder; the alert transcriptionist would realize that what the dictator meant was ''greater tuberosity.'' Or, the requisition slip could

ask for a left foot and the radiologist dictates **right** foot. In this case, the transcriptionist would know to check further which side was meant, since the doctor could have dictated the wrong side, **but** the person who filled out the request slip could just as easily have misread the attending physician's order. If the radiology transcriptionist still cannot determine which is the correct side, a blank should be left in the report and a note of explanation attached.

The professional radiology transcriptionist uses the requisition slip, an extensive reference library, other medical professionals, sales representatives, catalogs, magazines, newsletters, seminars, conventions, and a good dose of initiative to track down the elusive term, the garbled dictation, the new procedure. Doing so guarantees work far removed from the complaints of boredom I used to hear. Doing so also gives the radiology transcriptionist a real sense of the importance of a professional job professionally done.

Medical Readings

Basic Diagnostic Radiology

Part 1

by John H. Dirckx, M.D.

X-rays are a form of electromagnetic radiation having a wavelength between that of gamma rays and that of ultraviolet rays. The importance of x-rays in medicine arises from their ability to penetrate most of the tissues of the human body and to expose photographic film in a manner similar to light. Like gamma rays, x-rays have potentially harmful effects on living tissue, particularly actively growing or reproducing tissue. The power of x-rays to shrink or destroy certain kinds of tumor has been put to use in therapeutic radiology. Because x-rays are also capable of inducing tumors in certain tissues, and of damaging any tissue after excessive exposure, they must be used with the greatest caution and restraint.

In diagnostic radiology, x-rays are produced in a high-voltage electron tube (Coolidge tube) with equipment that controls the intensity of the beam, its direction and shape, and the duration of emission. X-rays pass through the part of the body under study and create an image on a sheet of film that is protected from light in a filmholder or cassette. Since no lenses are used to focus x-rays, the image is of about the same size as the subject, and correspondingly large sheets of film must be used.

X-rays can also be used with cinematographic equipment to make moving pictures of internal organs such as the heart, lungs, and digestive system. In fluoroscopy, a continuous stream of x-rays passing through a part of the body is made to create an image on a sensitive screen. Modern fluoroscopic equipment electronically enhances this image and projects it on a television screen so that the dose of radiation can be kept to a minimum.

The fact that x-ray images are made by rays that have passed through the subject accounts for several important differences between x-ray and conventional photography. Different tissues offer different amounts of resistance to the passage of x-rays and produce correspondingly light or dark images on film. When x-rays encounter little resistance, as in passing through a zone of gas in the bowel, they expose the film to a maximal extent. After developing, this area of the film will be dark gray or black. When x-rays are stopped, as by a bone or a metallic foreign body, the corresponding area on the film is left unexposed, and after developing appears white (translucent).

The radiologist can distinguish only four degrees of density in tissue: metal density (bone, gallstones, urinary calculi, metallic foreign bodies, orthopedic pins, screws, and wires); water density (body fluids and most soft tissues other than fat); fat density; and air or gas density (air in respiratory passages, gas in digestive passages, or either of these in inappropriate places). Shapes or outlines appear in an x-ray image *only* where two zones of contrasting density touch or overlap.

Radiologists can see the outline of a bone (which is of metal density) because it is silhouetted against surrounding soft tissues of water density. They can usually see a bubble of air in the stomach because it, too, is surrounded by water-density tissue. But where two structures of like density (e.g., two muscles, or the spleen and pancreas) are contiguous, no silhouette is produced, and the border or interface between them is not represented in the image.

This limitation of radiography has been overcome to some extent by the use of contrast media—solutions of metallic salts or iodides that are opaque to x-rays. Introduced into the body, they can outline a hollow structure such as the stomach or the colon, or a tubular system such as the circulation, the bile ducts, or the urinary tract. Contrast media can be swallowed, in-

jected, or introduced through a tube, catheter, or enema apparatus.

In light photography, a positive print is made from the film negative. In radiology, the film itself is used. For examination or "reading," the film is placed on a backlighted viewbox that provides bright, even illumination. Unlike a photograph, an x-ray picture gives no information about the depth or contours of the subject. An x-ray picture is literally a shadow or group of shadows. Everything is represented in an absolutely flat, two-dimensional image. An x-ray film of a right hand, when turned over, cannot be distinguished from an x-ray of a left hand. For this reason, an x-ray picture of any part of an extremity is normally labeled L or R at the time of exposure. A metal letter clipped to a corner of the filmholder becomes a part of the image.

When x-rays leave their source, they tend to radiate in all directions. Their direction and lateral spread can be controlled with metal housings, deflectors, and cones, but any x-ray beam (like any beam of light), no matter how narrow, will tend to spread out the further it gets from its source. This has an effect on the fidelity with which an x-ray picture reproduces the internal structures through which the rays have passed. The closer an object is to the source of x-rays (and the further from the film), the larger and less distinct it will appear. Hence for maximum clarity the zone of interest is placed as close to the x-ray film as possible. A standard chest x-ray is taken with the front of the patient's chest against the filmholder and the x-ray source behind the patient. (This is called a posteroanterior or PA view.) This technique gives maximum definition to the heart shadow while blurring and dulling the shadow of the spinal column. When the thoracic spine is the center of interest, the same part of the body is x-rayed with the patient's back nearest the filmholder (anteroposterior or AP view).

As x-rays pass through tissue, they tend to be deflected to some extent from their straight course, much as light waves are when passing through murky fluid. This phenomenon (soft-tissue scatter) causes a certain blurring of images, which may limit the value of a study performed on an obese subject or in certain body regions. In order to reduce soft-tissue scatter and the effects of lateral spreading (radiation), a Bucky grid may be placed between the subject and the film. This grid consists of very thin metal strips arranged in parallel with very narrow spaces between them. Rays that are still traveling comparatively straight after passing through the subject get through the grid and expose the film. Deflected (oblique) rays cannot get through to add their blurring effect to the image. During the fraction of a second that the film is being exposed, the grid is set in motion by an automatic mechanism so that the grid itself will not appear in the image.

Tomography is a technique for focusing on a particular site or level within the subject. While the subject remains stationary, the x-ray source and the filmholder rotate in an arc around him, in opposite directions, during exposure of the film. The point within the subject about which this rotation occurs will produce an image of maximum clarity on the film, while tissues closer to and further away from the film will be blurred or invisible. In effect, a tomogram is an x-ray of a narrow slice of the subject. Typically a series of tomograms or ''cuts'' are made, each focused at a different plane. Tomography is used primarily in defining and localizing abnormal masses and foreign bodies. This technique should not be confused with computer tomography (CT).

Radiology glossary. Following are some of the most commonly used radiology terms in dictation. The glossary of radiology terms continues in Lesson 25.

air-fluid level   A line representing the level of a collection of fluid seen in profile, with air or gas above it.

air-space disease   As seen on chest x-ray, disease or abnormality of lung tissue that encroaches on space normally filled by air.

ankle mortise   The normal articulation between the talus and the distal tibia and fibula.

blunted costophrenic angle   On chest x-ray, a costophrenic angle that is flattened or distorted by scarring or pleural fluid.

bony island   Benign developmental abnormality consisting of a localized zone of increased density in a long bone.

bowel gas pattern   (abdominal film) The normal radiographic appearance of gas in the intestine.

bridging osteophytes   Osteophytes on adjacent vertebrae that meet and fuse, forming a ''bridge'' across the joint space.

collateral vessels   Vascular channels newly formed from existing ones to maintain the circulation of a tissue or organ whose normal blood supply has been impaired by disease or injury.

collecting system   On an intravenous pyelogram (IVP), the nonexcretory portions of the kidney, which collect newly formed urine and conduct it to the ureter; the minor and major calices and the renal pelvis.

coned-down view   A study limited to a small area by the use of a cone that narrows and ''focuses'' the x-ray beam.

consolidative process   An abnormal process that increases the density of a tissue or region.

correlate radiographic findings clinically   Interpret x-ray appearance in the light of the patient's medical history and objective findings on physical examination and laboratory testing.

deglutition mechanism   The coordinated sequence of muscular contractions in the mouth, pharynx, and esophagus involved in normal swallowing, as demonstrated in a barium swallow or upper GI series.

demineralization   Reduction in the amount of calcium present in bone, due to disease or immobilization.

double contrast technique   A modification of the barium enema procedure. After the standard barium enema examination has been completed, the patient expels most of the barium, and the colon is then inflated with air. The coating of barium remaining on the surface may outline masses or defects not seen during the standard examination.

duodenal bulb   Onion-shaped dilatation of the duodenum immediately below its origin at the pylorus.

duodenal C-loop   C-shaped loop formed by the duodenum as it courses around the head of the pancreas.

duodenal sweep   The normal course of the duodenum, from the pylorus and around the head of the pancreas to the ligament of Treitz, as visualized with contrast medium in an upper GI series.

effacement   Abnormal flattening of the contour of a structure.

esophageal dysmotility   Seen on upper GI series; abnormality in the strength or coordination of peristaltic movements in the esophagus.

extravasation of contrast   Leakage of contrast medium from the structure into which it is injected through a perforation or other abnormal orifice.

filling defect   A zone within a tubular structure that is not filled by injected contrast medium (usually a tumor or abnormal mass).

fixation device   Any appliance placed surgically in or on a bone to stabilize a fracture during healing.

free air   Air or gas in a body cavity where it does not belong, usually after escape from the GI tract.

frogleg view   An x-ray of one or both hip joints for which the patient lies on his back with thighs maximally abducted and externally rotated and knees flexed so as to bring the soles of the feet together.

full-column barium enema Barium enema examination in which the contrast medium is injected into the colon under full pressure, by elevation of the barium reservoir to the maximum safe height.

gas density line A linear band of maximal radiolucency, representing or appearing to represent a narrow zone of air or gas.

gastroesophageal reflux Abnormal backflow of material from the stomach into the lower esophagus.

great vessels On chest x-ray, the major vascular trunks entering and leaving the heart: the superior and inferior venae cavae, the pulmonary arteries and veins, and the aorta.

hypoaeration Abnormal reduction in the amount of air in lung tissue.

hypokinesis Abnormal reduction of mobility or motility; reduced contractile movement in one or both cardiac ventricles.

ileus Small bowel obstruction due to failure of peristalsis.

impingement Contact or pressure, generally abnormal, between two structures.

interstitial markings The radiographic appearance of lung tissue, as opposed to the appearance of air contained in the lung.

interval change Change in the radiographic appearance of a structure or lesion in the interval between two examinations.

loculated effusion A collection of fluid in the pleural space whose distribution is limited by adjacent normal or abnormal structures.

low-dose screen-film technique A radiographic technique used in mammography to provide adequate imaging with less radiation than is used in conventional techniques.

lucent defect An abnormal zone of decreased resistance to x-rays.

lytic (for **osteolytic**) **lesion** A disease or abnormality resulting from or consisting of focal breakdown of bone, with reduction in density.

mammography Radiologic evaluation of the female breast, primarily to search for or evaluate abnormal masses that may be malignant. Special equipment and techniques have been devised to limit radiation exposure and enhance the diagnostic value of the procedure.

mass effect The radiographic appearance created by an abnormal mass in or adjacent to the area of study.

mass lesion Anything that occupies space within the body and is not normal tissue.

midline shift Displacement of a structure that is normally seen at or near the midline of the body, such as the pineal gland or the trachea.

opacification An increase in the density of a tissue or region, with increased resistance to x-rays.

open-mouth odontoid view A view of the odontoid process of the second cervical vertebra for which the x-ray beam is aimed through the patient's open mouth.

orthopedic hardware Wires, pins, screws, plates, and other devices of metal or other material that are implanted in or attached to bone in the course of a surgical procedure.

peribronchial cuffing Thickening of bronchial walls by edema or fibrosis, as seen in asthma, emphysema, cardiac failure, and other acute and chronic respiratory and circulatory disorders.

peristaltic wave A wave of muscular contractions passing along a tubular organ (such as the intestine), by which its contents are advanced.

plain film A radiographic study performed without contrast medium.

pleural effusion An abnormal accumulation of fluid in the pleural cvity.

pole of kidney The upper or lower extremity of a kidney.

portable film An x-ray picture taken with movable equipment at the bedside or in the emergency department or operating room when it is not feasible to move the patient to the radiology department.

posterior sulcus The groove formed by the intersection of the diaphragm and the posterior thoracic wall, as seen in a lateral chest x-ray.

pulmonary vascular markings As seen on chest x-ray, the normal radiographic appearance of the branches of the pulmonary arteries and veins about the hila of the lungs.

pulmonary vascular redistribution Increased prominence of upper pulmonary vessels and reduced prominence of lower pulmonary vessels at the lung hila in left ventricular failure and other disturbances of circulatory dynamics.

radiolucent Offering relatively little resistance to x-rays (by analogy with *translucent*).

radiopaque Resisting penetration by x-rays.

sacralization Abnormal bony fusion between the fifth lumbar vertebra and the sacrum.

skyline view of patella X-ray study of the knee region in which the patella is visualized above the distal femur and appears like a rising (or setting) sun.

small bowel transit time   The time required for swallowed contrast medium to pass through the small bowel and appear in the colon.

spurring   Formation of one or more jagged osteophytes, as in osteoarthritis.

strandy infiltrate   A pulmonic infiltrate that appears as strands or streaks of increased density.

stress cystogram   A radiographic study of the bladder intended to demonstrate stress incontinence. Contrast medium is instilled into the bladder and films are taken while the subject coughs and bears down.

subcutaneous emphysema   Air or gas in subcutaneous tissue.

subcutaneous fat line   The radiographic appearance of the subcutaneous fat layer.

suboptimal   Not as good as might have been expected; usually referring to technical factors in an x-ray study, such as positioning, film quality, and patient cooperation.

swimmer's view   An oblique view of the thoracic spine in which the arm nearer to the x-ray source hangs at the patient's side and the opposite arm is upraised.

tail of breast   A wedge-shaped mass of normal breast tissue extending toward the axilla.

takeoff of a vessel   The origin of a branch from a larger vessel, as demonstrated radiographically with injected contrast medium.

tenting of hemidiaphragm   On chest x-ray, a distortion of the diaphragm by scarring, in which an upward-pointing angular configuration (like a tent) replaces all or part of the normal curved contour of a hemidiaphragm.

tertiary contractions   Aberrant contractions of the esophagus, occurring after the primary and secondary waves of normal swallowing.

tibial plateau   A flattened surface at the upper end of the anterior aspect of the tibia.

upper GI series   Also known as barium swallow. Barium sulfate is given orally to outline the esophagus, stomach, and duodenum on x-ray films.

upper GI series and small bowel follow-through   An upper GI is done, and x-ray films are taken over a period of time to visualize the barium as it moves through the small bowel.

working orthopedic surgery film   A radiographic study done during the course of an operation, for example, to monitor the reduction of a fracture or the placement of a fixation device.

Anatomy/Medical Terminology

Medical Terminology Matching Exercise

Instructions: Match the term in Column A with its definition in Column B.

Column A	Column B
A. x-ray	____ x-ray of breast
B. barium	____ general term for any radioactive substance used in x-ray imaging
C. fluoroscopy	____ contrast medium used in studies of GI tract
D. intravenous pyelogram	____ uses sound waves to show differences in tissue density
E. myelogram	____ x-rays appear on a fluorescent screen rather than x-ray film
F. mammogram	____ image produced by a gamma camera after injection of a radionuclide
G. ultrasound	____ the image produced by ultrasound
H. sonogram	____ image produced after injection of a radionuclide that shows rates of tissue metabolism
I. radionuclide	____ roentgenogram
J. Tc-99m	____ x-ray of spinal cord using contrast medium
K. scan	____ chemical symbol for the radioactive contrast medium technetium
L. PET	____ x-ray of urinary system using contrast medium

Abbreviations Exercise

All abbreviations (except for laboratory test names) must be spelled out in the Diagnosis or Impression section of any report.

Instructions: Define the following radiology abbreviations and memorize the definitions to increase your speed and accuracy in transcribing.

AP view _____

BE _____

CAT _____

CT _____

CXR _____

DSA _____

IVP _____

KUB _____

MRI _____

PA view _____

PET _____

UGI _____

Directions Matching Exercise

Instructions: Match the directions in Column A with their definitions in Column B.

Column A   *Column B*

A. anterior   ____ further away from the
B. caudal   midline of the body
C. cranial   ____ further away from the
D. distal   center of the body or some
E. dorsal   other point of reference
F. inferior   ____ upper, upward
G. lateral   ____ lower, downward
H. medial   ____ higher in the body
I. posterior   ____ nearer to the center of the
J. proximal   body or some other point
K. superior   of reference
L. ventral   ____ lower in the body
                  ____ pertaining to or in the
                       direction of the front
                       surface of the body
                  ____ rear, toward the back
                  ____ front, toward the front
                       of the body
                  ____ pertaining to or in the
                       direction of the back
                  ____ nearer to the midline
                       of the body

Transcription Tips

1. Directions can be expressed as adverbs by adding the suffix *ly*.

Direction	*Adverb*
anterior	anteriorly
distal	distally
inferior	inferiorly
lateral	laterally
medial	medially
posterior	posteriorly
proximal	proximally
superior	superiorly

2. Two directions used together to designate a direction can be either hyphenated or combined into a single word. Notice the spelling changes in the combined form. Note: This is the physician's option, not the transcriptionist's. The transcriptionist should transcribe what is dictated.

anterior-posterior	*or*	anteroposterior
anterior-lateral	*or*	anterolateral
posterior-anterior	*or*	posteroanterior
posterior-lateral	*or*	posterolateral
superior-lateral	*or*	superolateral

3. The direction *transverse* is an adjective. Do not confuse it with the verb *traverse*, which means "to go across."

A transverse incision was utilized.
The scar traversed the entire abdomen.

4. The term *sagittal* is commonly misspelled. Remember that it has one *g* and two *t*'s.

5. Like many adjectives in medical terminology, the word *navicular,* meaning boat-shaped (from Latin *navicula* 'little boat'), is usually used without a noun, becoming in effect a noun itself. There are naviculars (navicular bones) in both the wrist and the ankle.

Prominent spurs are seen off the anterior surface of the talus and the navicular.

6. The term *x-ray* is written with a lowercase *x* and a hyphen. Occasionally you may see it written with a capital *X* in nonmedical publications; however, *x-ray* is the accepted medical style.

7. The term *x-ray* can be used as a noun (the photographic film) or a verb (the radiologic procedure).

   An x-ray was taken of the abdomen.
   The patient was x-rayed after admission.
   The patient was re-x-rayed on the second day.

8. Translate the following slang terms when encountered in dictation.

Slang	Translate to read:
C spine	cervical spine
echo	echocardiogram
LS spine	lumbosacral spine
T spine	thoracic spine
tib	tibia, tibial
fib	fibula, fibular

9. The following words have more than one acceptable spelling.

Preferred	Acceptable
annulus	anulus
distention	distension
disk	disc
transected	transsected

10. Some radiologists say ''full colon'' to indicate the colon as a mark of punctuation, so as to avoid confusion with the colon of the large bowel.

11. Radiologists often dictate in the present tense because they are interpreting the radiographic findings as they actually view the films. It is not unusual for them to switch from the present tense to past tense within the same report. As a general rule, the history is past tense and the findings are present tense.

    PA and oblique views were obtained, and they show a transverse fracture.

Terminology Challenge

Instructions: The following terms appear in the dictation on Tape 12A. Before beginning the medical transcription practice for Lesson 24, look up each word in a medical or English dictionary, and write out a short definition of each term.

air-fluid level
alveolar
ankle mortise
AP (anteroposterior)
bony island
bronchiectasis
cardiac silhouette
cardiomegaly
cervical rib
choroid plexus
condyle
consolidative
costophrenic angle
CVP (central venous
  pressure) line
demineralization
dextrorotoscoliosis
distention
disuse
duodenal bulb
duodenal sweep
dysmotility
dysplasia
enchondroma
epidural
esophagitis
falx
femur
fracture
  acute
  calcaneal
  comminuted
  fibular
  oblique
  phalangeal
  transverse
gastroenteritis
gastroesophageal reflux
genu varum
granulomata
greater tuberosity

hemidiaphragm
hemithorax
humeral head
ileus
KUB (kidneys, ureters,
  bladder)
lucency
mammogram
mass effect
medial compartment
  (of knee)
metacarpal
microcalcification
midline shift
navicular
nodular-like
oblique
obscures
opacification
osseous
osteochondritis dissecans
osteomyelitis
osteopenia
pedicles
peribronchial cuffing
perihilar
phalanx
pineal
PIP (proximal inter-
  phalangeal) joint
preliminary film
prosthesis
  acetabular
  femoral
region
  basal
  basilar
  hilar
  residual
  retroareolar
  ropy

Terminology Challenge *(cont.)*

sclerosis
sclerotic area
sinus
  ethmoid
  frontal
  maxillary
  sphenoid
sinusitis
spondylolisthesis
spondylolysis
spurring
static (adjective)
subchondral
swimmer's views

talus
tarsal
tertiary
tibial plateau
Towne's view
transfixing screw
tube
  ET (endotracheal)
  nasogastric
  thoracotomy
upper GI series
vascularity
vertebral body

Sample Reports

Sample radiology reports appear on the following pages.

Transcription Practice

After completing all the readings and exercises in Lesson 24, transcribe Tape 12A, Radiology. Use both medical and English dictionaries and your Quick-Reference Word List as resource materials for finding words. Proofread your transcribed documents carefully, listening to the dictation while you read your transcripts.

Transcribe (*NOT* retype) the same reports again without referring to your previous transcription attempt. Initially, you may need to transcribe some reports more than twice before you can produce an error-free document. Your ultimate goal is to produce an error-free document the first time.

ROCKY DOGGETT   #122541   9/13/92   DR. KATT

CHEST, PA AND LATERAL:

The heart is normal in size. Trachea is at midline. Normal pulmonary vascular markings. Opaque sutures are seen in the projection of the right upper chest, and there are minimal fibrotic changes in the right lung. Lungs are expanded, and no active infiltrate is otherwise seen.

IMPRESSION: Presence of opaque sutures in the projection of the right upper chest, and minimal fibrotic changes in the right lung. No active cardiopulmonary disease is otherwise demonstrated at this time.

LOUDEN BARKER, M.D.

LB:hpi
d&t:9/13/92

MARIA CONCEPCION   #111332   9/13/92   DR. BRIETZSCH

LOW-DOSE MAMMOGRAPHY USING EGAN'S TECHNIQUE:

CLINICAL HISTORY: There is no family history of breast cancer. Patient had onset of menses at age 12 years, and her LMP was at age 50 years. Patient is a gravida 4, para 3, ab 1. Currently asymptomatic. There is no history of previous breast surgery. Intermittent estrogen therapy.

Bilateral mammographic examination reveals atrophic breasts with minimal fibrocystic residuals, predominantly fibrotic. There are no dominant mass lesions. No abnormal calcifications are detected. Small intramammary lymph nodes are noted in the tail of each breast. The skin and subcutaneous fat lines appear smooth. Vascularity is normal and symmetrical.

IMPRESSION:
1. Atrophic breasts with minor fibrocystic residuals.
2. No evident malignant mass lesion.
3. Annual mammography is recommended in this age group.

IAN GREENSLEEVES, M.D.

IG:hpi
d&t:9/13/92

LIMITED SINUSES:

Upright Waters and Caldwell views demonstrate apparent air-fluid level in the left maxillary sinus, consistent with sinusitis. However, I certainly cannot exclude this representing a polyp or cyst. The remainder of the visualized paranasal sinuses, soft tissue, and bony structures are unremarkable.

IMPRESSION:
Demonstration of an apparent air-fluid level in the left maxillary sinus, consistent with sinusitis. Please correlate clinically.

CT SCAN OF THE SINUSES:

Multiple 4 mm sections at 4 mm intervals were taken in coronal projection without iodinated intravenous contrast. Air-fluid level is seen in the right maxillary sinus, suggesting a right maxillary sinusitis. No bony abnormality is seen about the paranasal sinuses. No soft tissue or bony abnormality is seen near the ostia of the maxillary sinuses. The soft tissues and bones of the face, which are also visualized, are grossly normal.

IMPRESSION:
Right maxillary sinusitis with no variation or abnormality seen.

VIEWS OF THE FOOT:

Views of the foot were obtained in this patient with a history of calcaneal fracture. Multiple pins are seen traversing the calcaneal fracture. No definite bony bridging is seen at this time. There is good approximation of the fracture fragments.

IMPRESSION:
Status post open reduction and internal fixation of calcaneal fracture.

VIEWS OF THE ELBOW:

Views of the elbow were obtained on this patient with a history of olecranon fracture. A compression plate and screws are seen traversing the olecranon fracture. Bony resorption is seen at the fracture site. There is good alignment of the fracture fragments. Some bony callus formation is evident anteriorly.

IMPRESSION:
Status post open reduction and internal fixation of the olecranon fracture.

KUB:

The spinous processes, transverse processes, and pedicles of the lumbar vertebrae are fairly well maintained. A minimal amount of degenerative disease is seen within the hips. A large amount of gas and feces is noted throughout the colon. Some gas is noted within small bowel. Calcified phleboliths are seen within the pelvis. There is also a large 2 x 4 cm mass of increased density in the midportion of the true pelvis.

IMPRESSION: Density within the midpelvis of undetermined etiology. In this first film on this patient, the possibilities include: (1) a suppository, (2) residual barium from a previous study, (3) a foreign body.

INTRAVENOUS PYELOGRAM:

The KUB study shows the 4 mm in diameter calcification in the lower midpole of the right kidney and is unchanged in the interval since our comparison study. The right kidney also appeared normal at that time. The left kidney showed exactly the same configuration on the outside study presented for review, with an irregular right upper pole and two small cystic changes lateral to the upper pole caliceal system, measuring 2.0 cm and 2.5 cm in diameter. The curvilinear displacement of the caliceal systems also suggests a larger cystic change in the parapelvic region, measuring approximately 5 cm in diameter. The compression of the renal pelvis and deviation of the left upper ureter are essentially the same as seen on our intravenous pyelogram. The bladder again appears normal with a minimal residual.

IMPRESSION: Right renal lithiasis and slight right nephroptosis on the upright study; otherwise normal-appearing right upper urinary tract and ureter. Deformity of the upper pole of the left kidney with some blunting of the caliceal system and the formation of cystic calices lateral to the main upper pole caliceal system suggests a pyelonephritis. Tuberculosis should be considered as an etiology. A larger peripelvic cyst is also noted, displacing the renal pelvis inferiorly and causing some deformity but no evident amputation of the middle or lower pole caliceal systems. The study is consistent with essentially the same findings as on our recent intravenous pyelogram.

ABDOMINAL SONOGRAM, OUTSIDE FILMS:

The abdominal sonogram performed is reviewed. The liver and gallbladder are normal in appearance with no evident stones. The abdominal aorta is normal in width with no aneurysmal dilatation. Calcified plaques are noted on the anterior aspect of the aorta. The right kidney is normal in size and appearance. The tiny calcification seen in the posterior midportion on IVP and CT scan studies is not demonstrated. The left kidney shows the large cystic structure in the pelvic portion of the left kidney with some distortion of the superior pole and a smaller cystic structure lateral to the upper pole caliceal system.

IMPRESSION: Abnormal left kidney with irregular margin of the superior cortex, with a small cystic lesion lateral to the upper pole caliceal system and a large parapelvic cyst in the midportion of the left kidney. The right kidney appears normal. The liver, gallbladder, aorta, and pancreas are generally within normal limits.

MRI OF THE CHEST:

An MRI of the chest was performed in this 43-year-old black female who has chest pain. T1 weighted coronal images were obtained as a scout. Then T1 weighted images were obtained at three different levels through the chest using cardiac gating and respiratory compensation. All images obtained were T1 weighted.

The lumen of the aorta does not show any evidence of a dissection. The ascending aorta is slightly enlarged at 4 cm in diameter. However, the descending aorta has a normal caliber. There is tissue around the descending aorta, which is somewhat unusual in appearance, but it most likely represents fat. There is a remote possibility that this could represent thrombus around a patent lumen, but this is felt to be unlikely. Since this is only on the slices through the lower part of the thorax, an ultrasound of the abdominal aorta up to the hiatus would be worthwhile to make sure the patient doesn't have an abdominal aortic aneurysm. The ventricles are normal in appearance.

IMPRESSION: MRI of the thorax showing no evidence of an aortic dissection.
The ascending aorta is slightly enlarged.

MRI OF THE PELVIS:

FINDINGS: MRI scan of the pelvis was performed in this patient who is 70 years old and had a large left labial mass which extends into the vagina. The study was done to determine the tumor extent. A T1 weighted coronal scout was obtained. Multi-echo sagittal images were then obtained. Multi-echo axial images through the pelvis and lower abdomen were obtained, and multi-echo coronal images were obtained to include the liver and periaortic area, as well as the pelvis. After two sequences, the patient was given 2 mg of glucagon I.V. to stop the bowel motion and improve the quality of the scans.

There is a mass lesion approximately 5 cm in diameter in the region of the left labia and distal vagina. This mass compresses the vagina at this level. On the sagittal images, especially images #18 and #20, there is a suggestion of a tongue of tissue extending from this mass behind the pubic symphysis toward the bladder. The mass is globular in shape and approximately 5 cm in diameter. The signal of the mass does not precisely match that of urine, but the mass does have a higher signal than most of the muscle and soft tissue around it. There is no evidence of nodes. The patient's uterus has been removed. The periaortic area and liver both appear to be free of abnormal structures.

IMPRESSION: A 5 cm mass of unknown etiology, with the suggestion of a tongue of tissue extending up toward the bladder.

Lesson 25. Radiology

Medical

- Discuss the purpose and technique involved in performing special radiology procedures.

Fundamentals

- Discuss how medical literacy is important to you as a medical transcriptionist.

Practice

- Accurately transcribe authentic physician dictation from the specialty of radiology.

A Closer Look

Medical Literacy

by Susan M. Turley, MA, CMT, RN

Recently I rediscovered a classic—*Cultural Literacy: What Every American Needs to Know* (Houghton Mifflin, 1987), by E. D. Hirsch, Jr. It created quite a stir in academic circles and among laypersons concerned with the state of education when it was published. As I reread it, some pertinent thoughts about medical transcription education came to mind that I would like to share with you.

Dr. Hirsch defines cultural literacy as "the grasp of background information that writers and speakers assume their readers and listeners already know. [This] is the hidden key to effective education" (p. xiii).

And yet, almost daily we hear of declining SAT scores; of students who believe Washington, D.C., is in Washington state; of students who cannot find Mexico on a world map; of students who cannot identify the century in which the Civil War occurred; of students, ready to graduate from college, who lack even the rudiments of effective oral and written communication skills; and of teachers who cannot pass eighth grade math tests.

Hirsch also notes that the level of literacy required to function in society has been rising steadily year by year. If the level of knowledge for cultural literacy has been rising, can the same be said of the level of knowledge needed for medical literacy? Absolutely.

The standard of medical literacy required of medical transcriptionists has risen dramatically over the years. For example, between 1980 and 1991, the FDA approved 270 new drugs. Considering that each drug has a generic name as well as a trade name, literacy in pharmacology could entail being conversant with, utilizing, and perhaps even memorizing the spelling of those approximately 540 new drug names. Not to mention the hundreds of surgical procedures, instruments, laboratory tests, and diagnostic tests which were also introduced during those same years.

Hirsch continues: "The complex undertakings of modern life depend on the cooperation of many people with different specialties. . . . The function of a national literacy is to foster nationwide effective communications. Where communications fail, so do the undertakings. Our chief instrument of communication over time and space is the standard national language, which is sustained by national literacy" (p. 2).

Suppose we were to substitute the word *medical* for *national* and *nationwide* in the above quotation. It would then read:

> The complex undertakings of modern medical care depend on the cooperation of many people with different specialties. The function of medical literacy is to foster effective medical communications. Where communications fail, so do the undertakings. Our chief instrument of communications over time and space is the standard medical language, which is sustained by medical literacy.

Which brings us face to face with the critical importance of a comprehensive education for medical transcriptionists. When transcriptionists are medically literate, they are able to send and receive technically complex communication, both orally and in writing. When they are medically illiterate, communication breaks down, misinformation is disseminated, and the medical process is ineffective.

Hirsch related an interesting research study in which the researcher first posed as a native of a particular city and asked directions of passersby. Later he stated he was a tourist and again asked for directions. Those who thought he was a native of the city gave very short, to-the-point directions. Those who thought he was a tourist with no knowledge of the city gave long directions, included a great deal of very basic information, and delivered their instructions slowly.

Hirsch concluded that if two people share a great deal of information in common, their communication can be brief, efficient, time-saving, and still very effective. If, however, they share little of the same knowledge, their communication is labored, inefficient, and must include much basic information before understanding occurs.

When physicians communicate with transcriptionists either face to face or through the dictated report, how much common information do they share? Can the dictation be of a highly technical, abstruse, or complex nature and still be conveyed accurately and with understanding if the transcriptionist is medically illiterate in some way?

When I began transcribing, I had seven years' nursing experience in pediatric and neonatal ICU care. Whenever I encountered dictation in those areas, I felt very comfortable. I took time to explain to my transcription co-worker the meaning of some of the specialized terms we were hearing, such as *heelstick hematocrit, bagged* (collecting a urine specimen or being ventilated by an Ambu bag), *gorky,* and *dusky.* However, as proficient as we were in pediatric transcription, we failed miserably when we encountered ophthalmology dictation. I remember we spent a great deal of time trying to find *cup-to-disk ratio* in our reference books, as well as other phrases like *cotton wool spots* and *cell and flare.* As far as ophthalmology dictation went, we were medically illiterate, just guessing at what we heard.

To be truly literate, we must understand a broad range of medical topics as well as information from related fields such as biology, chemistry, and English. Hirsch notes: "To know what somebody is saying, we must understand more than the surface meanings of words; we have to understand the context as well. . . . To grasp the words on a page we have to know a lot of information that isn't set down on that page" (p. 3).

Hirsch provides a familiar example of this phenomenon of incomplete literacy with the song "Waltzing Matilda," which is well known to Australians. Most Americans are aware of this song and some may even be able to sing the chorus. But a close examination of the lyrics reveals that, while we may attempt to reconstruct the meaning of the song, the particulars elude us because there are certain words for which we have no working definition.

> Once a jolly swagman camped by a billy-bong,
> Under the shade of a kulibar tree,
> And he sang as he sat and waited for his billy-boil,
> "You'll come a-waltzing, Matilda, with me."

As you read the lyrics, did you completely understand what was taking place? You probably recognized and knew the meaning of the majority of words, but the meaning of the whole hinged on those few words which you did not know. A Matilda is a kind of knapsack with which you go walking (waltzing). A swagman is a hobo, billy-bong is a brook, kulibar is eucalyptus, and billy-boil is coffee.

And so it is for medical transcriptionists. By knowing some, but not all, of the words they encounter, transcriptionists can fool themselves into thinking that they really understand the intended meaning when, in fact, they do not.

Unless we have been educated as to the exact meaning of medical root words, suffixes, and prefixes, we may try to guess the meaning of unknown words in a dictation by looking at the context, or we may assign an incorrect meaning, or we may assume we know the meaning when we do not, or we may be too embarrassed to admit that we cannot decipher the true meaning, or we may not know we have selected an incorrect meaning and may carry that with us from report to report. Reading medical journal articles or hearing continuing education lectures on new medical advances does not make one medically literate if the fund of basic medical knowledge is lacking.

Consider the following excerpt from a medical journal article. If we read the passage below without the prerequisite medical knowledge the authors assume we have, we can only guess at its meaning. Imagine how much useful information you would actually gather from this article if you brought a limited medical knowledge to its reading. Its essential content as understood would appear something like this:

** **, which account for about one-half of the 9,000 new cases of ** brain tumors reported in the United States each year, remain ** to treatment despite numerous attempts to provide effective forms of therapy. . . . The most effective agent, ** (**), has considerable ** ** and a short **-** in **. To ** these problems, a method has been developed for the local sustained release of ** ** by their incorporation into ** **.

Following is the same passage as it actually appeared in the medical journal article. Note the basic knowledge which the authors assume the reader possesses (as noted in brackets).

Malignant gliomas [medical terminology], which account for about one-half of the 9,000 new cases of primary [medical terminology] brain tumors reported in the United States each year, remain refractory [English terminology] to treatment despite numerous attempts to provide effective forms of therapy. . . . The most effective agent, BCNU (carmustine) [pharmacology], has considerable systemic toxicity [pharmacology] and a short

half-life [chemistry] in the serum [medical]. To obviate [English] these problems, a method has been developed for the local sustained release of chemotherapeutic agents [pharmacology] by their incorporation into biodegradable polymers [chemistry].

When I was in nursing school, medical terminology was not included in the curriculum as a separate and distinct course. We were never formally taught word roots, prefixes, and suffixes. It was assumed that we would encounter and develop an understanding of all medical and surgical terms just by working in the hospital around patients during our clinical times for each medical specialty. The faulty foundation that was laid hampered me immensely. Even while working in the ICU, I could not begin to break apart a word such as *choledocholithotomy* and define its word parts. This is medical illiteracy.

Do the vast majority of transcriptionists fare any better in their education? Undoubtedly most programs include a course in medical terminology, but what about pharmacology or laboratory procedures? Ignorance and lack of knowledge in these two areas are equally damaging. Two equally talented typists, grammarians, and formatters will never produce medical reports of equal excellence if one lacks a comprehensive background in medical knowledge.

Another important part of the picture to consider is *critical thinking skills*—the buzzword in educational circles today. The *AAMT Model Job Description: Medical Transcriptionist* (1990) includes the following two performance standards, among many, which demonstrate the need for critical thinking skills and medical literacy. A medical transcriptionist "applies knowledge of medical terminology, anatomy and physiology, and English language rules to the transcription and proofreading of medical dictation," and "recognizes, interprets, and evaluates inconsistencies, discrepancies, and inaccuracies in medical dictation, and appropriately edits, revises, and clarifies them without altering the meaning of the dictation or changing the dictator's style."

Medical transcriptionists desperately need critical thinking skills, but these can be exercised only if a broad base of medical knowledge has first been taught, memorized, and understood.

A transcriptionist friend who works at home called me some time ago to say that she had been called in for a meeting the following morning with the medical record director and the transcription supervisor to review errors in her work. She was understandably anxious and called me for advice. Since I knew her work was excellent, I told her to make sure that they provided her with copies of the actual reports in which her errors had occurred. She called the following night to report what had transpired at that meeting.

Aside from some spelling errors which my friend agreed to correct, there were two main points of contention. The medical record director pointed to a report in which my friend had typed *fascicle*. "What's wrong with that?" my friend asked. "There is no such word," she was told. "You must have misheard the doctor. The correct word here should have been *fascia*." My friend reviewed the context of the sentence and then showed them the definitions of both words in the medical dictionary she had brought to the meeting, thus proving that *fascicle* was correct. They protested, "But we never heard of that word."

Their second complaint was that she was not typing laboratory data correctly. "When the doctor dictates the bilirubin levels, you should be including that under the heading *electrolytes* along with the sodium and potassium," they said. My friend stated that she was fairly certain that bilirubin was not an electrolyte. They replied, "Of course it is. The doctors always dictate the bilirubin level right after the electrolytes; they say 'lights' when they mean electrolytes; and when the babies in the nursery are jaundiced they put them under bilirubin lights. So we know bilirubin is an electrolyte." Medical illiteracy.

A transcriptionist asked me for help in locating a word. "Is aminoglycoside a generic or trade name drug?" she inquired. "Neither," I answered. "It's a group or class of antibiotics." "Oh," she said, "I would never have thought of that." Medical illiteracy.

A few years ago I asked a college medical record program director about converting a pharmacology class for medical transcriptionists from the semester to the quarter system. She cut me short with the question, "Why would transcriptionists need to know anything about pharmacology?" Medical illiteracy.

What is the end result, then, of illiteracy and how does it impact on the medical transcription profession? Hirsch notes that illiteracy results in the "powerlessness of incomprehension." The illiterate cannot participate actively in the change process because they have not mastered the ability to communicate effectively.

It is critical for medical transcriptionists to master the ability to communicate effectively using medical language. As we strive to strengthen our position as members of the healthcare team, we cannot afford the luxury of medical illiteracy.

Medical Readings

Basic Diagnostic Radiology

Part 2

by John H. Dirckx, M.D.

This is a continuation of the radiology glossary begun in Lesson 24. Radiology special procedures, including angiography, tomography, radionuclide scans, MUGA scans, ultrasonography, and MRI scans, are briefly described, followed by definitions of terms related to the procedure.

Angiography (arteriography) is the radiographic study of arteries into which radiopaque medium has been injected. Still pictures may be taken immediately after injection, or motion pictures may be made showing the flow of blood and contrast medium through vessels.

iodinated contrast medium A contrast medium containing iodine rather than a metallic salt; used in angiography, intravenous pyelography, oral cholecystography, and other studies.

origin of a vessel The commencement of a vessel as it branches off from a larger vessel.

reconstitution Maintenance of flow in an artery beyond an area of narrowing or obstruction by establishment of collateral circulation.

runoff The flow of blood (and contrast medium) through the branches of an artery into which the medium has been injected.

takeoff of a vessel Same as *origin*.

Computed tomography. Computed tomography (CT) is an application of computer technology to diagnostic radiology. Instead of exposing a film after passing through the subject, x-rays are detected and recorded by a scintillation counter. The x-ray tube moves around the subject on a frame called a gantry, rotating through an arc and "cutting" across one plane of the subject. A series of scintillation counters are so placed that each detects the rays passing through the subject at a different angle. (Alternatively a single counter may rotate in perfect alignment with the x-ray source.)

Data on the amount of x-ray that penetrates the subject at each angle are collected from the counters, digitized, stored, and analyzed by a minicomputer programmed to generate a cross-sectional image of the subject corresponding to the plane cut by the moving x-ray beam.

Contrast medium may be injected into the circulation immediately before CT scanning. IV contrast enhances the sensitivity of CT scanning of certain structures and body regions and improves the visibility of some tumors.

contiguous images   A series of scans without intervals of unexamined tissue between them.

cut   A CT section or image; a scan.

reconstruction study   Generation of an image by computer processing of scan data.

resolution   The ability of an optical, radiographic, or other image-forming device to distinguish or separate two closely adjacent points in the subject. In CT, resolution is measured in lines per millimeter. The higher the resolution, the sharper and more faithful the image.

serial scans   A series of scans made at regular intervals along one dimension of a body region.

stacked scans   Same as *contiguous images.*

Radionuclide scans. The essence of any radioactive scan procedure is the introduction into the body of a radioactive substance whose distribution in tissues, vessels, or cavities can be detected and recorded by a device that senses radiation. A variety of radioactive substances (radionuclides, isotopes) are used in scanning procedures. In some cases the choice of material is governed by the tendency of certain organs or tissues to take up (absorb, concentrate) certain elements or compounds.

Radionuclides may be swallowed, inhaled, or injected into a body cavity or into the circulation. Scanning may be performed immmediately after the material is administered (as in studies of blood flow) or after an interval (as when absorption or concentration of a substance in an organ must occur first). The standard lung scan procedure includes two separate scans of the lungs, one after inhalation of a radionuclide and the other after injection of a second radionuclide into the circulation.

The scanning is done with a scintillation camera (scintiscanner, gamma camera) which creates a picture on film representing the distribution and intensity of gamma radiation emitted by the subject.

blood pool   The circulating blood, into which radionuclides are injected for various types of circulatory scans.

label   To render a substance radioactive by incorporating a radionuclide in it; also, to cause a tissue or organ to take up radioactive material.

radionuclide   A radioactive isotope; a species of atom that spontaneously emits radioactivity.

sensitize   To introduce radioactive material into a fluid, tissue, or space for purposes of performing a radioactive scan; essentially the same as *label.*

tag   Same as *label.*

uptake   Absorption or concentration of a radionuclide by an organ or tissue.

washout phase   Scintiscanning of the lungs at the conclusion of the inhalation phase of a lung scan, after an interval during which all inhaled radionuclide would be expected to have been exhaled.

Multiple-gated acquisition scan (MUGA). This is a study of cardiac shape and dynamics in which a radionuclide is introduced into the circulation. Radioactive emissions from the heart are electronically monitored, stored, and analyzed, resulting in a composite scan consisting of a series of successive images all taken at the same point in the cardiac cycle.

cine (for cinematograph) **view**   A moving picture of the cardiac cycle, constructed from individual frames, each of which is a composite image of one point in the cardiac cycle obtained by cardiac gating.

first pass view   An image or set of images obtained immediately after injection of radionuclide into the circulation, when its concentration in the blood pool is at its highest.

gated view   An image obtained by a technique synchronized with motions of the heart to eliminate blurring.

hypokinesis   Abnormally decreased mobility (as of a cardiac ventricle).

ventricular ejection fraction   That portion of the total volume of a ventricle that is ejected during ventricular contraction (systole); usually expressed as a percent rather than a fraction.

Ultrasonography. Ultrasonography is a means of visualizing internal structures by observing the effects they have on a beam of sound waves. The sound used for this procedure is at a higher frequency (pitch) than the human ear can detect. Ultrasound waves pass through air, gas, and fluid without being reflected. However, they bounce back from rigid structures such as bone and gallstones, creating an ''echo'' that can be detected by a receiver. Solid organs such as the liver and kidney partially reflect ultrasound waves in predictable patterns. Waves are also reflected from the interface between two structures.

Ultrasonography might be compared to taking a flash photograph. Light from the flashbulb bounces off the subject and comes back to create an image on film of the surface contours of the subject. In ultrasonography, however, the echo must be converted electronically to a visible image before it can be interpreted. Sophisticated electronic equipment permits ultrasound scanning of a body region with generation of a two-dimensional picture of internal structures.

In practice, the same device (a transducer) that generates the sound waves also acts as the receiver. Although it emits signals at a rate of 1000 per second, the transducer is actually functioning as a receiver 99.9% of the time.

acoustical shadowing Reflection of large amounts of ultrasound from the surface of structures or materials that are physically incompressible (bone, gallstones), with blockage of further transmission.

echo characteristics The frequency, intensity, and distribution of echoes produced by a structure or region.

echo pattern The ultrasonographic appearance of a structure as seen on a visual display.

full-bladder technique An ultrasonographic examination of the pelvic region performed while the subject's bladder is distended with urine. This is done to improve the recognition of the bladder outline, which cannot be distinguished adequately when the bladder is empty.

real-time examination Ultrasonographic examination performed by sweeping the ultrasound beam through the scan plane at a rapid rate, generating up to 30 images per second. The display of images at this frequency is in effect a motion picture, providing visualization of movement of internal structures as it actually occurs.

probe Ultrasound transducer.

sonolucent Offering relatively little resistance to ultrasound waves (as air or fluid) and hence generating few or no echoes.

Magnetic resonance imaging (MRI). Magnetic resonance imaging is a method of obtaining cross-sectional "pictures" of the human body electronically. It is based on physical principles altogether different from those used in x-ray and ultrasonography. Although the theoretical basis of magnetic resonance imaging is abstruse and complex, the practical applications and terminology can be grasped without difficulty.

As in an x-ray or ultrasound examination, this diagnostic technique depends on variations in the physical properties of tissues—for example, bone vs. muscle, and normal liver vs. neoplasm. However, instead of detecting varying resistances to penetration by x-rays or sound waves, the MRI technique detects varying concentrations or densities of hydrogen atoms (ions) from one tissue to another.

The attraction of a magnet for iron and iron-containing alloys is familiar to everyone. A magnet will attract, to some degree, any atoms which, like those of iron, have an unequal number of protons and neutrons in their nuclei. The degree to which such an atom will respond to magnetic attraction depends on its nuclear structure and is expressed as a physical constant called *spin*.

The simplest of all atoms is that of hydrogen, which, with but a single proton in its nucleus, possesses spin and responds to magnetic attraction. If the human body is placed in a static magnetic field of sufficient strength, its hydrogen atoms align themselves with this field like so many infinitesimal compass needles.

In a magnetic resonance examination, the patient is placed inside a static magnetic field generated by a large and powerful magnet. A pulse of radio waves (excitation pulse) is then used to create for a brief period of time a second magnetic field at a right angle to the static field. While this second field is present, the hydrogen ions (protons) change their orientation, and when the second field is removed, they go back to their previous orientation to the static magnetic field. In doing so they give off a stream of radiofrequency energy or "signal," which can be detected by a suitably placed receiving coil. The intensity of the signal given off by any tissue is proportional to its hydrogen concentration or proton density. Muscle emits a very high signal, bone a very low one, air almost none.

The time it takes for the protons to return to their former orientation after an excitation pulse is called T1. This time interval, a fraction of a second, is also in direct proportion to the hydrogen ion density of the sample. Purely by way of analogy, one might think of the time it takes a roomful of people to come back to order after a sudden disturbance as a measure of the number of people in the room.

When the excitation pulse is applied, all of the protons in the sample respond together, or in phase, in taking up their new orientation. After the excitation pulse ceases, but before the protons have all come back to their former orientation with the static magnetic field, they tend to get out of phase with each other because of the interaction of many adjacent molecules. Once the protons go out of phase, a signal can no longer be detected by the receiving coil. The time it takes for the protons to go out of phase is called T2.

Because both T1 and T2 vary in proportion to the proton density of the sample, they can be used by a computer to generate an image of it. However, direct measurement of T1 is not possible, since the signal is lost as soon as the protons go out of phase. There are also technical obstacles to precise measurement of T2. Some of these obstacles have been eliminated by the spin echo technique, in which the excitation pulse is followed, after a brief interval, by a second and stronger pulse. This results in the production of an echo signal from which T2 can be determined. The time that elapses between the first pulse and the appearance of the echo is called the echo time (TE).

In order to obtain cross-sectional images, it is necessary to modify the magnetic resonance system by adding yet a third magnetic field. This gradient magnetic field, created by a separate coil, introduces a positional element into the signals detected by the receiver. A computer decodes and analyzes the signals, generating two-dimensional cross-sectional images of the subject in much the same way that cross-sectional x-ray images are generated in computed tomography.

In practice, a number of different pulses and time intervals are used in predetermined series called pulse sequences, and the resulting spin echo signals are averaged. Repetition time (TR) is the interval between one pulse sequence and the next. An image generated with a pulse sequence using a relatively short TR is called a T1 weighted image because it reflects the T1 to a greater extent than the T2 of the specimen. An image generated with a longer TR is called a T2 weighted image.

high field strength scanner   A magnetic resonance imaging device using a static magnetic field of maximal intensity.

multi-echo images   A series of spin echo images obtained with various pulse sequences.

partial saturation technique   A magnetic resonance technique in which single excitation pulses are delivered to tissue at intervals equal to or shorter than T1.

signal intensity   The strength of the signal or stream of radiofrequency energy emitted by tissue after an excitation pulse.

spin echo image   A magnetic resonance image obtained by the spin echo technique. With this technique, T2 is determined indirectly, as a function of TE, the echo time.

surface coil   A simple flat coil placed on the surface of the body and used as a receiver.

T1   The time it takes for protons to return to their orientation to a static magnetic field after an excitation pulse.

T1 weighted image   A spin echo image generated by a pulse sequence using a short TR (0.6 seconds or less).

T2   The time it takes for protons to go out of phase after having been shifted in their orientation by an excitation pulse.

T2 weighted image   A spin echo image generated by a pulse sequence using a long TR (2.0 seconds or more).

TE   Echo time; the interval between the first pulse in a spin echo examination and the appearance of the resulting echo.

TR   Repetition time; the interval between one spin echo pulse sequence and the next.

Anatomy/Medical Terminology

Radiology Word Search

Instructions: Locate and circle the radiology terms hidden in the puzzle horizontally, vertically, and diagonally, forward and backward. A numeral following a term in the word list indicates the number of times it can be found in the puzzle.

```
N A C S B W A T E R S V X S R F I
B L L O B E I G R E P P U W N A G
R A D I O I S O T O P E L E O K D
A T R D N V I M A S S T F I I R E
D E A I Y G M A R G O N E V T L I
I R Q T U C F R A C T U R E A A F
O A M A M M O G R A M A D C I Y O
L L E S I O N O E J D X A H D R K
O I M A R G O L E Y M S R O A S H
G R O E N T G E N U C L E A R E N
I M K J L N H Y P A Q U E E Y G L
S C G S A I V P N E N I C K A A N
T L M L I F E N W O T A L U R E U
S O I I X D E J C X R N T B N R O
Y O P G A R E K A T P U Z U O P E
C P E U S S I T S A R T N O C E A
```

angle	IVP	reflux
axial	KUB	rib
barium	lateral	roentgen
bony	lesion	sac
cine	lobe	scan
C-loop	mammogram	scanner
coil	mass	tissue
Conray	MRI	Towne
contrast	myelogram	tracer
cut (2)	nuclear	UGI (2)
CXR	oblique	upper GI
cyst	PET (2)	uptake
disk	pyelogram	venogram
echo	rad (3)	view
film	radiation	views
fracture	radioisotope	Waters
Hypaque	radiologist	x-ray

Proofreading Skills

Instructions: Circle the errors in the report below. Identify misspelled and missing medical and English words and punctuation errors. Write the correct words and punctuation marks in the numbered spaces below the text.

```
1  AIRCONTRAST BARIUM ENEMA:
2
3  Under floroscopic control the Barium was
4  allowed to flow in a retrograde manner to fill
5  the cecam. Using a double-contrast technique
6  multiple fimms was attained. Several small
7  diverticuli are noted. There is some lateral
8  displacment of the sigmoid towards the left.
9  There is also some elevation of the small
10 bowl. A defuse soft tissue density is seen
11 within the lower adbomen. No mucosal
12 ulceratoins or polypiod lesions are identified.
13
14 IMPRESION:
15 Air contrast study shows displacment of bowel
16 sugestive of a pelvic mass. Posibility of an
17 enlraged bladder should be considered. No
18 evidence of polypiod lesoins or masses are
19 seen within the colon.
```

1. AIR CONTRAST _____
2. _____
3. _____
4. _____
5. _____
6. _____
7. _____
8. _____
9. _____
10. _____
11. _____
12. _____
13. _____
14. _____
15. _____
16. _____
17. _____
18. _____
19. _____

Terminology Challenge

Instructions: The following terms appear in the dictation on Tape 12B. Before beginning the medical transcription practice for Lesson 25, look up each word in a medical or English dictionary, and write out a short definition of each term.

8 mm sections
22-gauge spinal needle
99m-technetium sodium
   pertechnetate
acoustical shadowing
aneurysm
angiogram
avascular necrosis
axial
blood pool images
bone window
C1-2 level
cardiac gating
CAT scan
   (computerized axial
   tomography)
catheter introducer
celiac
cistern
collecting system
   (of kidneys)
contiguous
contrast column
cortex, cortices
dural sac
echo pattern
effacement
heparin
hydronephrosis
Hypaque-76
hyperdense
I-123
iliac
iliofemoral graft
immunoblastic
   lymphoma
impingement

intramedullary
Iohexol
mCi (millicuries)
meglumine diatrizoate
microcuries
morphologic
MRI (magnetic
   resonance imaging)
myelogram
perusal
plane
   coronal
   sagittal
popliteal vein
pubic symphysis
radioiodine
scoliosis
scout film
short-arm Grollman
   catheter
sodium iodide
sonography
stasis
sulci
T1 weighted images
T2 weighted images
T9-10
technetium-99m albumin
   colloid
tomograms
tract
vertex
V/Q scan (ventilation/
   perfusion)
   (Q = quotient)
white matter

Transcription Practice

After completing all the readings and exercises in Lesson 25, transcribe Tape 12B, Radiology. Use both medical and English dictionaries and quick-reference word books as resource materials for finding words. Proofread your transcribed documents carefully, listening to the dictation while you read your transcripts.

Transcribe (*NOT* retype) the same reports again without referring to your previous transcription attempt. Initially, you may need to transcribe some reports more than twice before you can produce an error-free document. Your ultimate goal is to produce an error-free document the first time.

1+ bacteria
1-second forced expiratory volume
  (FEV$_1$)
3+ (three plus)
3+ blood
4+ (four plus)
8 mm sections
10-channel EEG
18-gauge wire
22-gauge needle
22-gauge spinal needle
99m-technetium sodium pertechnetate
110 mm screw
150-degree four-hole plate
1700 hours

A

a.m. (morning)
A$_2$ heart sound (aortic valve closure)
abdominopelvic CT scan
abducens muscle
abduction pillow
Abraham contact lens
accessory respiratory muscles
acetabular
acoustical shadowing
Acufex rasp
Acufex tibial guide
acute abdomen series
ADA (American Diabetes Association)
  diet
ADH (antidiuretic hormone)
Advil
AFB (acid-fast bacilli)
air-fluid level
Aldoril
alpha activity on EEG
aluminum splint
Alupent
AML arthroplasty
AML hip prosthesis
AMLS (Master of Arts in Library
  Science)
amphotericin B
ampicillin
Amvisc
Ancef
androgen level
anesthesia
  general
  spinal
ankle mortise
annulotomy
antacid
anterior chamber
anterior cruciate ligament
anterior leaf of the broad ligament

anterior pack
anti-inflammatory
antianginals
antibody, IgE
antihypertensive
antiviral therapy
aortic root
AP (anteroposterior) diameter
AP (anteroposterior) study
apical aneurysm
ART (accredited record technician)
arteriolar narrowing
arteriosclerotic disease
artery
  left anterior descending (LAD)
  left circumflex coronary
  left internal mammary
  main circumflex coronary
  posterior descending coronary
artificial tears
ASA (acetylsalicylic acid [generic for
  aspirin]) or A.S.A. (trade name)
ASHD (arteriosclerotic heart disease)
aspiration trocar
aspirin
asthma, exercise-induced
Atarax
atherosclerotic heart disease
atrial rate
atropine
atypia
Augmentin
autostapler
AV (atrioventricular) block
aVF lead on EKG
aVL lead on EKG
axial weight loading
Axis I, II, III, IV, V (in psych reports)
Azulfidine

B

BA (Bachelor of Arts)
b.i.d. (twice daily)
bacitracin
bacteriostatic water
Bactrim DS
balloon angioplasty
band neutrophils
bands (banded neutrophils)
basal neck fracture
basilar skull fracture
Beaver blade
Benzagel
Betadine
Betadine ointment
Betadine scrub and solution
Betadine-impregnated

bethanechol
bibasilar
bicortical screw
bipolar affective disorder
bipolar cautery
BK (below-knee) amputee
bladder blade
bladder floor
bladder outlet
bladder suspension
blind vaginal pouch
blood gas
blood panel
blood pool images
blowing systolic murmur
Blue Cross
blunt trauma
bone cement
bone densitometry studies
bone window
bony island
bowel sounds
BPH (benign prostatic hypertrophy)
branch (of artery)
  diagonal
  first obtuse marginal
  second obtuse marginal
BRAT (bananas, rice cereal,
  applesauce, toast) diet
breath sounds
broad ligament
bronchial brushings and washings
bronchovesicular breath sounds
Bronkometer
BS (Bachelor of Science)
BS and U (Bartholin, Skene, and
  urethral) glands
BSS (balanced salt solution)
Bufferin
BUN (blood urea nitrogen)
Burow soaks
BUS (Bartholin, urethral, and Skene
  glands)
BVE (Bachelor of Vocational Education)
bypass surgery

C

C (cervical) spine or vertebrae
C-section (cesarean section)
C. (Clostridium) difficile
C1-2 interspace (spine)
C5-6 interspace (spine)
CABG (coronary artery bypass graft)
calcitonin
calcium
cancerization
Capoten

captopril
Carafate
carbon black
carcinoma, undifferentiated
cardiac enzyme
cardiac gating
cardiac silhouette
cardiomegaly
cardioplegia solution
Cardizem
CAT (computerized axial
    tomography) scan
catheter introducer
catheter
    5 French
    8 French
    18 French
    acorn-tipped
    angle-tipped
    Foley
    ureteral
cavitary mass
Cavitron AIS irrigating-aspirating
    needle
CBC (complete blood count)
cc (cubic centimeter)
CCU (Cardiac Care Unit)
Ceclor
Cefobid
cefoperazone
cell, infiltrating
cellulated
cervical myelogram
cervical os
cervical stump
chemistry panel
CHF (congestive heart failure)
Chlamydia enzyme test
chronic lead placement
CIN-3 (cervical intraepithelial
    neoplasia)
Clark's level 3
clefting
Clinoril
clonidine
cm (centimeter)
CMA-A (certified medical assistant—
    administrative)
CMT (certified medical transcrip-
    tionist)
CO_2 (carbon dioxide)
coagulase-negative staphylococcus
coarse rhonchi
codeine
Cogentin
Colace
cold nodule
collateral flow
collecting system (of kidneys)
colon, proximal
Compazine

concentrating defect
congestive heart failure
consolidative change (on chest
    x-ray)
contact sensitivity
contrast column
contrast media
    Hypaque-76
    meglumine diatrizoate
COPD (chronic obstructive pulmonary
    disease)
corneoscleral scissors
coronary artery
Cortef
cortical sensation
cortisone acetate
cosmetic removal
Coumadin
counterpressure
CPI Astra bipolar generator
CPK (creatine phosphokinase) enzyme
CPR (cardiopulmonary resuscitation)
CPR (computerized patient record)
crescendo angina pectoris
creviced
cross-clamped
crutch ambulation
cryptococcal antigen
CT (computerized tomography) scan
curettings
CVA (cerebrovascular accident)
CVA (costovertebral angle)
CVP (central venous pressure) line
cytologic features
Cytomel

D

D (dorsal) spine or vertebrae
D&C (dilatation and curettage)
D5W (5% dextrose in water)
Dalmane
Darvocet-N
Darvocet-N 100
DC (direct current) countershock
deciduoid reaction
deep venous thrombosis
DeLee trap
Demerol
Demulen
Depo-Medrol
description
    gross
    microscopic
deviated nasal septum
dextrorotoscoliosis
Di-Gel
DiaBeta
diastolic rumble

diet
    BRAT (bananas, rice cereal,
        applesauce, toast)
    clear liquid
    high-bulk
differential (on CBC)
digoxin
Dilantin
dipyridamole
discoid atelectasis
disk (disc) space
disk bulge
Donnatal
double-J stent
double-voided urine
dressing
    2 x 2
    collodion
    iodoform gauze
    Steri-Strips
DTRs (deep tendon reflexes)
duodenal sweep
dura
Dyazide
dysmotility
dysrhythmic

E

EB (Epstein-Barr) viral infection
ECG (electrocardiogram)
echo pattern
Ecotrin
ectasia
EEG (electroencephalogram)
EKG (electrocardiogram)
Elavil
electrolyte battery
electrolytes
    chloride
    carbon dioxide (CO_2)
    potassium
    sodium
emergently
EMG (electromyogram)
end-inspiratory wheeze
end-stage
end-to-side anastomosis
endobronchial
ENT (ears, nose, and throat)
EOMI (extraocular movements intact)
ependymal lining
epinephrine
ER (emergency room)
ERYC
ESWL (extracorporeal shock-wave
    lithotripsy)
ET (endotracheal) tube
Ethilon suture
Ex-Lax

examination
  ophthalmoscopic
  slit-lamp
Excedrin
Excedrin with codeine
exercise-induced asthma
exertional angina
exploratory laparotomy
external muscular fascia
external oblique
external oblique fascia
external otitis media
external rotation
extracapsular cataract extraction with
  lens implant
extracorporeal shock-wave lithotripsy
  (ESWL)
extradural defect
extraocular motility
extraocular movements

F

fascia lata
FEF-25 (or FEF$_{25}$)
FEF 25-75 (or FEF$_{25\text{-}75}$)
femoral condyle
ferrous sulfate
fetal distress
FEV$_1$ (or FEV-1) (forced expiratory
  volume in one second)
FEV$_1$/FVC (or FEV-1/FVC) ratio
fibromyomata
fine-needle aspiration
finger cot
finger dissection
fingerbreadths
first tracheal ring
Flagyl
flank pain
flat line EKG
Fleet enema
Flexeril
flight of ideas
Florinef Acetate
fluorescein
focal tenderness
forced vital capacity (FVC)
forceps blade
forceps
  angulated
  McPherson
formalin
Fox shield
fracture
  acute
  fibular
  phalangeal
frozen control
frozen section diagnosis
full-thickness
fundal height

fundus of disk
furosemide
FVC (forced vital capacity)

G

g (gram)
ganciclovir
Garamycin solution
genu valgum
glucose
Gore bit
Gore-Tex prosthesis
Gore-Tex tape
grade 2 hypertensive change
grade 2-3/6 blowing systolic heart
  murmur
graft occlusive disease
gram-negative cocci
gravity drainage
griseofulvin
gross description
gross examination
grumous (or grumose)
GTT (glucose tolerance test)
GU (genitourinary)
guide wires

H

h.s. (at hour of sleep)
Halcion
Haldol
Hastings frame
hCG (human chorionic gonadotropin)
Healon
heart disease, atherosclerotic
heart gallop
heart rub
HEENT (head, eyes, ears, nose, and
  throat)
Hemoccult card
Hemovac drain
heparin
Herplex
Hibiclens soaks
high-grade lesion
hilar aspect
HIV (human immunodeficiency virus)
HIV antibody
humeral head or neck
Humulin insulin
hydrochlorothiazide
hydrocortisone cream
hydrogen peroxide
Hypaque-76
hyperdense
hypertensive
hypertrophied
hypodense
hypothermia

I

I&D (incision and drainage)
I-123 (or I^{123})
I.M. (intramuscular)
I.V. (intravenous)
IDDM (insulin-dependent diabetes
  mellitus)
IgE antibody
iliofemoral graft
illicit
immunoblastic lymphoma
implant stimulator
incision
  thoracoabdominal
  Y-shaped
Inderal
indirect visualization
inflammatory reaction
insight and judgment
insulin
  Humulin
  NPH
  regular
  Ultralente
intellectual functioning
interdigital web space
interferon
internal rotation
interstitial pulmonary edema
intimal hyperplasia
intrinsic brain stem lesion
inverted
iodoform gauze
Iohexol
Iolab intraocular lens
irregularly irregular rhythm
Isordil
ITE (in-the-ear) hearing aid
IVP (intravenous pyelogram)

J

joint line
jugular venous distention
jugulodigastric areas
JV (jugular venous)

K

Kayexalate
Keflex
Kefzol
Kenalog
ketoconazole
kg (kilogram)
kidney architecture
Klonopin
Kocher clamp
Komed

Kondremul
KUB (kidneys, ureters,
     bladder) x-ray
kV (kilovolt) reading

L

L (lumbar) spine or vertebrae
L3-4 interspace (spine)
L4-5 interspace (spine)
L5 (spine)
L5-S1 interspace (spine)
labium minus
LAD (left anterior descending) artery
Lanoxin
laparotomy pad
laser
     coherent YAG
     YAG
Lasix
lateral epicondyle
LCD (generic for liquor carbonis
     detergens) or L.C.D. (trade
     name)
LDH (lactic dehydrogenase)
lead (EKG)
     I, I, III, IV
     anterolateral
     inferior
     V_1, V_2, V_3, V_4, V_5, V_6
left lower quadrant
left shift (on white blood count)
leiomyomata
lens cortex
lid speculum
lidocaine
lithium
liver panel
LMP (last menstrual period)
loading dose
lobular parenchyma
Lomotil
long leg immobilizer
long-standing
loose associations
Lotrimin cream
low cervical transverse C-section
lower pole calix
LS (lumbosacral) spine or vertebrae
lymphoid hyperplasia
lymphoid plaques

M

MA (Master of Arts)
Maalox
macular edema
main stem bronchi
main stem carina

manic phase
Marcaine
mass effect
Mayo scissors
MB fraction (a cardiac enzyme)
mCi (millicuries)
M.D. (doctor of medicine)
medications
     Advil
     Aldoril
     Alupent
     amphotericin B
     ampicillin
     Amvisc
     Ancef
     ASA (or A.S.A.)
     aspirin
     Atarax
     atropine
     Augmentin
     Azulfidine
     bacitracin
     bacteriostatic water
     Bactrim DS
     Benzagel
     Betadine
     Betadine ointment
     Betadine scrub and solution
     bethanechol
     Bronkometer
     BSS (balanced salt solution)
     Bufferin
     Burow soaks
     calcitonin
     calcium
     Capoten
     captopril
     Carafate
     cardioplegia solution
     Cardizem
     Ceclor
     Cefobid
     cefoperazone
     Clinoril
     clonidine
     codeine
     Cogentin
     Colace
     Compazine
     Cortef
     cortisone acetate
     Coumadin
     Cytomel
     Dalmane
     Darvocet-N
     Darvocet-N 100
     Demerol
     Demulen
     Depo-Medrol
     Di-Gel
     DiaBeta

medications (*continued*)
     digoxin
     Dilantin
     dipyridamole
     Donnatal
     Dyazide
     Ecotrin
     Elavil
     electrolyte solution
     epinephrine
     ERYC
     Excedrin
     Excedrin with codeine
     ExLax
     ferrous sulfate
     Flagyl
     Fleet enema
     Flexeril
     Florinef Acetate
     fluorescein
     formalin
     furosemide
     ganciclovir
     Garamycin solution
     glucose
     griseofulvin
     Halcion
     Haldol
     Healon
     heparin
     Herplex
     Hibiclens soaks
     Humulin insulin
     hydrochlorothiazide
     hydrocortisone cream
     hydrogen peroxide
     Inderal
     interferon
     Iohexol
     Isordil
     Kayexalate
     Keflex
     Kefzol
     Kenalog
     ketoconazole
     Klonopin
     Komed
     Kondremul
     Lanoxin
     Lasix
     LCD (or L.C.D.)
     lidocaine
     lithium
     Lomotil
     Lotrimin cream
     Maalox
     Marcaine
     methacholine
     Metamucil
     Mevacor
     Micro-K

medications *(continued)*
 milk of magnesia
 Minipress
 Moduretic
 Monocid
 morphine sulfate
 Mylicon
 Naprosyn
 Navane
 Neosporin
 Neutra-Phos
 niacin
 nitro patch
 Nitro-Dur II
 nitroglycerin SL
 nitroglycerin transdermal
 Nizoral
 normal saline
 NPH insulin
 Ocean spray
 penicillin
 penicillin V potassium
 pentamidine aerosol
 Pepcid
 Percodan
 Permax
 Pernox
 Persantine
 Phenergan
 phenobarbital
 Polysporin
 potassium
 potassium permanganate soaks
 prednisone
 Premarin
 Procardia
 promethazine
 Prostigmin
 Proventil
 Proventil inhaler
 Provera
 PTU (propylthiouracil)
 Quinaglute
 Quinidex Extentabs
 quinidine
 Reglan
 regular insulin
 Restoril
 saline
 saline gargle
 Saluron
 selenium
 Septra DS
 Slow-K
 sodium bicarbonate
 sodium iodide
 Solu-Cortef
 Spectazole
 Stadol
 Synthroid
 tacrine

medications *(continued)*
 Tagamet
 Tegretol
 Tenex
 Tenormin
 Tensilon
 tetracycline
 Theo-Dur
 thyroxine
 ticarcillin
 Timoptic
 tobramycin
 toluidine O
 Torecan
 triamcinolone cream
 Tylenol No. 3
 Valisone cream
 valproate
 valproic acid
 Vanceril
 Vasotec
 Versed
 Vicodin
 Viroptic
 Vistaril
 vitamin A
 vitamin D complex
 Voltaren
 Wydase
 Xanax
 Xylocaine
 zinc oxide
 Zantac
 Zovirax
medial aspect
medial compartment (of knee)
medial rectus recession
medial retinaculum
median sternotomy incision
medullary zone
meglumine diatrizoate
mental status
mEq/L (milliequivalents per liter)
mesenteric soft tissue
mesocolonic
mesocolonic fat
Metamucil
methacholine
methacholine challenge
Mevacor
mg/dl (milligrams per deciliter)
mg/kg (milligrams per kilogram)
MI (myocardial infarction)
micro ear forceps
Micro-K
microcalcification
microcuries
microscopic description
mid-pretibial area
midepigastric
midline shift

Mighty-Vac vacuum extractor
milk of magnesia
mitotic rate
mixed flora
mJ (millijoules)
ml or mL (milliliter)
MM fraction (cardiac enzyme)
mm (millimeter)
mmHg (millimeters of mercury)
Moduretic
mold spores
monitoring lines
Monocid
monos (monocytes)
morphine sulfate
morphologic
motor examination
motor status
MPA (Master of Public Administration)
MRI (magnetic resonance imaging) scan
multisystem
muscle
 inferior oblique
 inferior rectus
 medial rectus
 orbicularis
 superior rectus
musculoskeletal deficit
Mylicon

N

myocardial hypothermia
myoclonic-type movements
Naprosyn
Navane
needle suspension
Neosporin
nerve, posterior tibial
neuroleptic
neuropraxic
neuroradiologist
Neutra-Phos
NG (nasogastric) tube
niacin
nitro patch
Nitro-Dur II
nitroglycerin SL (sublingual)
nitroglycerin, transdermal
Nizoral
nodular-like
nonkeratinizing
nonproductive cough
nonpruritic
nonstress test (pregnancy)
nontender
normal saline
normocephalic
notchplasty
NP lead on EEG
n.p.o. (nil per os [nothing by mouth])

NSAID (nonsteroidal anti-inflammatory drug)
nuchal rigidity
nuclear-cytoplasmic ratio

O

O'Connor-O'Sullivan retractor
obscures
obstructing
occluded graft
Ocean spray
opacified
operative cholangiogram
operative field
operative leg holder
oral hypoglycemic agent
orbital aspect
ORIF (open reduction and internal fixation)
osteochondroplasty
osteochondritis dissecans
OU (each eye; both eyes)

P

P&A (percussion and auscultation)
p.o. (per os [by mouth])
p.r.n. (pro re nata [as needed])
P_2 heart sound (pulmonary valve closure)
PA and lateral chest x-ray
pacemaker capture
pacemaker failure to capture
pacemaker generator
pacemaker lead
pacemaker resistance
pacemaker sensitivity
painful stimuli
Panel A
parafollicular
paroxysmal supraventricular tachycardia
partial thromboplastin time (PTT)
patellar tilt
PCO_2 (partial pressure of carbon dioxide)
pelvic brim
pelvic relaxation
penicillin
penicillin V potassium
Penrose drain tourniquet
pentamidine aerosol
Pepcid
peptic ulcer disease
Percodan
percussion note
percutaneous transluminal coronary angioplasty (PTCA)
periareolar
peribronchial cuffing

peripheral edema
peripheral neuropathy
periumbilical area
PERL (pupils equal, reactive to light)
Permax
Pernox
PERRLA (pupils equal, round, reactive to light and accommodation)
Persantine
pH
Phalen's test
Phenergan
phenobarbital
PIE (pulmonary interstitial emphysema)
PIP (proximal interphalangeal) joint
pleural space
PND (paroxysmal nocturnal dyspnea)
PND (postnasal drip/drainage)
PO_2 (partial pressure of oxygen)
Polysporin
popliteal recess
position sense
position
    3 o'clock
    9 o'clock
    12 o'clock
    dorsal lithotomy
    lateral decubitus
postangioplasty (or post-angioplasty)
postcoital
posterior capsulotomy
posterior cervical nodes (neck)
posterior horn (of medial meniscus)
posthyperventilation period
postvoid residual
potassium permanganate soaks
PR interval
prednisone
preliminary film
Premarin
premature ventricular beat
pressure sponges
pretibial edema
Procardia
processus vaginalis
promethazine
prophylactic coverage
prostatic bed
prostatic chips
prosthesis
    acetabular
    femoral
Prostigmin
prothrombin time (PT)
Proventil
Proventil inhaler
Provera
provisional diagnosis
PT (prothrombin time)
PTT (partial thromboplastin time)
PTU (propylthiouracil)

pulmonary artery vent
pulmonary function studies
pulsatile perfusion
pupillary constriction
pyramids

Q

Q angle
q. (every); for example, q.12h. (every 12 hours)
q.a.m. (every morning)
q.h.s. (every evening)
q.i.d. (four times daily)
q.o.d. (every other day)
QRS (on EKG)
quadrilateral cartilage
Quinaglute
Quinidex Extentabs
quinidine

R

radialized
radiation cystitis
radiation therapy
RAST (radioallergosorbent test)
RBC (red blood cell)
RCA (right coronary artery)
reapproximated
rebound constipation
reciprocal change on ECG
referred tenderness
reflexes
    deep tendon
    pathological
refractile material
region
    basal
    hilar
Reglan
respiratory excursions
Restoril
retracting
retroareolar
retrobulbar block
retrocecal
retrograde pyelogram
revascularization procedure
reversible ischemia
Rh+ (Rh positive)
Rh- (Rh negative)
Richards screw
right lower quadrant
Robert Jones dressing
rongeur
    downbiting
    pituitary
    straight
    upbiting
round ligament

RPR (rapid plasma reagent)
rugous
Rush rod

S

S (sacral) spine or vertebrae
S-shaped configuration
S1 (first heart sound)
S2 (second heart sound)
S3 (third heart sound)
S4 (fourth heart sound)
S1 vertebra (spine)
saline
saline gargle
Saluron
sclerotic area
scope
    11.5 French
    22 French
    28 Storz
    ureteroscope
scout film
secondarily infected
secretory endometrium
segmented neutrophils
segs (segmented neutrophils)
Segura stone basket
seizure, generalized
selective coronary arteriogram
selenium
sensory examination
Septra DS
serum hCG (human chorionic
    gonadotropin)
serum RPR (rapid plasma reagent)
SGOT (laboratory test)
short-arm Grollman catheter
side-biting clamp
Silastic tapes
silver nitrate
Sinskey hook
sinus, sphenoid
sleep-deprived EEG
Slow-K
SMA-20
SMAC panel (laboratory test)
small bowel obstruction
smell hallucination
SOB (shortness of breath)
sodium bicarbonate
sodium iodide
Solu-Cortef
space-occupying lesion
Spectazole
spermatocytic
spine
    cervical (C)
    dorsal (D)
    lumbar (L)
    lumbosacral (LS)

spine *(continued)*
    sacral (S)
    thoracic (T)
    thoracolumbar
sponge and needle counts
spun hematocrit
spurring
ST elevation (on EKG)
ST segment (on EKG)
ST wave (on EKG)
ST-T wave changes (on EKG)
Stadol
stage D3 adenocarcinoma
staph (staphylococcus)
STD (sexually transmitted disease)
    screen
stereo acuity
stereognosis
stocking-glove distribution
stone basketing
stool culture
strep (streptococcus) screen
subendocardial myocardial infarction
submucosal tunnel
subtherapeutic
suicidal ideation
sulfa drug
superficial tenderness
superomedial
supravalvular aortogram
surgical clips
surgical staples
suture
    1-0 (or 0)
    2-0 (or 00)
    3-0 (or 000)
    4-0
    5-0
    6-0
    7-0
    10-0
    chromic
    dermal
    imbricating
    interlocking
    nylon
    plain
    Prolene
    silk
    subcutaneous
    traction
    Vicryl
    Z-type
suture-ligated
symphysis pubis
Synthroid

T

T&A (tonsillectomy and
    adenoidectomy)

T (thoracic) spine or vertebrae
T1 weighted (in MRI scan)
t.i.d. (three times daily)
T2 weighted (in MRI scan)
T3 (or T$_3$) thyroid hormone
T4 (or T$_4$) thyroid hormone
T9-10 interspace (spine)
TA-55 Roticulator
tacrine
Tagamet
TAH (total abdominal hysterectomy)
tandem walking
tbsp. (tablespoon)
technetium-99m albumin colloid
TDI (toluene di-isocyanate)
Tegretol
Tenex
Tenormin
TENS (transcutaneous electrical
    nerve stimulator) unit
Tensilon
test
    anterior drawer
    finger-to-nose
    four-dot
    heel-to-shin
    Lachman
    pivot shift
    Prostigmin
    psychometric
    TFTs (thyroid function)
    thallium treadmill stress
    Thayer-Martin
    thyroid function
testicle and cord
tetracycline
TFTs (thyroid function tests)
thallium treadmill stress test
Thayer-Martin test
Theo-Dur
third-degree complete heart block
thyroid function test
    T3
    T4
    TSH
thyroxine
ticarcillin
Tigan elixir
Timoptic
tinkling bowel sounds
TKO (to keep open)
tobramycin
toluene di-isocyanate (TDI)
toluidine O
tonsillar pillar
Torecan
total CPK
total serum protein
Towne's view
toxic digoxin level
tracheal hook
tracheostomy tube

transepithelial migration
transfixing screw
transit time
treadmill stress test
triamcinolone cream
trilobar
trocar plug
TSH (thyroid stimulating hormone)
tube
    right-angle
    straight chest
    thoracotomy
TURP (transurethral resection of the prostate)
Tylenol No. 3
Tzanck smear

U

ulnar deviation
undifferentiated carcinoma
unlabored
unremarkable
unresectable
unstable angina
upper GI (gastrointestinal) series
upper GI with small bowel series
upper respiratory infection
uptake scan
uremia
ureteroscopy
urethrovesical angle
URI (urinary tract infection)
urinary force
urinary hesitancy
urinary stream
urinary terminal dribbling
urinary urgency
urine catecholamines
urine dipstick

uterine descensus
uterine gutter
UTI (urinary tract infection)

V

V_1, V_2, V_3, V_4, V_5, and V_6 leads (on electrocardiogram)
vaginal cuff
vaginal vault
Valisone cream
valproate
valproic acid
valve cusps
valve leaflet
Van Lint lid block
Vanceril
Vasotec
vastus lateralis
VDRL (Venereal Disease Research Laboratory; a test for syphilis)
vein harvesting
ventilation tube
ventilation and perfusion lung scan
ventricular rate
Versed
vertebral body
vesical neck
vesicle
vesicouterine reflection
vessel loop
vibratory sense
Vicodin
Viroptic
vision
    20/200
    20/30
    20/40
    20/50+

Vistaril
visual acuity
vitamin A
vitamin D complex
VMO (vastus medialis obliquus)
Voltaren
VP (ventriculoperitoneal) shunt
V/Q (ventilation-perfusion) scan

W

wartlike lesion
watt-second shock
WBC (white blood cell)
weightbearing
well-differentiated epithelium
well-leg holder
well-oriented male
white count
wide margin resection
wide-complexed rhythm
Wydase

X, Y, Z

x 0 to 3 (0 to 3 times)
x 4 (four times)
x 12 (twelve times)
X-Acto knife
Xylocaine
YAG (yttrium-aluminum-garnet) laser
yeast infection
Zantac
Zeiss operating microscope
zinc oxide ointment
Zovirax

Aamodt, Elaine. "Promoting Wellness, Preventing Injury," *Perspectives on the Medical Transcription Profession* (Winter 1992-93, pp. 10-11). Publications assistant, Health Professions Institute.

Cadigan, Carolyn. "Transcribing Orthopedic Dictation," *Orthopedic Transcription Unit* (HPI, 1988), pp. xv-xviii. Medical transcriptionist, Baltimore, Maryland.

Campbell, Linda. "Confidentiality and the Patient Healthcare Record." Director of Development, Health Professions Institute, Modesto.

Diehl, Marcy. "Criticism," *Beginning Medical Transcription* (HPI, 1989), pp. 7-8. College instructor in medical assisting and transcription, San Diego, California. Co-author of *Medical Typing and Transcribing: Techniques and Procedures*, 3rd ed. (Saunders, 1991) and *Medical Transcription Guide: Do's and Don'ts* (Saunders, 1990).

Dirckx, John H., M.D. "A Brief Look at STDs in Women," *Perspectives* (Winter 1992-93, pp. 41-47); "Dictation and Transcription: Adventures in Thought Transference," *Perspectives* (Summer 1990, pp. 34-37). Director of the student health center at University of Dayton (Ohio) since 1968, and medical editor, Health Professions Institute, since 1987.

Dirckx, John H., M.D. *H & P: A Nonphysician's Guide to the Medical History and Physical Examination.* Modesto, Ca.: Health Professions Institute, 1991.

Dirckx, John H., M.D. *Laboratory Medicine: Essentials of Anatomic and Clinical Pathology.* Modesto, Ca.: Health Professions Institute, 1991.

Donneson, Kathy. "Professionalism and the Medical Transcriptionist," *Beginning Medical Transcription* (HPI, 1989), pp. 4-5. Management consultant for Health Professions Institute, 1982 president of the American Association for Medical Transcription, and former medical transcription service owner.

D'Onofrio, Elizabeth. "Curve Balls," *Perspectives* (Summer 1990, pp. 4-6); "Transcribing Lines in the Sand," *Perspectives* (Fall 1990, pp. 4-6). Medical transcriptionist, Tucson, Arizona, co-author of *Psychiatric Words and Phrases* (HPI, 1990), and former HPI publications assistant.

D'Onofrio, Mary Ann. "The ESL Physician and the Art of Medical Transcription," *Perspectives* (Fall 1992, pp. 29-31); "The Ophthalmology Medical Transcriptionist," *Perspectives* (Fall 1990, pp. 22-24). Independent medical transcriptionist, Tucson, Arizona, and co-author of *Psychiatric Words and Phrases* (HPI, 1990).

Drake, Ellen. Director of Education, Health Professions Institute, Modesto. Former college instructor in medical transcription, former medical transcription service owner, and co-author of *Saunders Pharmaceutical Word Book 1993* (Saunders, 1992).

Ellis, Michael A., M.D. "Orthopedic Practice and Surgery," *Orthopedic Transcription Unit* (HPI, 1988), pp. xi-xiii. Orthopedic surgeon, St. Agnes Hospital, Baltimore, Maryland.

Hinickle, Judy. "Employment Enigmas," *Perspectives* (Spring/Summer 1991, pp. 22-23); "The New Technology," adapted from "Using Technology to Improve Productivity," *Perspectives* (Spring/Summer 1992, pp. 31-34). Medical transcription service owner and consultant, Milwaukee, Wisconsin.

Largen, Thomas L., M.D. "A Surgeon's View of Gastroenterology," *Gastrointestinal Transcription Unit* (HPI, 1989), pp. xi-xv. General surgeon, Central Florida Regional Hospital, Sanford, Florida.

Marshall, Judith. *Medicate Me.* Illustrated by Cindy Stevens. Modesto, Ca.: Health Professions Institute, 1987. Selections by Judith Marshall were taken from *Medicate Me* and from *Perspectives on the Medical Transcription Profession.* Medical transcriptionist, Boston, Massachusetts, and Barton, Vermont, and former college instructor and medical transcription service owner.

O'Donnell, Michael J., M.D. "A Cardiologist's View," *Cardiology Transcription Unit* (HPI, 1989), pp. xi-xv. Cardiologist, Midwest Heart Specialists, Ltd., Lombard, Illinois.

Pitman, Sally C. "Humor in Medicine: Bloopers." Editor and Publisher, Health Professions Institute.

Pyle, Vera. "The Mind Behind the Machine." Editorial consultant, Health Professions Institute, and author of *Current Medical Terminology,* 4th ed. (HPI, 1992).

Rambo, Kathy. "Dizzy Gillespie, My Brother, and Me," *Perspectives* (Winter 1992-93, p. 8); "The Radiology Transcriptionist," *Radiology Transcription Unit* (HPI, 1987, rev. 1990), pp. xi-xiii; "Transcriptionists Are People, Too," *Perspectives* (Fall 1991, p. 25).

Taylor, Bron. "The Arms Race," *Perspectives* (Spring/Summer 1992, pp. 26-27); "Transcribing Gastroenterology Dictation," *Gastrointestinal Transcription Unit* (HPI, 1989), pp. xvii-xix. Medical transcriptionist, San Francisco, and former HPI research assistant.

Tennant, Bruce. "Medical Transcription Equipment," *Beginning Medical Transcription* (HPI, 1989), pp. 9-10. Former medical transcription service owner and college instructor, Long Beach, California.

Turley, Susan M. *Understanding Pharmacology.* Englewood Cliffs, NJ: Regents/Prentice Hall, 1991. Director of Curriculum Development, Health Professions Institute, Baltimore. Curriculum consultant, former nurse, and former college instructor in medical assisting and transcription.

Wear, Pamela K. "The Healthcare Record," *Beginning Medical Transcription* (HPI, 1989), pp. 11-13. Executive Director, American Health Information Management Association, Chicago, Illinois, since 1991.

Woods, Kathleen Mors. "Transcribing Cardiology Dictation," *Cardiology Transcription Unit* (HPI, 1989), pp. xvii-xix. Cardiac surgery coordinator, Johns Hopkins Hospital, Baltimore, Maryland.

Index

The Authors

Linda C. Campbell, CMT, Modesto, California, is Director of Development, Health Professions Institute. As Director of Education from April 1987 to May 1993, she coordinated the development of The SUM Program for Medical Transcription Training and co-authored *The SUM Program Student Syllabus* and *Teacher's Manual.* A former nursing student, she learned medical transcription on the job and is completing a B.S. degree in health management. She has 18 years of transcription experience in hospitals, transcription companies, and self-employment. She has written numerous articles for medical transcriptionists, teachers, and students, some of which have appeared in *Perspectives on the Medical Transcription Profession, Journal of American Health Information Management Association* (AHIMA), and *Journal of American Association for Medical Transcription* (AAMT). She works with medical facilities to implement medical transcription training programs and advises individuals in independent study. She has presented many seminars for medical transcription teachers and workshops in radiology and pathology transcription.

Ellen Drake, CMT, Modesto, California, joined Health Professions Institute as Director of Education in June 1993, having recently moved from Sanford, Florida, where she taught medical transcription in a community college, worked as a hospital medical transcriptionist, and owned a medical transcription service. She has a B.A. degree in education and taught high school English for four years and worked as a medical transcriptionist for 24 years. She co-authors the annual *Saunders Pharmaceutical Word Book* (Saunders, 1992) and the bimonthly newsletter, *The Latest Word*, published by Saunders, and she consulted on *Dorland's Medical Speller* (Saunders, 1992). She has presented many seminars and workshops for medical transcriptionists and teachers on grammar, punctuation, transcription practices, and newsletter production. Her articles on transcription practices and teaching techniques have been published in the *Journal of AAMT* and *Perspectives on the Medical Transcription Profession.*

Sally Crenshaw Pitman, MA, CMT, Modesto, California, is the owner of Health Professions Institute and editor and publisher of numerous books, periodicals, and educational materials for medical transcriptionists, teachers, and business owners. She owned a medical transcription service for ten years (until 1982), having previously taught English in a community college for five years. She was a founding director of AAMT (1978-1984), editor and publisher of AAMT publications for eight years (until 1986), and co-author of the *Style Guide for Medical Transcription* (AAMT, 1984). Since 1985 she has owned and operated Prima Vera Publications and Health Professions Institute, serving exclusively the medical transcription educational market through seminars and conferences for teachers, business owners, and transcriptionists, The SUM Program for Training Medical Transcriptionists, a wide selection of textbooks and reference books, and the quarterly magazine, *Perspectives on the Medical Transcription Profession.*

Susan M. Turley, MA, CMT, RN, Baltimore, Maryland, is an experienced medical transcriptionist, nurse, and college instructor, having taught medical transcription, terminology, pharmacology, and clinical laboratory procedures in a community college. As Director of Curriculum Development for Health Professions Institute since March 1987, she has participated in the development of the medical transcription curriculum, reference materials, and transcription units in The SUM Program for Medical Transcription Training. She has presented many seminars and workshops to teachers and medical transcription practitioners on the local and national level, and provides curriculum consulting services for schools and medical facilities. She has written many articles which have been published in the *Journal of AAMT, Perspectives on the Medical Transcription Profession,* and *Journal of AHIMA.* She has a master's degree in adult education, is the author of *Understanding Pharmacology* (Regents/Prentice Hall, 1992), and co-author of *The SUM Program Student Syllabus* and *Teacher's Manual.*